Advanced Cosmetic Otoplasty

Melvin A. Shiffman
Editor

Advanced Cosmetic Otoplasty

Art, Science, and New Clinical Techniques

Springer

Editor
Melvin A. Shiffman, M.D., J.D.
Tustin, California
USA

ISBN 978-3-662-52166-3 ISBN 978-3-642-35431-1 (eBook)
DOI 10.1007/978-3-642-35431-1
Springer Heidelberg New York Dordrecht London

Softcover reprint of the hardcover 1st edition 2013

Printed on acid-free paper

Springer is part of Springer Science+Business Media (www.springer.com)

Foreword

It gives me great pleasure and privilege to write a foreword to this book titled *Advanced Cosmetic Otoplasty: Art, Science, and New Clinical Techniques*. Having been involved with cosmetic surgery for over 30 years, I find that very little has been focused on the aesthetic otoplasty in facial rejuvenation, and details of various techniques are lacking. The ears are a vital part in the beauty and symmetry of the face, and it is often forgotten or neglected. Over the years, children and adults can have a huge complex about their ears. It also varies with trends, as adults sometimes wear their hair short, or with career moves, for instance, if a person goes into the army. Also children are often teased at school because of their ears.

Otoplasty (Greek ōtoûs, ear + plassein, to shape) denotes the surgical and nonsurgical procedures for correcting the deformities and defects of the pinna (external ear).

All those who practice otoplasty surgery are very aware that this seemingly simple surgery is far from straightforward. In fact, it is very difficult to achieve consistently good results. Any text to improve the knowledge of otoplasty is welcomed. If you as a surgeon sometimes feel overwhelmed to organize the fundamental concepts of certain fields, it is great to have one book at hand, as an invaluable resource to enlarge your knowledge and practice.

Very little advances have been noted over the years since otoplasty was developed in ancient India, in the fifth century BC by Sushruta, the ayurvedic physician. He developed otoplastic and other plastic surgical techniques and procedures at that time. Then in the nineteenth century Johann Friedrich Dieffenbach (1794–1847) reported the first surgical approach for the correction of prominent ears. This was a combination otoplasty procedure that featured the simple excision (cutting) of the problematic excess cartilage from the posterior sulcus (back groove) of the ear and the subsequent affixing, with sutures, of the corrected pinna to the mastoid periosteum, the membrane covering the mastoid process at the underside of the mastoid portion of the temporal bone, at the back of the head.

In 1920, Harold D. Gillies (1882–1960) first reproduced the pinna by burying an "external-ear support framework," made of autologous rib cartilage, under the skin of the mastoid region of the head, which reconstructed the pinna. He then separated this from the skin of the mastoid area by means of a cervical flap. In 1937, Dr. Gillies also attempted a similar pediatric ear reconstruction with a pinna support framework fabricated with maternal cartilage. That otoplasty correction technique proved inadequate, because of the problems inherent to the biochemical breakdown and elimination (resorption) of the cartilage tissue by the patient's body. After this came the Mustardé technique for creating an antihelical fold, the Merck method technique, and the incisionless Fritsch otoplasty. As you can see, after that period very little advancements have been made in this field, hence the importance of this book.

The trend of the last century is to look younger. This is due to many factors: improved technology and emphasis on beauty – we have become a society of "appearance."

This book is aimed at all types and ages of surgeons, to help them to choose the best technique that works for them, and the preoperative and postoperative management.

A big thank you to Dr. Shiffman on this book for imparting his time and knowledge in this field.

The format is splendid. The heading and the text are richly articulate and it is a pleasure to read. Dr. Shiffman has helped to create a beautiful surgical text book, for all surgeons interested to learn about otoplasty, at all levels of expertise. This book delivers to the reader basic principles, advanced techniques, and innovations. This book is an essential tool for the contemporary surgeon. It defines what we do, how we do it, and, most importantly, why we do it.

Congratulations to Dr. Shiffman on such hard work. I wish the book every success.

Mr. (Dr.) Anthony Erian, M.D., FRCS (Lon), FRCS (Edin)
Consultant Plastic Surgeon
President of the International Board of Cosmetic Surgery
President of the European Society of Aesthetic Surgery

Wimpole, Cambridge, UK Anthony Erian, M.D.

Preface

There are only a few books on rhinoplasty and most are limited to the editor's techniques or those of a few contributors. These give restricted information on the variety of procedures that are available and are mainly for teaching the inexperienced and somewhat experienced surgeons how to do rhinoplasty and possibly stay out of trouble.

This book on Advanced Aesthetic Otoplasty: Art, Science, and New Clinical Techniques gives a history of otoplasty and a detailed analysis of the newer techniques that are available in otoplasty. National and international experts of newer procedures report on subjects covering ear embryology and anatomy, surgical techniques of otoplasty, the possible risks and complications of otoplasty, and outcomes in otoplasty. This concept of gathering new techniques from international experts is not present in any other book on otoplasty, and the information is extensive and quite different from even recent books on otoplasty. The book is for the inexperienced, experienced, and the very experienced surgeon doing rhinoplasties.

The editor wishes to present advanced technology and clinical techniques in otoplasty from unique contributors experienced with these procedures that are modified or original procedures. The contributors are inventive and eloquent in presenting to the reader a way to progress from inexperienced or experienced surgeons in rhinoplasty to better understanding that there is more than following simplified techniques as a template to performing a procedure that is fraught with possible risks and complications.

All cosmetic surgeries are potential problems if the patient is not properly evaluated preoperatively, not only physically but also mentally. This is most true with the patient considering otoplasty. However, the satisfaction of the patient who has a good result is inestimable.

Tustin, CA, USA — Melvin A. Shiffman, M.D., J.D.

Contents

Part I

Anatomy

Embryology and Anomalies of the External Ear

1

Jeremiah C. Tracy, Arnold S. Lee, Andrew R. Scott, and Collin S. Karmody

Introduction

A basic knowledge of normal ear development allows for an understanding of the full spectrum of congenital auricular abnormalities. The embryology of the ear provides insight into the fundamentals of surgical reconstruction and support to the concepts that guide our approaches to complete excision of redundant elements. The external ear develops from ectodermal and mesodermal elements of the first and second branchial arches. Anomalies of the ear may therefore reflect abnormal development of either first or second arch structures. Accurate recognition of syndromic ear anomalies also allows for the potential detection of other systemic conditions.

Embryology

Overview

The external ear is divided broadly into three components: auricle, cartilaginous external auditory canal (EAC), and bony EAC. These structures are formed over the course of fetal development, predominantly in weeks 5 through 20. The structures of the external and middle ear are made up of endodermal, mesodermal, and ectodermal elements of the first and second branchial arches. The external auditory canal is itself the physiologic remnant of the first branchial cleft.

In brief, inner ear structures develop from the otic placode. This ectodermal structure is first

J.C. Tracy, M.D. (✉)
Department of Otolaryngology,
Tufts University School of Medicine,
800 Washington Street,
Boston, MA 02111, USA

Department of Otolaryngology,
Tufts University School of Medicine,
116 Harrison Avenue, Boston,
MA 02111, USA
e-mail: jtracy@tuftsmedicalcenter.org

A.S. Lee, M.D.
Facial Plastic & Reconstructive Surgery,
Otolaryngology-HNS,
Tufts University School of Medicine,
Tufts Medical Center, 860 Washington Street, South 1,
Boston, MA 02111, USA
e-mail: alee2@tuftsmedicalcenter.org

A.R. Scott, M.D.
Department of Otolaryngology – Head & Neck Service,
Tufts Medical Center, 800 Washington St.,
Box 850, Boston, MA 02111, USA

Department of Otolaryngology Pediatries,
Tufts University School of Medicine,
Boston, MA, USA

Divisions of Pediatric Otolaryngology
and Facial Plastic & Reconstructive Surgery,
Tufts Medical Center,
Boston, MA, USA

Cleft Lip and Palate Team,
Floating Hospital for Children,
Tufts Medical Center,
Boston, MA, USA
e-mail: ascott@tuftsmedicalcenter.org

C.S. Karmody, M.D.
Department of Otolaryngology,
Tufts University School of Medicine,
116 Harrison Avenue, Boston, MA 02111, USA
e-mail: ckarmody@tuftsmedicalcenter.org

M.A. Shiffman (ed.), *Advanced Cosmetic Otoplasty*,
DOI 10.1007/978-3-642-35431-1_1, © Springer-Verlag Berlin Heidelberg 2013

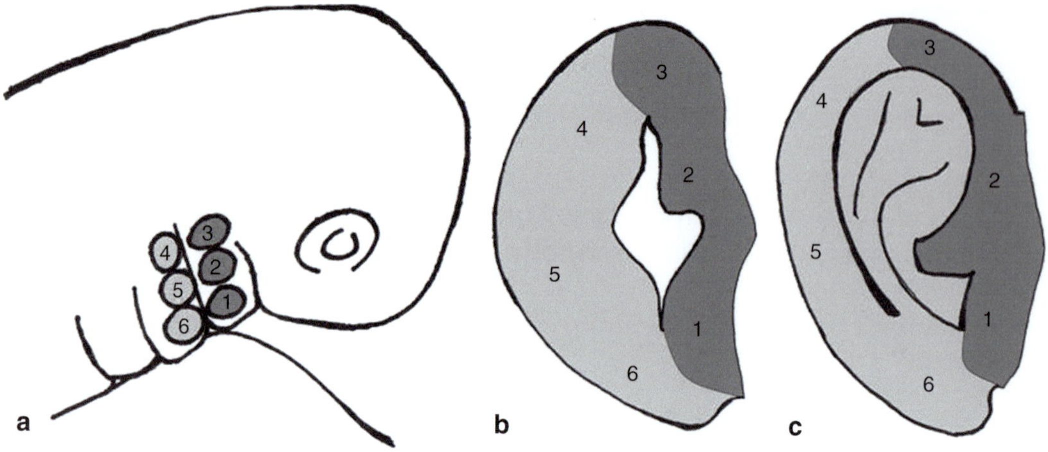

Fig. 1.1 Auricular development. (**a**) Hillocks 1–3 are derived from the first branchial arch and 4–6 from the second. (**b**) Fusion of the hillocks begins to form the auricle in the seventh week of gestation. (**c**) Contributions of the hillocks of His to the fully formed ear

visible in the embryo at week 3, and as development proceeds, it invaginates medially. By week 4, this structure has lost its connection with the ectodermal surface and has migrated medially, forming what is termed the otocyst. This structure will give rise to all inner ear structures with the significant exception of the stapes footplate [1].

It is therefore notable that inner ear structures develop independent of middle ear and outer ear elements and that critical periods of development occur at different times. This is why children with inner ear malformations may have normal external anatomy and children with markedly abnormal surface anatomy may in fact have perfectly normal inner ear structures.

The development of the external ear is generally complete by 20 weeks' gestation and always complete by birth. Through childhood, the external ear and EAC will grow in size but in relative proportion to the scale present at birth. In contrast, the middle and inner ear are fully formed and of adult size at birth and do not grow significantly with the child.

Auricle

Development of the external ear begins at about the fifth week of fetal growth. The first stages of auricular development manifest in the form of small mesenchymal prominences around the first branchial cleft, an ectodermal groove that will eventually develop into the external auditory canal. There are six discrete prominences, which are termed the hillocks of His. It is generally accepted that hillocks 1–3 develop from first branchial arch mesoderm (rostral to the first branchial cleft) and hillocks 4–6 develop from the second branchial arch, just caudal to the cleft. As development proceeds, the relative contribution of cells from the first arch decreases, such that second branchial arch derivatives contribute about 85 % of the mature external ear (Fig. 1.1) [2–5].

Some recent studies have questioned this classic division of the hillocks of His, indicating that only the first hillock is derived from the first branchial arch and that hillocks 2–5 are second branchial arch derivatives [6].

The hillocks of His achieve maximal prominence by the end of week 6. In the seventh week of fetal development, the hillocks undergo directional growth such that they fuse and begin to form the shape of the auricle. Hillock 1 gives rise to the tragus. Hillocks 2 and 3 form the crus of the helix and the helix proper. Cells of hillock 4 and 5 constitute the anti-helix; and the anti-tragus and lobule are formed from hillock 6 [3]. These assignments are general and there almost certainly is overlap in terms of the primordial contributions to the developed ear (Fig. 1.1).

The formation of the auricle centers on the growth and migration of the hillocks of His.

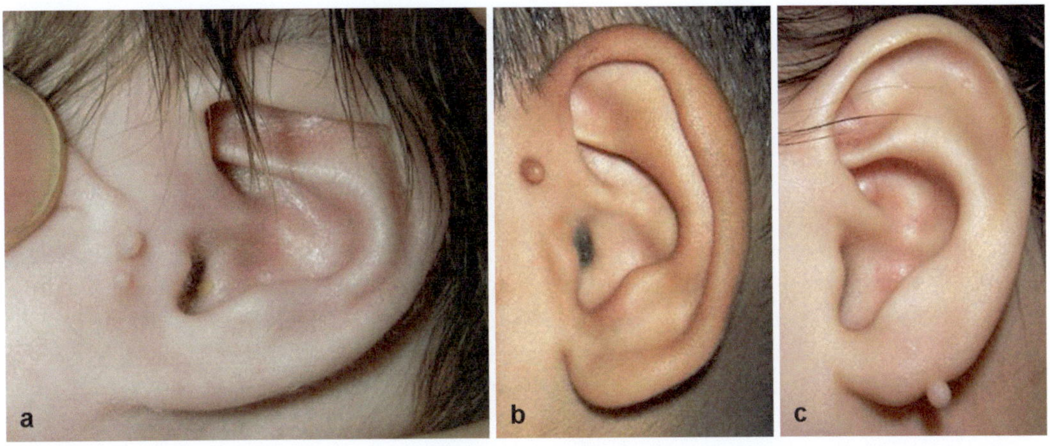

Fig. 1.2 Auricular appendages representing duplications of the hillocks of His. (**a**) Three preauricular appendages likely representing a duplication of the 1–3 hillocks. (**b**) Auricular appendage at the root of the helix likely representing a duplication anomaly versus failure of incorporation of the second hillock into the mature auricle. (**c**) An auricular appendage at the lobule likely representing a duplication anomaly of the sixth hillock

Failure of fusion, or duplications of the hillocks can be observed in the form of auricular appendages (Fig. 1.2). The earliest event is the fusion of hillocks 2 and 3 and the growth of these tissues in a caudal direction, eventually creating the auricular helix. The fusion of hillocks 4 and 5 begins shortly thereafter, and then growth of the antihelix continues concurrently with that of the helix. The overall migration of the developing auricle is cephalad relative to other first and second branchial arch derivatives. This is reflected in the sensory innervation of the mature auricle, which is predominantly from branches of the cervical plexus, with only minor contributions from cranial nerves V, VII, IX, and X. Additionally, syndromic children with first arch anomalies will often exhibit posteriorly rotated, low-set ears.

The dimensions of the external ear are well characterized, and knowledge of the appropriate proportions is essential to the clinician. The height of the adult ear is 5.5–6.5 cm. On average the width of the ear is 55 % that of the height. The overall angle of the auricle seen laterally is about 25–30 % from the vertical. Normal protrusion from the mastoid is about 2 cm (or an angle of 15–25°). The ear at birth is about 66 % of the total size of the adult ear, although, as noted above, the proportions at birth remain unchanged throughout life. Adult ear size is generally achieved in adolescence at about 13–15 years of age, though the majority of growth is complete by 5–7 years of age.

External Auditory Canal

The development of the cartilaginous and bony EAC is not so well-defined. The EAC itself is the remnant of the first branchial cleft, and mesenchymal elements of the canal are derived from the first branchial arch. The cartilaginous canal is in continuity with the cartilage of the auricle and likely develops and fuses with the cartilaginous elements of the hillocks of His at the time of auricle formation.

The canal itself forms as the first branchial cleft extends medially. Eventually, the endodermal lining of the first branchial pouch is in close proximity to the ectoderm of the cleft. In this location the mesoderm thins to a single translucent layer, contributing the fibrous middle layer of the mature tympanic membrane. At this point in development of the EAC, the entire canal is cartilaginous. At about week 12 of development, ossification of the medial-most aspect of the canal begins, forming the bony tympanic annulus and (more laterally) the bony canal [3, 7].

Dysmorphogenesis of the Auricle

Congenital deformities of the ear may be secondary to genetic abnormalities or through sporadic developmental anomalies. The second category is believed to be the more common cause, although twin studies have indicated that genetic contributions are important as well [8]. Further, it is estimated that about 50 % of external ear anomalies are associated with other congenital abnormalities [9]. Sporadic anomalies are most commonly assumed to be related to fetal malposition or vascular insults in development.

Dysmorphogenesis has been broadly classified as agenesis, hypoplasia, hyperplasia, dysplasia, heterotopia, or duplication. In the case of the auricle, the terms anotia, microtia, and macrotia are used. The term microtia is often used broadly to refer to auricular anomalies representing hypoplasia, dysplasia, and perhaps inappropriately, heterotopia as well. Duplication of the auricle is an extremely rare event.

The development of the ear allows for a broad range of different anomalies, and classification can be a challenge. Further, as noted above the auricle, canal, and middle ear all develop concurrently and from tissues of the first and second branchial arches. Therefore, congenital anomalies frequently involve more than one part of the ear. Anomalies of the external ear will be categorized based on clinical appearance.

Auricular Pits, Cysts, and Sinuses

Preauricular pits, cysts, and sinuses represent a spectrum of congenital ear anomalies. The underlying developmental problem is a failure of fusion of two of the hillocks of His. The most common location is at the anterior aspect of the root of the helix, indicating a residual sinus tract or cyst between the second and third hillocks. These anomalies (as a group) make up the most common congenital anomaly of the ear, with an incidence of 0.3–0.9 %. They are most commonly found as isolated anomalies, in individuals with no other congenital malformations. However, there is a documented increased incidence of auricular pits, cysts, and sinuses in many different syndromes including branchio-oto-renal syndrome, Beckwith-Wiedemann syndrome, and mandibulofacial dysostosis. Isolated, non-syndromic preauricular pits are inherited in an autosomal dominant fashion.

Because these defects are a result of failure of fusion of the hillocks, they generally extend down to mesenchymal elements, namely, auricular perichondrium or cartilage. The course of this condition may be marked by recurrent infections, and surgical excision is recommended for symptomatic cases. Complete removal of the cyst or sinus tract requires following it to the auricular cartilage and removing it en bloc with a small cuff of normal tissue and cartilage (Fig. 1.3). Incomplete excision has been shown to result in unacceptable levels of recurrence.

Microtia

Microtia refers to hypoplasia and sometimes dysplasia of the auricle. This anomaly is the result of abnormal development or fusion of the hillocks of His (as described above). Microtia may be bilateral in the case of syndromic or genetic clinical presentations; however, it is most often unilateral. There have been many classification systems described; perhaps the most commonly utilized is the Marx classification of microtia types I–IV (Fig. 1.4) [10]:

Type I: All anatomic subunits are present but slightly dysmorphic in proportions.

Type II: Some identifiable auricular subunits present, but not all of them. The auricle is generally smaller than usual with abnormal, often thickened appearing cartilage. Lobule is present.

Type III: There are no identifiable auricular subunits. Cartilage is present but in an abnormal, often cylindrical configuration.

Type IV: Anotia.

Microtia occurs in 1:12,500 live births [11]. It is more common in males and for unknown reasons the right side is more commonly affected than the left [12]. Type III microtia is the most common form.

Anomalies of the Antihelical Cartilage

"Lop ear" refers to deformity of the auricle, causing the superior helix and sometimes antihelix to fall inferiorly. This is secondary to cartilaginous

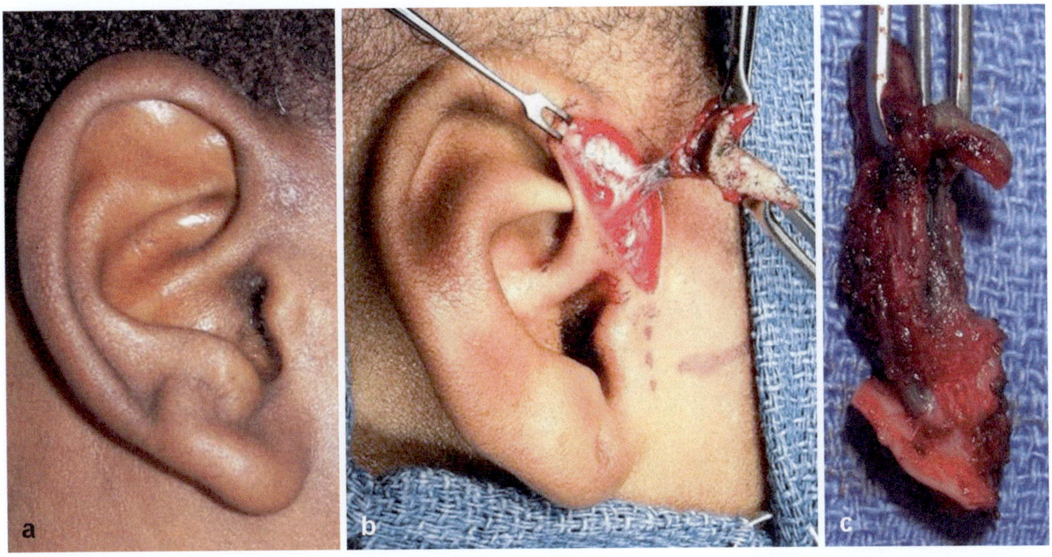

Fig. 1.3 Preauricular sinus. (**a**) Preoperative view demonstrates a small preauricular pit with some overlying skin change. (**b**) Dissecting along the sinus tract down onto helical perichondrium. (**c**) Surgical specimen including a small cuff of normal tissue and helical cartilage, a probe stents the sinus tract, which has been stained with methylene blue

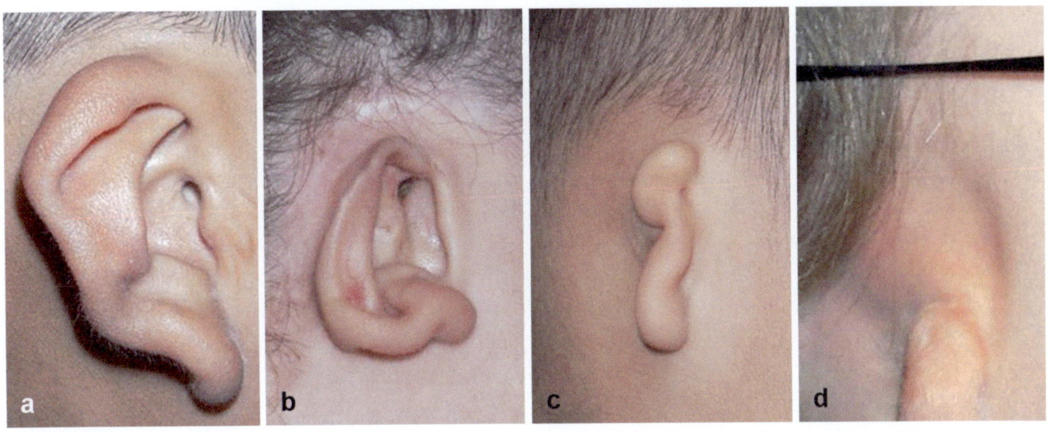

Fig. 1.4 Microtia. (**a**) Type I – All anatomic subunits are present but slightly dysmorphic in proportions. (**b**) Type II – Some identifiable auricular subunits present, but not all of them. The auricle is generally smaller than usual with abnormal, often thickened appearing cartilage. Lobule is present. (**c**) Type III – There are no identifiable auricular subunits. Cartilage is present but in an abnormal, often cylindrical configuration. (**d**) Type IV: Anotia

abnormality. Specifically, a loss of the convex anterior surface of the antihelix will result in this deformity. Involvement that is isolated to the part of the antihelix superior to Darwin's tubercle results in a mild form of this deformity. The resultant appearance of the ear is almost normal, however, with slightly decreased superior to inferior length. When the cartilage of the antihelix inferior to Darwin's tubercle is involved, the appearance is more abnormal. This condition leads to a widening of the auricular angle, giving the appearance of proptosis.

When this cartilaginous abnormality involves the entire antihelix down to the rise of the antitragus, the term "cup ear" is applied. In this case, the lack of convexity of the antihelix to balance the anteriorly concave structures of the helix and concha results in abnormal anterior positioning

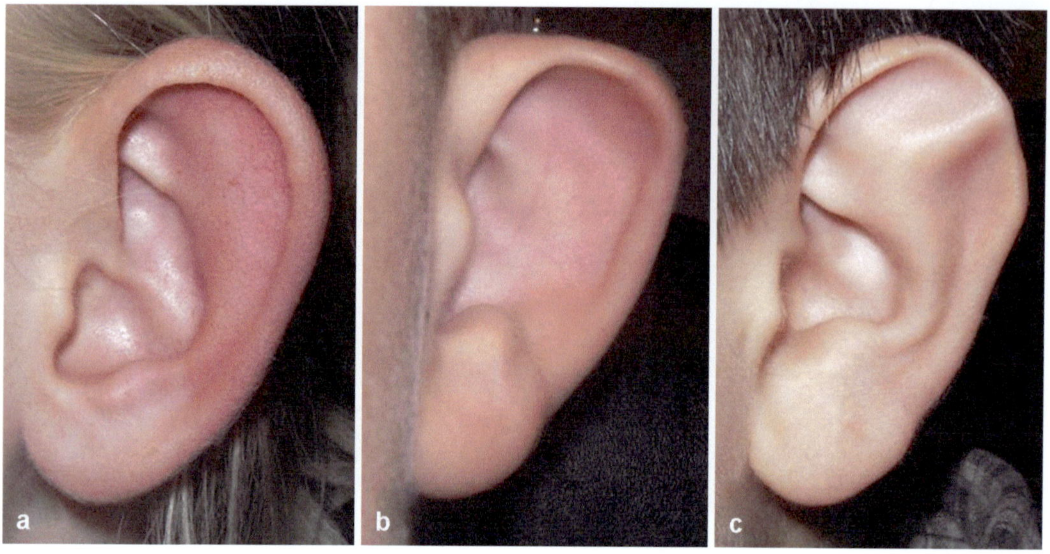

Fig. 1.5 Helical cartilage dysmorphology. (**a**) Lop ear. (**b**) Cup ear. (**c**) Stahl ear

of the helix. In such cases the helical and conchal cartilages are often abnormally formed as well.

The term Stahl ear describes a similar congenital abnormality of the antihelical cartilage. In this case there is an additional cartilaginous fold of the antihelix, oriented in a vertical direction. The resultant loss of the scaphoid depression gives the pinna a pointed appearance (Fig. 1.5).

Protruding Ears

A variety of anomalies may lead to the appearance of protruding ears. Although many patients with such anomalies may complain of having "big ears," the majority of such cases are the result of abnormal position of the ear or auricular subunits. Dysplasia of the helix or antihelix may cause the appearance of protruding ears. As noted above, loss of the normal antihelical roll will result in this appearance.

Often the cause is related to the size and shape of the conchal cartilage and its position relative to the mastoid and other auricular subunits. The normal auricle projects from the mastoid at an angle of 15–20°. It has been observed that, in a normal appearing ear, the distance on posterior view from mastoid to the lateral extent of the auricle should be about 2 cm. In assessing the patient with protruding ears, it is essential to determine the exact anatomic cause of protrusion (Fig. 1.6) [6].

Cryptotia

Cryptotia is a rare congenital ear anomaly in which the cartilage of the auricle is tethered to the temporal portion of the head. This is the result of a deficiency of skin. There is a loss of the usual skin over the posterior aspect of the helix. The cartilage in cryptotia is normally formed. This condition occurs almost entirely in individuals of Japanese descent, indicating a likely genetic contribution.

Anomalies of the External Auditory Canal

Anomalies of the EAC may be categorized as aplasia, atresia, stenosis, or duplication. In assessing an abnormality of the auricle, it is important to diagnose a concurrent EAC or middle ear abnormality.

The distinction between aplastic and atretic anomalies lies in the position of the condyle relative to the mastoid. In a case of true EAC aplasia, there is complete lack of development of a canal and the glenoid itself is displaced posteriorly. The

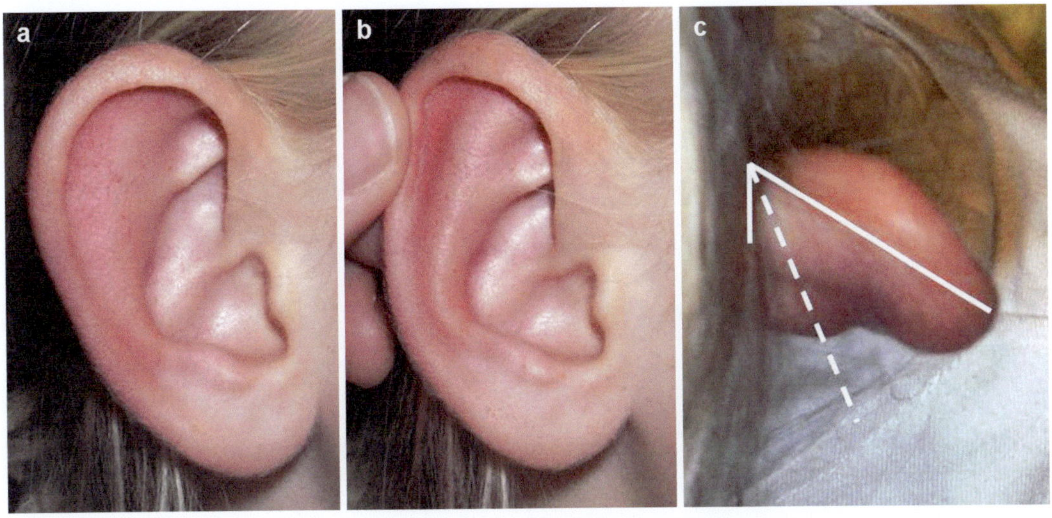

Fig. 1.6 Protruding ears. (**a**) Loss of normal antihelical fold, causing a lop ear defect. (**b**) Manual recreation of normal antihelical fold. (**c**) Significantly widened auricular angle (normal angle of 20° illustrated by *dotted line*)

mandibular condyle essentially articulates with the anterior surface of the mastoid. In EAC aplasia, there may be a minimal remnant of the first branchial cleft represented by a sinus or fistula tract.

EAC atresia refers to a canal that has developed normally to a point, but has not been successfully canalized. That is, the EAC is occluded by bony or fibrous tissue. This condition is more common than EAC aplasia. Jahrsdoerfer has presented a set of criteria in order to evaluate the likelihood of improving hearing through surgical repair of EAC atresia. These criteria include the presence of a normal stapes, oval window, and round window; articulation between the malleus-incus and incus-stapes; facial nerve anatomy; the appearance of the auricle; and pneumatization of the mastoid and middle ear space [13, 14].

Stenosis of the EAC may occur along the cartilaginous or bony canal. In most cases of canal stenosis, the TM and middle ear structures are normal. Canal stenosis must be severe in order to contribute to hearing deficits. However, patients with severe stenosis (less than 2 mm) are at high risk of developing canal cholesteatomas (Fig. 1.7) [15].

Duplication of the EAC may occur. This is more commonly termed a first branchial cleft anomaly. These are categorized as work types I or II. Work type I anomalies represent an EAC duplication that extends from the preauricular skin and runs parallel to the EAC, often opening into the middle ear space. Type I anomalies are made up of ectodermal tissue only. A work type II anomaly is a fistulous tract extending from the skin (or possibly from a subcutaneous cyst), typically overlying or just inferior to the angle of the mandible. Type II first branchial cleft anomalies generally open into the EAC itself, at the bony cartilaginous junction. Work type II anomalies are made up of both ectodermal and mesodermal elements (contain cartilage) and are notoriously involved with the facial nerve [16].

Syndromic Ear Anomalies

The majority of congenital abnormalities of the ear occur in otherwise normally developed individuals. However, there are many genetic syndromes that are associated with an increased incidence of certain congenital ear anomalies. Identification of such patterns can be important in diagnosing additional, systemic abnormalities.

Oculo-Auriculo-Vertebral syndrome (OAV), also known by the eponym Goldenhar's syndrome, is a congenital syndrome characterized by defects of the first and second branchial arches. OAV has an incidence of about 1/3,000 live births. It is most commonly sporadic, although occasional familial clusters indicate a genetic predisposition. This syndrome presents with abnormalities of the mandible and palate, limbal dermoids, and cervical vertebrae. It is generally unilateral although bilateral cases have been reported. OAV is associated with unilateral microtia, often severe (grade II or IV). This syndrome is also associated with preauricular appendages, which represent either duplications of the hillocks of His or tissue from hillocks that failed to fuse normally (Fig. 1.8) [17, 18].

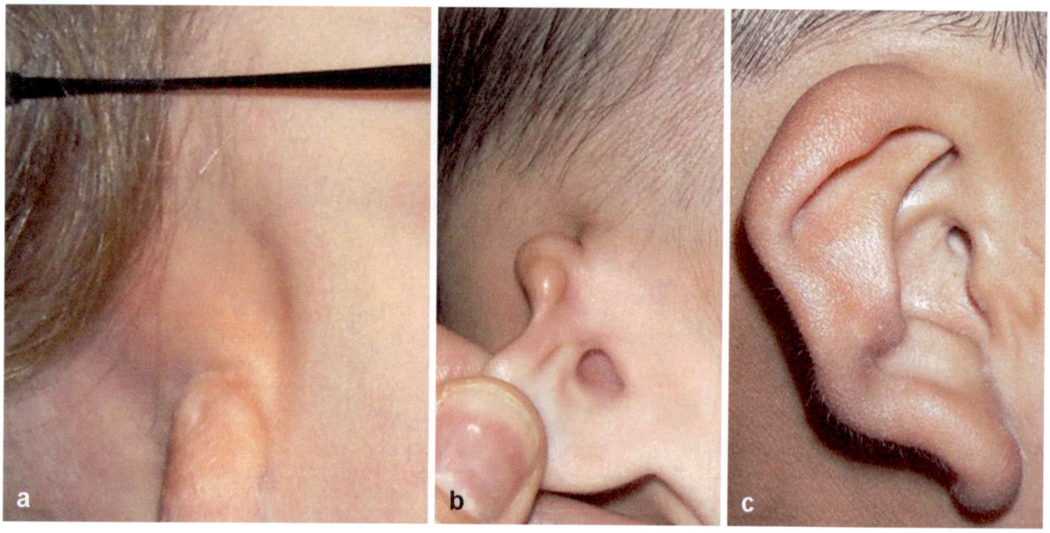

Fig. 1.7 EAC abnormalities. (**a**) Canal atresia. (**b**) Atresia of the bony canal with patent cartilaginous portion. (**c**) Canal stenosis

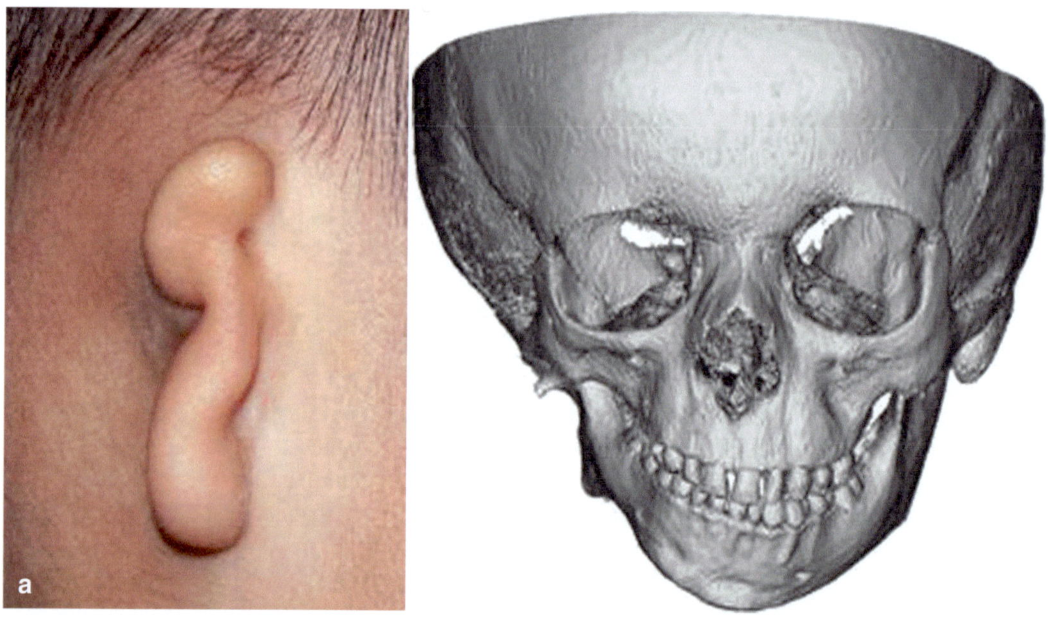

Fig. 1.8 Syndromes associated with external ear anomalies. (**a**) OAV syndrome with hypoplastic right midface and loss of normal mandibular height shown in 3D reconstruction. Grade III microtia. (**b**) BWS with characteristic lobular clefting. Macroglossia. (**c**) CHARGE syndrome with variable presentation of ears, generally hypoplastic or absent lobule. Coloboma of the eye

Fig. 1.8 (continued)

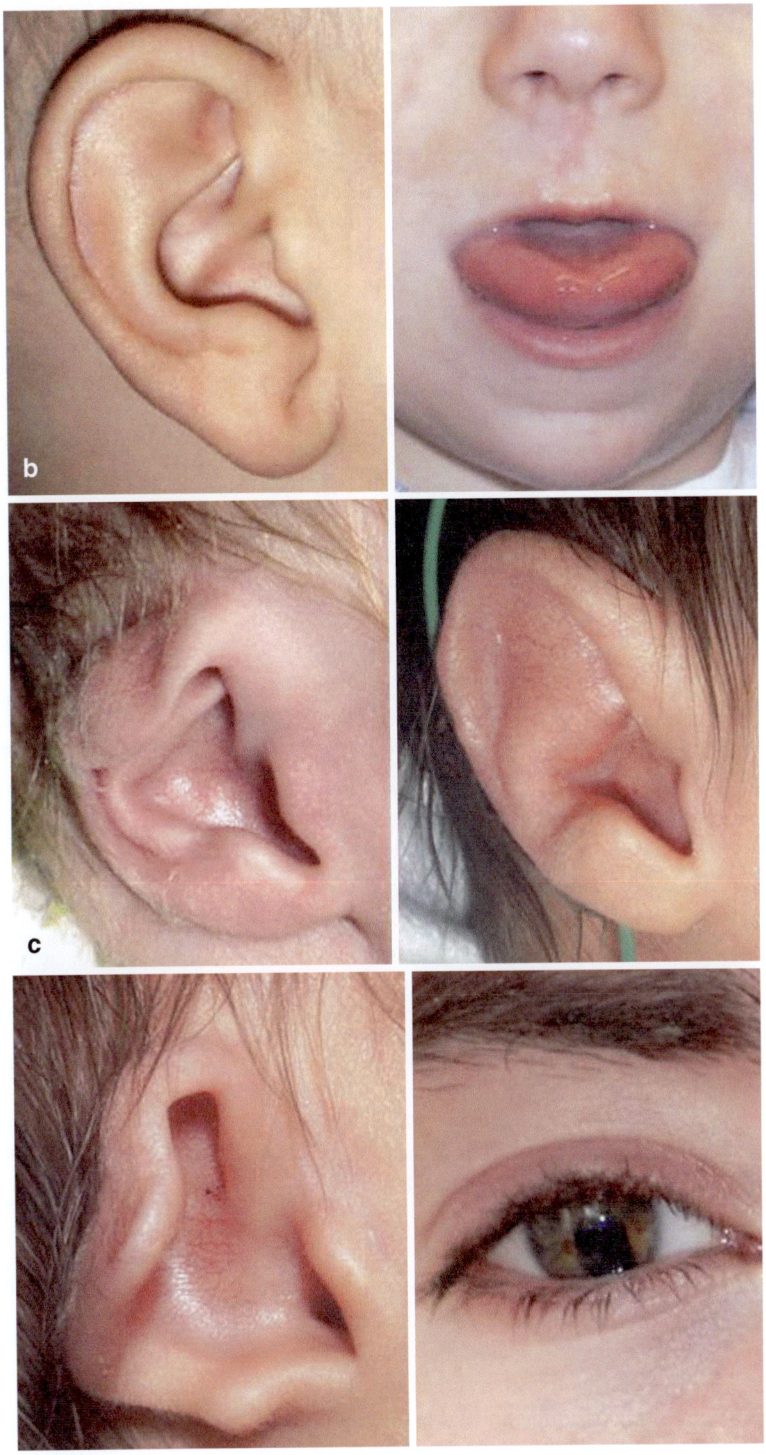

Beckwith-Wiedemann syndrome (BWS) is a congenital syndrome characterized by exomphalos (a congenital abdominal wall defect), macrosomia, macroglossia, and neonatal hypoglycemia. This syndrome is most commonly sporadic, although familial cases have been identified, with a common mutation on the short arm of chromosome 11 [19]. BWS is associated with characteristic lobular clefts (or dimples) as well as posterior helical pits. Patients with this disorder have a significantly increased risk of developing childhood cancers including Wilm's tumor and hepatoblastoma (Fig. 1.8) [20].

CHARGE syndrome (formerly CHARGE association) is characterized by coloboma of the eyes, heart defects, atresia of the nasal choanae, retardation of growth/development, genitourinary abnormalities, and ear anomalies. This condition was previously known as an association of congenital abnormalities. Recent studies have identified an associated mutation of the CHD7 gene on chromosome 8 in 60–70 % of patients with this phenotype, and as such it is now termed a genetic syndrome. CHARGE is associated with dysmorphology of the external, middle, and inner ear. The auricle of patients with CHARGE often has an absent lobule, although there is an increased prevalence of other abnormalities as well (Fig. 1.8) [21, 22].

Conclusions

The external ear develops from ectodermal and mesodermal elements of the first and second branchial arches, primarily during the 5th–20th weeks of gestational development. Six hillocks of His are formed initially and the fusion of these structures forms the auricle as well as cartilaginous EAC. An understanding of the normal development of the ear is essential in order to understand the various congenital anomalies that may develop. Accurate recognition of congenital ear anomalies allows for the appropriate management of these conditions and also the potential recognition of other congenital abnormalities.

References

1. Rodríguez-Vázquez JF. Development of the stapes and associated structures in human embryos. J Anat. 2005;207(2):165–73.
2. His W. Anatomie Menschlicher Embryonem Part III. Leipzig: FCW Vogel; 1885. p. 211.
3. Karmody CS, Annino Jr DJ. Embryology and anomalies of the external ear. Facial Plast Surg. 1995;11(4):251–6.
4. Rogers BO. Anatomy embryology and classification of auricular deformities. In: Tanzier RC, Edgerton MT, editors. Symposium on reconstruction of the auricle. St. Louis: CV Mosby Co.; 1974. p. 3–11.
5. Bowden RE. Development of the middle and external ear in man. Proc R Soc Med. 1977;70(11): 807–15.
6. Papel ID, Frodel JL, Larrabee WF, Holt GR, Nachlas NE, Park SS, et al. Facial plastic and reconstructive surgery. 3rd ed. New York: Thieme Medical Publishing; 2002.
7. Lucente FE. Anatomy, histology, and physiology. In: Lucente FE, Lawson W, Novick NL, editors. The external ear. Philadelphia: WB Saunders Co.; 1995. p. 1–16.
8. Artunduaga MA, Quintanilla-Dieck Mde L, Greenway S, Betensky R, Nicolau Y, Hamdan U, et al. A classic twin study of external ear malformations, including microtia. N Engl J Med. 2009;361(12): 1216–8.
9. Alasti F, Van Camp G. Genetics of microtia and associated syndromes. J Med Genet. 2009;46(6): 361–9.
10. Marx H. Beitrag zur morholgie und genese der mittelohrmissbildungen mit gehorgangsatresie. Z Hals Nasa Ohrenheilkd. 1922;2:230.
11. Karmody CS. A classification of the anomalies of the first branchial groove. Otolaryngol Head Neck Surg. 1979;87(3):334–8.
12. Klockars T, Rautio J. Embryology and epidemiology of microtia. Facial Plast Surg. 2009;25(3): 145–8.
13. Jahrsdoerfer RA, Hall III JW. Congenital malformations of the ear. Am J Otol. 1986;7(4):267–9.
14. Shonka Jr DC, Livingston 3rd WJ, Kesser BW. The Jahrsdoerfer Grading Scale in surgery to repair congenital aural atresia. Arch Otolaryngol Head Neck Surg. 2008;134(8):873–7.
15. Cole RR, Jahrsdoerfer RA. The risk of cholesteatoma in congenital aural stenosis. Laryngoscope. 1990; 100(6):576–8.
16. Work WP. Newer concepts of first branchial cleft defects. Laryngoscope. 1972;82(9):1581–93.
17. Passos-Bueno MR, Ornelas CC, Fanganiello RD. Syndromes of the first and second pharyngeal arches: a review. Am J Med Genet A. 2009;149A(8): 1853–9.

18. Rosa RF, da Silva AP, Goetze TB, Bier Bde A, de Almeida ST, Paskulin GA, et al. Ear abnormalities in patients with oculo-auriculo-vertebral spectrum (Goldenhar syndrome). Braz J Otorhinolaryngol. 2011;77(4):455–60.
19. Pettenati MJ, Haines JL, Higgins RR, Wappner RS, Palmer CG, Weaver DD. Wiedemann-Beckwith syndrome: presentation of clinical and cytogenetic data on 22 new cases and review of the literature. Hum Genet. 1986;74(2):143–54.
20. DeBaun MR, Tucker MA. Risk of cancer during the first four years of life in children from The Beckwith-Wiedemann Syndrome Registry. J Pediatr. 1986;132(3 Pt 1):398–400.
21. Lalani SR, Safiullah AM, Fernbach SD, et al. Spectrum of CHD7 mutations in 110 individuals with CHARGE syndrome and genotype-phenotype correlation. Am J Hum Genet. 2006;78(2):303–14.
22. Vissers LE, van Ravenswaai CM, Admiraal R, Hurst JA, de Vrie BB, Janssen IM, et al. Mutations in a new member of the chromodomain gene family cause CHARGE syndrome. Nat Genet. 2004;36(9):955–7.

Anatomy of the External Ear

2

Peter M. Prendergast

Introduction

The external ear comprises the auricle and the auditory canal. The fibrocartilaginous auricle funnels sound waves from the environment into the auditory canal to the tympanic membrane. This convoluted shell-like pliable structure is functionally but also aesthetically important. Deviations from the norm or aberrations in position, shape, size, or in the architecture of the auricle are noticeable and undesirable. Careful surgical correction or reconstruction can restore the beauty of the ear and a harmonious appearance with the face. Aesthetic otoplasty techniques are elegant and often intricate and rely on a complete understanding of anatomy. As well as knowing the muscles, nerves, and vessels supplying the auricle, every groove, fold, concavity, and convexity of the ear should be clearly imprinted in the mind of any surgeon embarking on aesthetic otoplasty and reconstruction of the auricle.

Auricle

The auricle is the irregularly shaped part of the external ear that protrudes from the face at the level of the temporal bone (Fig. 2.1). It consists of an elastic, convoluted cartilaginous plate covered in skin. The auricle is tilted posteriorly somewhat so that the long axis creates an angle of approximately 8° with the retromandibular line. The superior aspect of the auricle is ideally located on a vertical plane with the brow [1]. Normal projection from the mastoid is about 10 or 17–20 mm from the mastoid to the free border of the helix. Normal projection varies between races, with a greater mastoid to helix distance seen in Asians. In children, the auricle is wider and shorter. The height-to-width ratio increases as the ear grows, reaching about 7:4 in adulthood. Depending on the position of the auricle, its surfaces can be described as anterior or lateral, and posterior or medial [2]. As the ear comes into view, it is easy to appreciate the eminences and cavities of the anterior auricular surface. On frontal view, the helix should be visible 2–5 mm laterally behind the antihelix [3].

Anterior (Lateral) Auricular Surface

The outline or margin of the auricle is formed by the helix, an incompletely folded tube that creates a gutter or scaphoid fossa along most of its length. The helix starts anteriorly, emerging from the cavity or concha of the auricle as the helical crus. It passes anterosuperiorly first, then posterosuperiorly, posteroinferiorly, and anterosuperiorly, creating a smooth, rounded arc. A small dimple marks the point where the helical tail merges with the lobule. Often, a small

P.M. Prendergast, M.D., MB, BCh, MRCSI
Venus Medical,
Heritage House, Dundrum Office Park,
Dundrum, Dublin 14, Ireland
e-mail: peter@venusmed.com

M.A. Shiffman (ed.), *Advanced Cosmetic Otoplasty*,
DOI 10.1007/978-3-642-35431-1_2, © Springer-Verlag Berlin Heidelberg 2013

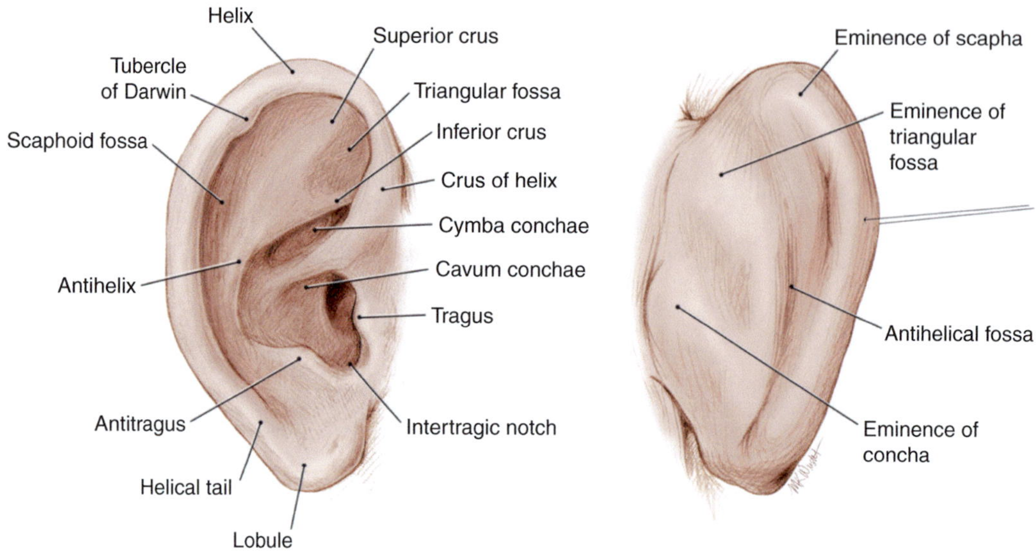

Fig. 2.1 Auricle surface. (*Left*) Anterior. (*Right*) Posterior

protuberance or tubercle, known as Darwin's tubercle, exists where the helix superior meets the helix posterior (Fig. 2.1).

Inside the helix lies the antihelix, making up part of the floor of the auricle and circumscribing the concha. Superiorly, the antihelix has two elevations, superior and inferior crura, between which lies the triangular fossa. Inferiorly, the antihelical tail joins the antitragus at the posterior auricular sulcus. Both the helix and antihelix are visible in a frontal view, but the antihelix protrudes more as it passes from superiorly to inferiorly, creating an angle of approximately 20° between the helical and antihelical planes [4]. The inferior crus of the antihelix is oriented more superiorly in taller people with longer ears. In those with shorter ears and in children, the inferior crus is oriented more horizontally.

The concha is an incomplete cavity that leads into the auditory canal. The sharp superior edge of the concha is formed by the inferior crus of the antihelix, the inferior edge by the sharp edges of the tragus and antitragus, which overhang the concha and make it appear smaller. In contrast, the lateral edge is smooth and rolled and formed by the antihelix. The tragus projects from the face to partially cover the anteroinferior part of the concha, whereas the antitragus projects superiorly rom the lobule to cover part of the inferior region of the concha. A prominent, sharp-edged, intertragic notch lies between the tragus and antitragus. In older patients, a tuft of hair—barbula hirci—often protrudes from this notch.

The lobule is the only part of the auricle without an underlying cartilaginous framework. About one-third of its perimeter is attached anteriorly to the cheek, with the remainder dangling as a free border. Above, an antitragal gutter or depression separates the lobule from the antitragus.

The skin of the anterior auricular surface is closely adherent to the underlying perichondrium, with almost no fat between them. Vessels and nerves lie within a slip of fascia that separates the skin and perichondrium. Sebaceous and sudoriparous glands are present in the triangular fossa and around the external auditory meatus, respectively. Ceruminous glands predominate in the auditory canal. The integument of the postauricular surface differs greatly from the tightly bound, fat-free skin found on the anterior auricular surface. In contrast, the posterior surface is characterized by skin that can wrinkle and glide over the underlying cartilage. There are two layers of fat that allow this, a superficial dense layer

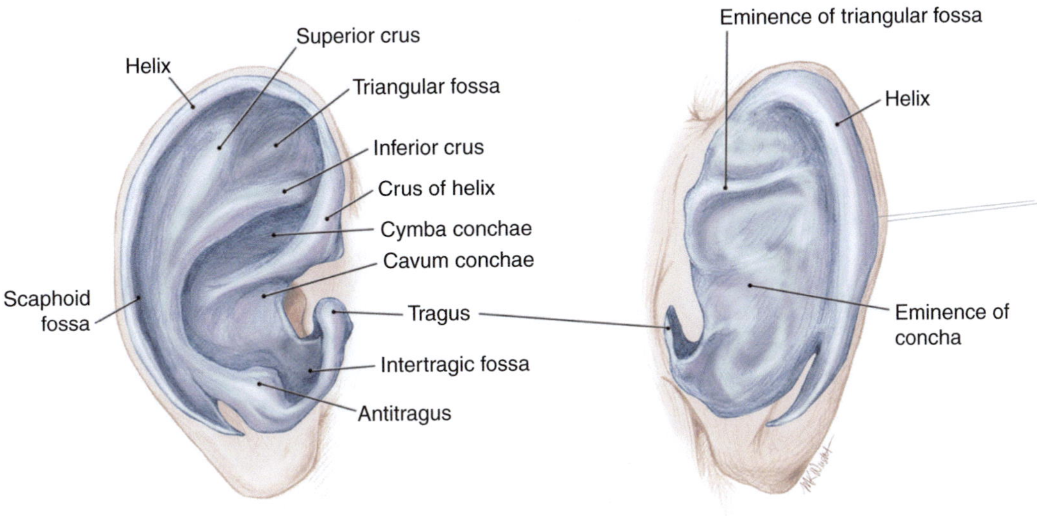

Fig. 2.2 Cartilage of the auricle. (*Left*) Anterior. (*Right*) Posterior

and a looser deep layer. A layer of fascia between the superficial and deep layers of adipose tissue envelopes the nerves, vessels, and lymphatics that supply and innervate the posterior surface of the auricle [4]. A subdermal vascular network also exists more superficially. This subdermal architecture extends over the helical margin to the helical rim where the transition from one type of integument to the other occurs. The lobule contains firm trabecular fat and a network of subdermal and deep vessels and is covered in fine hairs. Over the inferior aspect of the auricle, the transition from skin that is adherent to that which glides is less sharp but occurs from the posterior auricular sulcus, antitragus, tragus, and anterior auricular sulcus.

Posterior (Medial) Auricular Surface

The posterior auricular surface is mostly hidden from view since the auricle projects only 10 mm from the mastoid. The surface is characterized by prominences and sulci in an inverse pattern to that seen on the anterior auricular surface (Fig. 2.1). The main eminences are formed by the scapha, the concha, and the triangular fossa. The antihelical fossa lies between these eminences.

Cartilage

The auricle obtains its shape, appearance, and flexibility from the underlying convoluted cartilaginous plate. The entire auricle, except for the lobule, has cartilage as its framework. The unique structure of the auricle, including creases and folds in the cartilage, allows it to be bent, folded, and compressed without discomfort or consequence. A thin, very adherent, layer of perichondrium covers the cartilage of the auricle.

The anterior/lateral surface of the cartilage greatly resembles the auricle itself since it is covered only in a thin layer of skin (Fig. 2.2). The helix curves anterosuperiorly from the crus and then backward to form the cartilaginous margin of the auricle. The scapha represents the valley between the helix and antihelix. The cartilaginous tragus and antitragus are separated by the intertragic notch. The concha and tragus continue medially to form the cartilaginous part of the external auditory canal. This cartilaginous part fits into and fuses with the socket of the bony part of the external auditory canal. The posterosuperior part of the helix and the scapha are peppered with numerous tiny openings [5]. Otherwise, the lateral cartilaginous plate of the auricle is smooth.

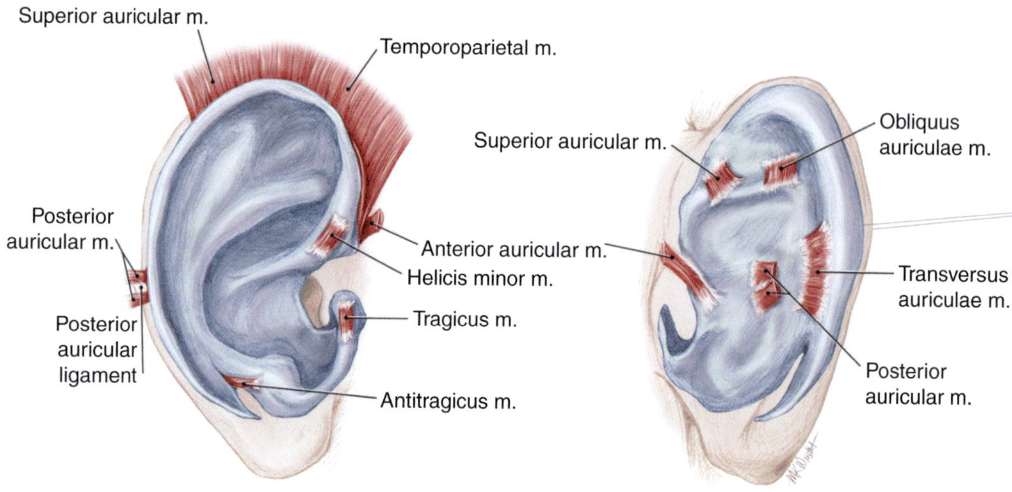

Fig. 2.3 Extrinsic and intrinsic muscles of the auricle

Foramina that transmit vessels and nerves are present throughout the cartilage of the auricle, particularly in the scapha, triangular fossa, and concha.

The medial surface of the cartilage of the auricle appears as fossae and eminences in a reverse pattern to its lateral counterpart (Fig. 2.2). The cartilage is almost uniform in thickness throughout the auricle, so the triangular fossa and concha appear as eminences on the medial surface of the auricle. Similarly, the antihelix appears as an antihelical fossa on the medial surface. Parts of the antihelix and concha on the medial surface are rough in texture where external auricular muscles attach.

The lobule hangs from the auricle inferiorly and has no underlying structural cartilaginous support. The entire cartilaginous auricle fits into the socket of the cartilaginous external auditory canal and is supported by ligaments and muscles.

Muscles

The small extrinsic muscles and ligaments of the ear provide anchorage and support for the auricle, holding it firmly in place over the bony skull. The resting tone of the tiny rudimentary intrinsic muscles provides structural support for the auricle and contributes to its characteristic convoluted and folded configuration (Fig. 2.3).

The extrinsic muscles consist of the posterior, superior, and anterior auricular muscles. The posterior muscle comprises a superior and inferior slip, supported by the posterior auricular ligament. Posteriorly, the muscles arise from the mastoid periosteum. The superior part attaches to the eminentia cymba, the upper part of the conchal eminence. The inferior part of the posterior auricular muscle inserts into the cartilage of the ponticulus, the lower part of the conchal eminence. The posterior auricular ligament reinforces the posterior auricular muscle and runs parallel to the two slips of muscle from the mastoid periosteum to the conchal eminence. These muscles are innervated by the posterior auricular branch of the facial nerve and supplied by posterior auricular vessels. The superior auricular muscle is a short but strong muscle arising from the epicranial aponeurosis above and inserts into the eminence of the triangular fossa on the posterior auricular surface. It is enveloped in layers of the superficial temporal fascia and receives innervation from temporal branch of the facial nerve. The superior auricular muscle receives its blood supply from small branches of the superficial temporal vessels. The anterior auricular muscle provides further support for the auricle anteriorly.

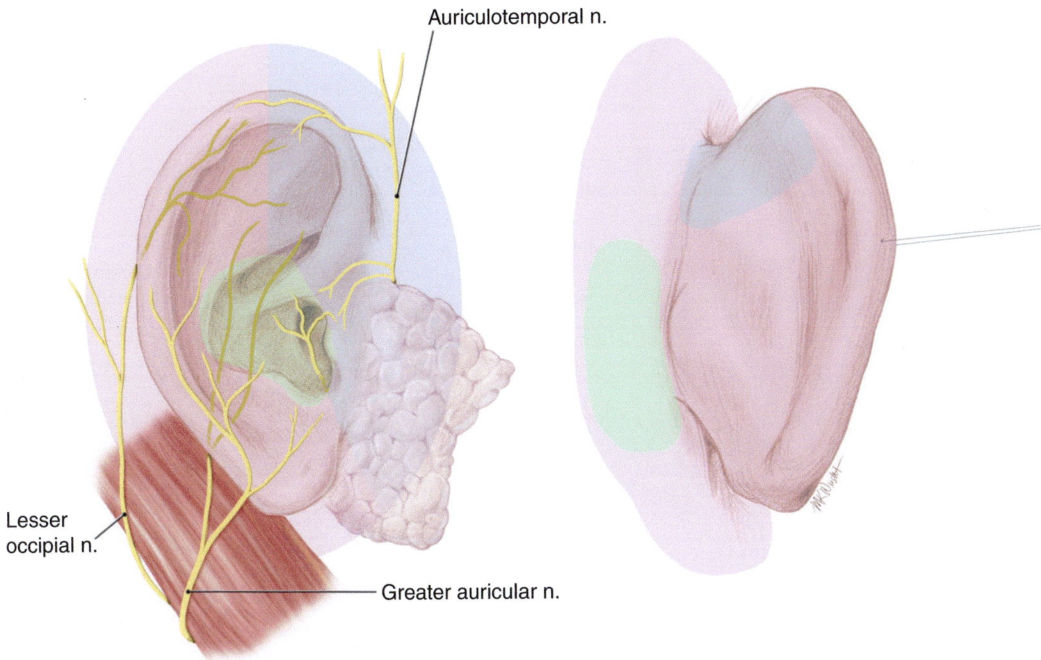

Fig. 2.4 Sensory innervation of the auricle

It passes from the zygomatic arch and epicranial aponeurosis anteriorly to the spine of the helix posteriorly. It is supplied by branches of the superficial temporal vessels and receives innervation from the auriculotemporal nerve and temporal branch of the facial nerve. The anterior auricular muscle is supported by a ligament of the same name that tethers the tragus and helical spine to the zygomatic arch and epicranial aponeurosis.

The intrinsic muscles consist of tiny anteriorly and posteriorly arranged slips that connect and bridge the convexities and concavities of the auricle (Fig. 2.3). Anteriorly, the helicis major, helicis minor, tragicus, and antitragicus muscles are arranged around the concha. They are not under voluntary control and are essentially remnants of what was once a sphincter controlling sound entry. Posteriorly, there are four main intrinsic ligaments as well as vertically and horizontally arranged muscle fibers connecting and supporting the cartilaginous convolutions of the auricle.

Nerves

The auricle receives innervation from branches of the greater auricular nerve, lesser occipital nerve, auriculotemporal nerve, facial nerve, and vagus nerve (Fig. 2.4). Most of these are sensory, with some vasomotor and secretory fibers arising from the facial nerve [6].

The greater auricular nerve provides most sensory innervation of the auricle. It arises from fibers of the second and third cervical nerves. It emerges onto the posterior border of sternocleidomastoid as a root, between the sternocleidomastoid fascia and platysma. The nerve passes in this plane toward the ear and divides into anterior and posterior branches below the auricle. The anterior branch pierces the lobule and sends sensory branches to the inferior, posterior, and superior parts of the lateral auricular surface. The posterior branch of the greater auricular nerve passes under the lobule and supplies the cranial surface of the auricle. The greater auricular nerve also innervates the anterior and superior walls of the external auditory

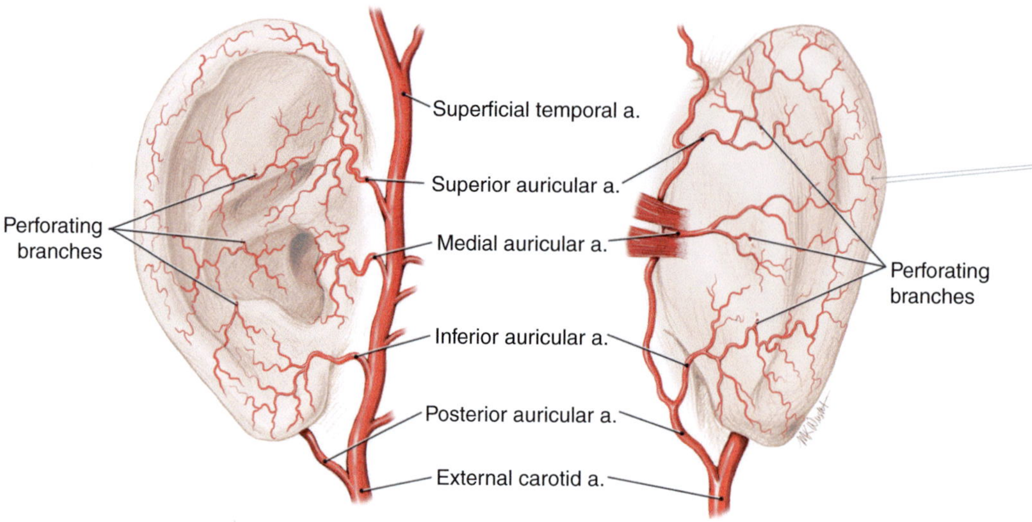

Fig. 2.5 Arterial supply of the auricle

canal. The lesser occipital nerve also arises from fibers of the second, and sometimes third, cervical nerves. It courses along the posterior border of sternocleidomastoid, behind the auricle, to innervate the scalp as well as the superior part of the cranial auricular surface.

The auriculotemporal nerve is a branch of the posterior trunk of the mandibular branch of the trigeminal nerve. Although it is mainly a sensory nerve, it also carries sympathetic and parasympathetic fibers and ganglionic branches that communicate with the otic ganglion. Its two roots encircle the middle meningeal artery and then unite behind the artery and pass superficially to lie between the external acoustic meatus and temporomandibular joint. The auriculotemporal nerve passes superiorly with the superficial temporal vessels, over the zygomatic arch toward the temple. Sensory branches from the auriculotemporal nerve supply the tragus, inferior crus of the antihelix, anterosuperior part of the scapha and helix, and crus of the helix. It also innervates the posterior wall of the auditory canal and tympanic membrane.

The auricular branch of the vagus nerve arises from the superior ganglion below the jugular foramen. It passes through the temporal bone and exits the tympanomastoid fissure at the opening of the external acoustic meatus. It divides into two branches, one supplying the concha and cymba conchae of the auricle and the other anastomosing with the posterior auricular branch of the facial nerve. The auricular branch of the vagus nerve, or nerve of Arnold, also innervates the floor of the external auditory canal.

Motor branches of the facial nerve innervate the extrinsic and intrinsic auricular muscles. After emerging from the parotid capsule, the temporal branch of the facial nerve passes beneath the superficial musculoaponeurotic system and anterosuperiorly toward the temporal area and lateral canthus. During its course, it gives off several branches that innervate tragicus, helicis major, helicis minor, and anterior auricular muscle. More superiorly, branches innervate the superior auricular muscle, and others continue to supply the posterior auricular muscle and the tiny intrinsic muscles of the posterior auricular surface. Autonomic sympathetic fibers traveling with the facial nerve provide vasomotor and secretory function to the vessels and glands of the auricle.

Vascular Supply

The external ear receives its arterial supply through branches of the superficial temporal artery anteriorly and posterior auricular artery posteriorly (Fig. 2.5). The superficial temporal artery arises within the parotid as the anterior branch of the external carotid artery. It emerges from the parotid capsule and runs superiorly toward the temporal area, about 1 cm anterior to the auricle and beneath the anterior auricular muscle and deep to the superficial temporal vein. As it travels superiorly, it sends three main branches posteriorly toward the auricle: inferior, medial, and anterosuperior auricular arteries. These vessels form a richly branching and anastomosing network between the skin and perichondrium of the anterior auricular surface. The caliber of these vessels varies, but there are fairly consistent perforating vessels that pass from the regions of the antitragus, cymba conchae, and triangular fossa to the posterior auricular surface.

The posterior auricular artery arises as the posterior branch of the external carotid artery. It courses below the greater auricular nerve toward the mastoid process. A mastoid branch supplies the skin in this area. The main posterior auricular artery continues behind the auricle and passes superiorly behind the posterior auricular muscles. Three main branches supply the posterior (cranial) auricular surface: inferior, medial, and posterosuperior auricular arteries. These arteries form a superficial anastomotic arcade just below the skin and a deeper subcutaneous vascular layer. The latter is ensheathed in fascia that separates the fat on the posterior auricular surface into a superficial trabecular layer and deep layer. The posterior auricular artery branches also perforate the auricular cartilage to anastomose with the anterior vessels.

The anterior and posterior auricular veins follow the arteries, although there is often more than one vein per artery. The veins are slightly larger in diameter, up to 2 mm. Posteriorly, the posterior auricular vein drains the posterior surface of the auricle and runs inferiorly between the posterior auricular artery and greater auricular nerve to drain into the external jugular vein.

References

1. Adamson PA, Litner JA. Aesthetic parameters and specific deformities. In: Litner JA, Adamson C, Adamson PA, editors. Aesthetic otoplasty, connecticut. People's Medical Publishing House, Beijing, China. 2011. p. 15.
2. Weerda H. Anatomy of the external ear. In: Weerda H, editor. Surgery of the auricle. Tumors, trauma, defects, abnormalities. Stuttgart: Georg Thieme; 2007. p. 1.
3. Wright WK. Otoplasty goals and principles. Arch Otolarygol. 1970;92(6):568–72.
4. Davis J. Surgical artistry and the levels of otoplasty. In: Davis J, editor. Aesthetic and reconstructive otoplasty. Berlin: Springer; 1987. p. 61.
5. Vidic B, O'Rahilly R. Lateral surface of isolated cartilage of auricle. In: Vidic B, O'Rahilly R, editors. An atlas of the anatomy of the ear. Philadelphia: Saunders; 1971.
6. Gilroy AM, MacPherson BR, Ross LM. External ear and auditory canal. In: Gilroy AM, McPherson BR, Ross LM, editors. Atlas of anatomy. New York: Thieme; 2008. p. 529.

Anatomy, History, and Utility of the Posterior Auricular Fascia in Otoplasty

3

Kayvan Shokrollahi and James P. Taylor

Historical Perspective

The anatomy of the fascia posterior to the ear, often referred to as the "retroauricular" or "superficial mastoid" region, is interesting due to its variety of applications within plastic surgery in general and more specifically in otoplasty. Its versatility relates to a number of factors including a defined and complex blood supply [1] and its thin but strong constitution [2, 3]. This fascia has been used in a variety of indications ranging from lip enhancement [4] and repairs of nasal [5] and auricular defects [2] to an adjunct in the management of congenital or acquired defects including microtia-atresia [1, 6].

In relation to otoplasty specifically, the post-auricular fascia gained recognition as a useful entity when used as cover for suture knots in Mustarde-style otoplasty [7], with the purpose of reducing recurrence and palpability or extrusion of permanent suture material. This flap is based posteriorly and sutured with fine absorbable sutures back up towards the helical rim after placement of chondral sutures. The posteriorly based flap is demonstrably useful for this indication [8], although it has minimal mechanical value in terms of shaping the ear or correcting the deformity.

Subsequently, the fascia was used as an intrinsic part of the otoplasty technique to give a natural look with minimal recurrence by raising it based anteriorly on the helical rim itself and suturing it to the mastoid [9]. Through its attachments along the helical rim, the fascia-mastoid juxtaposition creates a natural ear contour difficult to achieve with sutures alone while maintaining suture cover and removing tension from Mustarde sutures. It was suggested [9] that the fascia-to-mastoid suture alone could correct the prominent ear, and this was partially confirmed by other authors subsequently [10], who described a similar technique. However, these authors [10] still used a permanent conchomastoid (Furnas) suture and advocated overcorrection as part of the procedure. The results were presented as "A total of 72 patients (87.8 %) underwent a single procedure. In ten patients, there was an excessive loss of medialization of the upper pole, 2 bilaterally, leading to a total of 12 reoperated ears (7.41 %). In seven ears (4.34 %) there was a partial extrusion of the suture thread, in its conchal portion, which was

K. Shokrollahi, M.D., BSc, MB, ChB, MSc, LLM, MRCS(Eng), FRCS(Plast) (✉)
Mersey Regional Burns and Plastic Surgery Unit, Ward 4D, Whiston Hospital, Warrington Rd, Liverpool L35 5DR, UK
e-mail: kshokrollahi@hotmail.com

J.P. Taylor, MA (Cantab), MBBChir, MRCS (Eng)
Core Surgical Trainee, Guys and St Thomas' NHS Foundation Trust, St Thomas' Hospital, Westminster Bridge Road, London, UK
e-mail: jamesptaylor23@gmail.com

M.A. Shiffman (ed.), *Advanced Cosmetic Otoplasty*,
DOI 10.1007/978-3-642-35431-1_3, © Springer-Verlag Berlin Heidelberg 2013

removed in the office and did not require additional corrections" [10].

It therefore remains inconclusive as to whether fascial repair alone can truly, reliably, symmetrically, and aesthetically correct prominent ears in the long term without sutures. We believe that for consistent and symmetrical results with minimal recurrence, Mustarde sutures are still required in the form of what is best termed fascia-augmented otoplasty and are not associated with high extrusion and revision rates [9] as experienced with Furnas sutures [10]. Overcorrection as an intrinsic part of this or any procedure is not desirable as it does not allow sufficient surgical control of the end result or sufficient control over final symmetry.

A further advantage of augmenting suture-based otoplasty with a de-tensioning anteriorly based fascial flap is that it works synergistically with our technique of glue instead of head bandages as postoperative splints [9, 11–13], allowing patients to wash their hair and for girls to hide all stigmata of surgery beneath long hair. The utility of this strategy has been reviewed recently [12]. The glue is used to affix the ear temporarily to the side of the head and usually lasts for up to 2 weeks but depends on the brand of glue.

Based on our own anatomical studies, we describe herein the macro- and microscopic detail of the fascia. The auriculocephalic sulcus demarcates the region previously described as the postauricular, or retroauricular, fascia from the fascia directly adherent to the posterior surface of the ear. The authors have termed these the extrinsic postauricular fascia (EPF) and intrinsic postauricular fascia (IPF), respectively.

Anatomy of the Postauricular Region

Our anatomical cadaveric studies have elucidated that the anatomy of the IPF, from superficial to deep, comprises the skin, subcutaneous fascia and fat, blood vessels and nerves, perichondrium, and finally cartilage (Figs. 3.1 and 3.2). Auricularis posterior, when present, is enveloped by the fascia. The IPF, in comparison to the tough fibrous tissues of the superficial peri-mastoid fascia of the EPF, is less fibrous and is not in

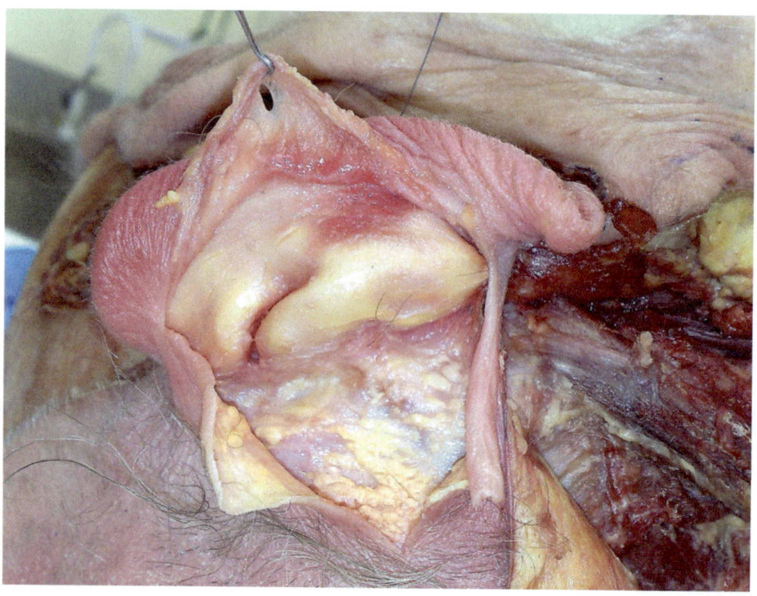

Fig. 3.1 Access incision with intrinsic fascia removed

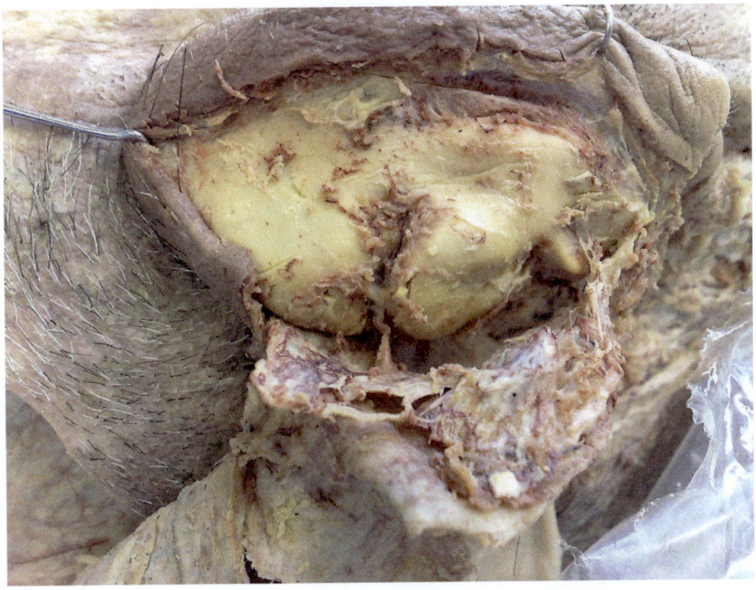

Fig. 3.2 Dissection of the IPF off the cartilage

direct continuity with any convincing muscle mass, except via those attachments to auricularis posterior.

Injection studies of the cadavers revealed that the IPF has a codominant blood supply mirroring that of the auricle itself, which arises from the superficial temporal artery and the posterior auricular artery (Fig. 3.3). One of the main reasons for the IPFs' excellent potential for use in plastic surgery is due to this rich vascular network (Fig. 3.4). This intricate labyrinth of vessels consists of multiple anastomoses (Fig. 3.5), which makes it an ideal candidate as a bed for skin grafts when used as a recipient flap. The EPF itself, in contrast, receives its main blood supply via the occipital artery and auricular branches of the posterior auricular artery. Its nerve supply hails from the greater auricular and lesser occipital nerves [1].

The auriculocephalic sulcus corresponds to the junction of the EPF and IPF, which we term the auricular fascial incisura (AFI) (Fig. 3.6). There is a clear and apparent change in the nature and quality of the fascia: the thin fascia of the IPF, which is adherent to the ear, becomes layered and fibrous up to and beyond the mastoid. Datta et al. [2] have previously described the layers of the mastoid fascia (EPF): below the skin and subcutaneous tissue, there exist three fascial layers. Firstly and most caudally, a strong, heavy, thick fibrous fascia exists which was previously referred to as the superficial mastoid fascia. More cranially, the previously described superficial temporal fascia exists, which is more elastic and less fibrous in consistency. Finally, the deep mastoid fascia exists below the superficial mastoid fascia, which is thinner and more fibrous than its superficial counterpart. This layer of fascia then attaches to the periosteum of the petrous temporal bone, while its cranial continuation is termed the innominate fascia. This separates the deep and superficial temporal fascia, which is the deep layer directly covering the temporal muscles (Fig. 3.7).

The IPF is thinner and less fibrous than its extrinsic counterpart. It is unique in that it lies between the posterior auricular skin and the perichondrium of the ear and possesses vessels and fine nerves within. If the skin and cartilage of the ear are excised, all that remains is the IPF, perichondrium, fibro-fatty tissue, nerves, and vessels.

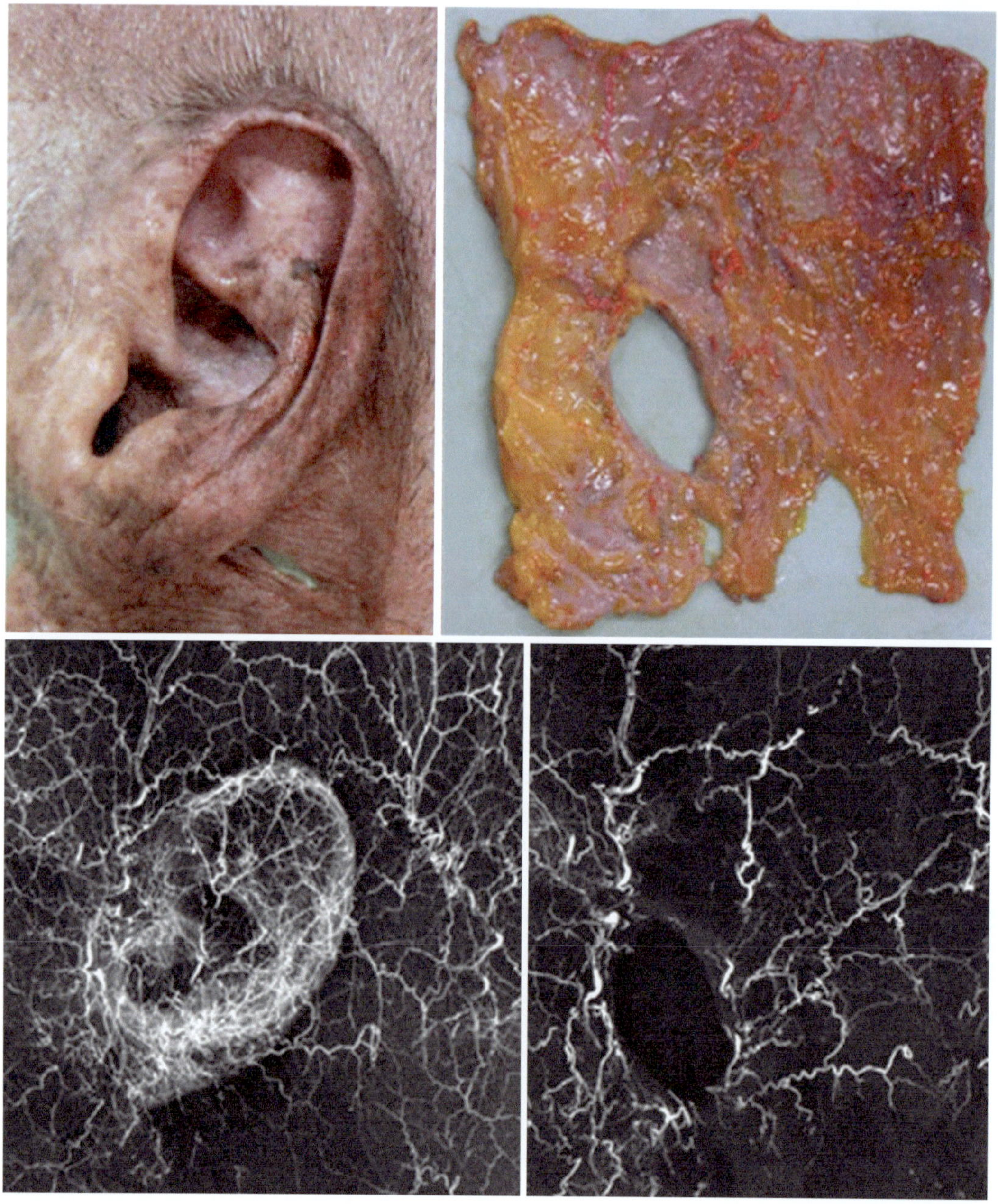

Fig. 3.3 Continuity of vascular anastomosis between head, neck, and ear

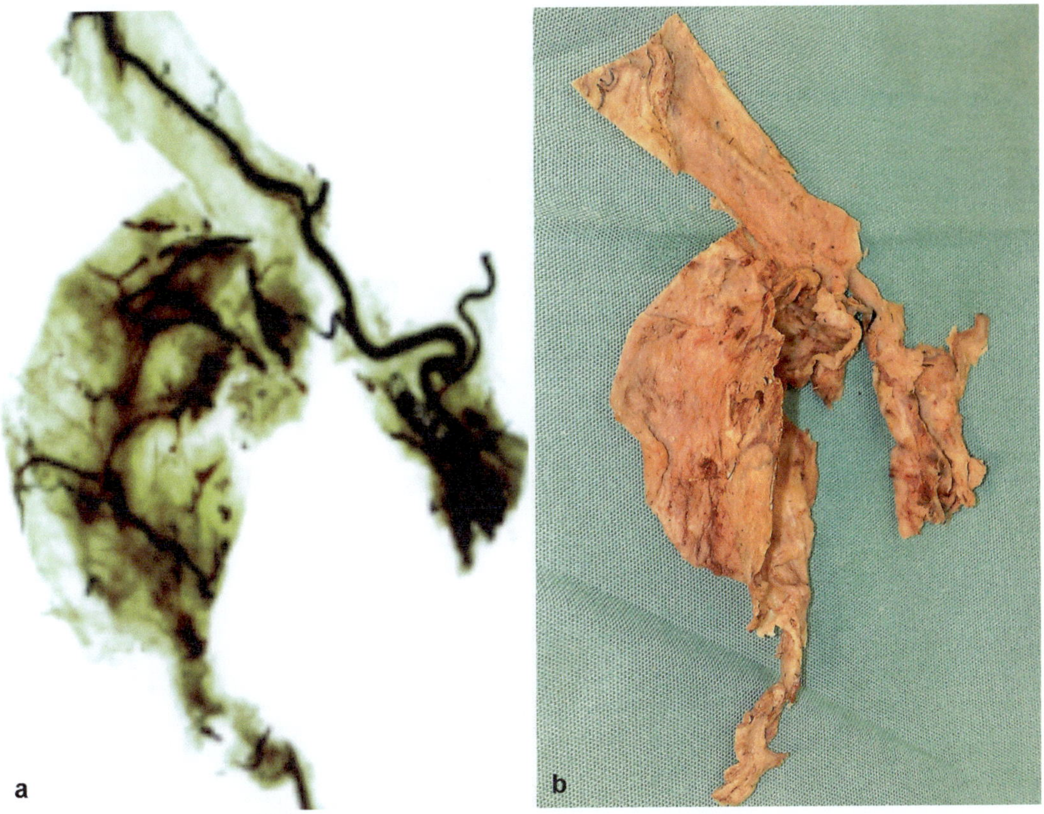

Fig. 3.4 Cleared and anatomical dissection of postauricular fascia

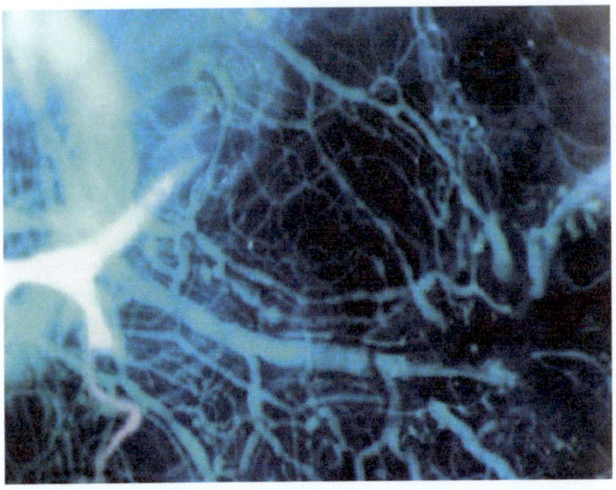

Fig. 3.5 High-power microscopy of vascular network in IPF

Clinical Applications

Thanks to the codominant bloody supply, rich vascular network (Figs. 3.3, 3.4, and 3.5), and inherent elasticity, the IPF has potential for both reconstructive flaps as well as acting as a free graft.

The IPF has the potential to reconstruct helical defects of the ear as demonstrated (Figs. 3.8 and 3.9) for defects of approximately 30 % of the pinna using IPF alone or greater with an extended flap using the EPF as well (Fig. 3.10).

There is potential to tunnel the fascia through the ear to reconstruct conchal defects (Fig. 3.11), and it may be feasible to roll the fascia to reconstruct or define the crura of the antihelix (Fig. 3.12). If the entire postauricular fascia is raised on a single or dual pedicle, it should cover most of the ear (Fig. 3.13) or reach as far as the zygoma (Fig. 3.14) or beyond.

By raising the IPF distally as a flap and suturing it to the mastoid, it is possible to provide correction of ear deformities for pinnaplasty [9]. Suture tension is relieved thanks to the fascia's attachment to the underlying helical cartilage acting as an "internal scaffold"

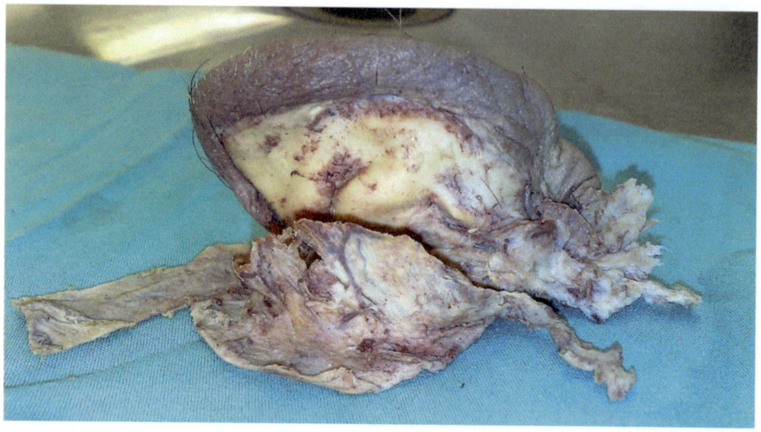

Fig. 3.6 The auricular fascial incisura: the meeting point of the thin intrinsic postauricular fascia directly adherent to the posterior surface of the ear and the thicker extrinsic postauricular fascia overlying the mastoid which is continuous with the thick fascia of the occipital musculature

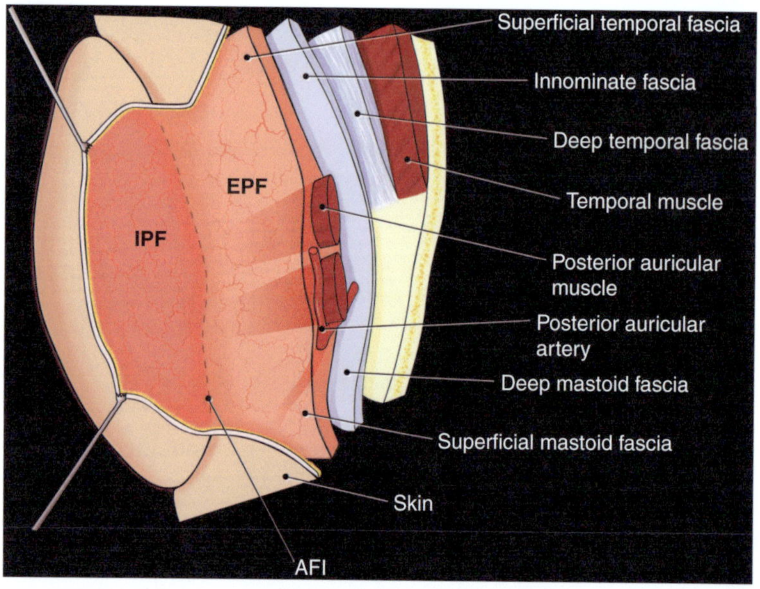

Fig. 3.7 Anatomy of the intrinsic (*IPF*) and extrinsic (*EPF*) postauricular fascia

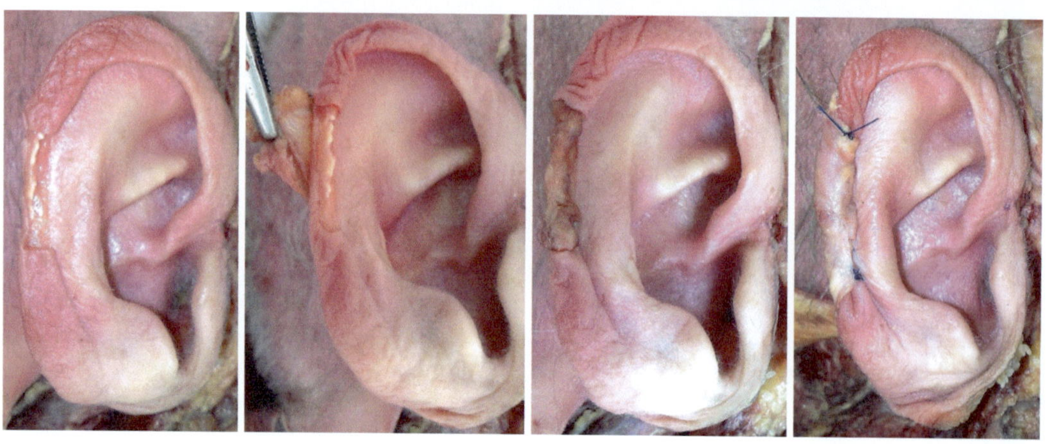

Fig. 3.8 Proposed helical repair utilizing the IPF in a cadaveric model

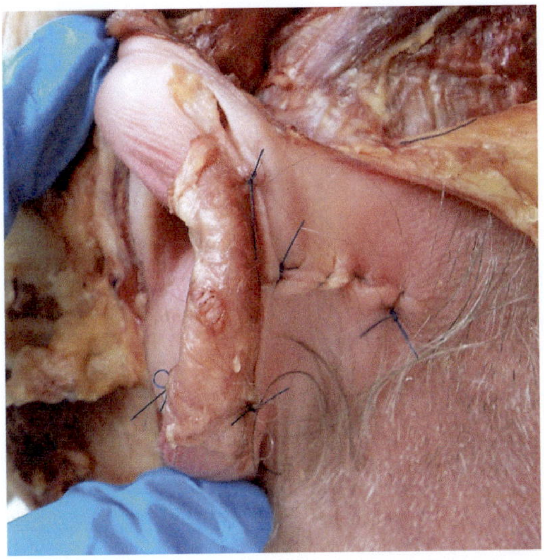

Fig. 3.9 Helical repair, highlighting incisions utilized and suture positions

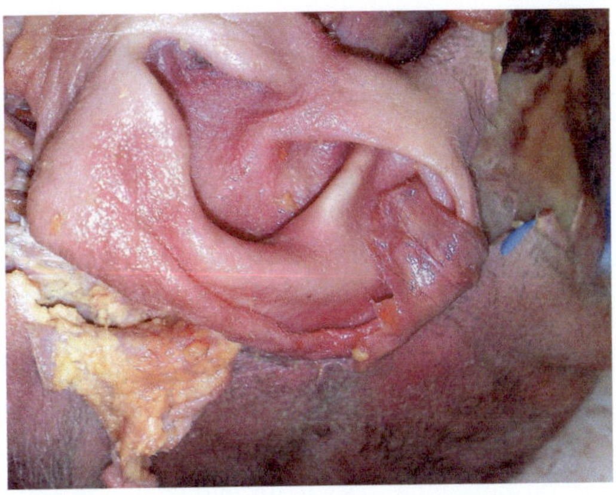

Fig. 3.10 Helical cover – an extended flap

(Figs. 3.15, 3.16, and 3.17). This technique, combined with the use of skin glue for postoperative splinting [14], makes head bandages obsolete and enables patients to not only wash their hair the day after surgery but also escape the stigma of the surgery (this is especially useful in girls who wear their hair long as all signs of surgery can be hidden) (Figs. 3.18 and 3.19).

It is also plausible that the fascia might be suitable for microtia reconstruction [1]. Cikelair produced a set of goals for reconstruction of the external ear, which included provision of skin of appropriate thickness and texture, in addition to

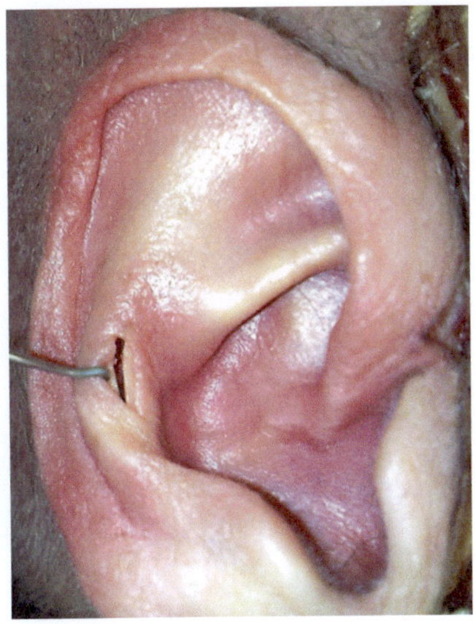

Fig. 3.11 Tunneling the IPF

the insertion of a framework for support. The IPF would theoretically act as a suitable scaffold. Similarly, major ear reconstructions using prosthetic materials may benefit from additional (fascial) soft-tissue cover to limit the high rates of extrusion.

In addition to its use in ear reconstruction, the superficial temporal fascia (STF) has been successfully utilized on a long pedicle to repair lower nasal defects [5]. The technique reported by Ying et al. involved marking the course of the superficial temporal artery with methylene blue on the skin, in conjunction with an ultrasound Doppler probe. Subsequently, the STF is exposed through careful dissection and the flap is raised. The flap is then transposed into the defect in question via a subcutaneous tunnel.

In complex rhinoplasty cases, where the skin is very thin or scar tissue has tethered the skin to underlying bone or cartilage (such as in revision rhinoplasty), the IPF can act as an excellent adjunct. Figure 3.20 shows success utilizing the IPF for protection of overlying fragile skin in a case complicated by a fracture. This is an excellent and autologous alternative to AlloDerm (Lifecell Corp.), Permacol (Covidien Surgical), or other synthetic or tissue-derived products. Other potential applications include bony

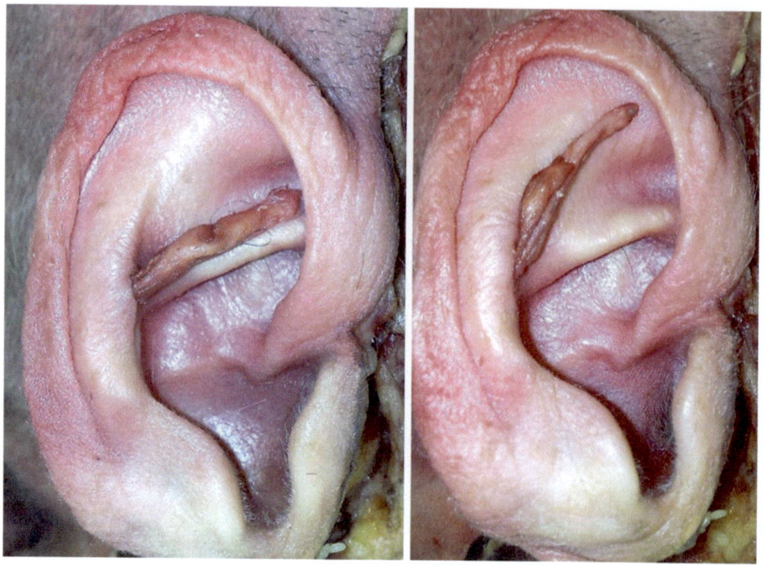

Fig. 3.12 Repairing the crura of the antihelix

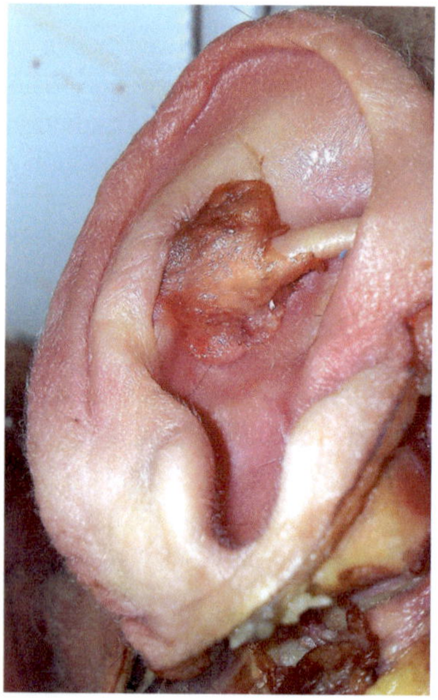

Fig. 3.13 Repair of the concha

remodeling – especially if the perichondrium is included in the flap, skin protection, and camouflage. The ear via a posterior approach is the commonest site for cartilage grafts in rhinoplasty and nasal reconstruction, and hence, the postauricular fascia is already accessible in such cases.

In addition to repairs of the nose and ear, the postauricular fascia has also been recruited for aesthetic augmentation of the lip [4]. In the referenced study, a comparison was made between an autologous musculoaponeurotic system tissue and the postauricular fascia, in conjunction with lip advancement. Despite the study being limited in patient number, the highest postoperative scores were recorded for the group undergoing the postauricular fascial lip augmentation with lip advancement.

Several techniques exist for lip augmentation, including injection of specific materials, implants, grafts, and local flaps. Sternocleidomastoid muscle and fascial grafts have been utilized by Agarwal et al. [13]. Other potential tissues for lip procedures or augmentation have included eyelid tissue [15], conchal cartilage [16], orbicularis oculi muscle [17], free dermis-fat grafts [18, 19], and even tissues as distant from the lip as the palmaris longus tendon [20].

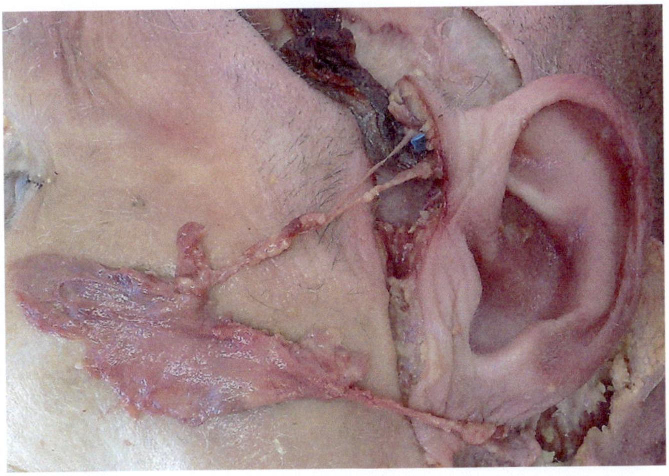

Fig. 3.14 Bipedicle IPF flap extending to the zygoma

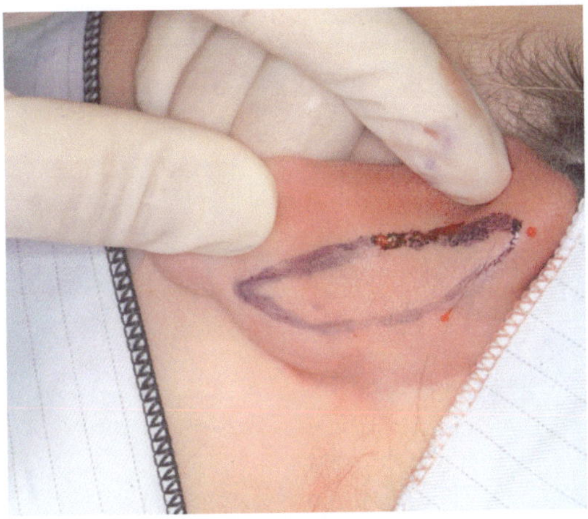

Fig. 3.15 Preoperative markings: fascia-augmented otoplasty

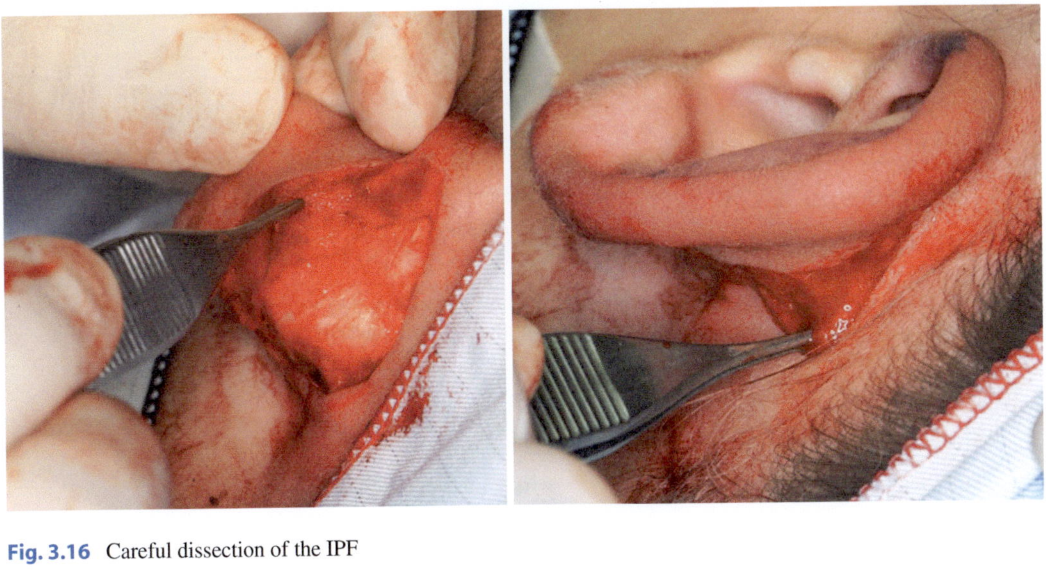

Fig. 3.16 Careful dissection of the IPF

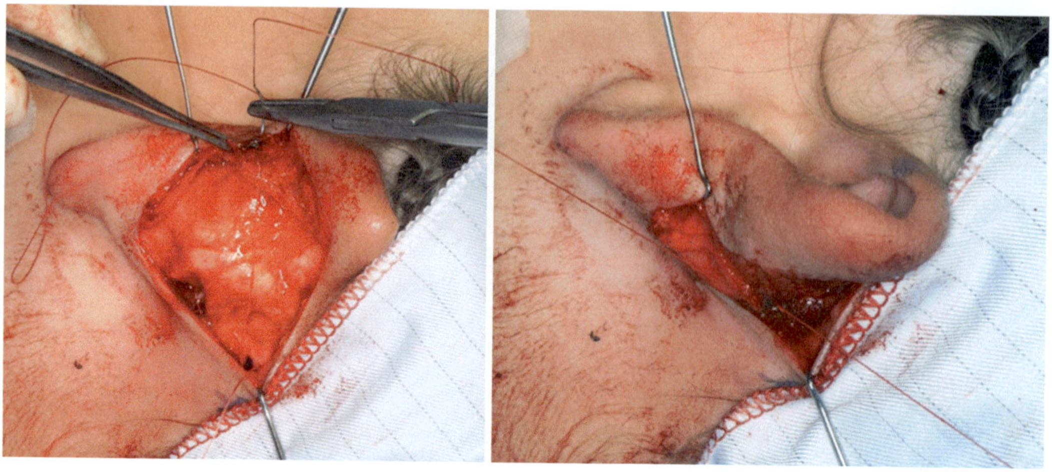

Fig. 3.17 Suture of IPF to mastoid

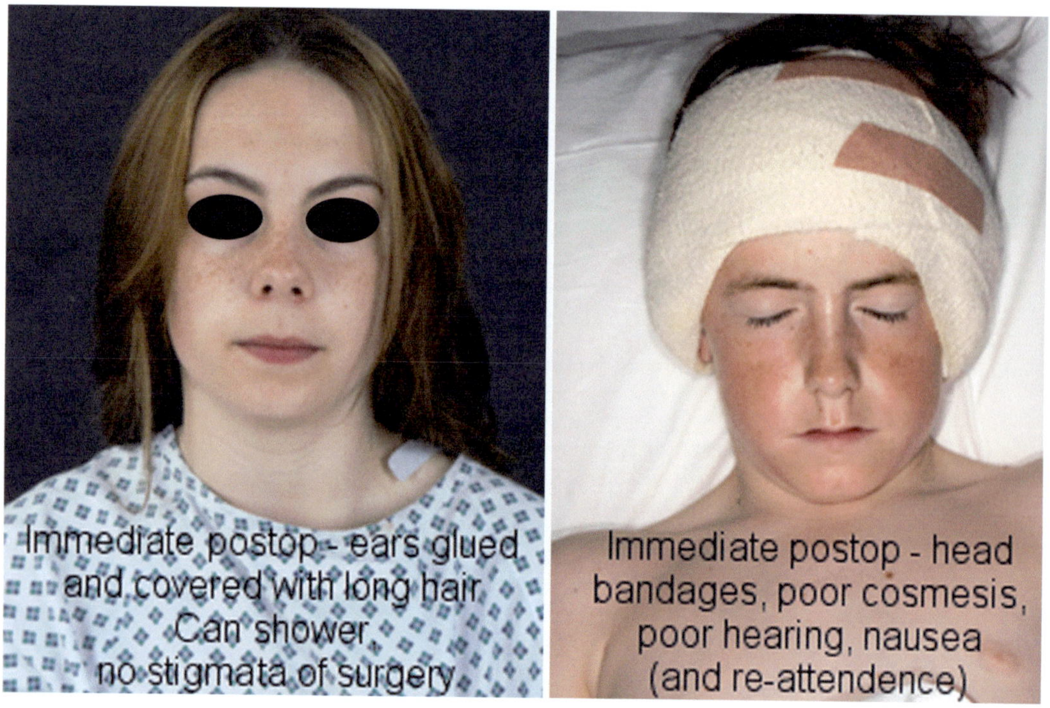

Fig. 3.18 Postoperative fascia-augmented otoplasty [9]. (*Left*) Using glue as postoperative splint. Immediate postop – ears glued and covered with long hair; can shower, no stigmata of surgery. (*Right*) Instead of head bandages. Immediate postop – head bandages, poor cosmesis, poor hearing, nausea (and re-attendance) [14]

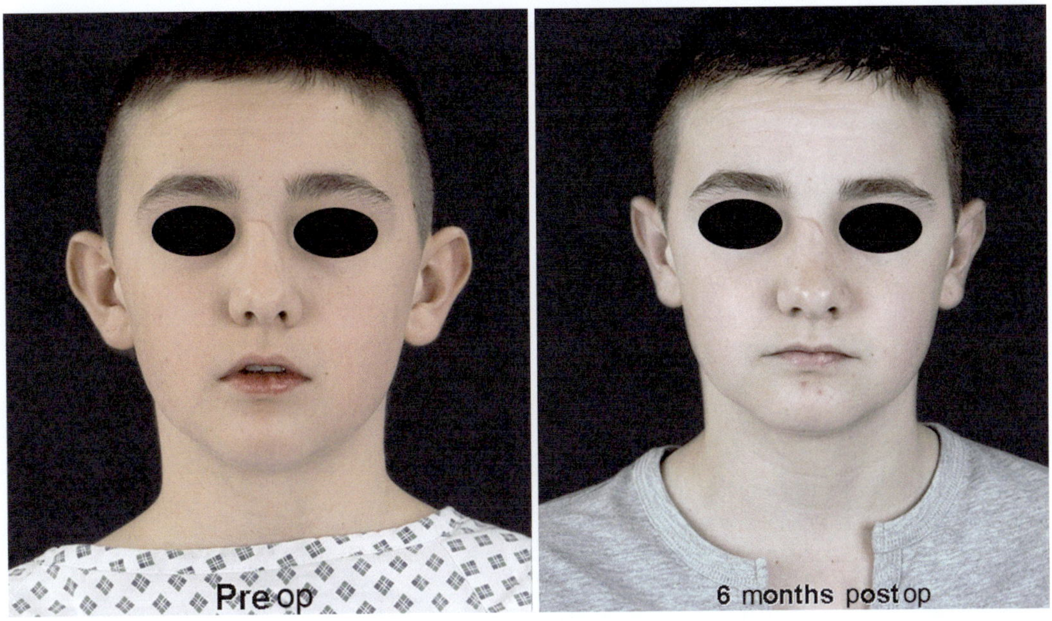

Fig. 3.19 (*Left*) Preoperative. (*Right*) Postoperative after otoplasty technique using the anteriorly based fascial flap showing good symmetry and natural "virgin ear" results [9]

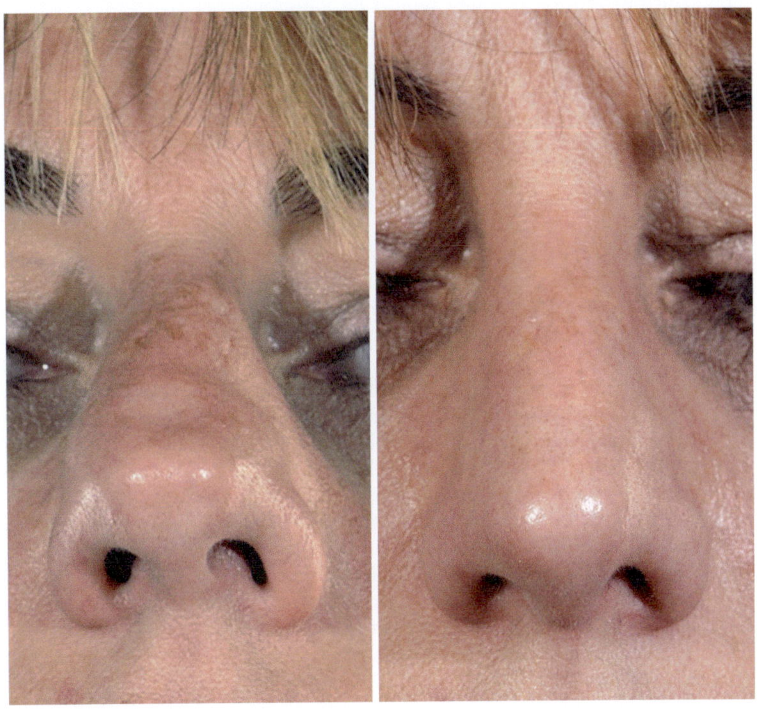

Fig. 3.20 Use of the IPF in rhinoplasty as a graft beneath thin skin (Courtesy of Professor Nicholas Jones, Queens Medical Centre, Nottingham, UK)

Conclusions

The anatomy of the posterior auricular fascia has been distinguished in detail, and a clear distinction has been made between the fascia overlying the mastoid continuous with the scalp musculature and the fascia adherent to the ear itself anterior to the auricular fascial incisura. The IPF is a thin and elastic fascial layer bound superficially by the skin and deeply by the cartilage of the ear, continuous with the perichondrium; it is a separate entity from the multilayered and more fibrous EPF and simply consists of the thin subcutaneous tissue directly adherent to the posterior side of the ear itself. Its potential and actual clinical applications have been demonstrated, though its use in reconstructive and aesthetic procedures is still in its infancy. The versatility of the tissue, thanks to its vascular network, hidden donor site, accessibility, and elastic properties, provides an excellent tool for the surgeon in reconstructive or aesthetic practice.

Further clinical studies would be valuable to highlight the areas where the IPF can be of greatest benefit as well as its limitations.

References

1. Wang Y, Zhuang X, Jiang H, Yang Q, Zhao Y, Han J, et al. The anatomy and application of the postauricular fascia flap in auricular reconstruction for congenital microtia. J Plast Reconstr Aesthet Surg. 2008;61 Suppl 1:S70–6.
2. Datta G, Carlucci S. Reconstruction of the retroauricular fold by 'nonpedicled' superficial mastoid fascia: details of anatomy and surgical technique. J Plast Reconstr Aesthet Surg. 2008;61 Suppl 1:S92–7.
3. Park C, Lee TJ, Shin KS, Kim YW. A single-stage two-flap method of total ear reconstruction. Plast Reconstr Surg. 1991;88(3):404–12.
4. Recupero WD, McCollough EG. Comparison of lip enhancement using autologous superficial musculoaponeurotic system tissue and postauricular fascia in conjunction with lip advancement. Arch Facial Plast Surg. 2010;12(5):342–8.
5. Ying Z, Jianlin F, Guoxian Z, Min W, Wei W, Zuoliang Q. Ultralong pedicled superficial temporal fascia island flaps for lower nasal defect. J Craniofac Surg. 2009;20(3):864–7.
6. Romo 3rd T, Morris LG, Reitzen SD, Ghossaini SN, Wazen JJ, Kohan D. Reconstruction of congenital microtia-atresia: outcomes with the Medpor/bone-anchored hearing aid-approach. Ann Plast Surg. 2009; 62(4):384–9.
7. Horlock N, Misra A, Gault DT. The postauricular fascial flap as an adjunct to Mustarde and Furnas type otoplasty. Plast Reconstr Surg. 2001;108(6):1487–90.
8. Schaverien MV, Al-Busaidi S, Stewart KJ. Long-term results of posterior suturing with postauricular fascial flap otoplasty. J Plast Reconstr Aesthet Surg. 2010; 63(9):1447–51.
9. Shokrollahi K, Cooper MA, Hiew LY. A new strategy for otoplasty. J Plast Reconstr Aesthet Surg. 2009; 62(6):774–81.
10. Frascino LF. The use of a retroauricular fascioperichondrial flap in the recreation of the antihelical fold in prominent ear surgery. Ann Plast Surg. 2009;63(5): 536–40.
11. Vetter M, Foehn M, Wedler V. A new postoperative otoplasty dressing technique using cyanoacrylate tissue adhesives. Aesthetic Plast Surg. 2010;34(2):212–3.
12. Patel AJ, Price RD. The use of tissue glue in prominent ear correction surgery. Aesthetic Plast Surg. 2011;35(2):245–7.
13. Agarwal A, Gracely E, Maloney RW. Lip augmentation using sternocleidomastoid muscle and fascia grafts. Arch Facial Plast Surg. 2010;12(2):97–102.
14. Shokrollahi K, Tanner B. "Glue Ear": beginning of the end for head bandages after prominent ear correction? J Plast Reconstr Aesthet Surg. 2008;61(9):1077.
15. Fezza JP, Cartwright M, Mack W, Flaharty P. Lip augmentation using eyelid tissue from upper blepharoplasty surgery. Ophthal Plast Reconstr Surg. 2003; 19(3):225–8.
16. Saha SS, Kumar V, Khazanchi RK, Agarwal A. Correction of the nose in patients with unilateral cleft lip with composite grafts. Scand J Plast Reconstr Surg Hand Surg. 2005;39(6):344–8.
17. Tarallo M, Monarca C, Rizzo MI, Scuderi N. Upper-lip augmentation by graft of preseptal orbicularis oculi muscle through blepharoplasty. Aesthetic Plast Surg. 2010;34(2):167–71.
18. Patel IA, Hall PN. Free dermis-fat graft to correct the whistle deformity in patients with cleft lip. Br J Plast Surg. 2004;57(2):160–4.
19. Niechajev I. Lip enhancement: surgical alternatives and histologic aspects. Plast Reconstr Surg. 2000; 105(3):1173–83.
20. Trussler AP, Kawamoto HK, Wasson KL, Dickinson BP, Jackson E, Keagle JN, et al. Upper lip augmentation: Palmaris longus tendon as an autologous filler. Plast Reconstr Surg. 2008;121(3):1024–32.

Part II

Preoperative

4 The Timing of Otoplasty

Patrick M. Spielmann and Michel Neeff

Introduction

Nonsurgical and surgical otoplasty may be indicated in the prevention or treatment of psychosocial issues resulting from prominent ears in children. It is a successful and well-tolerated intervention to correct prominent ears, but counseling a parent as to the optimum age for their child to undergo correction can be a difficult process. This chapter will present the literature regarding the timing of otoplasty; the evidence in this chapter is based on a literature search performed in March 2012.

There are common scenarios when children are brought for consideration of otoplasty: Firstly a parent may request correction for a young child to prevent future teasing and psychological harm. Secondly a child perceives the deformity and requests correction (often after they have been bullied or stigmatized). Finally, corrective surgery may be requested in adulthood. Three relevant areas must be considered: the anatomical aspects of ear cartilage and growth, the psychosocial functioning of the child, and the practical considerations of surgery.

P.M. Spielmann, M.D. (✉)
Department of Otolaryngology,
Ninewells Hospital and University of Dundee,
Dundee DD1 9SY, UK
e-mail: patrickspielmann@nhs.net

M. Neeff, M.D.
Department of Otolaryngology,
Auckland City Hospital and Starship Children's Hospital,
Auckland, New Zealand
e-mail: micheln@adhb.govt.nz

Anatomical

Cartilage remains pliable for a short time after birth, probably due to the influence of maternal estrogens [1, 2]. This allows effective splinting to correct protruding ears within the first 3–6 weeks but ideally within the first week of life [3–6]. Some authors advocate splinting beyond this age but before 3 months [1, 7]. Splints have to be applied for longer, and outcomes are less favorable in older patients as cartilage becomes progressively less pliable [1, 5].

Adamson et al. [8] studied the growth of normal ears and found that 85 % of full size had been achieved by the age of 3 years. In contrast Farkas [9] reported that 85 % of full size was achieved only by 6 years of age. Balogh and Milesi [10] examined ear growth after otoplasty in a cohort of 76 cases using cartilage-cutting techniques including children aged 5–8 years: They identified no significant growth differences between the operated ears and controls. Songu [11] reported satisfactory outcomes in 10 children undergoing otoplasty aged 4–5 years with no observed growth restriction at 1 year follow-up. Furthermore, Gosain et al. [12] followed 12 children undergoing otoplasty under 3 years of age (youngest 9 months) and also observed no significant differences between ears in the three unilateral cases

M.A. Shiffman (ed.), *Advanced Cosmetic Otoplasty*,
DOI 10.1007/978-3-642-35431-1_4, © Springer-Verlag Berlin Heidelberg 2013

with at least 39 months follow-up. No growth restriction was observed in the bilateral cases with median 41 months follow-up.

These authors comment that cartilage at young age is more pliable, so repositioning techniques rather than cartilage weakening and cutting techniques are utilized, and an incision rather than excision of postauricular skin is made. These factors may explain why there is no significant change in growth characteristics following this minimally "destructive" surgery, if there is an influence of surgery on cartilage growth at all. While the numbers studied are small and the follow-up does not continue to adulthood, there is some evidence to suggest that otoplasty can be performed at a very young age without adversely affecting future growth.

In the management of prominent macrotic ears, where potential growth restrictions due to surgery may be advantageous, otoplasty in patients as young as 2 years has been performed.

Psychological

Being teased is a common experience of childhood; however, children with prominent ears experience more teasing than their peers. This difference was present up to but not beyond the age of 13 years in a study of 30 children undergoing otoplasty [13]. Gasques [14] identified many anxiety traits and substantial distress in children with prominent ears, all of which improved following otoplasty. The level of distress experienced appears independent of the degree of prominence [13]. Children with microtia are aware of their own deformity from an early age – Jiamei [15] demonstrated that the majority of children recognized their deformity at 3 or 4 years of age. However, teasing or ridicule does not usually begin until a few years later; thus, while they themselves are aware, other children either do not notice or have the motivation to tease. On the other hand, Songu [11] asserts that psychological pressures in the preschool age group are often underestimated and that increasing socialization outside the family home exposes the child to early stigmatization, but there is insufficient evidence to confirm this. Bradbury et al. reported onset of self-consciousness in children with prominent ears anywhere between 4 and 13 years of age [13]. After the onset of psychosocial problems due to prominent ears, otoplasty has been shown to substantially reduce and in many cases eliminate bullying, improving psychosocial functioning and health-related quality of life [13, 14, 16–19]. But it is difficult to predict whether a child will become self-conscious of their ears and if so at what age. The adage "prevention is better than cure" may not apply to the surgical correction of prominent ears in some children. While parents wish to prevent their children suffering at a formative stage in their socialization and development, they may submit their child to an unnecessary cosmetic procedure. If the child becomes self-conscious or a victim of bullying, a successful and well-tolerated intervention is available. There is no evidence to suggest that early otoplasty results in less psychological distress than delayed surgery.

While teasing and bullying for prominent ears appear to be less prevalent in adolescence [13], self-image and confidence may be adversely affected and thus a strong motivator for surgery. Adolescents are able to provide informed consent for surgery and comply with postoperative care. Kamburoglu [19] concludes that appropriately selected adolescents are good candidates for a variety of cosmetic procedures including otoplasty as they are motivated and experience significant improvements in self-esteem, body image, and life satisfaction. Adults who underwent surgery in early childhood reported resentment and anger (towards their caregivers) after unfavorable outcomes of aesthetic surgery. An engaged and motivated child would likely be more accepting of an unfavorable result or complication.

Practical

Psychosocial complications of prominent ears can be prevented by correction of prominent ears using splinting techniques in the neonatal period. The practical aspects of undergoing surgery must be considered: These include the child's ability to cooperate with the aftercare, the fact that the surgery is purely cosmetic and carries risks of complications and worsening of the appearance of the ears. Unfortunately very young children are often unable to comply with the postoperative care required, particularly prolonged head bandaging as required by some techniques. Thus, a young or unmotivated child will find the postoperative course stressful and unpleasant. Songu et al. [11] advocate surgery in children aged 4 or over and report a series of ten children with satisfactory outcomes but noted that all had returns to hospital for repeated head bandaging and a single revision procedure due to the children getting fingers underneath the bandage. There is no prospective series comparing outcomes of surgery (including recurrence rates) performed in very young compared with older children.

Current Practice

Surveys of surgeon practice have been performed in the USA and UK: 174 members of the American Association of Aesthetic Plastic Surgeons responded to a postal survey (a 37 % response rate), and 57 % of respondents routinely performed surgery over the age of 5 years [12]. The commonest reasons cited for performing surgery at this age were near-adult size of the ear (38 %), greater patient cooperation (25 %), and increased peer ridicule (19 %). One hundred and twenty members of the British Association of Plastic, Reconstructive and Aesthetic Surgeons responded to a similar but independent survey (a 65 % response rate), and 79 % felt that the optimum age to perform surgery was over 6 years. The majority of parents (79 %) and child psychologists (63 %) surveyed also agreed that 6 years or older was the preferred age for surgery. The most important factors cited by all three groups were the child's awareness of prominent ears, the child suffering bullying, and school absence due to embarrassment [20]. The studies concur that most surgeons tend to favor performing the surgery when the child has reached a level of maturity firstly to express concern over their ears and secondly to cope with the postoperative aftercare required. Interestingly although surgery appears to be feasible in the younger age group, the majority of surgeons responding to these surveys prefer to delay surgery.

Conclusions

The timing of otoplasty should therefore take into account child's wishes, the psychosocial burden of the perceived deformity, and the maturity/motivation of the child to cooperate with the postoperative care.

References

1. Tan ST, Abramson DL, MacDonald DM, Mulliken JB. Molding therapy for infants with deformational auricular anomalies. Ann Plast Surg. 1997;38(3):263–8.
2. Kenny FM, Angsusingha K, Stinson D, Hotchikiss J. Unconjugated estrogens in the perinatal period. Pediatr Res. 1973;7(10):826–31.
3. Van Wijk MP, Breugem CC, Kon M. A prospective study on non-surgical correction of protruding ears: the importance of early treatment. J Plast Reconstr Aesthet Surg. 2012;65(1):54–60.
4. Smith W, Toye J, Reid A, Smith R. Nonsurgical correction of congenital ear abnormalities in the newborn: case series. Paediatr Child Health. 2005;10(6):327–31.
5. Park C, Yoo Y-S, Hong ST. An update on auricular reconstruction: three major auricular malformations of microtia, prominent ear and cryptotia. Curr Opin Otolaryngol Head Neck Surg. 2010;18(6):544–9.
6. Byrd HS, Langevin CJ, Ghidoni LA. Ear molding in newborn infants with auricular deformities. Plast Reconstr Surg. 2010;126(4):1191–200.
7. Porter CJ, Tan ST. Congenital auricular anomalies: topographic anatomy, embryology, classification, and treatment strategies. Plast Reconstr Surg. 2010;115(6): 1701–12.
8. Adamson JE, Horton CR, Crawford HH. The growth pattern of the external ear. Plast Reconstr Surg. 1965;36(4):466–70.
9. Farkas LG. Growth of normal and re-constructed auricles. In: Tanzer RC, Edgerton MT, editors. Symposium on reconstruction of the auricle. St. Louis: Mosby; 1974. p. 24–31.
10. Balogh B, Millesi H. Are growth alterations a consequence of surgery for prominent ears? Plast Reconstr Surg. 1992;89(4):623–30.
11. Songu M, Adibelli H. Otoplasty in children younger than 5 years of age. Int J Pediatr Otorhinolaryngol. 2010;74(3):292–6.
12. Gosain AK, Kumar A, Huang G. Prominent ears in children younger than 4 years of age: what is the appropriate timing for otoplasty? Plast Reconstr Surg. 2004;114(5):1042–54.

13. Bradbury ET, Hewison J, Timmons MJ. The psychological and social outcome of prominent ear correction in children. Br J Plast Surg. 1992;45(2):97–100.
14. Gasques JA, de Godoy JM P, Cruz EM. Psychosocial effects of otoplasty in children with prominent ears. Aesthetic Plast Surg. 2008;32(6):910–4.
15. Jiamei D, Jiake C, Hongxing Z, Wanhou G, Yan W, Gaifen L. An investigation of psychological profiles and risk factors in congenital microtia patients. J Plast Reconstr Aesthet Surg. 2008;61 Suppl 1:S37–43.
16. Cooper-Hobson G, Jaffe W. The benefits of otoplasty for children: further evidence to satisfy the modern NHS. J Plast Reconstr Aesthet Surg. 2009;62(2):190–4.
17. Braun T, Hainzinger T, Stelter K, Krause E, Berghaus A, Hempel JM. Health-related quality of life, patient benefit, and clinical outcome after otoplasty using suture techniques in 62 children and adults. Plast Reconstr Surg. 2010;126(6):2115–24.
18. Niemelä BJ, Hedlund A, Andersson G, Wahlsten VS. Prominent ears: the effect of reconstructive surgery on self-esteem and social interaction in children with a minor defect compared to children with a major orthopedic defect. Plast Reconstr Surg. 2008;122(5):1390–8.
19. Kamburoglu HO, Ozgur F. Postoperative satisfaction and the patient's body image, life satisfaction, and self-esteem: a retrospective study comparing adolescent girls and boys after cosmetic surgery. Aesthetic Plast Surg. 2007;31(6):739–45.
20. Spielmann PM, Harpur RH, Stewart KJ. Timing of otoplasty in children: what age? Eur Arch Otorhinolaryngol. 2009;266(6):941–2.

Part III

Techniques

History of Otoplasty: Review of Literature

5

Melvin A. Shiffman

Introduction

To appreciate how far we have gone to develop the treatment of the prominent ear, we must understand the historical development of otoplasty. Ear repair began with flaps for repair of injuries and distortions. Ultimately the repairs extended to the prominent ear for cosmetic improvement. Myriads of techniques and modifications have been reported.

History

Sushruta, in Sushruta Samhita, described various reconstructive methods or different types of defects like release of the skin for covering small defects, rotation of the flaps to make up for the partial loss, and pedicle flaps for covering complete loss of skin from an area such as earlobe reconstruction [1]. In 30 A.D., Aulus Cornelius Celsus in De Medicina [2] referred to repair of mutilated ears with advancement quadrangle flaps [3]. Gaspari Tagliacozzi (1597), in his treatise De Curtorum Chirurgia per Institutionem, instructed surgeons on how to reconstruct ears [4].

Dieffenbach [5] attempted to correct the protruding, or lop ear, deformity with postauricular skin excision in the auriculocephalic sulcus with conchomastoidal fixation. The correction of protruding (large) ears (macrotia) was by means of triangular excisions taken from the auricle described by de Martino in 1856 [6]. In 1968, Rogers [7] claimed that the origins of otoplasty for the prominent ear were by Eli [8] who described prominent ear correction that consisted of postauricular skin excision, conchomastoidal fixation, and conchal strip excision. Keen [9] removed a narrow, V-shaped section of cartilage from the posterior surface of the auricle after a large section of skin had been excised. Monks [10] described removal of skin from the back of the ear, but if the cartilage was stiff, then excision of some cartilage. Cocheril [11] modified the original techniques by adding incision and excision of various parts of the conchal cartilage to improve the results. Haug [12] reported removal of triangular wedges of cartilage along with excision of the skin on the posterior surface of the auricle. In 1896, Joseph [13] divided protruding ears into two types: the soft and the hard cartilage types. For ears of the soft cartilage type, he advised excision of skin at the auriculomastoid angle. For the hard cartilage type, he advised resection of cartilage from the region along with excision of skin. The prominent ear in children was corrected by DeSchweinitz and Randall [14] by attaching the auricle to the skull surface with glue or collodion and bandaging it firmly union the union was secure. In adults skin excisions were made on the back of the ear and over the mastoid, but no cartilage was excised.

M.A. Shiffman, M.D., J.D.
Section of Surgery, Newport Specialty Hospital,
17501 Chatham Drive, 92780-2302 Tustin, CA, USA
e-mail: shiffmanmdjd@gmail.com

M.A. Shiffman (ed.), *Advanced Cosmetic Otoplasty*,
DOI 10.1007/978-3-642-35431-1_5, © Springer-Verlag Berlin Heidelberg 2013

Gersuny [15] sutured the perichondrium to the mastoid periosteum. Morestin [16] bent the cartilage and held it in place with nonabsorbable sutures. He believed that the incision through the cartilage must extend well up to the upper and lower borders of the cartilage. Payr [17] embedded a cartilage flap under the periosteum. Miller [18] described his experience in the correction of various facial deformities including "outstanding" ears. Goldstein [19] described an operation similar to Morestin, but he sutured the cartilage to the mastoid periosteum.

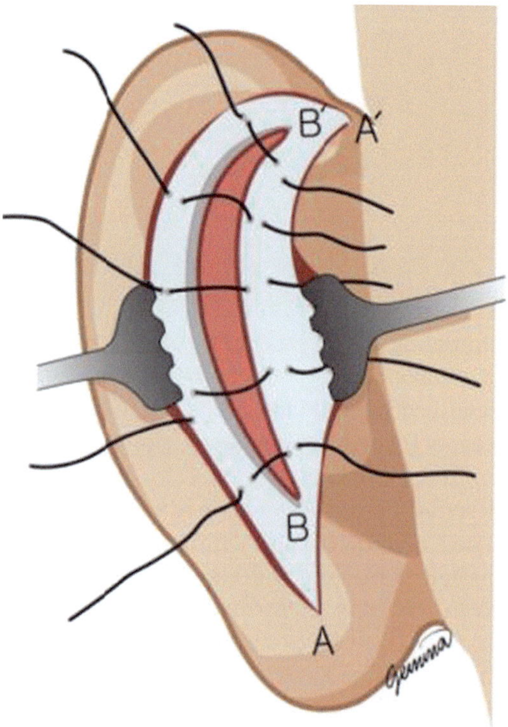

Fig. 5.1 Luckett's technique (1910) [20]. Excision of cartilage along predetermined site of the antihelix with sutures in place. *A* to *A′*: Skin closure, *B* to *B′*: Cartilage closure

Luckett [20] (Fig. 5.1) resorted to a cartilage-breaking technique consisting of crescent medial skin and cartilage excision along the entire vertical length of the antihelical fold to restore the antihelical fold. However, this produced a sharp outline to the antihelical fold in some cases. Luckett attempted to alleviate this problem with several horizontal mattress sutures, as adapted from Lembert, that allowed the flat surfaces of the concha and the antihelix to be apposed, not the edges of each, as the sutures were tied tightly.

Modifications of Luckett's technique include: Barsky [21] beveled the borders and kept an intact segment of cartilage over the cartilage incisions by suturing the cut edges under a bridge, Baxter [22] made parallel incisions of the cartilage instead of a single one, Young [23] prolonged the cartilage incision to break the spring and avoid suturing, Farina (Fig. 5.2) [24] varied the skin incision and cartilage resection (Fig. 5.3), Vidaurre [25] added an incision for the anterior crus, and Seltzer [26] gave a lengthy description

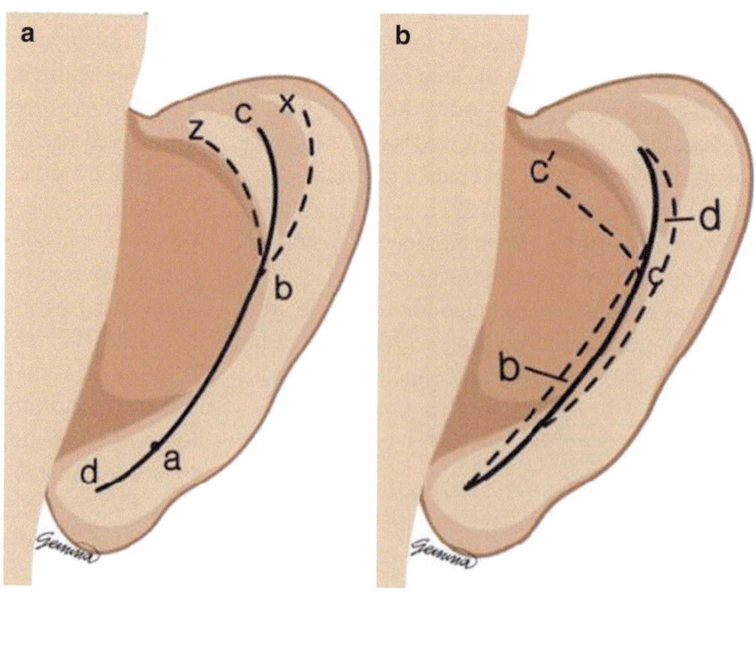

Fig. 5.2 Farina's technique (1951) [24]. (**a**) *dabc*: Cutaneous incision. *ab*: Trunk of antihelix. *bx*: Superior ramus of antihelix. *bz*: Inferior ramus of antihelix. (**b**) Elliptical cartilaginous excision. *a*: Portion of scapha removed. *b*: Portion of concha removed. *cc′*: Incision of inferior ramus of antihelix

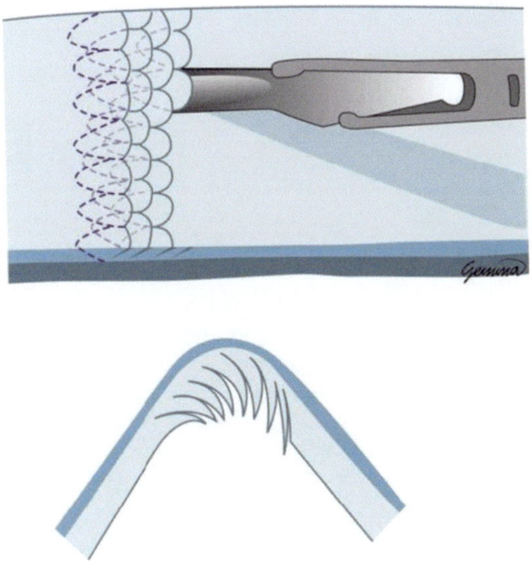

Fig. 5.3 Holmes' technique (1959) [29]. A method of breaking cartilage spring using a special gouge. Point of blade should come just through the cartilage on the anterior surface

of his technique, including obliterating the postauricular sulcus, modifying Luckett's technique. Hatch [27] modified Luckett's procedure by removing three separate, though continuous, crescent-shaped pieces of tissue: two of which are cartilage, and one of which is cartilage and fat in the lobule. This repositioning allowed the ear to open out in three separate and opposing directions simultaneously to produce anatomic and aesthetic normality; Jones [28] excised a wider cartilage strip in order to decrease the sharpness of the antihelical ridge; Holmes [29] used a special gouge to make fish-like scales up and down the proposed antihelix (Fig. 5.3); Cloutier [30] divided the cartilage from the top of the ear to the lobule and the skin overlying the anterior surface of the cartilage dissected off the cartilage approximately 3/8 in. on each side. The upper and lower ends of one edge of the cartilage are grasped with forceps and turned back so that the anterior side of the cartilage faces the operator. The edge of the cartilage is beveled with a razor blade. The edge of the cartilage will curl, and the width of the curl will depend on the width of the beveled edge. The proper width should be made on the first attempt. A similar procedure is carried out on the other edge of cartilage. The cartilage does not require suturing; McDowell [31] made a precise placement of the main cartilage incision from the posterior surface while continuously observing the marked line to follow on the anterior surface of the ear (Fig. 5.4). The knife point goes through the cartilage, and its continuing path is easily seen under the anterior skin. This method allows for a quicker and more accurate incision than does the use of perforating needles.

Ruttin [32] anchored the cartilage with fascia lata strips. Kolle [33] corrected protruding (macrotia) ears with excision of skin and an elongated ellipse of cartilage (Fig. 5.5). Alexander [34] corrected ear prominence due to a high concha by incising and overlapping the posterior wall of the concha. Frühwald [35] removed a wedge of tissue with scissors at the junction of the upper and middle thirds of the helix extending into the cavity of the concha. This was then closed by approximating the edges of the wound. Demel [36] advised the removal of a large section of conchal cartilage to be turned on itself and pedicled beneath a bridge of periosteum over the mastoid region. Eltner [37] tried to eliminate the wrinkling of skin on the anterior surface that occurred with the Joseph and Morestin techniques, by excising two triangles of cartilage with a common base from the region of the concha. The skin and perichondrium were incised horizontally and then undermined before excision of the cartilage. Davis and Kitlowski [38] described the use of needles passed through and through the auricle to mark the antihelix. They recommended dipping the needles in a dye and then marked the cartilage with a series of puncture points to assist in the incision and remodeling of the auricular cartilage. MacColumm [39] and Young [40] combined the Luckett technique of antihelical correction with earlier techniques of conchal reduction that now forms the foundation for most of the modern otoplasty techniques for correcting the prominent ear deformity.

New and Erich [41] described a technique of external stay sutures that permitted an easy and flexible method of modeling the antihelix fold and maintaining the infolding of the cartilage in position during healing.

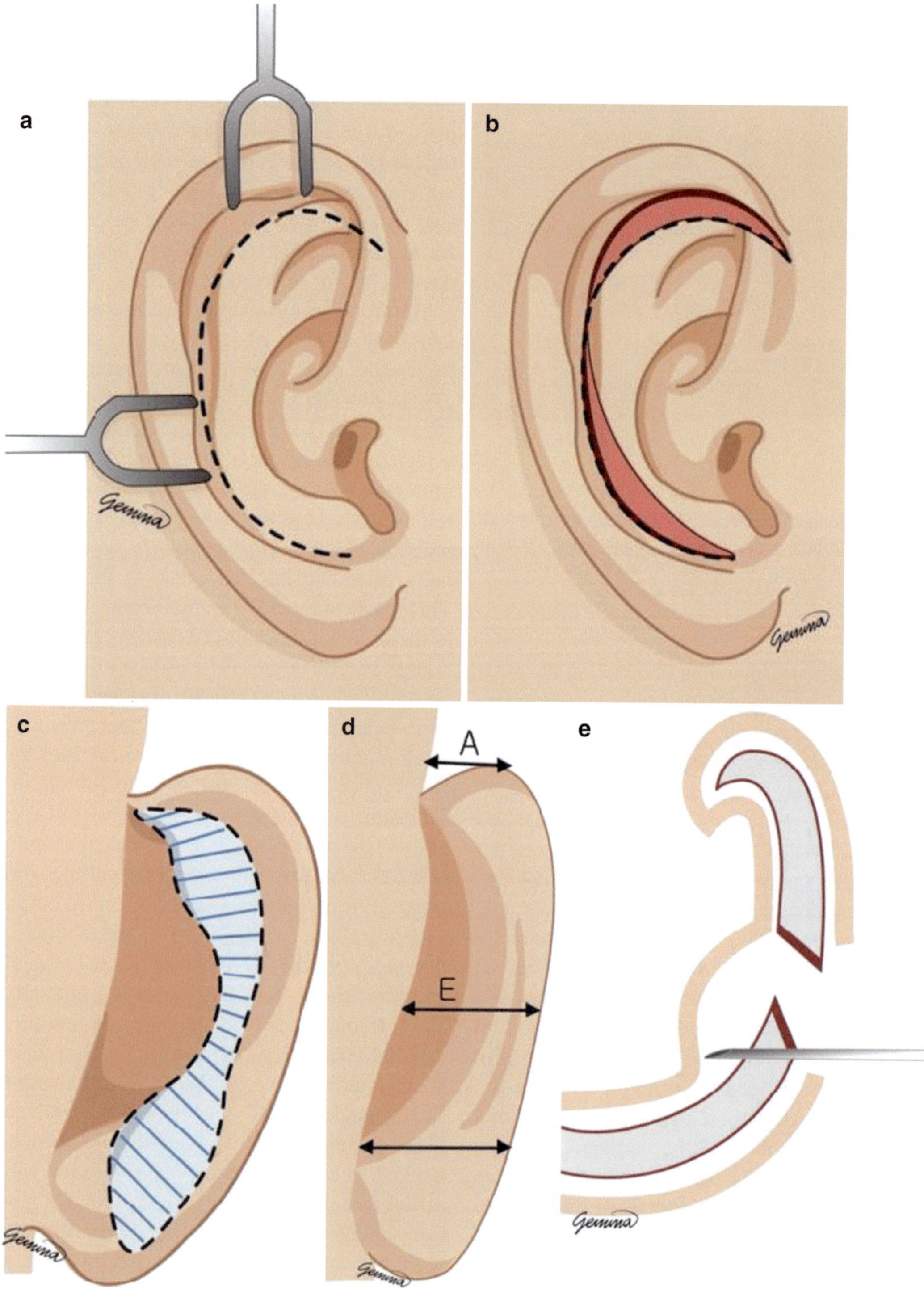

Fig. 5.4 McDowell's technique (1968) [31]. (**a**) Line of main cartilage incision marked on anterior surface. Note exaggerated curvature in line for new superior crus. (**b**) *Shaded areas* show approximate scope and location of cartilage excision as related to the initial cartilage incision. (**c**) *Cross-hatched area* shows skin marked for excision. An elongated dumbbell pattern provides for 1–3 mm excision in mid-portion but several mm at each end. (**d**) Corrected ear: Distance from outer border of helix to mastoid skin should be 10–12 mm at *top*, 16–18 mm in mid-portion, and 20–22 mm in lower third. (**e**) After main cartilage excision is completed, the edges should be trimmed square or else beveled only in the direction advocated by Cloutier. (**f**) Careful trimming of cartilage edges does much toward avoiding sharpness of the new antihelix. Slight subluxation of scaphal cartilage does not spoil the antihelix crest and helps the overall correction

Fig. 5.4 (continued)

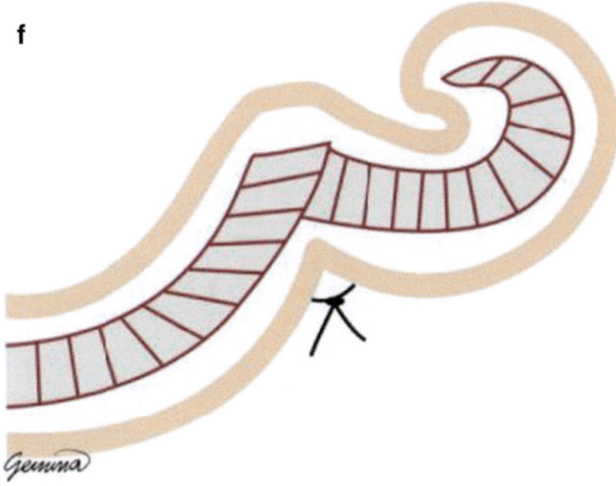

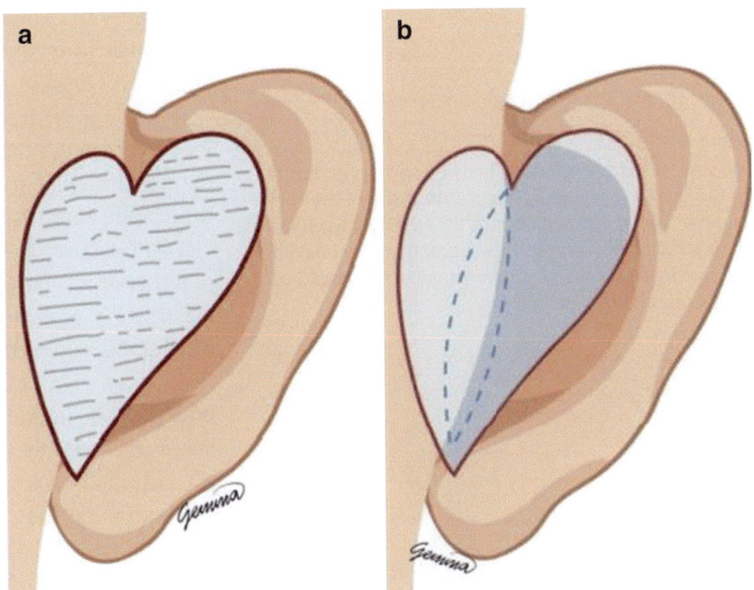

Fig. 5.5 Kolle's technique (1911) [33]. (**a**) An incision is made along the whole back of the ear as far down as the sulcus, where the retroaural integument joins that of the neck. The skin incision is ¾ to ½in. from the outer border. Oozing blood from the skin is impressed on the skin by pressing the ear backward on the bare skin of the head, leaving an imprint. A second incision is made along this line, fiving the total heart-shaped outline. (**b**) The skin is removed and an elongated ellipse of cartilage excised. Catgut sutures are placed through the conchal cartilage and deeper tissue back of the ear. A continuous running suture is used in the skin

Fishman and Fishman [42] used a through-and-through excision after premarking (Fig. 5.6). The outer or lateral portion followed the curve of the helix closely extending beyond the crural of the antihelix at the upper end and into and through the length of the fossa of the concha at the lower end. The medial incision was in accordance with the amount of skin and cartilage required to be excised. Subsequent modifications were described by Pierce et al. [43], Dufourmental [44], and Paletta et al. [45].

Borges [46] felt that Young's technique had the disadvantage of the middle ridge and the superior crus being too sharp and does not conform to the normal ear. He modified the technique by not excising the elliptical strip of cartilage from the concha but just incising and crisscrossing it while excising the inferior and internal strip from the concha (Fig. 5.7) so that it may give bulk and roundness to the superior crus and medial part of the antihelix.

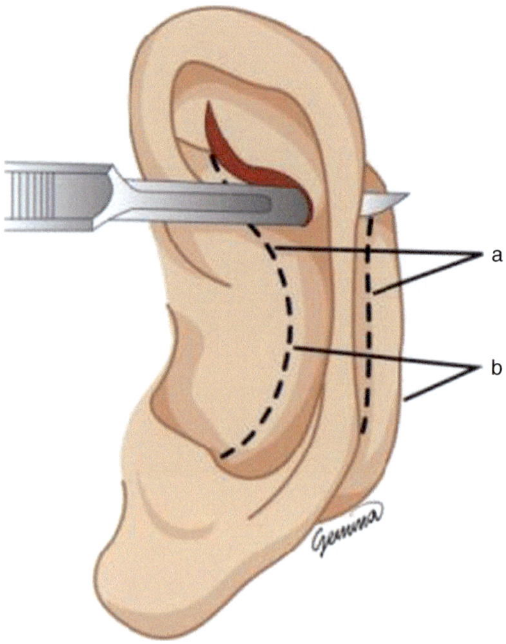

Fig. 5.6 Fishman and Fishman [42] technique. Lines of incision. (*a*) Outer or lateral incision following the curve of the antihelix extending beyond the crura of the antihelix at the *upper* end and through the length of the fossa of the concha at the *lower* end. (*b*) Second incision medial to the first in accordance with the amount of skin and cartilage required to be excised

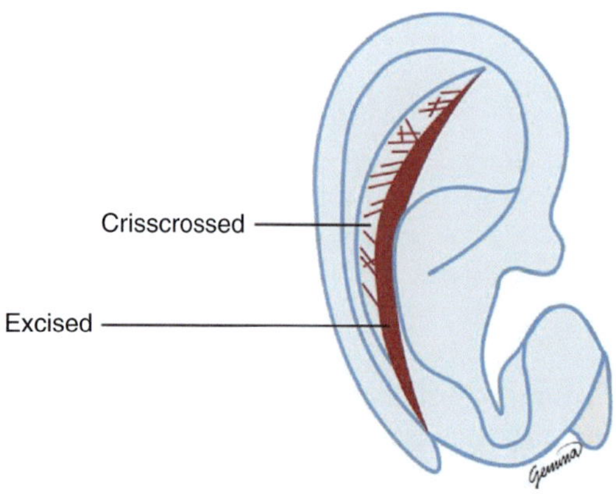

Fig. 5.7 Borges' [46] technique. The superior and external strip of cartilage from the scapha is incised and crisscrossed while the inferior and internal strip from the concha is excised

McEvitt [47] used multiple parallel antihelical incisions to soften the hard-edge contours of the corrected antihelical fold (Fig. 5.8). He also divided protruded ears into types:

Type 1: Ears of normal size with moderate protrusion caused by underdevelopment of the normal fold of the antihelix. The concha and fossae are approximately normal size, and their ratio to one another is correct. The antitragus is not overprominent.

Type 2: Large ears usually with marked protrusion, underdevelopment of the fold of the antihelix, overprominence of the antitragus, and wide scapha (fossa of the helix).

Type 3: Long narrow ears with little or no evidence of the antihelix. The structure seems curled forward. The concha and fossae form a continuous hollow giving the ear almost the appearance of a shell. They tend to be wide at the top and taper toward the lobule being roughly triangular.

Weaver [48] modified the technique of New and Erich (1940).

Becker [49] described a procedure with an incision through the skin and perichondrium in the postauricular region of the margin between the scapha and the concha, in the fossa antihelicis, and extended at the superior portion to the junction of the ear and temporal region, while at the inferior portion it is extended down to the base of the antitragus close to the mastoid region (Fig. 5.9). The skin and perichondrium are undermined laterally almost to the mastoid angle and to the beginning rim of the helix. The ear is folded back against the head to show the new antihelix. Skin and cartilage are pierced by a needle and the posterior surface of the cartilage marked with methylene blue. The double row of marks delineates the posterior and anterior borders of the antihelix and superior crus. Two incisions are made through the cartilage along the markings and a section of cartilage removed from the antihelix. The skin is undermined laterally for a few millimeters on the anterior surface of the auricle. The sulcus antihelicis transversus is incised completely through extending the incision into the previously incised cartilage of the antihelix that breaks the spring of the inferior crus. The cauda helicis is completely removed and the superior crus crosscut by incisions to weaken the spring of the cartilage. A small transverse section of cartilage

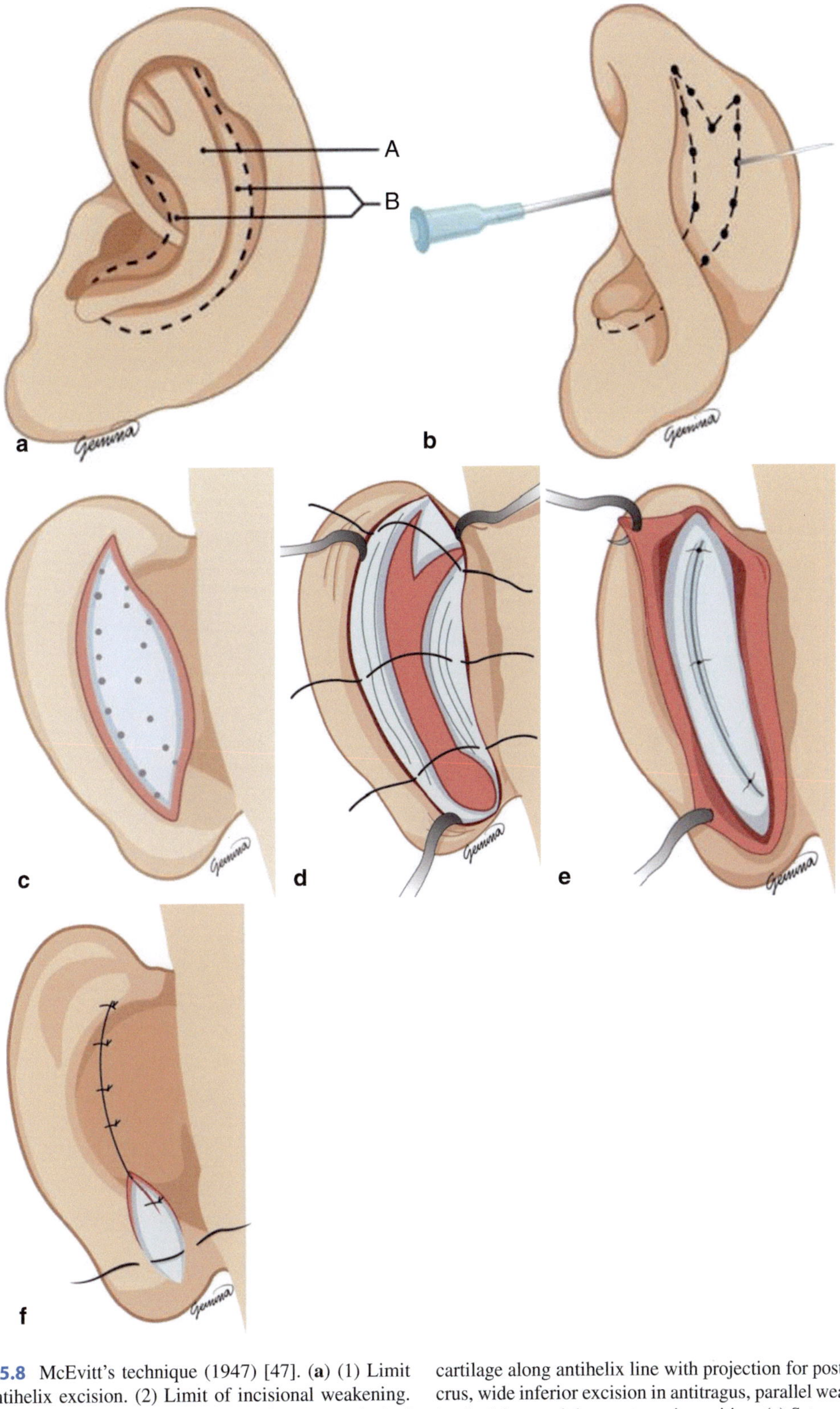

Fig. 5.8 McEvitt's technique (1947) [47]. (**a**) (1) Limit of antihelix excision. (2) Limit of incisional weakening. (**b**) Transfer of outline to posterior surface by method of Davis and Kitlowski. (**c**) Ellipse of skin excised showing needle marks on the underlying cartilage. (**d**) Excision of cartilage along antihelix line with projection for posterior crus, wide inferior excision in antitragus, parallel weakening incision, and three sutures in position. (**e**) Sutures tied forming antihelix. (**f**) Closure of skin with interrupted silk sutures

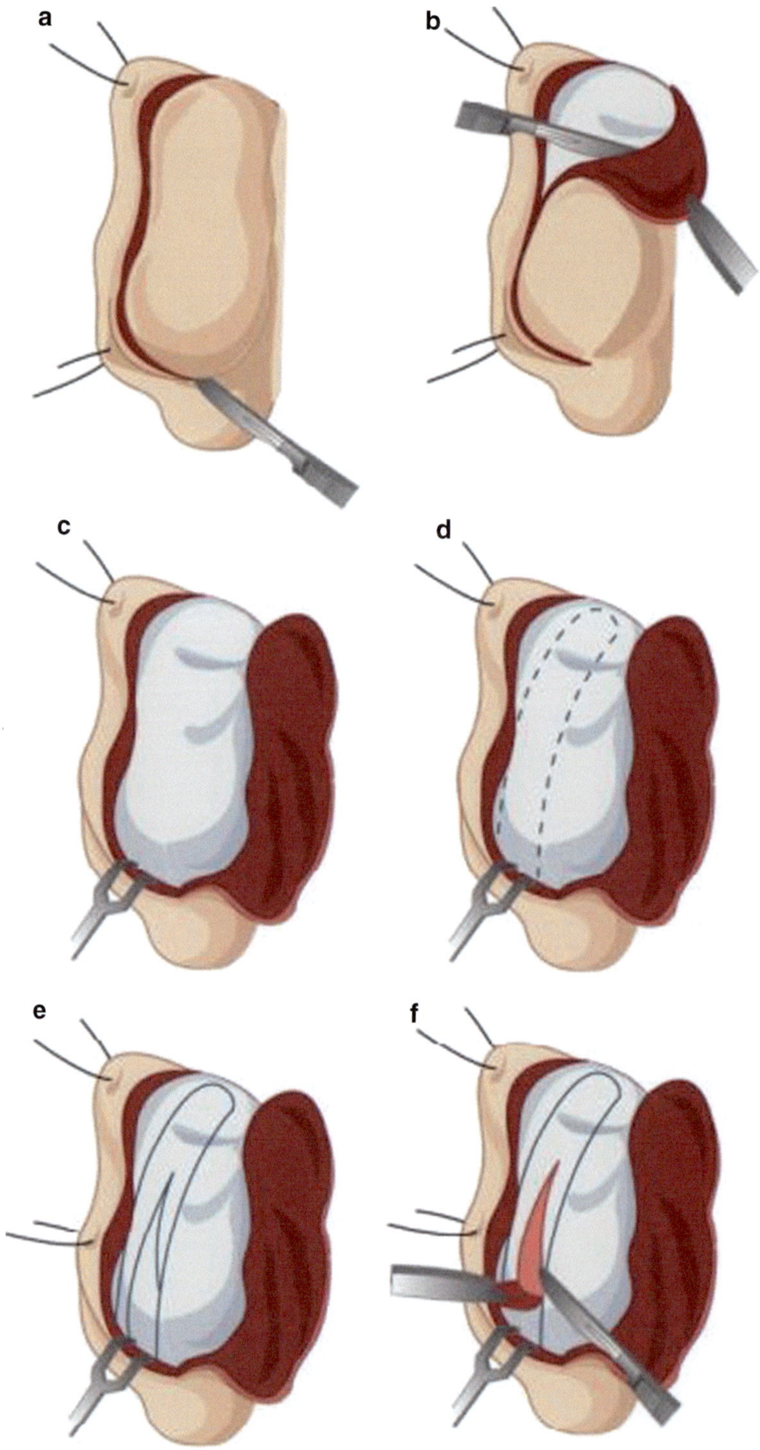

Fig. 5.9 Becker's technique (1949) [49]. (**a**) Incision through skin and perichondrium on the posterior surface of the auricle in the region of the fossa antihelicis. (**b**) Undermining of the skin and perichondrium almost to the auriculmastoid angle. (**c**) Complete exposure of the posterior surface of auricle, revealing all landmarks; undermining of the skin anteriorly to expose the cauda helicis and fissure antitragohelicis. (**d**) Outlining of the new antihelix

Fig. 5.9 (continued)

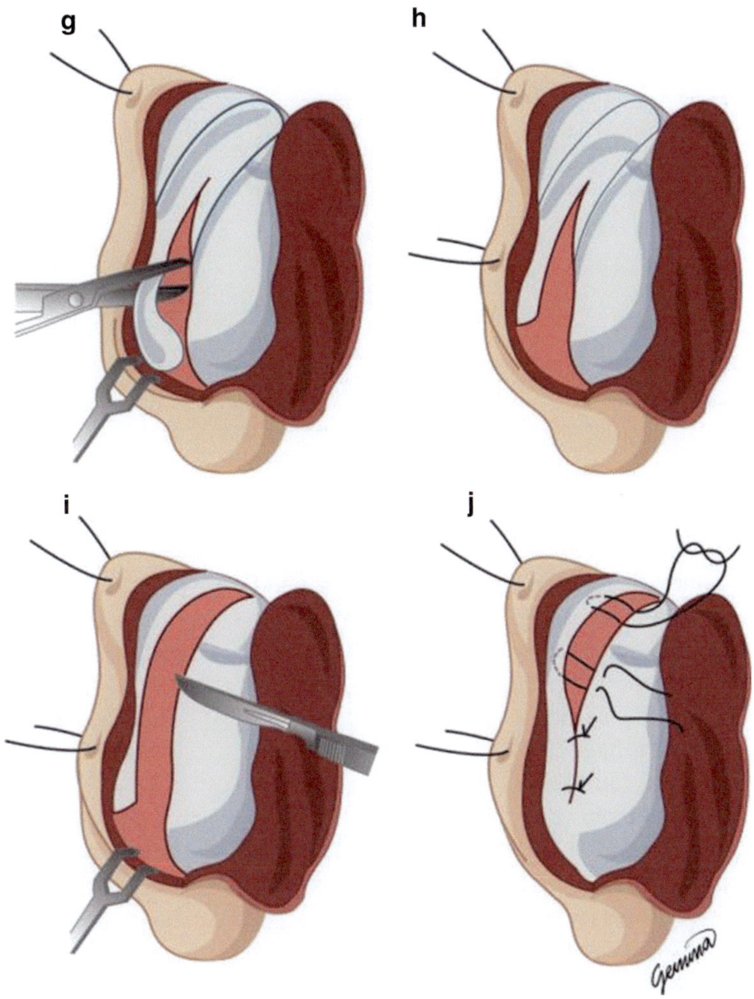

and its posterior crus. When the ear is folded back, the new antihelicis is noted on the anterior surface of the auricle. The skin is punctured through from the anterior surface with a fine needle along the outer and inner borders of the new antihelix and superior crus. Each point is marked on the posterior surface of the auricular cartilage with methylene blue to delineate the cartilage incision. No markings are necessary to outline the inferior crus since the sulcus antihelicis transversus is usually visible. (**e**) Incision made along the markings down to the fissure antitragohelicina. An incision is also made through the sulcus antihelicis transversus to form the inferior crus. A diamond-shaped section of cartilage is the outlined, which extends up to the inferior crus. (**f**) Section of cartilage removed. The width of the excision carries with the amount of spring found in the cartilage. (**g**) Cauda helicis exposed and removed. This procedure is necessary in the majority of cases. An incision is made at the upper end of the superior crus for removal of a section of cartilage. This incision is located under the helix and is usually necessary to break completely the spring of the cartilage. (**h**) The cartilage removed. (**i**) Partial crosscutting of the remaining cartilage that forms the superior crus. These incisions are made to weaken the spring of the cartilage and must not pass completely through the cartilage. In cases in which the cartilage is soft and pliable, crosscutting is not necessary. In other cases, thinning of the cartilage by shaving is sufficient to weaken the spring. A section of antitragus is removed in most cases of extreme cupping of the lower portion of the ear. (**j**) Surgical gut fixation sutures inserted. The sutures are tied only tight enough to form a smooth antihelix and superior crus. External mattress sutures tied over cotton rolls, instead of surgical gut sutures, have been used to good advantage in many cases. If the cartilage is soft and pliable, allowing the ear to fall back easily, no fixation sutures are necessary. Excess skin is trimmed, and *black* silk sutures are used to close the incision

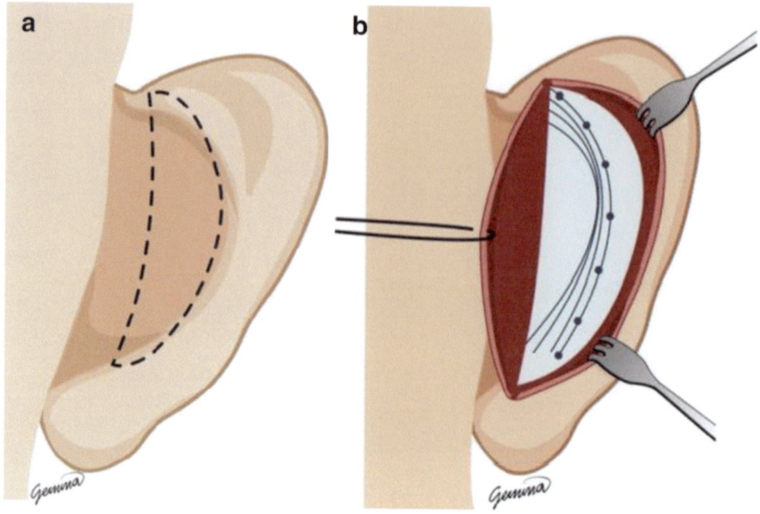

Fig. 5.10 Kristensen's technique (1952) [52]. (**a**) Postauricular skin excision. (**b**) Parallel incision in the cartilage

is removed from the upper end of the superior crus to completely break the spring of the antihelix and superior crus. Three or four surgical gut mattress sutures are inserted in the perichondrium along the margins of the original incisions in the cartilage and tied to form the new antihelical fold. Excess skin is excised and the skin sutured closed.

Jayes and Dale [50] modified the Luckett technique by also using antihelical incisions. Also, they classified the prominent ear into types:

Type 1: The antihelix is formed but is not folded back as sharply as in a normal ear, and the scapho-conchal angle is widened. The ear is small and it will not be abnormally prominent, but if large, it will definitely "stick out."

Type 2: Superior crus of the antihelix is absent. The upper part of the scapha looks abnormally wide owing to the absence of the dividing ridge. The whole upper part of the ear turns forward and tends to droop as it lacks the stiffening support of the superior crus.

Type 3: The whole of the antihelix is poorly formed, and the scapho-conchal angle is widely obtuse. The superior crus is absent. The inferior crus and the lower part of the antihelix, though visible, are very much flattened. The ear stands sharply out from the head at a right angle.

Type 4: The antihelix is totally absent. The ear is of the fetal type curving smoothly outward and forward from the head in the pane of the concha. This type of deformity is sometimes associated with microtia or relative shortness of the helix.

Sercer [51] resected the anterior spine of the helix, thinned the back of the conch, and excised an ellipse or myrtle-leaf piece of the retroauricular skin. Kristensen [52] devised variations in skin resection and cartilage incisions (Fig. 5.10). Becker [53] described parallel antihelical incisions held together by permanent sutures to produce conical antihelical tubing in order to soften the external contour of the corrected prominent ear. This was refined by Converse et al. [54] and further elaborated by Converse and Wood-Smith [55] (Fig. 5.11) and Wood-Smith and Converse [56].

Straith [57] corrected unpleasant effects of otoplasty (Fig. 5.12) by (1) running a cutaneous 0000 nylon suture just back of the cut edges of the concha and helix; (2) predetermining the correct height of concha and antihelix by folding the ear back and placing needles, after which the needles are removed and the ear folded back to determine the amount of cartilage to be determined and excised accordingly; and (3) predetermining the formation of a normal curve of the antihelix by folding the ear back and placing the needles along the edges of the concha and triangular fossa.

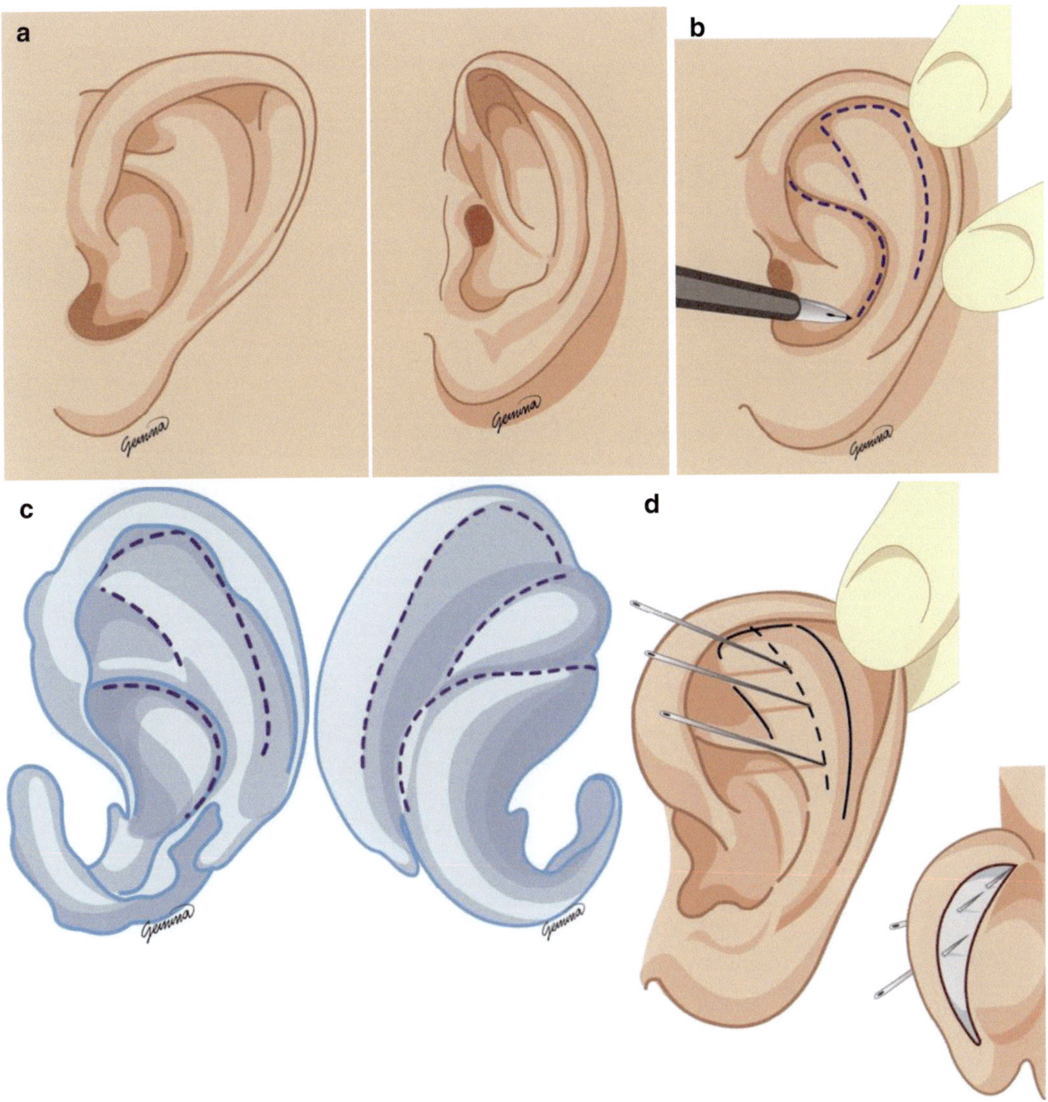

Fig. 5.11 Converse and Wood-Smith technique is a cartilage-breaking technique applicable to severe prominent ear deformities in all age groups. (**a**) Prominence of the ear with conchal excess, lack of an antihelical fold, and obliqueness of the conchoscaphal angle. (**b**) While pressing medially on the prominent ear helix, several linear markings are drawn on the anterior surface. These markings surround the superior crus on three sides and include the superior rim of the triangular fossa, the upper border of the superior crus, and the junction of the scapha with the helix. The conchal rim is marked by its full length. (**c**) Markings are visualized on both anterior and posterior auricular surfaces. (**d**) By passing a straight Keith cutting needle through the ear, the exact location of the posterior auricular skin excision is determined. The skin is excised down to the cartilage, excising all soft tissue and perichondrium from the posterior auricular cartilage. (**e**) The straight Keith needles are passed through the previous anterior marking so that the anterior cartilage markings can be transposed to the posterior surface of the cartilage. (**f**) Transference of all markings requires that the posterior skin and perichondrium be dissected off the cartilage to the rim of the helix. Full-thickness breaks in the cartilage can then be made with care to preserve the anterior skin of the ear. (**g**) Tubing of the antihelix is performed with several permanent white sutures placed in mattress fashion. The sutures are tied simultaneously with enough tension to provide for the proper amount of tubing of the antihelix. (**h**) The amount of conchal cartilage excess is estimated by pressing inward on the newly folded antihelix. (**i**) The conchal excess is excised from the conchal rim, usually performed in elliptical fashion. Variations may be required depending on the deformity. (**j**) The edges of the newly formed antihelix and freshly contoured conchal rim are approximated with several well-placed 4-0 permanent *white sutures* placed in mattress fashion. The sutures are tied with enough tension to provide the intended end result and are placed in such a fashion that the edges of the cartilage do not evert

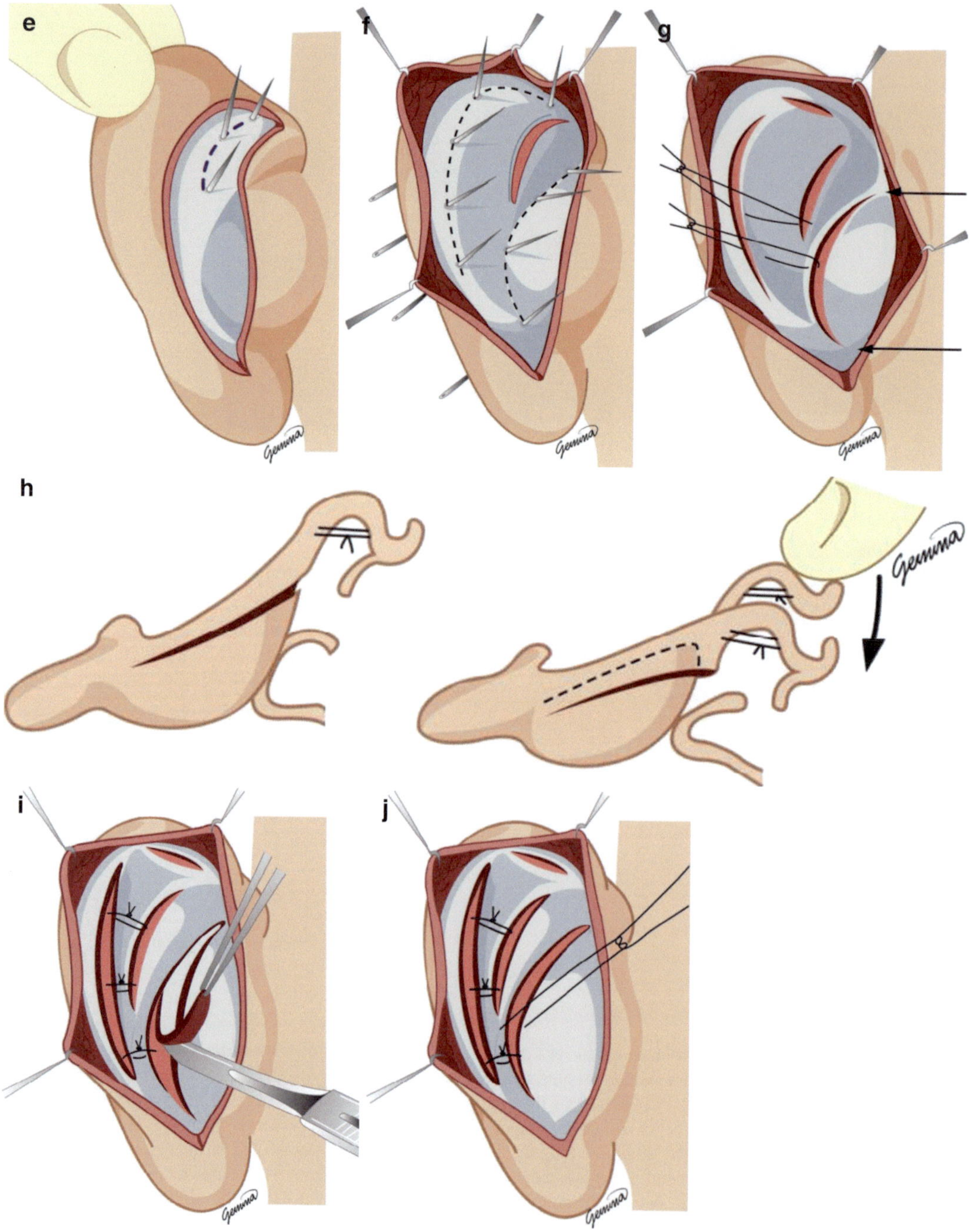

Fig. 5.11 (continued)

Usually a strip no more than 2 mm wide is excised to give a normal appearance.

Surgical abrasion of the antihelix was described by Stark and Saunders [58]. Mustarde (1963 [59], 1967 [60], 1971 [61]) simplified these techniques by creating a conical antihelical tubing with permanent conchoscaphal mattress sutures (Fig. 5.13). These sutures, placed full

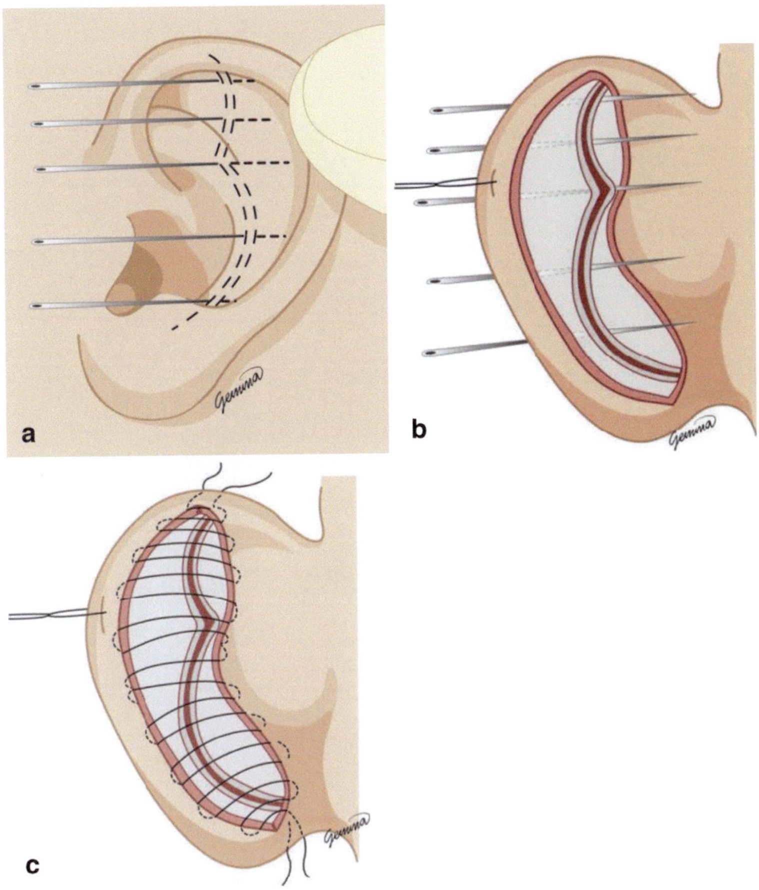

Fig. 5.12 Straith's technique (1953) [57]. (**a**) By normal pressure the helix is forced back into a normal position and the height and shape of the antihelix determined. The ear is pierced by needles approximately 1 cm below the desired antihelical rim (after the method of Davis and Kitlowski). (**b**) An incision is made just above the needles that are then removed, and the ear is folded back for examination. The excess cartilage as seen anteriorly can then be removed to the desired shape and height of the antihelix and posterior crus. (**c**) A subcuticular suture is started at one end. Four-millimeter bites are taken in alternate edges of the under surface of the antihelix approximately 1 mm back from the edges. At the center of the antihelix, these sutures are brought out to the surface to facilitate easy removal in two sections. The ear is folded back, the sutures pulled taut, and the antihelix is examined from the lateral side. If a sharp antihelix ridge is present, the suture should be removed and placed closer to the surface or farther away, as the case may be, to correct the deformity

thickness through the cartilage of the concha and scapha in mattress fashion without piercing the lateral skin, are particularly successful to treat the pliable cartilage of children. All cartilage tubing techniques depend on scarring to fill the tube and lock the sculpted framework into position.

Tamerin and Mirehouse [62] noted the tendency of the auricular cartilage in the region of the helix to curl backward when it is incised near the free edge of the ear and when it is separated from its anterior lining perichondrium. Farrior [63] used the smallest dermabrader to remove parallel concave troughs similar to the full-thickness wedges removed in the current technique. The strips that remain between the troughs give body and resilience to the ear. He used a method of three incisions and an overriding cartilage strip in the reconstruction of the antihelix proper. He did not join the superior crus and conchal rim incisions but left an

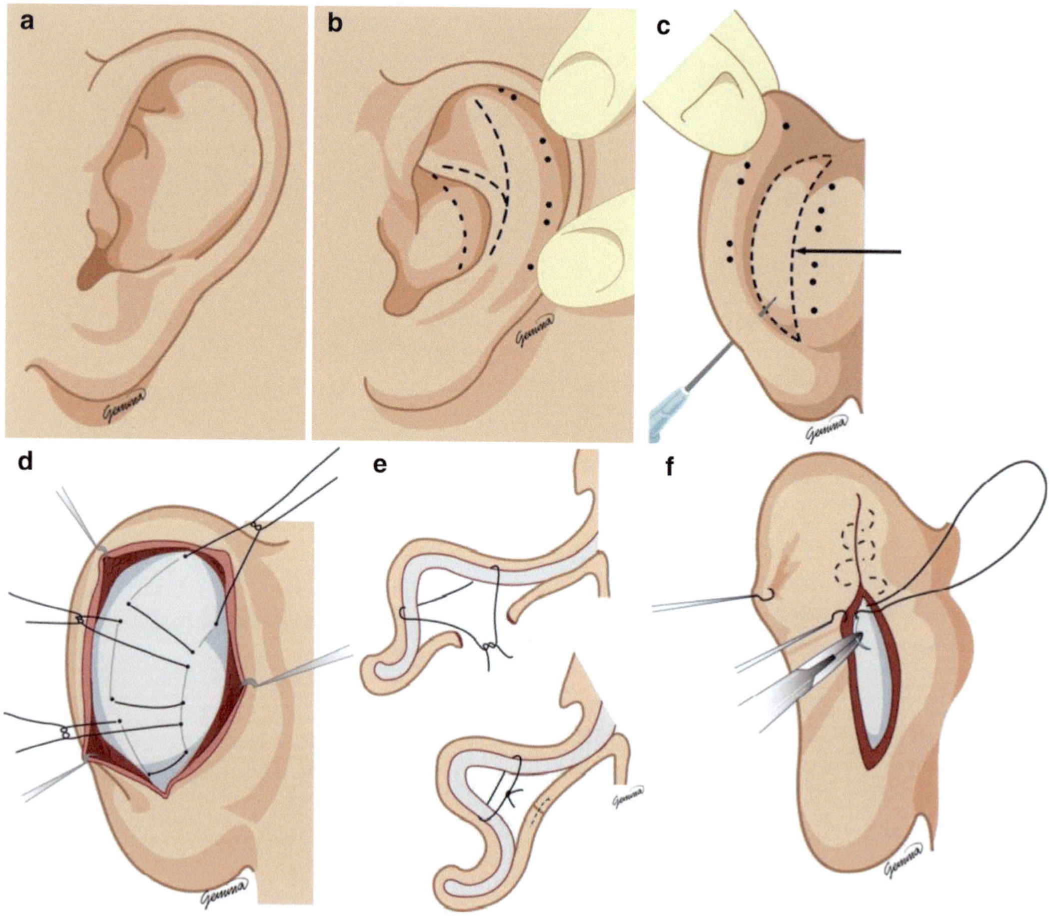

Fig. 5.13 Mustarde's cartilage molding technique. (**a**) Best used in children with a pliable nature of the cartilage. (**b**) While pressing medially on the helix of the ear, several pairs of ink marks are made on the conchal and outer aspect of the antihelix. These pairs of *marks* precisely mimic the position of the mattress sutures to be used in the repair. (**c**) Several 25-gauge needles dipped in ink are used to transfer the pairs of *ink marks* to the postauricular skin. A postauricular skin excision is marked between the rows of transferred ink marks. (**d**) The skin excision is carried down to the cartilage, excising all soft tissue and perichondrium from the posterior auricular cartilage. Several permanent white 4-0 sutures are placed through the full thickness of cartilage, making certain that the perichondrium of the anterior auricular cartilage is pierced. (**e**) The sutures are tied simultaneously, not under full tension. (**f**) A subcuticular or over-and-over running 4-0 nylon suture is used for closure

isthmus of cartilage at the junction of the crura as in Straith's [57] method.

Pitanguy and Rebello [64] used an island technique to cover visible cartilage ridges. Gibson and Davis [65], Chongchet [66] (Fig. 5.14), and Stenströem [67] introduced lateral cartilage weakening techniques to take advantage of the unique ability of a sheet of cartilage to warp away from the injured surface. In the Chongchet technique, the lateral scaphal cartilage is scored with a scalpel to form an antihelix. In the Stenströem technique, postauricular incision is used so that a short-tined rasp could be used to "blindly" scar the antihelix. Morcellation of the antihelix through a direct lateral incision was advocated by Ju et al. [68].

Crikelair and Cosman [69] described a new technique for the prominent ear with combined concha and antihelix deformity (Fig. 5.15). A postauricular incision parallel to the free border

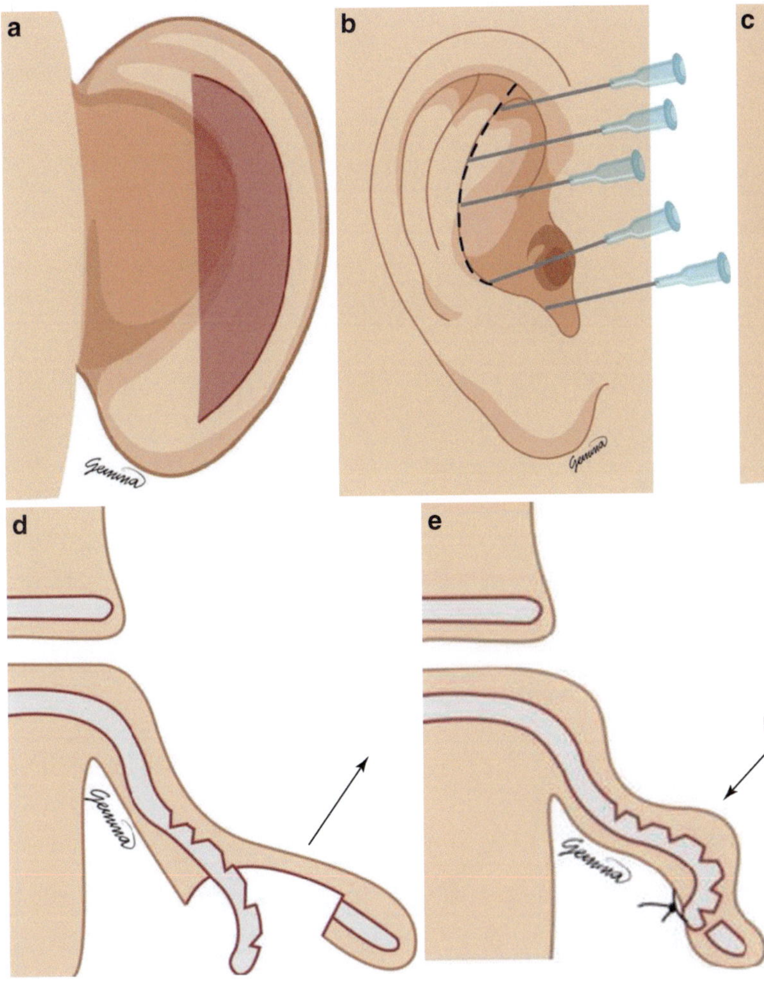

Fig. 5.14 Chongchet's technique (1963) [66]. (**a**) Excision of skin. Undermining toward the free border. (**b**) Marking of new antihelix. (**c**) Anterior scoring of the cartilage. (**d**) Curling of the cartilage. (**e**) Overlapping of cartilage

of the helix and 1 cm from the border is extended from the cephaloauricular angle superiorly to the fleshy lobule inferiorly. An ellipse of skin can be excised using the incision line as the outer border. Needles are passed posteriorly from the anterior surface of the ear just beneath the helix overhang, tipped with methylene blue and then withdrawn. The wound edges are slightly undermined and the methylene blue markings identified on the cartilage. The auricular cartilage is cut through along this line from superiorly at the cephaloauricular angle inferiorly to where the tail of the helix begins. This separates the rim of the ear from the major ear cartilage. The auricular cartilage is freed subchondrally on its anterior surface and the anterior dissection carried forward in the upper part of the ear until the inferior crus of the helix is exposed. The middle and lower portion of the ear, the edge of the cavum concha, is similarly exposed. The anterior cartilage surface is lightly striated (not through the full thickness of the cartilage) in at least three or four directions. The cartilage will bend back on itself forming the smooth roll of the antihelix. The acuteness of the roll can be increased by increasing the number and decreasing the spacing of the striations. The redundant auricular cartilage can be trimmed. The amount to be

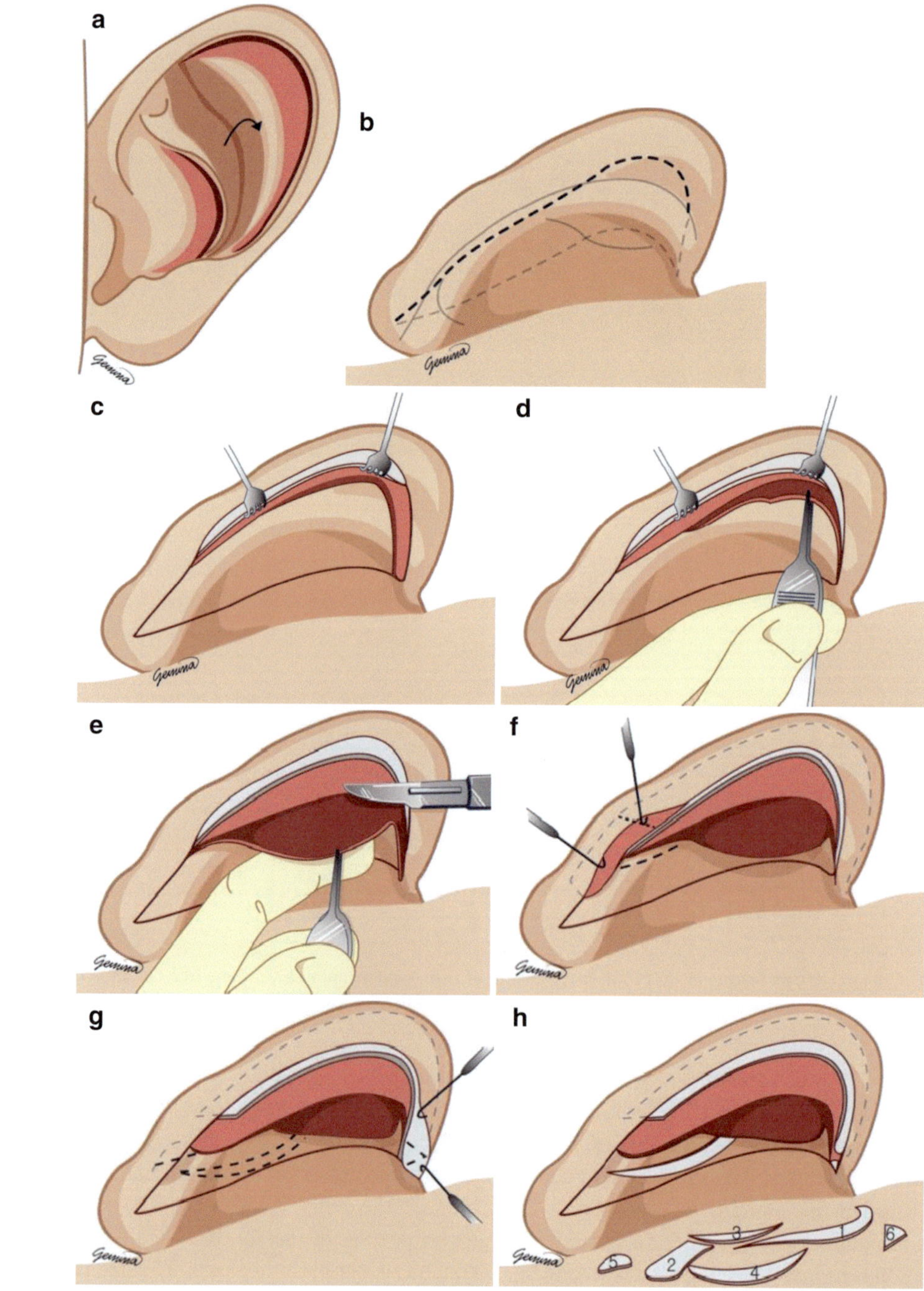

Fig. 5.15 Crikelair and Cosman technique (1964) [69]. (**a**) Prominent ear with combined concha and antihelix deformity. The darkened ellipses indicate desirable reductions in size. The *arrow* indicates the antihelix with superior crus to be constructed. (**b**) Posterior incision in *dark dashes*. Possible elliptical skin excision in *light dashes*. (**c**) Auricular cartilage cut through to anterior surface. (**d**) Subepichondrial auricular cartilage dissection on the anterior surface. (**e**) Striation of anterior surface of cartilage. (**f**) Trimming of auricular cartilage and concha edge to be carried out as indicated by heavy *dark lines*. Tail of the helix excision is also indicated. (**g**) Tail of helix excised. Tentative excisions of superior helix, concha ellipse, and antitragus prominence indicated by heavy *dash line*. (**h**) Pieces of cartilage excised in maximum reduction. 1 through 3 are usual excisions, 4 through 6 are excisions dictated by the individual case. *1* Auricular cartilage edge. *2* Tail of helix. *3* Edge of concha. *4* Ellipse of concha. *5* Antitragal prominence. *6* Helix wedge. (**i**) Cutaway view showing effect of cartilage excisions with formation of free helix bucket handle

i

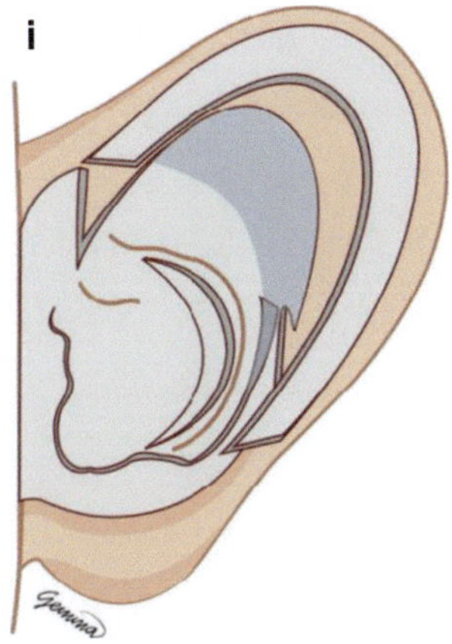

Fig. 5.15 (continued)

excised can be determined by replacing the helix over the auricular cartilage and observing the excess from behind. The width removed affects the width of the new scaphoid fossa. The amount trimmed from the superior pole affects the vertical length of the ear. The edge of the cavum concha is trimmed, and the tail of the helix is dissected free and excised. The anterior skin flap is replaced on the cartilage and molded into its new contours. The postauricular incision is closed.

In 1966, Barnes and Morris [70] reported use of the Stenströem technique by elevating the skin from the postauricular skin excision site and freeing tail of the helix from the conchal cartilage and the skin anteriorly. Half of a Brown-Adson tissue forceps was introduced into the subcutaneous tunnel to make multiple superficial scratches along the antihelix and its crura. The ear can then be folded back quite easily and held in its new position by simply closing the elliptical skin defect. Kaye [71] developed a combination of the Stenströem technique of antihelical rasping and the Mustard concept of permanent mattress suture fixation to maintain the proper amount of antihelical roll after a lateral rasp of the antihelix. Permanent sutures are introduced through tiny lateral incisions along the conchal crest, which are carried across the antihelical fold and tied on the lateral side.

Further contributions of the Ely technique with conchomastoidal sutures include Owens and Delgado [72] and Furnas [73]. Spira et al. [74] combined conchomastoidal suturing with conchoscaphal suturing with good results (Fig. 5.16). Webster [75] stated that regardless of the skill of the operator or the technique of the operation, however, one falls short of the ideal appearance in every case. Perfection is impossible of attainment. He used a combination of ideas of many authors plus individual interpretation (Fig. 5.17). The essential concept is thinking of the concha as one entity and the rest of the ear, including the helix and antihelix area, as another unit. Wood-Smith [76] reported on correction of prominent lobules when the lower third of the ear protrudes with a modified fishtail excision (Fig. 5.18).

Weerda [77], in cases of thick auricular cartilage with low elasticity, used a diamond drill to weaken the auricular cartilage immediately above and below the intended new antihelical fold and the antihelical crus through a retroauricular access. Full-thickness mattress sutures of slowly absorbable suture material are placed at the positions with the corresponding markings to fix the helix in the intended position.

Wegener [78] stated that the procedure that combined correction of protruding ears with reduction of hyperplastic auricles had been developed by the author more than 30 years previously. During the postauricular removal of the prominent cartilage in a layer-by-layer fashion, the scalpel is used tangentially following the outline of the individual crural curvature to the antihelix margin and the auricle base. Falciform excision of the cartilage of the superior helix is performed starting from the anterior fold of the auricle peripherally toward the scapha. After an anterior skin sickle excision, a new helix margin is created by eversion of the still intact skin of the posterior helix wall. The operation is finished by a wedge-shaped skin-cartilage excision of the superior part of the helix.

Horlock et al. [79] described a postauricular fascial flap in otoplasty. Scuderi et al. [80] reported on a posterior auricular muscle flap in otoplasty.

An excellent algorithm was developed by Stal and Hatef [81] for the analysis and treatment of the prominent ear.

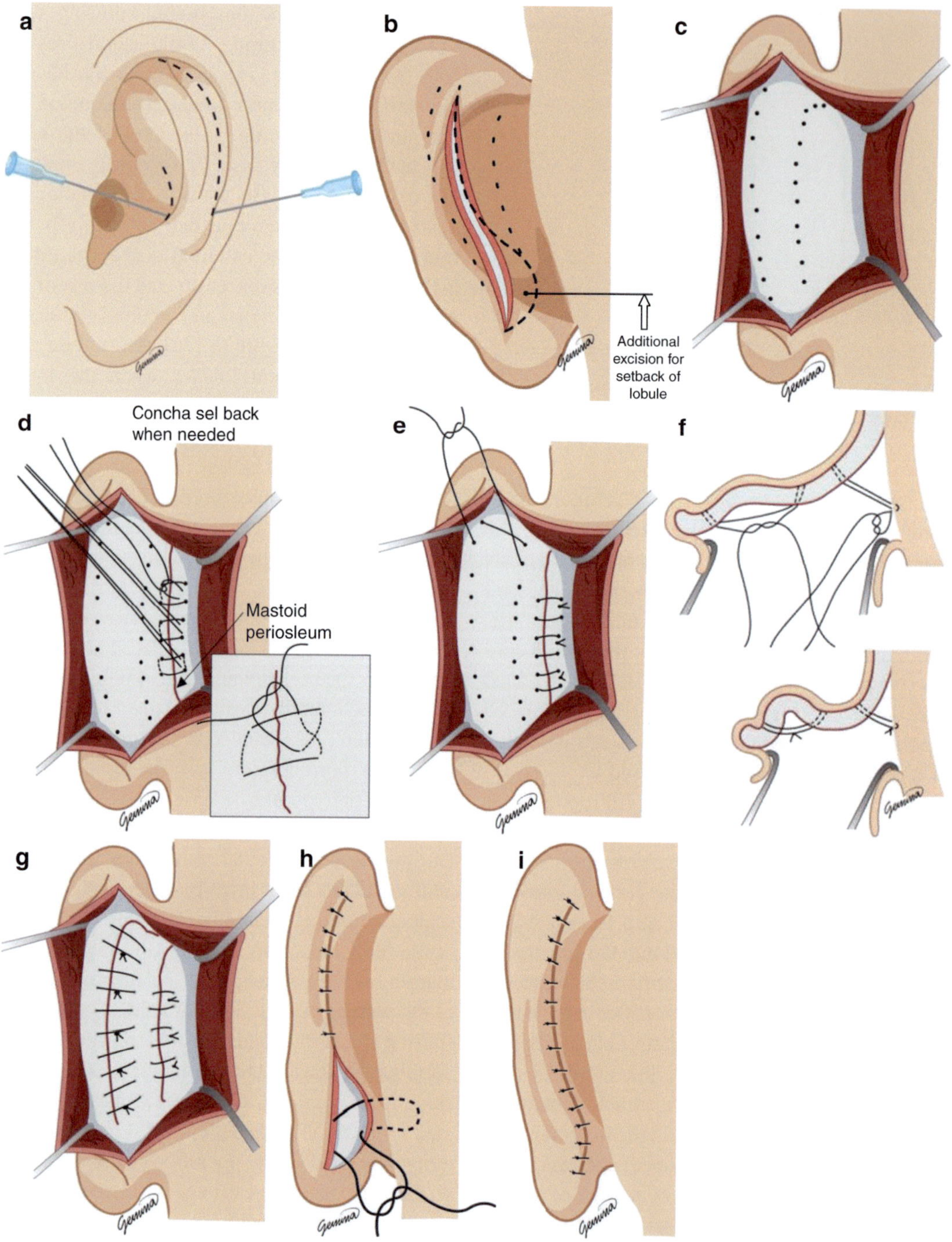

Fig. 5.16 Spira's technique (1969) [74]. (**a**) Creating outline for insertion of sutures by depressing helix to create normal contour. (**b**) Dye marks on posterior ear. Skin excisions. (**c**) Cartilage exposed. (**d**) Concha setback when needed. (**e**) Sutures forming antihelical fold inserted and tied. (**f**) Sutures in position. (**g**) Internal closure complete. (**h**) Dermis to periosteum suture repositioning lobe. (**i**) Closure completed

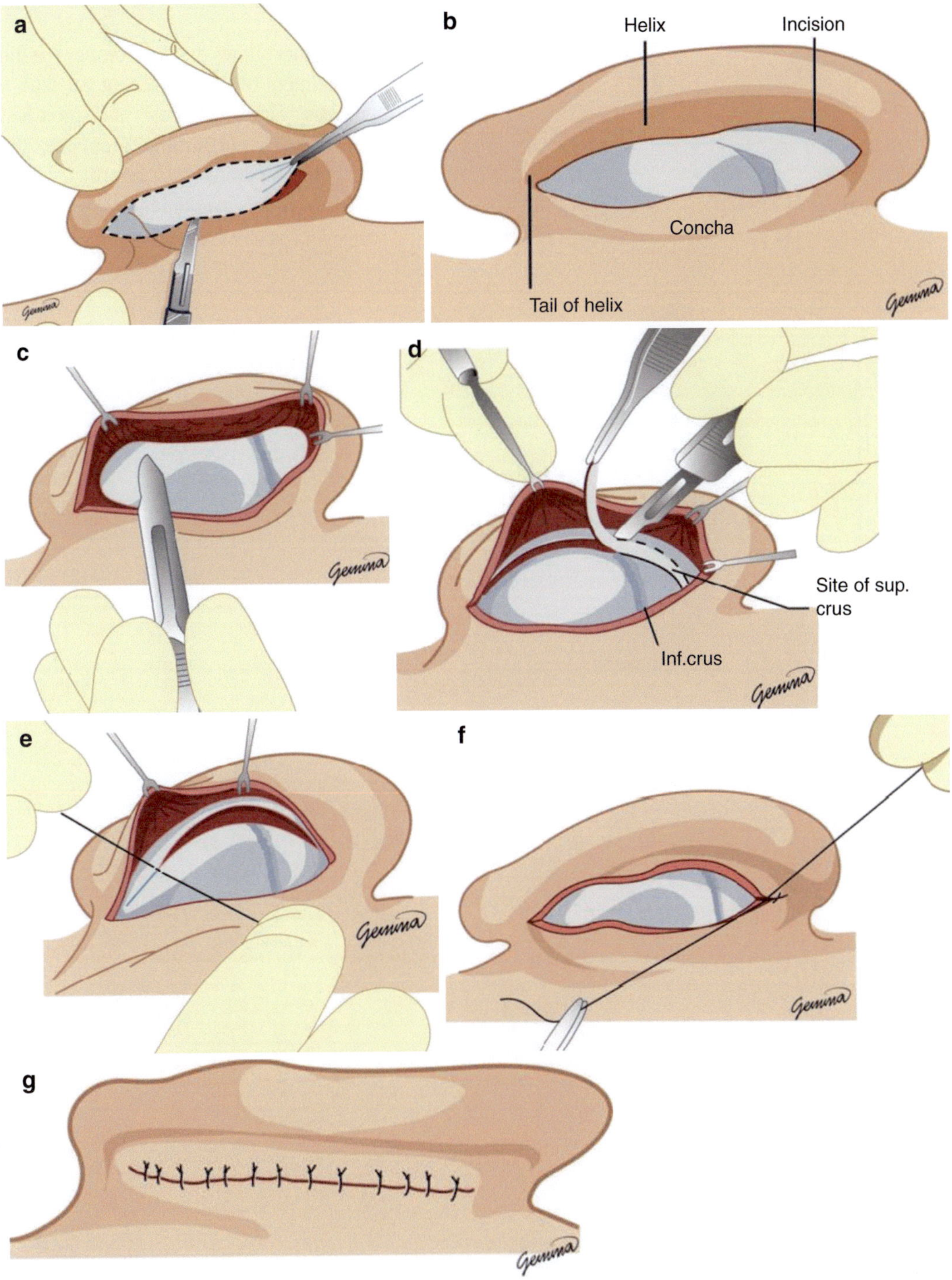

Fig. 5.17 Webster's technique (1969) [75]. (**a**) Outline of slipper-shaped incision. (**b**) After resection of skin. Note width of the skin resection is widest opposite the superior and lower portions of the ear. (**c**) Undermining skin and subcutaneous tissues. (**d**) Resection of redundant concha continuing into strip resection at level of new antihelical fold. (**e**) Replacement of the tail of the helix on the concha. This 4-0 plan catgut suture is the only buried suture used. (**f**) Skin closure with 4-0 silk (for easier removal). (**g**) Completed everting closure. (**h**): Location of through-and-through mattress sutures of 4-0 plain catgut for fixation of reconstructed antihelical fold. Base of each *arrow* describing the structure

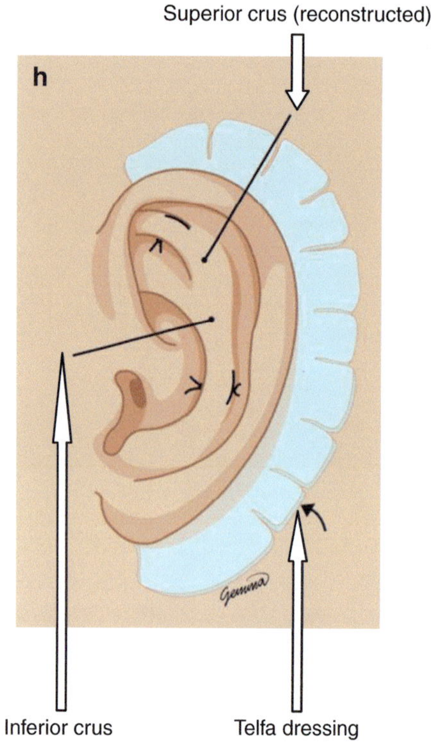

Fig. 5.17 (continued)

Conclusions

Otoplasty history shows the development of the surgical treatment of the prominent ear with a multitudinous variety of new and modified techniques. When performing otoplasty, the surgeon should be thoroughly informed of the variety of procedures available.

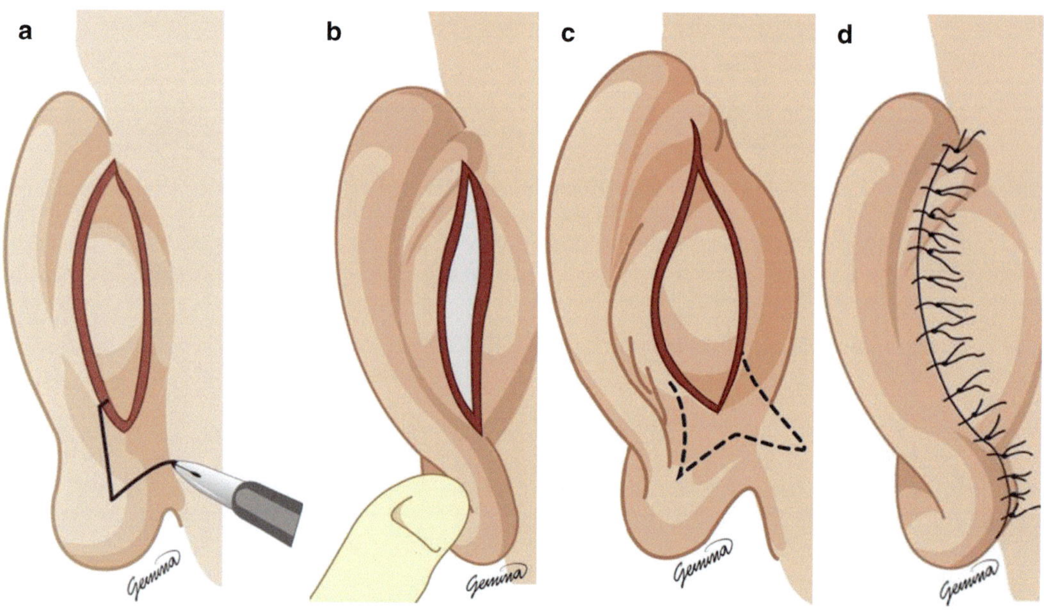

Fig. 5.18 Wood-Smith technique. (**a**) The skin is excised over the concha, and a V extension of the excision is drawn on the posterior surface of the lobule. (**b**) While the ink is wet, the lobule is pressed against mastoid skin. (**c**) The mirror impression of the V is transposed to the mastoid skin. Excision of all the skin within the borders of the modified fishtail design is carried out. (**d**) Closure is with 4-0 nylon suture

References

1. Saraf S, Parihar RS. Sushruta: the first Plastic Surgeon in 600 B.C. Internet J Plast Surg. 2007;4(2):4
2. Rufus Cornelius Celsius. http://www.answers.com/topic/celcus-aulus-cornelius. Accessed 15 Jan 2011.
3. Cornelius Celsius Biography. http://www.bookrags.com/tandf/aulus-cornelius-celsus-tf/. Accessed 15 Jan 2011.
4. De Curtorum Chirurgia. http://beckeerexhibits.wustl.edu/rare/collections/ball.html. Accessed 15 Jan 2011.
5. Dieffenbach JE. Die operative Chirurgie. Leipzig: Brockhaus; 1845.
6. de Martino G. Anomalie de pavillon de l'oreille et proced d'otomisie. Bull Acad Imperiale Méd. 1856;22:647. 810.
7. Rogers BO. Ely's 1881 operation for correction of the protruding ear. A medical "first". Plast Reconstr Surg. 1968;42(6):584–6.
8. Ely ET. An operation for prominence of the auricles. Arch Otolaryngol. 1881;10:97.
9. Keen WW. New method of operating for relief of deformity of prominent ears. Ann Surg. 1890;11:49.
10. Monks GH. Operation for correcting the deformity due to prominent ears. Boston Med Surg J. 1891;124:84.
11. Cocheril R. Essai sur la Restauration du Pavillon de l'Oreille. Lille, Paris Theses; 1894.
12. Haug R. Eine einfache neue plastische method zur rücklagerung hochgradig abstehender ohrmuschelu. Deutsche Med Whnschr. 1894;20:776.
13. Joseph J. Eselsohren, Verhandl. Berl Med Gesellsch. 1896;27:206.
14. DeSchweinitz GE, Randall BA. Affections of the external ears. In: DeSchweinitz GE, Randall BA, editors. American text-book of diseases of the eye, ear, nose, and throat. Philadelphia: WB Saunders Co; 1899. p. 691.
15. Gersuny R. Uber einige kosmetische operationen. Wien Med Wochenschr. 1903;53:2253–7.
16. Morestin H. De la reposition et du plissement cosmétiques du pavillon de l'oreille. Rev Orthop. 1903;4:394.
17. Payr E. Plastische operationen an der ohren (stellungsverbesserung, verkleinerung). Langenbeck's Arch. 1906;87:919. Arch Klin Chir 1906;78:918.
18. Miller CC. The correction of featural imperfections. Chicago: Oak Printing Co; 1907.
19. Goldstein MA. The cosmetic and plastic surgery of the ear. Laryngoscope. 1908;18:826–52.
20. Luckett WH. A new operation for prominent ears base on the anatomy of the deformity. Surg Gynecol Obstet. 1910;10:365–7.
21. Barsky AJ. Plastic surgery. Philadelphia: WB Saunders; 1938.
22. Baxter H. Plastic correction of prominent ears in children. Can Med Assoc J. 1941;45(3):217–20.
23. Young F. Correction of abnormally prominent ears. Surg Gynecol Obstet. 1944;77:541.
24. Farina R. Protruding ears: Luckett's otoplasty. Hospital (Rio J). 1951;39(4):563–9.
25. Vidaurre S. Protruding ears, another method of treatment. Plast Reconstr Surg. 1952;10(1):39–45.
26. Seltzer AP. Plastic surgery of the prominent auricle. AMA Arch Otolaryngol. 1954;69(3):1316–33.
27. Hatch MD. Common problems of otoplasty. J Int Coll Surg. 1958;30(2):171–8.
28. Jones EH. Operation for the correction of protruding ears. South Med J. 1959;52:1967–71.
29. Holmes EM. A new procedure for correcting outstanding ears. AMA Arch Otolaryngol. 1959;69:409.
30. Cloutier AM. Correction of outstanding ears. Plast Reconstr Surg Transplant Bull. 1961;28:412–6.
31. McDowell AJ. Goals in otoplasty for protruding ears. Plast Reconstr Surg. 1968;41(1):17–27.
32. Ruttin E. Eine methode zur korrektur abstehender ohren und zumverschluss retroaurikulärer offnumgen. Monastsschr Ohrenh. 1910;44:196.
33. Kolle FS. Plastic and cosmetic surgery. New York: D. Appleton and Co; 1911.
34. Alexander G. Zur plastischen korrektur abstehender ohrmuscheln. Wien Klin Wochenschr. 1928;41:1217.
35. Frühwald V. Plastic surgery of the nose, ear, and face. Vienna: Wilhelm Maudrich; 1932.
36. Demel R. Eriolge der beseitung der abstehenden ohren. Wien Klin Wchnschr. 1935;48:1185.
37. Eltner E. Eine einfachemethod korrektur abstehender ohrer. Wien Klin Wchnschr. 1937;50:1185.
38. Davis JS, Kitlowski EA. Abnormal prominence of the ears; a method of readjustment. Surgery. 1937;2:835–48.
39. MacColumm DW. The lop ear. J Am Med Assoc. 1939;110:1427.
40. Young F. The correction of abnormally prominent ears. Surg Obstet Gynecol. 1944;78:541.
41. New GB, Erich JB. Protruding ears. A method of plastic correction. Am J Surg. 1940;48:385–90.
42. Fishman LZ, Fishman VP. Plastic surgery for outstanding ears: a simple surgical procedure. Bull Pract Ophthalmol. 1946;16(1):19–21.
43. Pierce GW, Klabunde EH, Bergeron VL. Useful procedures in plastic surgery. Plast Reconstr Surg. 1947;2(4):358–61.
44. Dufourmental C. The free tubular cutaneous graft; new technical method for reflection of the helix during reconstruction of the pavilion of the ear. Ann Chir Plast. 1958;3(4):311–5.
45. Paletta FX, Ship AG, Vannorman RT. Double spring release in otoplasty for prominent ears. Am J Surg. 1963;106:506–10.
46. Borges AF. Prominent ears: modification of Dr. Forrest Young's technic. Plast Reconstr Surg. 1946;12(3):208–10.
47. McEvitt WG. The problem of the protruding ear. Plast Reconstr Surg. 1947;2(5):481496.
48. Weaver DF. Correction of prominent ears. Arch Otolaryngol. 1947;42(2):205–8.
49. Becker OJ. Surgical correction of the abnormally protruding ear. Arch Otolaryngol. 1949;50(5):541–60.
50. Jayes PH, Dale RH. The treatment of prominent ears. Br J Plast Surg. 1951;4(3):193–201.

51. Sercer A. Einige worte über die ursache und die korrektur abstehender ohren. Pract Otorhinolaryng. 1951;13(1):9–16.
52. Kristensen HK. Korrektion af udstående ører. Ugeskr Laeger. 1952;114(17):517–25.
53. Becker OJ. Correction of protruding deformed ear. Br J Plast Surg. 1952;5(3):187–96.
54. Converse JM, Nigro A, Wilson FA, Johnson N. A technique for surgical correction of lop ears. Plast Reconstr Surg. 1955;15(5):411–8.
55. Converse JM, Wood-Smith D. Technical details in the surgical correction of the lop ear deformity. Plast Reconstr Surg. 1963;31:118–28.
56. Wood-Smith D, Converse JM. The lop ear deformity. Surg Clin North Am. 1971;51(2):417–27.
57. Straith RE. Anti-helix reconstruction in the protruding ear operation. Plast Reconstr Surg. 1953; 12(6):454–9.
58. Stark RB, Saunders DE. Natural appearance restored in the unduly prominent ear. Br J Plast Surg. 1962;15:385–97.
59. Mustardé JC. The correction of prominent ears using simple mattress sutures. Br J Plast Surg. 1963; 16:170–8.
60. Mustardé JC. The treatment of prominent ears by buried mattress sutures: a ten-year survey. Plast Reconstr Surg. 1967;39(4):382–6.
61. Mustardé JC. Plastic surgery in infancy and childhood. Churchill-Livingstone: Edinburgh; 1971.
62. Tamerin J, Mirehouse O. Reconstruction of the antihelix and scapha in selected cases of protruding ears. AMA Arch Otolaryngol. 1959;70:597–605.
63. Farrior RT. A method of otoplasty: normal contour of the antihelix and scaphoid fossa. AMA Arch Otolaryngol. 1959;69(4):400–8.
64. Pitanguy I, Rebello C. Ansiform ears. Correction by "island" technique. Acta Chir Plas. 1962;4:267–77.
65. Gibson T, Davis W. The distortion of autogenous cartilage grafts: its cause and prevention. Br J Plast Surg. 1958;10:257.
66. Chongchet V. A method of antihelix reconstruction. Br J Plast Surg. 1963;16:268–72.
67. Stenstroem SJ. A "natural" technique for correction of congenitally prominent ears. Plast Reconstr Surg. 1963;32:509–18.
68. Ju DM, Li C, Crikelair GF. The surgical correction of protruding ears. Plast Reconstr Surg. 1963;32:283–93.
69. Crikelair GF, Cosman B. Another solution for the problem of the prominent ear. Ann Surg. 1964; 160(2):314–24.
70. Barnes WE, Morris Jr FA. Otoplasty: an improved technic. South Med J. 1966;59(6):681–4.
71. Kaye BL. A simplified method for correcting the prominent ear. Plast Reconstr Surg. 1967;40(1): 44–8.
72. Owens N, Delgado DD. The management of outstanding ears. South Med J. 1965;58:32–3.
73. Furnas DW. Correction of prominent ears by conchal mastoid sutures. Plast Reconstr Surg. 1968; 42(3):189–93.
74. Spira M, McCrea R, Gerow FJ, Hardy SB. Analysis and treatment of the protruding ear. Transactions of the Fourth International Congress of Plastic Surgeons. Amsterdam: Excerpta Medica; 1969. p. 1090.
75. Webster GV. The tail of the helix as a key to otoplasty. Plast Reconstr Surg. 1969;44(5):455–561.
76. Wood Smith D. Otoplasty. In: Rees T, editor. Aesthetic plastic surgery. Philadelphia: WB Saunders; 1980. p. 833.
77. Weerda H. Remarks about otoplasty and avulsion of the auricle. Laryngol Rhinol Otol (Stuttg). 1979;58(3): 242–51.
78. Wegener HE. Correction of protruding ears in combination with reduction surgery of hyperplastic auricles. Aesthetic Plast Surg. 1981;5(1):57–62.
79. Horlock N, Misra A, Gault DT. The postauricular fascial flap as an adjunct to Mustardé and Furnas type otoplasty. Plast Reconstr Surg. 2001;108(6): 1487–90.
80. Scuderi N, Tenna S, Bitonti A, Vonella M. Repositioning of posterior auricular muscle combined with conventional otoplasty: a personal technique. J Plast Reconstr Aesthet Surg. 2007;60(2):201–4.
81. Stal S, Hatef DA. Prominent ears. In: Marsh JL, Perlyn CA, editors. Decision making in plastic surgery. St. Louis: Quality Medical Publishing, Inc; 2010. p. 68–9.

Current Trends in Otoplasty

6

Rajanya S. Petersson

Introduction

The incidence of prominent ears is 5 % in the Caucasian population, with the most common abnormality being an unfurled antihelix, and the second most common, a deep conchal bowl [1]. Often, these abnormalities coexist and both must be addressed. Over 200 techniques have been described for the surgical correction of prominent ears, suggesting that no single "best" technique exists and that techniques and modifications will continue to evolve [2]. Otoplasty techniques can typically be divided into two broad categories: cartilage-cutting and cartilage-sparing. Cartilage-cutting techniques aim to eliminate the inherent elastic spring of the cartilage and improve the longevity of surgical results; these include cartilaginous incisions, wedge excisions, scoring, and abrasion of either the posterior or anterior auricular surfaces. Cartilage-sparing techniques emerged in an attempt to prevent anterior pinna irregularities that can arise with cartilage-cutting techniques. Suturing, rather than cutting, is used to create the desired auricular contours, thereby preserving cartilaginous support and minimizing contour irregularities. However, elements of both categories are often used in conjunction. Here, historical techniques will be reviewed and discussed, as well as more recent modifications and techniques found in the literature, paying particular attention to the last 5 years.

R.S. Petersson, M.D.
Division of Pediatric Otolaryngology,
Virginia Commonwealth University,
1200 East Broad Street, West Hospital,
12th Floor, South Wing, Suite 313,
Richmond, VA 23298, USA
e-mail: rajpetersson@gmail.com

Pertinent Anatomy

A thorough understanding of the anatomy of the normal and prominent ear is essential for correct analysis prior to surgical correction of the defect. The pinna is composed of fibroelastic cartilage that is covered by thin skin. The anterior skin is quite adherent to the perichondrium, but on the posterior aspect, there is a layer of loose areolar tissue between the skin and cartilage. The pinna is defined by the contours of the lobule, the helix, the antihelix, the superior and inferior crura, the fossa triangularis, the scapha, and the helical crus (Fig. 6.1). The conchal bowl is divided into two concavities, the concha cavum inferiorly and the concha cymba superiorly. Several intrinsic and extrinsic muscles and ligaments stabilize the auricular cartilage. The intrinsic muscles are the helicis major, helicis minor, tragicus, antitragicus, transversus auriculae, and obliquus auriculae muscles; the extrinsic muscles are the anterior auricular, superior auricular, and posterior auricular muscles. Auricular blood supply is derived from branches of the external carotid artery and includes the superficial temporal, posterior auricular, and occipital arteries. The posterior auricular, external jugular, superficial temporal, and retromandibular veins provide venous drainage.

M.A. Shiffman (ed.), *Advanced Cosmetic Otoplasty*,
DOI 10.1007/978-3-642-35431-1_6, © Springer-Verlag Berlin Heidelberg 2013

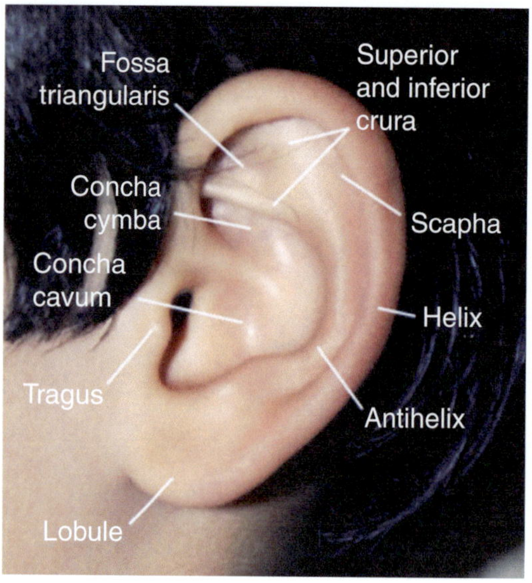

Fig. 6.1 Anatomy of the pinna

Sensory innervation is through the auriculotemporal nerve (cranial nerve V3), the great auricular nerve, and branches of cranial nerves VII (temporal and posterior auricular branches), IX, and X (Arnold's nerve).

Eighty-five percent of auricular growth is completed by age 3, and 90–95 % of adult size is achieved by age 5 [1]. Vertical length of the auricle measures approximately 5–6 cm, and the width should be approximately 55 % of the length. The long axis of the ear should be inclined about 20° posteriorly. The helical rim usually protrudes 1–2 cm from the mastoid skin, and the angle of protrusion should be between 21 and 30° [1, 3].

Timing of Repair

Prominent ears can be surgically repaired when children are aged 3–6 years, when most of the growth of the ear has been completed [2]. However, most surgeons seem to perform the surgery at about 5 or 6 years of age, with the hope of correcting the malformation prior to socialization in school in order to minimize ridicule by peers [4]. Significant psychosocial distress due to the deformity has been documented in the literature, as have improvements in many psychosocial parameters after otoplasty [5–7]. Performing otoplasty in children aged 5–8 years old does not seem to affect further growth and development of the ear [8]. In fact, Gosain et al. showed that otoplasty could be performed safely, without growth arrest or alteration, in children younger than 4 years and as young as 9 months [4, 9]. They assert that an important advantage of performing otoplasty at these younger ages is increased malleability of the auricular cartilage, allowing for the effective use of cartilage-sparing techniques and decreasing the need for cartilage-cutting techniques.

Goals of Correction

The goals of otoplasty are to restore normal anatomic features and anatomic position of the auricle in a permanent and aesthetically acceptable fashion. These were summarized by McDowell in 1968 [10], are still the guiding principles used for otoplasty today, and are as follows:

1. All trace of protrusion in the upper 1/3 of the ear must be corrected.
2. From front view, the helix of both ears should be seen beyond the antihelix.
3. The helix should have a smooth and regular line throughout.
4. The postauricular sulcus should not be markedly decreased or distorted.
5. The ear should not be placed too close to the head – posterior measurement from the outer edge of the helix to the mastoid should be 10–12 mm at the top, 16–18 mm in the middle 1/3, and 20–22 mm in the lower 1/3.
6. The position of the two ears should match fairly closely – to within 3 mm at any given point.

Treatment

Treatment of prominent ears includes nonsurgical as well as surgical methods. Surgical methods can be divided largely into two groups: cartilage-cutting and cartilage-sparing. These techniques are often utilized in combination.

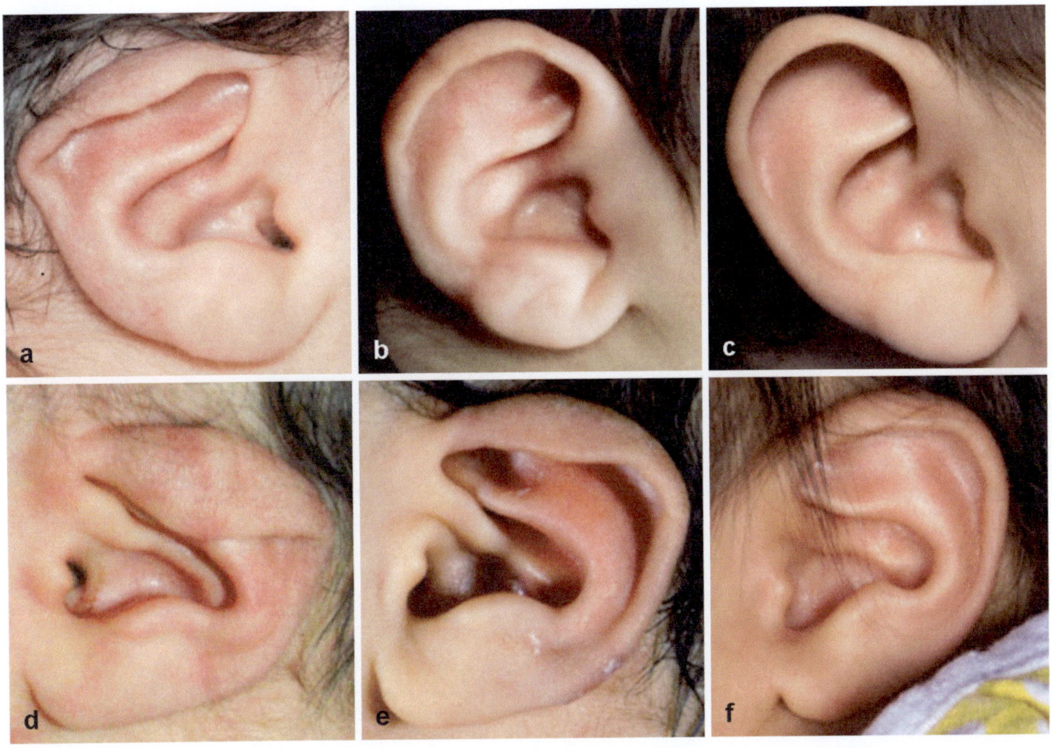

Fig. 6.2 Cup ears. The first infant (**a–c**) underwent 1.5 weeks of splinting. (**a**) Before splinting, (**b**) 2 weeks after splinting initiated, (**c**) 3 months after splinting initiated. The second infant (**d–f**) underwent 2 weeks of splinting and 2 weeks of taping. (**d**) Before splinting, (**e**) 1 week after splinting initiated, (**f**) 4 weeks after splinting initiated

Nonsurgical Correction

Several reports, mostly in the Japanese and British literature in the 1980s and 1990s, have shown that molding the deformed ear, especially if started within the first 3 days of birth, can lead to excellent correction [11–15]. Auricular molding has been reported to be a simple, effective, and inexpensive treatment for correction of congenital auricular deformities, particularly when initiated within the first 3 days of birth when the auricular cartilage is soft and lacks elasticity [11]. High maternal estrogen levels during this period cause the auricular cartilage to be highly malleable by external forces [12]. The author's own experience with these techniques has shown excellent results [16], especially for cup (Fig. 6.2) and Stahl's ear deformities (Fig. 6.3); results are variable for prominent ears, especially if a deep conchal bowl is present (Fig. 6.4). The author's preference is to fashion a splint by inserting 24-guage copper wire through a small (6- or 8-Fr) silicone feeding tube (Fig. 6.5). This is measured to fit between the helical rim and newly created antihelical fold and is then secured in place with Steri-strips® (Fig. 6.5). Dermabond® is then applied over the entire taped area to allow for waterproofing and ease of care.

In early 2012, van Wijk et al. [17] prospectively studied 209 ears in 132 babies treated with ear splinting using the commercially available Earbuddies® system. They noted fair or good results in 66.7 % of those who followed up if splinting was started before 6 weeks of age. Older babies also had longer splinting times required in addition to more variable results. It should also be noted that these techniques are best suited for reshaping the antihelical fold, but do not reliably treat a deep conchal bowl. These molding techniques are worth considering, especially in the neonatal period, as they are noninvasive, carry minimal morbidity, and surgical correction may be prevented in many cases.

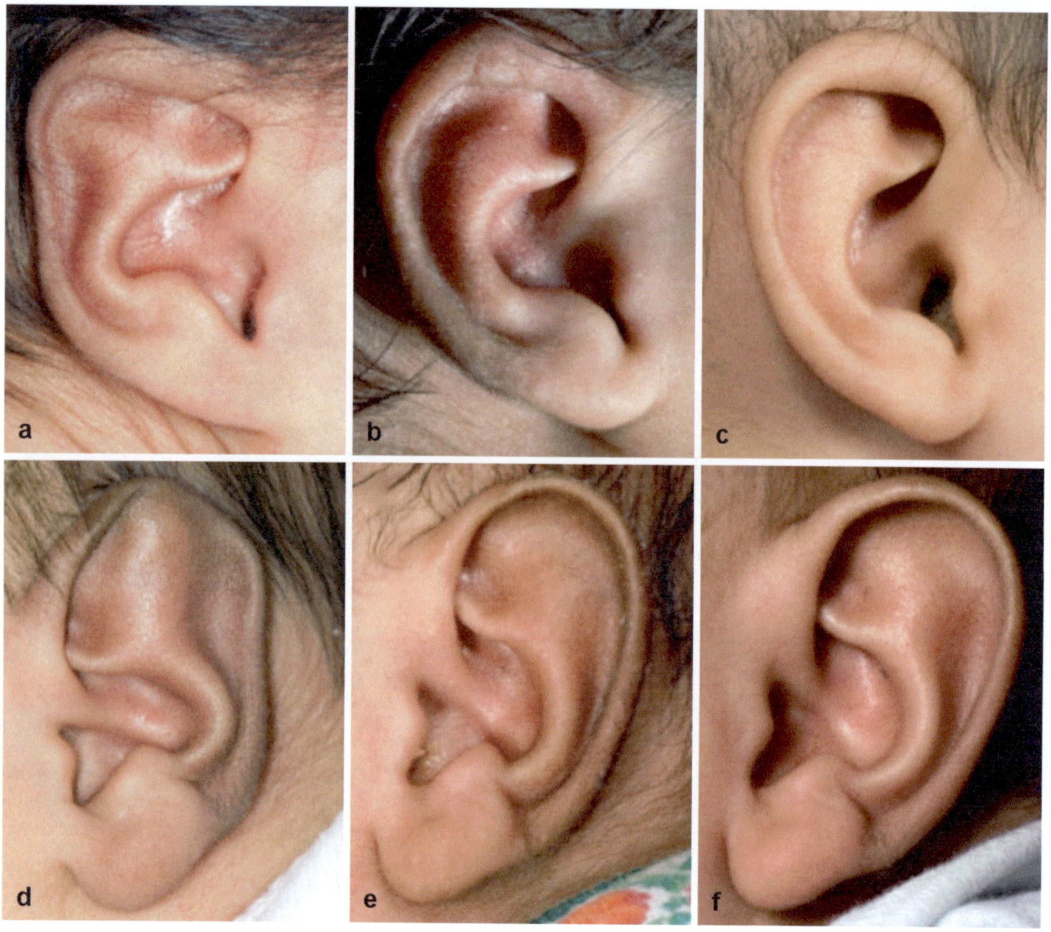

Fig. 6.3 Stahl's ears. The first infant (**a**–**c**) underwent 1 week of splinting. (**a**) Before splinting, (**b**) after 1 week of splinting, (**c**) 2 weeks after splinting initiated. The second infant (**d**–**f**) underwent 4 weeks of splinting. (**d**) Before splinting, (**e**) after 2.5 weeks of splinting, (**f**) after 4 weeks of splinting

Cartilage-Cutting Techniques

The first aesthetic otoplasties described by Ely in 1881 [18] and Luckett in 1910 [19] were examples of cartilage-cutting techniques. Luckett [19] noted the importance of recreating an underdeveloped antihelical fold in prominent ear surgery. Cartilage-cutting techniques were advanced in the 1950s and 1960s by surgeons including Becker [20], Converse [21, 22], Farrior [23], and Pitanguy [24]. These techniques are most appropriate for stiff, thick cartilage that requires disruption in its inherent elasticity to maintain results. Cartilage may be incised either partial or full thickness and either anteriorly or posteriorly. Portions of cartilage may also be excised, scored, or abraded in order to help reshape it. With any cartilage-cutting technique, there is the risk of creating visible contour irregularities and sharp edges, which may limit the aesthetic acceptability of the results.

The technique described by Converse is an example of a classic, yet complicated, cartilage-cutting technique [21, 22]. Parallel, full-thickness cartilaginous incisions are made along the conchal rim and the desired antihelical fold to form an island of cartilage, which is then tubed and secured with sutures to create the new antihelical fold. Becker's technique also involves incisions through the cartilage.

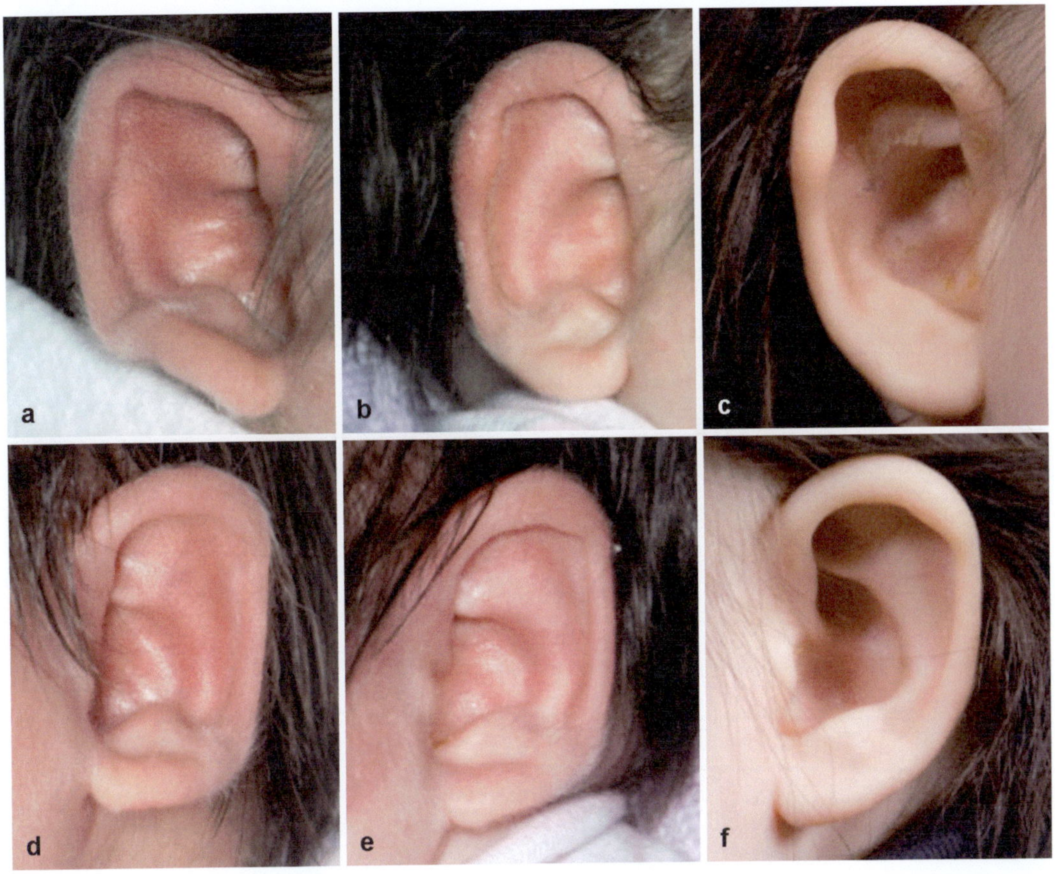

Fig. 6.4 Prominent ears. The right (**a–c**) and *left* (**d–f**) ears of one infant with prominent ears are shown after 4 weeks of splinting. (**a** and **d**) Before splinting, (**b** and **e**) after 2 weeks of splinting, (**c** and **f**) after 4 weeks of splinting. This infant is continuing with molding therapy, as full correction has not been achieved after 4 weeks, although there has been some improvement in recreating the antihelical fold

Farrior's [23] technique involves removing longitudinal wedges of cartilage at the superior crus without through-and-through cartilaginous incisions and along the entire antihelix; through-and-through incisions are then made at the borders of the antihelical fold to create an overriding island that widens from inferior to superior, giving a gentle bend to the antihelix. Pitanguy [24, 25] described a simpler technique that involves the formation of a smaller cartilage island by parallel incisions in the region of the desired antihelical fold; this island is then projected forward to create an antihelical fold by approximating the under-riding cartilage with mattress sutures. This technique effectively reconstructs the antihelix and forms a new triangular fossa.

In 2007, Werdin et al. [26] reviewed their results in 278 patients, who underwent 551 otoplasty operations from 1991 to 2006 using a modification of Pitanguy's island technique. The original technique involved a conchal-mastoid suture for conchal hyperplasia [25], which is known to risk posterior constriction of the external auditory canal. The modification used by Werdin et al. involves the resection of a rim of conchal cartilage to avoid this complication [26]. Complications were seen in 41 patients (7 %), of whom 24 (4 %) required reoperation. In 2010, Maricevich et al. [27] reviewed the experience with the island technique at the Ivo Pitanguy Clinic, where 111 patients underwent otoplasty with this technique between 1990 and 2008. These patients also underwent reconstruction of

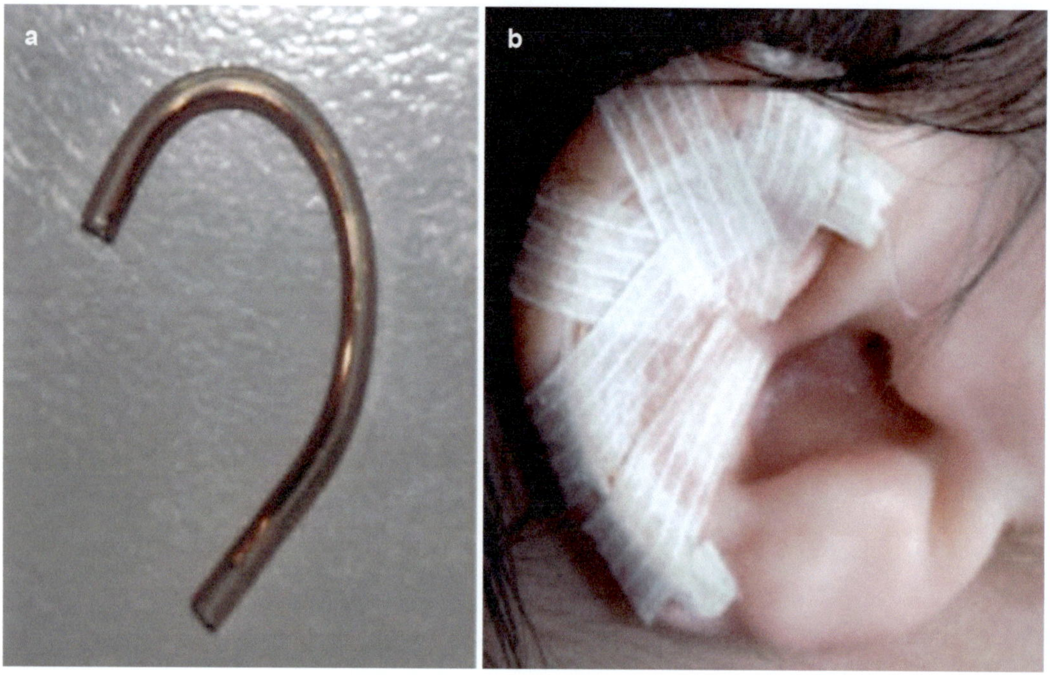

Fig. 6.5 Ear splint. (**a**) Splint made from 6 French silicone feeding tube with 24-gauge copper wire core. (**b**) Splint applied to newborn ear with Steri-Strips

the concha with conchal-mastoid sutures with or without excision of conchal cartilage as necessary. Two patients experienced early complications, which were hematoma development in one patient and wound dehiscence in another, for a rate of 1.8 %. The total late complication rate was 10.8 % and included five patients (4.5 %) whose antihelical folds appeared "operated" on, three patients (2.7 %) with asymmetry, one patient with both of the above complications (0.9 %), and three patients (2.7 %) with undercorrection. No patient showed recurrence of the defect. Overall, Pitanguy's island technique seems to have good, predictable aesthetic results in these authors' hands.

Cartilage-Sparing Techniques

Cartilage-sparing, or suture, techniques were developed to address potential contour irregularities that may develop with cartilage-cutting techniques. Suture techniques are most appropriate for thin or pliable cartilage. No contour irregularities are created, as the cartilage is not incised. However, in cases of stiffer cartilage, these techniques may not achieve adequate, long-term correction, as the elastic spring of the cartilage would remain intact. Mustardé first described the use of multiple horizontal mattress sutures to recreate the antihelical fold in 1963 [28]. In 1968, Furnas [29] introduced the use of conchal-mastoid mattress sutures to decrease the projection of a deep conchal bowl. As a pediatric otolaryngologist and facial plastic surgeon that sees only pediatric patients, the author primarily uses the following techniques.

Once the patient is prepped and draped, preoperative measurements are taken at three points: the superior pole, the middle third, and the lobule. A ruler is gently held against the scalp and measurements taken to the lateral aspect of the helical rim at each of the above points (Fig. 6.6). These measurements are recorded. The helical rim is then folded back towards the mastoid to visualize the line of the new antihelix, which is marked (Fig. 6.7). A dumbbell-shaped postauricular skin excision is centered on the postauricular

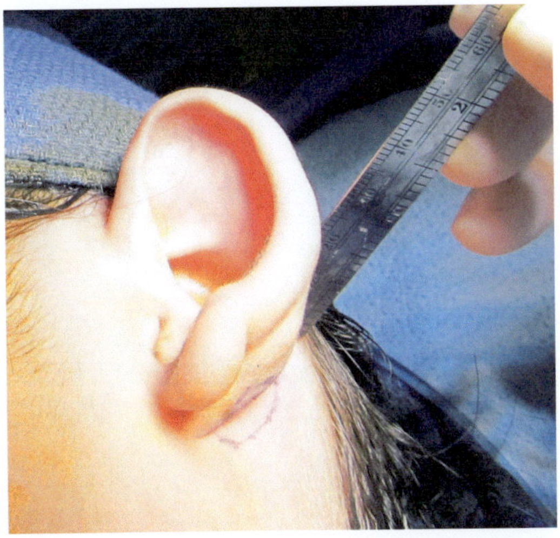

Fig. 6.6 Measurement of distance from mastoid scalp to helical rim

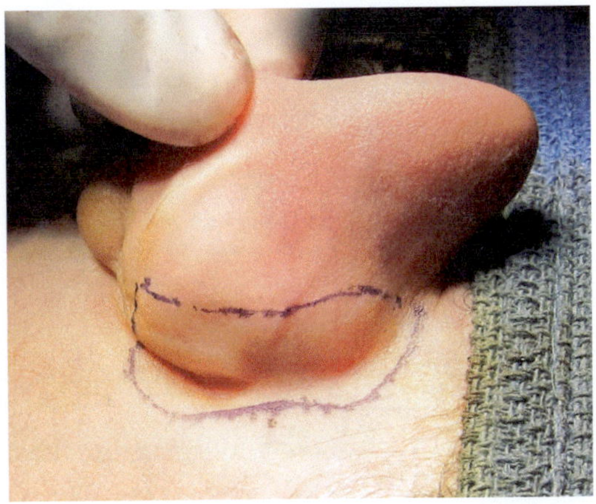

Fig. 6.8 Planned dumbbell-shaped postauricular skin excision

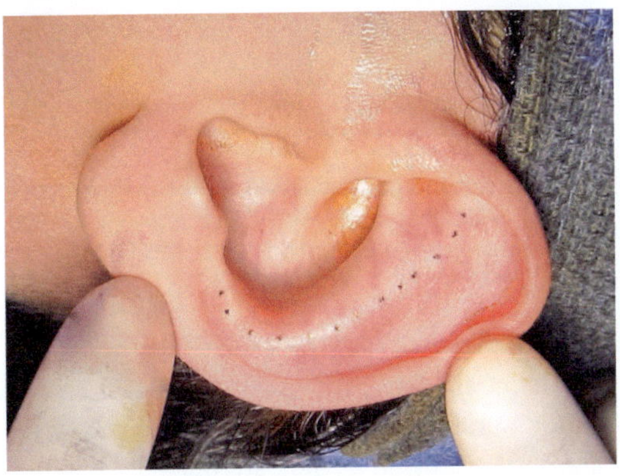

Fig. 6.7 Digital manipulation to create antihelical fold, which is marked along its apex

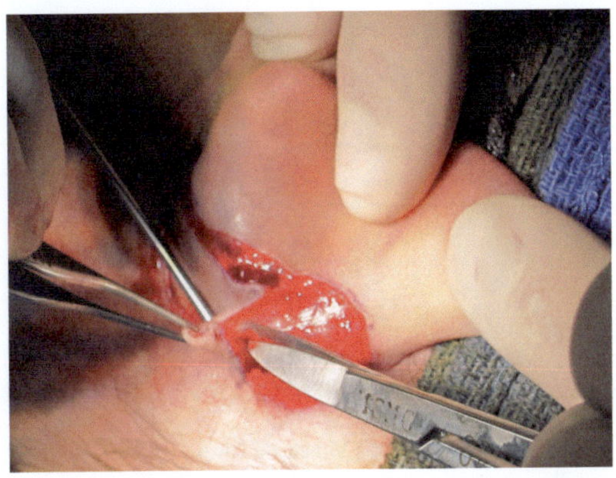

Fig. 6.9 Postauricular skin excision

sulcus (Fig. 6.8). This may also be placed entirely on the postauricular surface, which allows for ease of dissection, but the author's preference is to center it on the postauricular sulcus to better hide the incision. The purpose of the skin excision is to help support the cartilaginous reconstruction in the healing phase and should not be relied upon for enduring results, as the skin will relax over time. The skin is incised with a 15 blade, and then curved iris scissors are used to resect the skin and underlying subcutaneous tissue (Fig. 6.9).

Following this, dissection of the postauricular skin is carried to the helical rim in a subperichondrial plane, allowing for adequate exposure for placement of Mustardé-type sutures to recreate the antihelical fold. The ear is turned back to visualize the location of the markings for the antihelix. Using digital pressure, the antihelix is created, and a 27-guage free needle is placed through-and-through the newly created antihelix in the middle portion, taking care not to catch the elevated postauricular skin, which is held away from the cartilage with a retractor (Fig. 6.10). Digital pressure is removed, and the curvature of the newly created antihelical fold at the needle site is maintained and observed. If deemed acceptable, a Mustardé horizontal mattress suture is placed. Either 4-0 Mersilene® or 4-0 clear nylon suture can be used. Each bite with the needle is

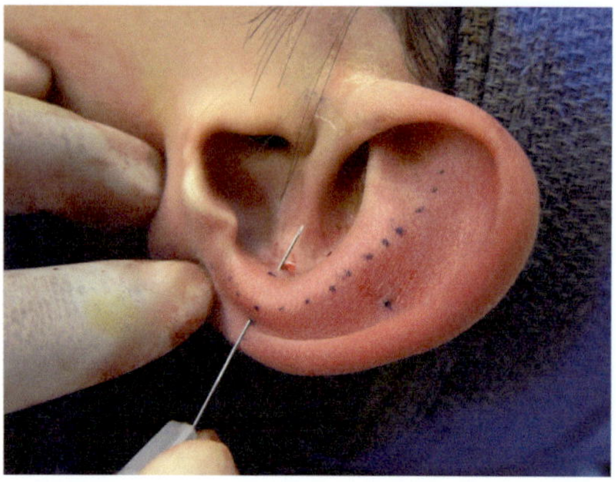

Fig. 6.10 27-gauge-free needle used to mark suture placement to create antihelical fold

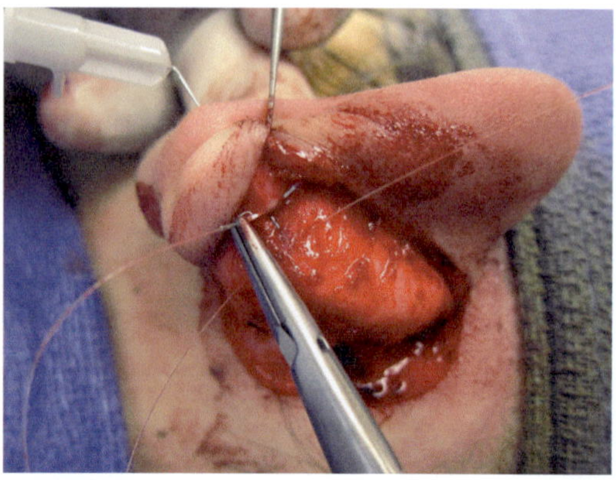

Fig. 6.11 Placement of Mustardé sutures using 27-gauge needle for guidance

placed perpendicular to the 27-guage hollow needle, and is through the cartilage, into the subcutaneous plane underlying the anterior skin, but not through the anterior skin (Fig. 6.11). A finger is placed on the anterior skin to feel for the needle, and just before fully driving the needle through posteriorly, the anterior ear is examined to ensure the needle is not visualized. The more lateral bite spans a slightly greater distance than the medial to account for the curvature of the antihelical fold. The suture is then tied down to appropriate tension to give a natural-appearing antihelical fold. Mustardé sutures are placed superior and inferior to this point as needed, following the above steps. Usually three or four sutures are needed to adequately create the antihelical fold, superior crus, and define the fossa triangularis (Fig. 6.12). The author's preference is to tie each suture down to appropriate tension as they are placed. However, all sutures can be placed and then tied down in succession.

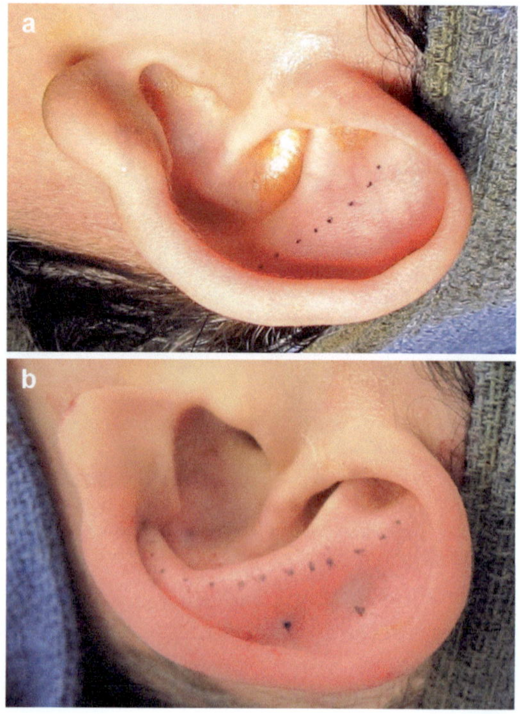

Fig. 6.12 Creation of antihelical fold. (**a**) Preoperative marking of antihelical fold with digital pressure released. (**b**) Newly created antihelical fold after Mustardé sutures placed

The conchal bowl is addressed next, if necessary, with conchal-mastoid setback sutures. Dissection is carried posteriorly to the mastoid periosteum. Typically, two horizontal mattress sutures are placed through the conchal bowl cartilage (again taking care not to penetrate the anterior skin) and mastoid periosteum. The more lateral the suture, the greater the setback. However, placing the sutures too laterally may cause narrowing of the external auditory canal, which must be avoided. In very deep conchal bowls with excess cartilage, it can be beneficial to shave or partially resect conchal bowl cartilage from the posterior aspect to ease the setback.

Once all of the cartilaginous work has been completed, and prior to skin closure, measurements are repeated. It is these measurements that are expected to be maintained long term. The skin incision is then closed using 4-0 Vicryl in a deep, inverted, interrupted manner in the subcuticular plane. Steri-strips® are then applied. Measurements are then repeated, and there may be further setback noted after skin closure, but this should be expected to decrease over time as the skin relaxes.

In 2001, Horlock et al. [30] described a postauricular fascial flap used in conjunction with the traditional Mustardé and Furnas suture otoplasty techniques. After performing a standard postauricular dumbbell skin excision, dissection is carried to the helical rim in the dermal subcutaneous tissue junction plane. That is, the subcutaneous tissue is left on the posterior aspect of the auricular cartilage. This subcutaneous tissue is then elevated from the cartilage as a separate fascial flap, and dissection carried to the mastoid. Mustardé and Furnas sutures are then placed, taking care not to catch the fascial flap. The flap is then advanced back over the sutures and secured to the posterior helical rim, and the skin closed. Complications of suture erosion and irritation from buried sutures are prevented by this technique. They did notice a recurrence rate of 8 %, which is lower than most described suture only techniques.

A study of the same technique by Schaverien et al. in 2010 [31] reviewed 57 ears in 30 patients (ages 4–14 years, mean 8.5 years) over a mean 3.9 year follow-up period. The recurrence rate was 4.5 %, and six minor complications were observed. These included wound dehiscence in one, bleeding in one, suture extrusion in one, and painful/palpable suture in three patients. Compared to previously reported recurrence rates with suture techniques alone, the recurrence rate of 4.5 % is favorable. Sinha and Richard [32] reviewed their experience with the technique in 227 patients over an 8-year period, with a recurrence rate of 3.67 %. Ten complications were observed, including suture extrusion in 6 (2.64 %), keloid formation in 3 (1.32 %), and infection and anterior skin necrosis in 1 each (0.44 %). They concluded that the postauricular fascial flap seems to prevent suture extrusion and reduces the risk of recurrence as evidenced by their low complication rate.

Although cartilage-scoring techniques are injurious to cartilage, they will be considered here with the cartilage-sparing techniques as no full-thickness cartilaginous incisions are performed. After Gibson and Davis showed the ability of injured cartilage to bend away from the side of injury in 1958 [33], Stenströem [34] described scoring of the anterior auricular cartilage to create an antihelical fold. Through a postauricular approach, he created a tunnel along the anterior aspect of the planned antihelix and then scored the anterior perichondrium and cartilage to allow it to bend posteriorly, creating an antihelical fold. Various instruments through various approaches have been used for scoring, including scalpels, rasps, abraders, diamond burr drills, Adson-Brown forceps, and hypodermic needles [35]. Scoring techniques are often combined with other approaches.

Incisionless Otoplasty and Cartilage Reshaping

The success of cartilage-sparing suturing techniques has led to the development of incisionless otoplasty, first described by Fritsch in 2004 [36] and then updated in 2009 [37]. The anterior surface of the planned antihelical fold is first scored percutaneously using a 20-gauge hypodermic needle. Three to four Mustardé-type sutures are then placed percutaneously to create an antihelical fold. For successful placement of these sutures, the needle must reenter the skin at exactly the same point from where it exited to ensure that no skin is buried subcutaneously. The needle never emerges through the anterior skin. A deep conchal bowl is addressed first by removing soft tissue between the conchal bowl and mastoid using needle-tip monopolar electrocautery through a small postauricular sulcus incision and then placing Furnas-type sutures percutaneously. It is noted that this technique is not useful for infants because their auricular cartilage is too soft, and the sutures cause accordion-like folding, rather than smooth curving.

There has been recent interest in incisionless ear reshaping using a 1,450-nm diode laser. In

2009, Holden et al. [38] performed a controlled animal study on rabbit ears in which nine right-sided rabbit ears, which have similar skin and cartilage thickness as human ears, underwent laser treatment with a 1,450-nm diode laser with cryogen skin cooling followed by splinting for 1, 3, or 4 weeks. The left ears served as controls and were splinted only. Shape change was noted in all nine laser-treated ears, with no change in the splinted controls. Reshaped ears were stiffest after 4 weeks of splinting. There was no skin injury or signs of postprocedural pain. Histologic analysis showed an expanded chondrocyte population in the laser-treated area, as well as perichondrial thickening and fibrosis of the deep dermis. These results echoed a similar rabbit ear study by Mordon et al. in 2004 [39] in which the same laser was used.

Three clinical studies by Mordon's group have since been published between 2006 and 2011 [40–42]. In all three studies, the entire helix and concha were treated with a 1,540-nm Er:glass laser with an integrated cooling device. The laser was set at 12 J/cm^3 per pulse. Seven stacked pulses (3 ms, 2 Hz-84/cm^2 cumulative fluence) were applied with a 4-mm spot size. Due to the integrated cooling device, no anesthesia was required. Immediately following treatment, a mold was made using a silicone elastomer typically used for dental impressions to stabilize the desired antihelical contour. The mold was left in place for 15 days, and the patients followed up. In the 2006 study, Trelles and Mordon performed the procedure on 12 ears in 8 patients [40]. Only one mild recurrence was noted, with a follow-up period of 6 months. In this study, 3 mm punch biopsies were performed at 1, 2, 3, and 4 weeks after the procedure. At 1 week, an inflammatory reaction was noted within the dermis. At 2 weeks, a thickening of the perichondrium and cartilage was observed. At 3 and 4 weeks, thickening was confirmed with an intact matrix, and the chondrocytes were viable and functional. The thickening appears to be responsible for the permanent shape change.

In the latter two studies, no major complications were noted, and overall stable results achieved [41, 42]. A few patients did suffer contact dermatitis from the ear molds and did not see improvement in the shape of their ears if the molds were discontinued. Advantages of this procedure are that no hypertrophic scars or keloids were observed, anesthesia was avoided, and the procedure could be completed in 15–20 min as an outpatient. However, the recurrence rate in the 2010 study was relatively higher than for other otoplasty techniques, with 3 out of 25 ears showing severe recurrence and 6 out of 25 showing moderate recurrence [41].

Combined Approaches

Many surgeons combine cartilage-cutting techniques with cartilage-sparing techniques to achieve the desired results. In 2007, Salgarello et al. [43] performed a retrospective review of such a technique, in which anterior auricular cartilage scoring with the Stenström otoabrader is combined with the placement of Mustardé-type horizontal mattress sutures through a posterior approach; if a deep conchal bowl is present, it is treated with a full-thickness conchal rim cartilage excision. No skin excision is performed. One hundred and thirty-five patients who underwent primary otoplasty between 1995 and 2005 were included in the study. No major complications were seen, and minor complications were observed in 20 ears. Aesthetic results were assessed by the surgeon, an independent plastic surgeon observer, and the patient. A four-level grading system was used: very good, good, satisfactory, and poor. Ninety-five percent of the cases received grades of very good or good, while the rest of the cases were graded satisfactory. It appears that this technique results in a high success rate with low morbidity.

Farrior's technique [23, 44, 45] is an effective approach to prominent ear surgery. The Farrior technique, which has been updated from its original description in 1959, combines elements of cartilage sculpting, suturing, and conchal setback techniques in a graduated approach that is based on anatomical demand [45]. After proper evaluation, the simplest methods are used first to achieve the desired contour. For example, a lack of an antihelical fold in a patient with thin, pliable cartilage may be amenable to treatment with mattress sutures alone. If a deep conchal bowl is the only deformity, a conchal reduction is performed with an elliptical excision of cartilage along the conchal rim, with or without conchal-mastoid sutures. Sometimes, the cartilage must be scored to break its resilient spring, and this is performed in conjunction with suturing. Farrior's description of cartilage scoring for the creation of an antihelical fold involves multiple incisions made through the cartilage along the axis of the antihelical fold placed perpendicularly to the direction of the antihelical fold. Subsequently, longitudinal, partial-thickness wedge excisions of cartilage may be made at the level of the superior crus and antihelical fold, with horizontal mattress sutures placed for reinforcement. Trimming of the cauda helicis may help reverse a protuberant lobule.

In 2007, Scharer et al. [45] published a retrospective analysis of the Farrior technique in 144 ears in 75 patients over a 15-year period. The main outcome measures of the study were satisfactory correction of the auricular deformity, incidence of postoperative complications, and degree of patient satisfaction. The most frequently used operation was a combination of conchal cartilage reduction, cartilage scoring, and mattress suturing. No major complications (large hematoma, tissue necrosis, gross deformity, and significant infection) were documented. Forty minor complications were observed in 29 patients. The most common were persistent auricular protrusion and suture extrusion. Eleven of the 75 patients underwent successful revision surgery. Patient satisfaction was assessed with a survey questionnaire consisting of ten questions, which showed overall high satisfaction. The authors conclude that the Farrior technique has been successful and reliable in their hands.

In 2009, Valente [46] reported on another concept in otoplasty in which the helix is separated from the antihelix to break the cartilaginous spring. A postauricular approach is used with a dumbbell-shaped skin excision. The posterior side of the cartilage is exposed, revealing the previously marked antihelical fold with methylene blue. The auricular cartilage is then incised with a 15 blade along the entire superior and posterior border of the antihelical fold, beginning at the fossa triangularis and extending to the tail of the helix, thus disconnecting the helix from the antihelix. The antihelix is then dissected free from the anterior skin and then shaped with horizontal mattress sutures. Because the cartilaginous spring is broken, no scoring is needed to mold the antihelical fold. The concha is then addressed if necessary. During the 10-year study period, 6 of 60 (10 %) patients experienced complications: two (3.3 %) small hematomas that did not require drainage, epidermolysis in two cases (3.3 %), hypertrophic scar in one case (1.7 %), and unnatural appearance in one case (1.7 %). There were discrete recurrences in the superior pole in six ears (10 %) requiring reoperation, and no major recurrences.

More recently in 2010, Ragab [47] described the use of a carbon dioxide (CO_2) laser to assist in reshaping the auricular cartilage into a well-defined antihelical fold. Thirty-two ears underwent surgery on patients aged 4–7 years. Average follow-up was 2.4 years, and no ears required revision surgery. A postauricular approach was used, and after a skin excision was performed on the posterior auricle, supraperichondrial dissection was carried out to the helical rim to expose the entire cartilaginous aspect. The posterior (scaphal line) and anterior (conchal line) borders of the planned antihelical fold were marked with methylene blue after needles were placed from the anterior surface through the cartilage posteriorly. The CO_2 laser controlled by a micromanipulator with a focal length of 200 mm, mounted on an operating microscope, was used to evaporate perichondrium and partial-thickness cartilage from the posterior surface between the markings of the planned antihelical fold. Defocused laser beam settings for this were 5 W, 0.5 s pulse, and 2-mm spot size. The beam was then focused to 0.8-mm spot size, 8 W, 0.5 s pulse to incise the scaphal and conchal lines. Pressure and cooling with wet gauze allowed curling of the antihelical fold and superior crus. 4-0 Vicryl sutures were then placed in a mattress fashion to stabilize the newly created antihelical fold. Advantages cited for the use of a laser in this application included the observation that laser incisions can be healed by formation of fibrosis-free young cartilage yielding permanent shape change; scalpel incision cartilaginous healing consists mostly of fibrosis.

Minimally invasive surgery is often appealing for patients, and de la Fuente and Sordo [48] reviewed their results with minimally invasive otoplasty in 2011. They reviewed 100 otoplasties between 2005 and 2009, and techniques used included conchal-mastoid sutures (in 81 % of patients), scapha reduction (76 %), antihelical folding (70 %), conchal reduction (53 %), and earlobe correction (19 %). Average follow-up was 12.4 months, and 84 % of patients were very satisfied, while 15 % were satisfied. Three patients experienced partial recurrence requiring revision, one patient experienced partial upper pole pressure necrosis from the dressing, and three experienced mild skin discoloration and epidermolysis lasting less than 10 days. Preoperative evaluation determined the needs to be addressed and included conchal cartilage hypertrophy, lack of antihelical fold, auriculocephalic angle, hypertrophic scapha, and hypertrophic lobule. They developed a specific surgical order by which to address these needs, but only operated on the relevant needs. If all of the above require surgery, scaphal reduction is addressed first via an incision placed at the most superior aspect of the anterior surface of the scapha at the junction of the helix. Subperichondrial dissection is performed, and the soft tissues are released inferiorly. This leaves a crescent-shaped segment of scaphal cartilage that extends beyond the cutaneous junction and guides the amount to be resected. The skin is then reapproximated. The hypertrophic concha is addressed next through a curved incision at the most superior aspect of the anterior concha at the border of the antihelical fold, where the incision will be camouflaged. Again, subperichondrial dissection is performed, and the cartilage incised. The ear is then set back to its desired location, causing the cartilage to overlap, which guides a crescent-shaped excision. The skin is then reapproximated. The antihelix is then address via a stab incision at the antihelical root, and a subperichondrial tunnel overlying the desired antihelical fold is made. An ophthalmic knife is then inserted and passed downwards several times to score the cartilage. That incision is then closed. A narrow 3–5 mm ellipse of skin is then removed from the postauricular sulcus, and tunnels are bluntly dissected to the mastoid periosteum at the superior, middle, and inferior aspects. Subcutaneous tissue and perichondrium that form the posterior auricle are then sutured to the mastoid periosteum through the tunnels, thus maintaining the desired position of the ear. If the lobule is hypertrophic, reduction is performed via a wedge excision and primary closure. The postauricular incision is then closed.

Thus far, only techniques that address the auricular cartilage itself for correction have been discussed. Smith and Takashima [49] postulated that a displaced insertion of the posterior auricular muscle lengthens its effective movement, thus leading to protrusion of the ear. In addition, Guyuron and DeLuca [50] demonstrated that a proximally displaced insertion of the posterior auricular muscle would lead to greater projection of the auricle. In 2007, Scuderi et al. [51] described repositioning of the posterior auricular muscle to reduce the increased cephaloauricular angle. The technique is appropriate only for cases of mild or moderate conchal projection. Essentially, the posterior auricular muscle is raised as a chondromuscular flap and then advanced and secured more peripherally, thus narrowing the cephaloauricular angle. The antihelix is addressed with cartilage scoring and suturing for mild to moderate antihelical hypoplasia, and with a cartilage-cutting island technique for severe defects. This technique was performed in 103 ears in 55 patients, with no skin necrosis or suture extrusion observed. Three ears in two patients required a further procedure to improve symmetry. Overall, the correction of the cephaloauricular angle was satisfactory, although pre- and postoperative measurements were not discussed.

There are many techniques utilized in otoplasty, all to accomplish similar goals. It appears from a review of the most current literature that most surgeons employ a combination of techniques to achieve the desired results. The training and experience of the surgeon, as well as patient factors (the particular deformity, nature of the cartilage, patient expectations), drive the choice of techniques used.

Postoperative Dressings

Various head bandages are commonly used after otoplasty, but the type and duration of these vary greatly depending on surgeon preference [52]. There have been no studies directly comparing the type of dressings used. A formal mastoid-type dressing is typically applied at the end of surgery and kept in place from 1 to 10 days, followed by various protocols for wearing an elastic headband over the ears. Some surgeons advocate wearing the headband day and night for a period of time (e.g., 2–3 weeks), followed by nighttime-only protection for another variable period of time (up to 6 months) [52]. Ramkumar et al. [52] addressed the length of time the bandage should be worn in a randomized controlled trial in children following otoplasty. Their previous protocol had been to leave the head bandage in place for 10 days postoperatively, but they noted an average of 1.5 unscheduled office visits per patient due to a slipped bandage. There previous protocol had been to leave the postoperative bandage in place for 10 days. This study randomized children undergoing anterior scoring technique otoplasty into two groups; the control group wore the head bandage for 10 days postoperatively, while the trial group wore it for 24 h postoperatively. All children wore a tubigrip headband at night for 4–6 weeks after the bandage was removed. Outcome measures (lateral ear projection, complications, unscheduled visits, and patient satisfaction) were recorded during scheduled follow-up visits at 10 days and 2 months postoperatively. There were no statistical differences in any of the outcome measures recorded, and the authors concluded it is safe to remove the head bandage after 24 h.

A few studies have questioned the need for any head bandage after otoplasty. Powell [53], using an anterior scoring technique, and Wong and Sylaidis [54], using posterior scoring and suturing techniques, showed no increased risk of hematoma formation or early recurrence in patients in whom a head bandage was not used. In fact, it has been noted that a padded head dressing may contribute to anterior skin necrosis, especially if applied incorrectly [53, 55]. The tendency for head dressings to slip or fall off often eliminates its potential utility [52, 56].

Recent studies have looked at the use of cyanoacrylate tissue glues as an alternative to the head bandage. In 2008, Shokrollahi and Tanner [57] reported on 15 patients in whom tissue glue was used over the suture line and to hold the pinna against the mastoid scalp. They noted that the glue released after approximately 3 weeks in children and that the ears did not require extra protection during this period. No complications were noted. In 2009, Bovill et al. [58] retrospectively compared the use of a conventional head dressing to Dermabond®. Twenty consecutive patients had conventional head dressings placed, and the next 17 had Dermabond® placed to seal the postauricular wound. The Dermabond® group was given an elastic headband to wear 24 h a day for the first week and then at night only for the second week. Of the head-dressing group, 30 % (12/40 ears) experienced complications, including a 10 % recurrence rate that required reoperation. They noted three patients in this group had unscheduled visit for problems with the dressing, two with suture granulomas, one with mild asymmetry, and two with formation. The Dermabond® group had a 9 % (3/33 ears) complication rate with a single recurrence, one superficial infection that responded to antibiotics, and one hypertrophic scar. No hematomas were reported in either group.

In 2010, Vetter et al. [59] described their method of applying cyanoacrylate tissue glue in a similar manner. They also place a flat piece of cotton wool padding over the ear and secured it with adhesive tape to give some compression to prevent hematoma formation. The cotton wool dressing is removed after 4–6 days, and the bonding removed after 10–14 days. They found this dressing to be convenient and comfortable for the patients and without adverse effects.

Also in 2010, Tang and Ponsky [60] described dressing three patients' ears that have undergone otoplasty with a silicone-based occlusive dressing (DiamondSeal®). After the procedure, wet cotton is placed in the external auditory canal to protect it from the silicone-based dressing; this is removed at the end. A bolster cotton piece is placed in the conchal bowl to eliminate any dead space and secured with a single dissolvable suture. The DiamondSeal®, a medical-grade silicone and a catalyst mixed into a single delivery tube, is then applied to the ear and spread evenly, and the ear is molded into the desired contour. The product is delivered as a gel that solidifies to a flexible membrane within 5–10 min. The authors leave the dressing on for 5 days, after which is easily removed by peeling. None of the three patients had any complications.

The traditional mastoid-style head dressing is bulky and difficult to keep in place, especially in the pediatric population. The above-described options seem to be an effective replacement of the traditional head dressing. At the very least, if a traditional head dressing is placed, there appears to be equal benefit to keeping the dressing in place for 24 h instead of a longer period of time.

Complications

Complications of otoplasty have been well described in the literature and can be divided into early and late categories [1, 61–63]. Early complications occur within hours to days and include hematoma, infection, and skin and cartilage necrosis. Late complications manifest themselves in weeks to months and include patient dissatisfaction, suture complications (e.g., extrusion, granuloma), recurrence or residual deformity, unacceptable scarring (e.g., keloid, hypertrophic scar), and hypoesthesia. Fortunately, overall complication rates are low, and when they do occur, tend to be minor. Devastating major complications, such as chondritis, necrosis, and large hematomas, are rarely seen today. Limandjaja [64] performed a literature review of 20 articles published between 2000 and 2007 to assess the complication rates associated with otoplasty. Though they could not directly compare the included articles, given variable reporting means, overall they noted early complication rates of 0–8.4 % and late complication rates of 0–47.3 %. However, late complication rates at the higher end of the spectrum did not necessarily correlate with reoperation rates of the same magnitude. Complications vary depending on the technique used and the experience of the surgeon.

Conclusions

Without good studies that directly compare cartilage-cutting and cartilage-sparing techniques, it is difficult to ascertain which methods are superior, and it may be that there is no one superior method. With several techniques to choose from, satisfactory and reliable results with low complication rates can be achieved, as long as the surgeon is proficient with the chosen techniques. It seems that an approach that utilizes a combination of techniques, based on careful preoperative evaluation and the anatomical needs of the patient, leads to optimal results. Techniques are constantly being refined, and large studies are important in identifying shortcomings, allowing otoplasty surgeons to make appropriate modifications. In addition, the future may hold a greater role for nonsurgical correction if effective screening programs can be implemented for early identification and treatment, especially during the immediate neonatal period.

References

1. Adamson PA, Galli SKD. Otoplasty. In: Cummings CW, editor. Otolaryngology – head and neck surgery. 4th ed. Philadelphia: Elsevier Mosby; 2005. p. 853–61.
2. Kelley P, Hollier L, Stal S. Otoplasty: evaluation, technique, and review. J Craniofac Surg. 2003;14(5): 643–53.
3. Farkas LG. Anthropometry or normal and anomalous ears. Clin Plast Surg. 1978;5(3):401–12.
4. Gosain AK, Kumar A, Huang G. Prominent ears in children younger than 4 years of age: what is the appropriate timing for otoplasty? Plast Reconstr Surg. 2004;114(5):1042–54.
5. MacGregor FC. Ear deformities: social and psychological implications. Clin Plast Surg. 1978;5(3):347–50.
6. Bradbury ET, Hewison J, Timmons MJ. The psychological and social outcome of prominent ear correction in children. Br J Plast Surg. 1992;45(2):97–100.
7. Horlock N, Vögelin E, Bradbury ET, Grobbelaar AO, Gault DT. Psychosocial outcome of patients after ear reconstruction: a retrospective study of 62 patients. Ann Plast Surg. 2005;54(5):517–24.
8. Balogh B, Millesi H. Are growth alterations a consequence of surgery for prominent ears? Plast Reconstr Surg. 1992;89(4):623–30.
9. Gosain AK, Recinos RF. Otoplasty in children less than four years old: surgical technique. J Craniofac Surg. 2002;13(4):505–9.

10. McDowell AJ. Goals in otoplasty for protruding ears. Plast Reconstr Surg. 1968;41(1):17–27.
11. Tan ST, Abramson DL, MacDonald DM, Mulliken JB. Molding therapy for infants with deformational auricular anomalies. Ann Plast Surg. 1997;38(3):263–8.
12. Matsuo K, Hirose T, Tomono T, Iwasawa M, Katohda S, Takahashi N, et al. Non-surgical correction of auricular deformities in the early neonate: a preliminary report. Plast Reconstr Surg. 1984;73(1):38–50.
13. Brown FE, Colen LB, Addante RR, Graham Jr JM. Correction of congenital auricular deformities by splinting in the neonatal period. Pediatrics. 1986;78(3): 406–11.
14. Matsuo K, Hayshi R, Kiyono M, Hirose T, Netsu Y. Nonsurgical correction of congenital auricular deformities. Clin Plast Surg. 1990;17(2):383–95.
15. Tan ST, Shibu M, Gault DT. A Splint for correction of congenital ear deformities. Br J Plast Surg. 1994;47(8): 575–8.
16. Petersson RS, Recker CA, Martin JR, Driscoll CL, Friedman O. Identification of congenital auricular deformities during newborn hearing screening allows for non-surgical correction: a Mayo Clinic pilot study. Int J Pediatr Otorhinolaryngol. 2012;76(10): 1406–12.
17. van Wijk MP, Breugem CC, Kon M. A prospective study on non-surgical correction of protruding ears: the importance of early treatment. J Plast Reconstr Aesthet Surg. 2012;65(1):54–60.
18. Ely ET. An operation for prominence of the auricles. Arch Otolaryngol. 1881;10:97–9.
19. Luckett WH. A new operation for prominent ears based on the anatomy of the deformity. Surg Gynecol Obstet. 1910;10:635–7.
20. Becker OJ. Correction of the protruding deformed ear. Br J Plast Surg. 1952;5(3):187–96.
21. Converse JM, Nigro A, Wilson FA, Johnson N. A technique for surgical correction of lop ears. Plast Reconstr Surg. 1955;15(5):411–8.
22. Converse JM, Wood-Smith D. Technical details in the surgical correction of lop ears. Plast Reconstr Surg. 1963;31:118–28.
23. Farrior RT. A method of otoplasty; normal contour of the antihelix and scaphoid fossa. AMA Arch Otolaryngol. 1959;69(4):400–8.
24. Pitanguy Y, Rebello C. Ansiform ears – correction by "island" technique. Acta Chir Plast. 1962;4:267–77.
25. Pitanguy I, Muller P, Piccolo N, Ramalho E, Solinas R. The treatment of prominent ears: a 25-year survey of the island technique. Aesthetic Plast Surg. 1987; 11(2):87–93.
26. Werdin F, Wolter M, Lampe H. Pitanguy's otoplasty: report of 551 operations. Scand J Plast Reconstr Surg Hand Surg. 2007;41(6):283–7.
27. Maricevich P, Gontijode Amorim NF, Duprat R, Freitas F, Pitanguy I. Island technique for prominent ears: an update of the Ivo Pitanguy Clinic experience. Aesthet Surg J. 2010;31(6):623–33.
28. Mustarde JC. The correction of prominent ears using simple mattress sutures. Br J Plast Surg. 1963;16:170–8.
29. Furnas DW. Correction of prominent ears by conchamastoid sutures. Plast Reconstr Surg. 1968; 42(3):189–93.
30. Horlock N, Misra A, Gault D. The postauricular fascial flap as an adjunct to Mustarde and Furnas type otoplasty. Plast Reconstr Surg. 2001;108(6): 1487–90.
31. Schaverien MV, Al-Busaidi S, Stewart KJ. Long-term results of posterior suturing with postauricular fascial flap otoplasty. J Plast Reconstr Aesthet Surg. 2010; 63(9):1447–51.
32. Sinha M, Richard B. Postauricular fascial flap and suture otoplasty: a prospective outcome study of 227 patients. J Plast Reconstr Aesthet Surg. 2012;65(3): 367–71.
33. Gibson T, Davis W. The distortion of autogenous cartilage grafts: its cause and prevention. Br J Plast Surg. 1957–1958;10:257–74.
34. Stenstroem SJ. A "natural" technique for correction of congenitally prominent ears. Plast Reconstr Surg. 1963;32:509–18.
35. Petersson RS, Friedman O. Current trends in otoplasty. Curr Opin Otolaryngol Head Neck Surg. 2008; 16(4):352–8.
36. Fritsch MH. Incisionless otoplasty. Facial Plast Surg. 2004;20(4):267–70.
37. Fritsch MH. Incisionless otoplasty. Otolaryngol Clin North Am. 2009;42(6):1199–208.
38. Holden PK, Chlebicki C, Wong BJ. Minimally invasive ear reshaping with a 1450-nm diode laser using cryogen spray cooling in New Zealand white rabbits. Arch Facial Plast Surg. 2009;11(6): 399–404.
39. Mordon S, Wang T, Fleurisse L, Creusy C. Laser cartilage reshaping in an in vitro rabbit moedl using a 1.54 micron Er:glass laser. Lasers Surg Med. 2004; 34(4):315–22.
40. Trelles MA, Mordon SR. Correction of ear malformations by laser-assisted cartilage reshaping. Lasers Surg Med. 2006;38(7):659–62.
41. Leclere FM, Petropoulos I, Mordon S. Laser-assisted cartilage reshaping (LACR) for treating ear protrusions: a clinical study in 24 patients. Aesthetic Plast Surg. 2010;34(2):141–6.
42. Leclere FMP, Trelles M, Mordon SR. Cartilage reshaping for protruding ears: a prospective long term follow-up of 32 procedures. Lasers Surg Med. 2011; 43(9):875–80.
43. Salgarello M, Gasperoni C, Montagnese A, Farallo E. Otoplasty for prominent ears: a versatile combined technique to master the shape of the ear. Otolaryngol Head Neck Surg. 2007;137(2):224–7.
44. Farrior RT. Otoplasty for children. Otolaryngol Clin North Am. 1970;3(2):365–74.
45. Scharer SA, Farrior EH, Farrior RT. Retrospective analysis of the Farrior technique for otoplasty. Arch Facial Plast Surg. 2007;9(3):167–73.
46. Valente ASC. Separating the helix from the antihelix: a new concept in prominent ear correction. Aesthet Surg J. 2009;30(2):139–53.

47. Ragab A. Carbon dioxide laser-assisted cartilage reshaping otoplasty: a new technique for prominent ears. Laryngoscope. 2010;120(7):1312–8.
48. de la Fuente A, Sordo G. Minimally invasive otoplasty: technical details and long-term results. Aesthetic Plast Surg. 2011;36(1):77–82.
49. Smith D, Takashima H. Protruding auricle: a neuromuscular sign. Lancet. 1978;1:747.
50. Guyuron B, DeLuca L. Ear projection and the posterior auricular muscle insertion. Plast Reconstr Surg. 1997;100(2):457–60.
51. Scuderi N, Tenna S, Bitonti A, Vonella M. Repositioning of posterior auricular muscle combined with conventional otoplasty: a personal technique. J Plast Reconstr Aesthet Surg. 2007;60(2): 201–4.
52. Ramkumar S, Narayanan V, Laing JH. Twenty-four hours or 10 days? A prospective randomised controlled trial in children comparing head bandages following pinnaplasty. J Plast Reconstr Aesthet Surg. 2006;59(9):969–74.
53. Powell BW. The value of head dressings in the postoperative management of the prominent ear. Br J Plast Surg. 1989;42(6):692–4.
54. Wong MC, Syladis P. Head dressing for pinnaplasty: a tradition not supported by evidence. Br J Plast Surg. 2001;54(1):81–2.
55. Patel AJ, Price RD. The use of tissue glue in prominent ear correction surgery. Aesthetic Plast Surg. 2011;35(2):245–7.
56. Jeffrey SL. Complications following correction of prominent ears: an audit review of 122 cases. Br J Plast Surg. 1999;52(7):588–90.
57. Shokrollahi K, Tanner B. "Glue ear": beginning of the end for head bandages after prominent ear correction? J Plast Reconstr Aesthet Surg. 2008; 61(9):1077.
58. Bovill ES, Boulton R, Wharton S. Use of Dermabond as a dressing for prominent ear correction: a sound alternative to head dressings. J Plast Reconstr Aesthet Surg. 2010;63(6):1065–6.
59. Vetter M, Foehn M, Wedler V. A new postoperative otoplasty dressing technique using cyanoacrylate tissue adhesives. Aesthetic Plast Surg. 2010;34(2): 212–3.
60. Tang CJ, Ponsky DC. Seal it and reveal it: postoperative otoplasty care using a silicone-based occlusive dressing. Otolaryngol Head Neck Surg. 2010;142(4): 621–3.
61. Janis JE, Rohrich RJ, Gutowski KA. Otoplasty. Plast Reconstr Surg. 2005;115(4):60e–72.
62. Adamson PA, Litner LA. Otoplasty technique. Otolaryngol Clin North Am. 2007;40(2):305–18.
63. Emery BE. Otoplasty. Facial Plast Surg Clin North Am. 2001;9(1):147–57.
64. Limandjaja GC, Breugem CC, Mink van der Molen AB, Kon M. Complications of otoplasty: a literature review. J Plast Reconstr Aesthet Surg. 2009;62(1): 19–27.

Hair Preparation in Otoplasty

7

Esta S. Bovill

Introduction

The perpetual problem of hair interference in ear and scalp surgery is a particular menace during otoplasty. In spite of traditional surgical drapes or stockinet [1], hair is easily caught in Mustarde and postauricular skin sutures, causing intraoperative aggravation and risking infection. Heden [2] first described the use of elastic bands in hair restraint, similar to the recent utilization of hemorrhoid bands during facelift procedures [3]. Long hair may be simply braided to keep the bulk out of the operative field [4], but it is the fine periauricular hair that often evades such restraint. Antibacterial gels, or prep agents, applied by hand or comb, may be used to both control and improve the sterility of hair in the immediate vicinity, but are messy and leave a sticky residue unacceptable to many patients, compounding frustration at being unable to wash the hair and contributing to sub-bandage itch. None of these techniques fully seals the operative field allowing blood to seep onto the hair-bearing scalp, which is difficult and time consuming to remove.

For use where the incisions are limited to the postauricular region, such as during otoplasty, the use of a swimming hat has been described as a quick and cost-effective solution [5]. The patient is helped to put on a latex or silicone swimming hat in the anaesthetic room. Hair is tucked into the hat behind the ears. Any area of hat that may be exposed at the edge of the drapes is prepped alongside the ears as normal. As good hair retention is inherent to the design and material of a swimming hat, ears are kept free of hair interference for the duration of the procedure, while the hair is kept completely clean from blood or prepping agent. The hat is easily removed at the end of the procedure allowing the surgeons choice of dressing to be applied. Such swimming hats are available commercially for less than $1.

The application of a swimming hat, however, is easier with awake-patient contribution and may not be appropriate for younger children. This illustrates the fact that while there is no single panacea for hair preparation in otoplasty, a solution usually exists for a particular patient and their hair type. Preoperative discussion with the patient regarding putative methods of preparation will often yield greater participation and acceptance, saving time in the operating room (Figs. 7.1 and 7.2).

E.S. Bovill, M.D., MBBS, Ph.D.
Department of Plastic and Reconstructive Surgery,
Royal Devon & Exeter Hospital,
Exeter EX2 5DW, UK
e-mail: ebovill@doctors.net.uk

M.A. Shiffman (ed.), *Advanced Cosmetic Otoplasty*,
DOI 10.1007/978-3-642-35431-1_7, © Springer-Verlag Berlin Heidelberg 2013

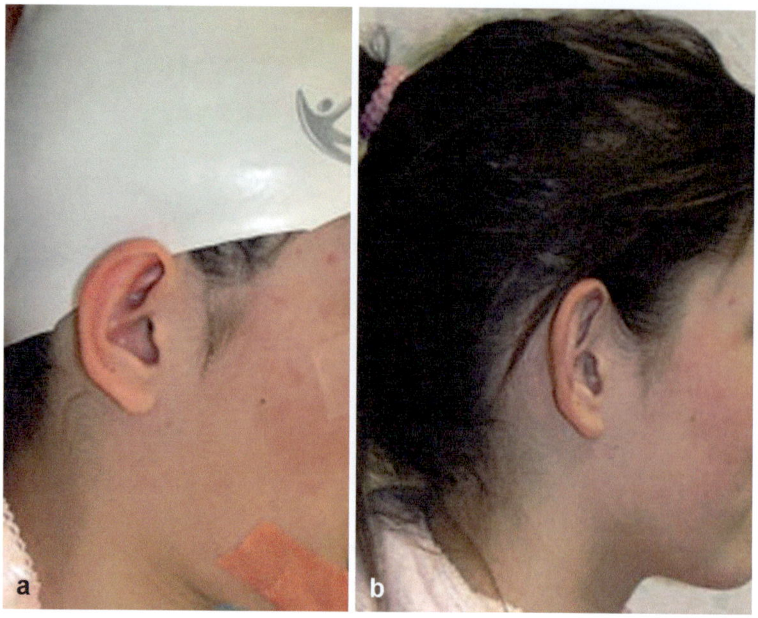

Fig. 7.1 (**a**) Preoperative appearance: routine otoplasty. (**b**) Prior to skin preparation. Hair is kept clean and free from gel, preparatory agent, and blood

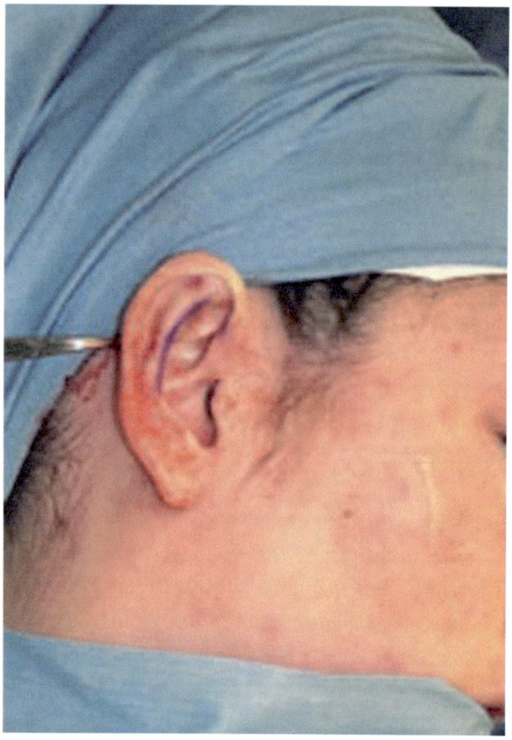

Fig. 7.2 Immediate postoperative appearance. Hair is clean, dry, and away from sutures

References

1. Burningham AR, Stucker FJ. Otoplasty technique: how I do it. Facial Plast Surg Clin North Am. 2006;14: 73–7.
2. Heden P. A new and simple way to clear the hair from operating fields in the scalp. Plast Reconstr Surg. 1992;89:144–6.
3. O'Neill JK, Stone CA. A novel method of hair control during face-lift surgery – haemorrhoid bands. Br J Plast Surg. 2005;58(5):741–2.
4. Knight RJ, Majumder S. A helpful adjunct to otoplasty surgery. Plast Reconstr Surg. 2005;116(6):1819.
5. Bovill ES, Wharton S. Not a hair out of place: a neat method of otoplasty preparation. J Plast Reconstr Aesthet Surg. 2009;62(12):e627–8.

Practical Perioperative Otoplasty Preparation

8

Richard A.J. Wain

Introduction

This chapter aims to provide practical advice on the more subtle aspects of preparing your patient for otoplasty in the perioperative setting. These tips have been used in clinical practice and provide a range of solutions to problems encountered during patient positioning, application of drapes, hair preparation, and marking. The intention is to equip you with various techniques to tackle these issues and allow you to find the methods that work best in your hands.

Positioning

Traditionally patients are positioned supine on the operating table. Varying amounts of "head-up" are used depending on surgeon preference, and it is uncommon to position patients completely flat. The use of a gel-filled head ring permits better access to the postauricular region and allows the head to be turned more easily than with a standard pillow.

R.A.J. Wain, MBChB, MRCS(Eng), MSc(Res)
Department of Plastic & Reconstructive Surgery,
Royal Preston Hospital, Lancashire Teaching
Hospitals NHS Foundation Trust,
Sharoe Green Lane, Fulwood, Preston,
Lancashire PR2 9HT, UK
e-mail: richwain@doctors.org.uk

Alternatively, the prone position has been suggested by Manushakian et al. [1]. In this method, the patient is lying face down on the operating table with a pillow supporting the patient's chest (Fig. 8.1). This method allows the operator to visualize both posterior sulci simultaneously and eliminates the need to turn the head intraoperatively. Figure 8.2 demonstrates the ease of access using this alternative method.

Draping

Following appropriate skin preparation, the standard method for draping involves a turban-style head drape held in place with towel clips (Fig. 8.3). This provides a sterile environment for the procedure and attempts to keep stray hairs from entering the operative field. A modification

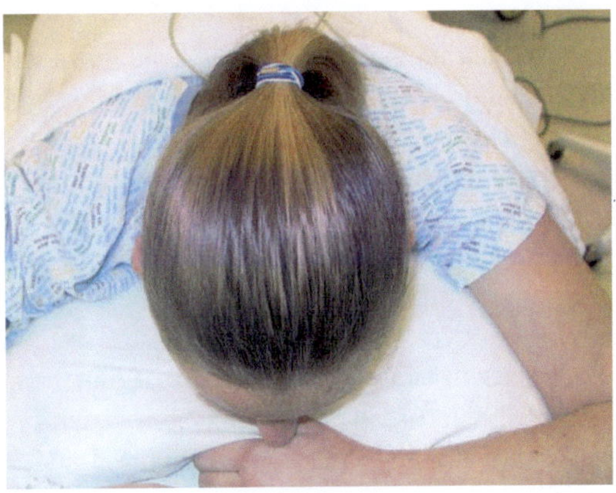

Fig. 8.1 Prone positioning of the patient prior to draping

M.A. Shiffman (ed.), *Advanced Cosmetic Otoplasty*,
DOI 10.1007/978-3-642-35431-1_8, © Springer-Verlag Berlin Heidelberg 2013

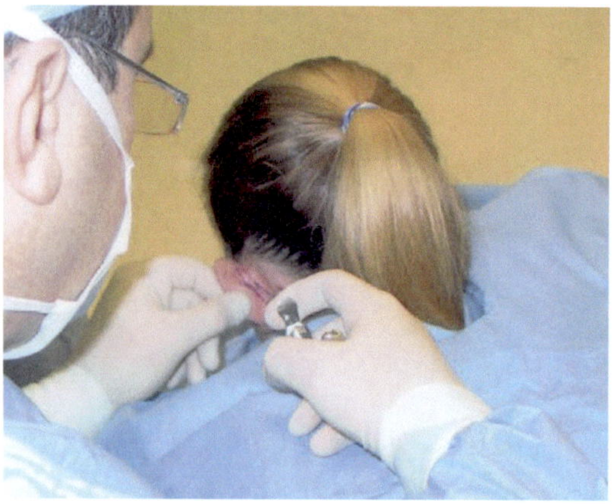

Fig. 8.2 Prone position demonstrating the ease of access

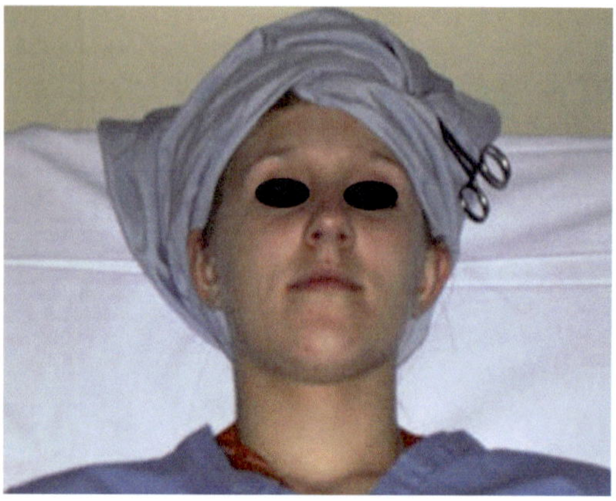

Fig. 8.3 The traditional turban-style head drape in position

of this technique has been proposed by Masud and Gilbert [2], which involves securing the drape with sterile gauze and adhesive tape in the post-auricular region (Fig. 8.4). It helps to prevent slippage during movement of the head, however, in the author's experience, is quite bulky and limits surgical access.

Drape slippage can be a problem during head movement. As well as being an inconvenience, it also can potentially lead to contamination of the surgical site. Georgeu [3] describes the use of 3½ in steri-strips (3M Healthcare, Neuss, Germany) to aid in the security of the head drape. The steri-strip positioning, above each eye and above the nose, is shown in Fig. 8.5 and is excellent at preventing slippage.

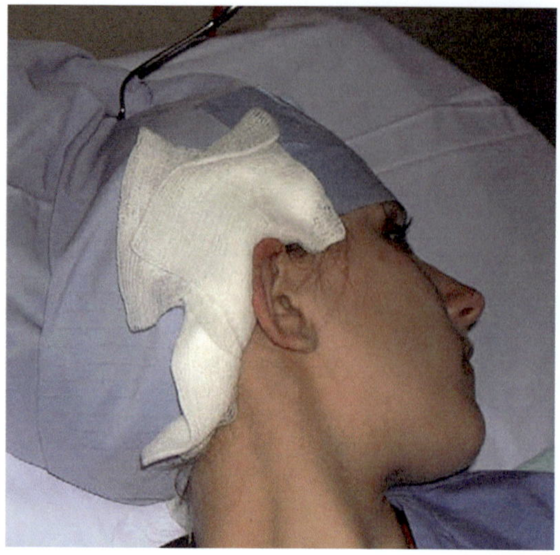

Fig. 8.4 Secure head drape using sterile gauze and adhesive tape

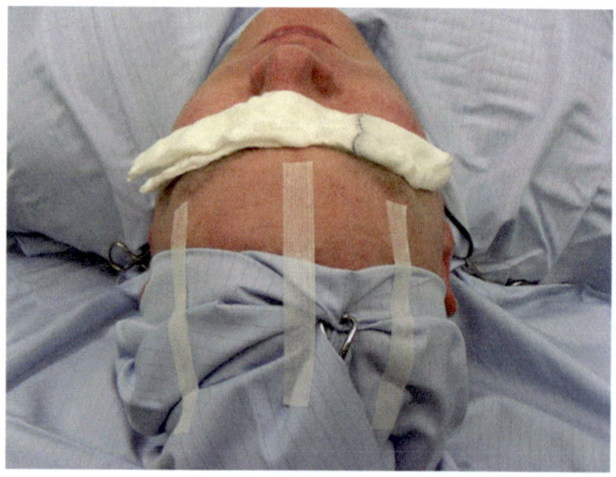

Fig. 8.5 Steri-strips in position to prevent drape slipping

Hair Preparation

One of the common obstacles in otoplasty surgery is that of stray hairs entering the surgical field. They can interfere with dissection, become entwined with sutures, and also contaminate the sterile operative area. Many techniques exist to prevent this, and several are detailed in this section.

The most traditional methods include simply wetting the hair, applying a water-based lubricant, or using surgical skin preparation solution to hold the hair in place. A straightforward alternative

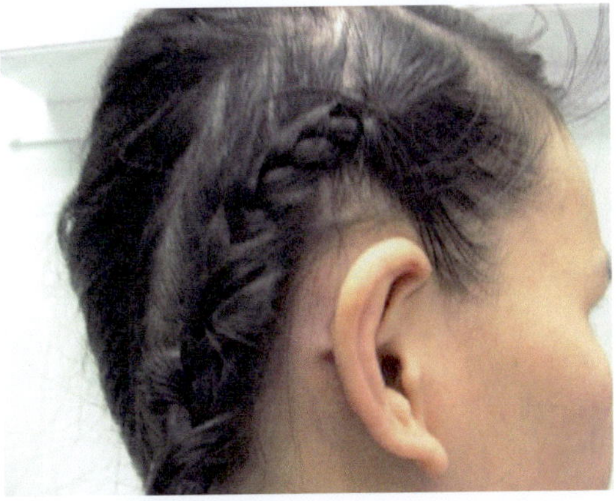

Fig. 8.6 Parallel helical plaiting of the hair

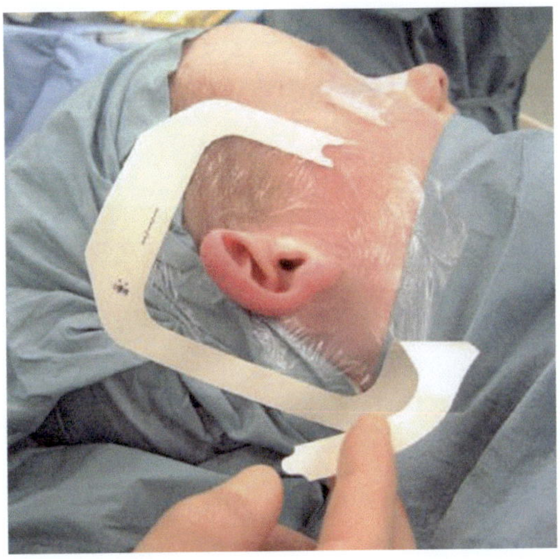

Fig. 8.7 Application of a clear adherent dressing to the pinna

employs parallel helical plaiting to prevent long hairs from obstructing the visual field (Fig. 8.6) [4]. This simple and economical technique, however, is only applicable to patients with hair of sufficient length and must be carried out prior to the patient arriving in the operating room.

Clear adhesive dressings are another option and can be applied directly to the ear to keep hairs out (Fig. 8.7) [5]. A longitudinal slit is cut into the sheet and the entire pinna passed through it. The dressing is then secured to the pre- and postauricular skin.

The use of a swimming cap has also been described to aid the surgeon in the quest for a hairless operating field [6]. The latex or silicone

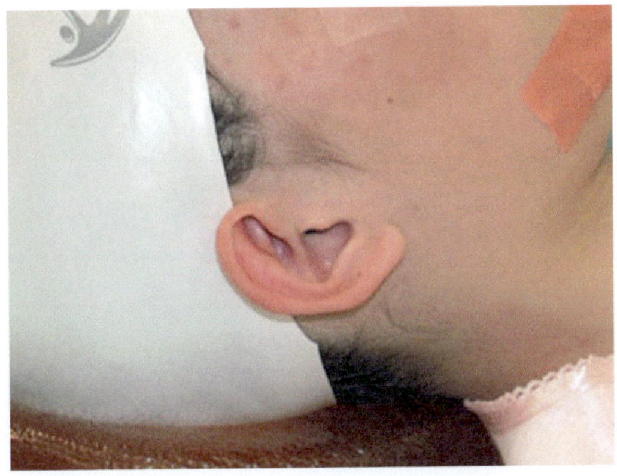

Fig. 8.8 Use of a latex swimming cap to prevent loose hair

cap is applied prior to skin preparation and stray hairs tucked beneath it (Fig. 8.8). The advantage of this system is that all of the patient's hair is protected from skin preparation agents and any blood. A potential disadvantage though is that you rely on the patient bringing the cap to hospital or the theater having an available supply.

The author's preferred technique reduces contamination and obstruction by stray hairs in the operative field while maintaining adequate access, at no added cost. Sterile paraffin gauze, such as Jelonet (Smith & Nephew UK Ltd., London), is often used in postoperative otoplasty dressings. The author utilizes the otherwise wasted protective paper sheets to create a clean and hairless surgical site [7]. A curve is cut across one of the corners of the dressing to fit the contour of the postauricular region. The protective paper sheet is removed and applied behind the ear on top of any loose hairs, paraffin side down, and slid 1–2 cm posteriorly. The remaining paraffin on the paper helps to hold it in position while preventing hairs from entering the surgical site. A sterile linen drape then is applied in a traditional turban style and secured with towel clips (Figs. 8.9 and 8.10). The shape and orientation of the cutout section of the paper can be modified to cover troublesome hairs anterior to the tragus if required. The patient now has a sterile, unobstructed operative field with a clear white background, making the procedure cleaner and wound closure less challenging. The second protective paper sheet can be used for the contralateral procedure if necessary.

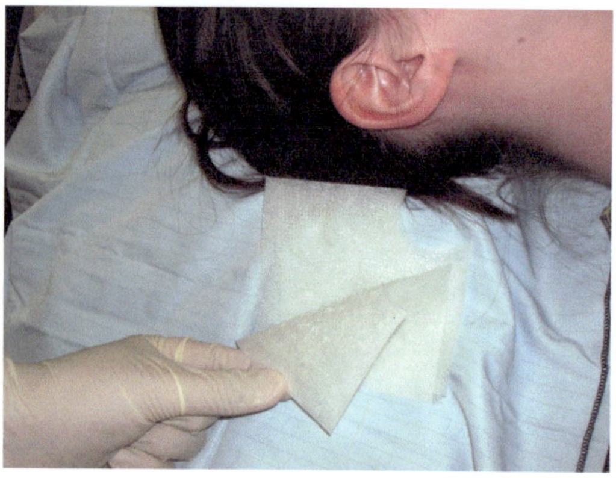

Fig. 8.9 Paraffin dressing cut to shape with protective sheet being removed

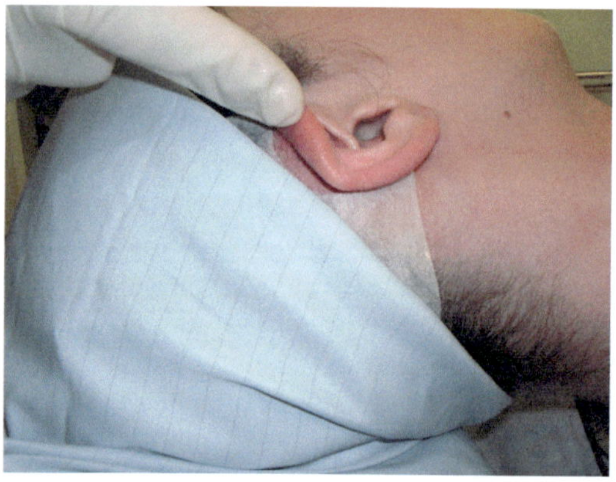

Fig. 8.10 Patient fully draped, with paper sheet in position demonstrating a clear unobstructed operative field

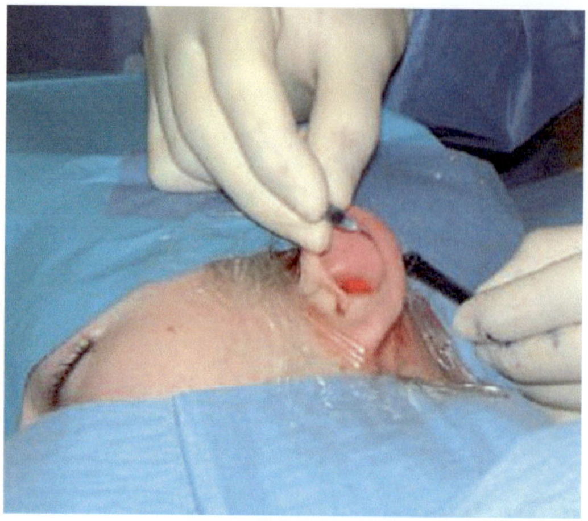

Fig. 8.11 Use of the needle sheath to apply dye when tattooing

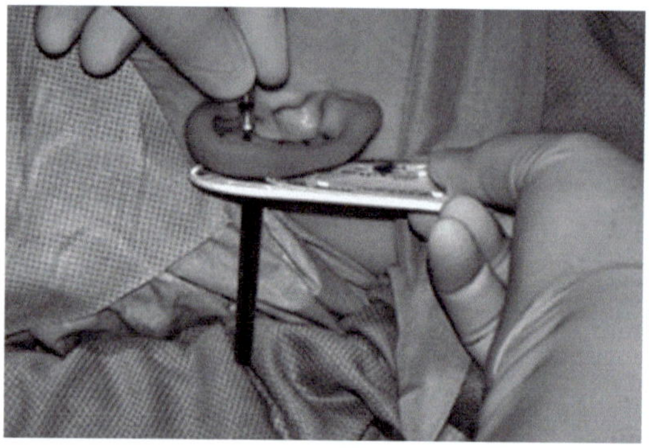

Fig. 8.12 Demonstrating the needle sheath held by the suture packet

Marking

It is common practice during otoplasty to tattoo the ear cartilage at the position of the antihelical fold to aid orientation of the correction. A 23-gauge hypodermic needle along with blue dye is the usual means of creating this tattoo. Removal of the silicone coating on the needle has been described to improve the capacity of the needle to hold the blue dye [5]. The needle is dipped in the dye, passed through the pinna at the desired point, re-dipped in the dye, and then withdrawn through the same point. Dye can be applied to the needle tip in a number of ways, but a particularly versatile method is using the needle sheath or cap filled with dye (Fig. 8.11). A potential drawback of this technique of course is the risk of needle stick injury. O'Neill et al. have proposed a safer variation on this with the use of a plastic suture packet [8]. The needle sheath is still used, but is held by the plastic suture packet, thereby reducing the risk of a needle stick injury (Fig. 8.12). The author's preferred technique is to apply dye to the needle tip using a sterile cotton bud dipped in the dye.

Conclusions

Otoplasty can be a challenging procedure, even for the most accomplished surgeons. The technical tips in this chapter aim to provide useful, practical advice on the preparation of your patient in the perioperative setting. Issues such as patient positioning, application of drapes, hair preparation, and marking techniques have been addressed. It is the author's intention to demonstrate the variety of methods available and allow the reader to choose those that will benefit their individual practice.

References

1. Manushakian HS, Wilson PA, De Souza BA, McGrouther DA. The prone position in otoplasty. Plast Reconstr Surg. 2005;115(3):963–4.
2. Masud D, Gilbert P. Secure sterile head drape for head and neck surgery. J Plast Reconstr Aesthet Surg. 2009; 62(1):143–4.
3. Georgeu GA. Stopping surgical drapes from slipping during pinnaplasty using steri-strips. Aesthetic Plast Surg. 2007;31(5):604–5.
4. Knight RJW, Majumder S. A helpful adjunct to otoplasty surgery. Plast Reconstr Surg. 2005;116(6):1819.
5. Bhatti AF, Chapman TWP, Orlando A. Practical tips for otoplasty. Plast Reconstr Surg. 2006;117(1):329–30.
6. Bovill ES, Wharton S. Not a hair out of place: a neat method of otoplasty preparation. J Plast Reconstr Aesthet Surg. 2009;62(12):e627–8.
7. Wain RAJ, Shah SHA. Practical perioperative pinnaplasty preparation. Aesthetic Plast Surg. 2011;35(2): 281–2.
8. O'Neill JK, Gnanajebamani A, Beach R, Khandwala AR. A safer method for inking the tattoo needle for pinnaplasty. Clin Otolaryngol. 2006;31(6):564–5.

Practical Tips for Otoplasty

9

Ahmad F. Bhatti and Antonio Orlando

Introduction

Otoplasty is a commonly performed operation both in adults and children by a variety of surgical specialists. There are minor technical difficulties encountered while performing this procedure which are more of a nuisance than anything else. These include intrusion of hair into the operative field, disappearance of ink marks after tattooing the cartilage, and difficulty in application of the dressing with its tendency to slip postoperatively to name the most common ones.

Although quite minor, these difficulties are frequently associated with increased operating time and may compromise the end results. The authors describe a few simple tips that have help in our practice to overcome these difficulties and have helped to improve our outcome.

A.F. Bhatti, M.D. (✉)
Department of Plastic and Reconstructive Surgery, Frenchay Hospital, Bristol, UK
e-mail: afbhatti1@yahoo.co.uk

A. Orlando, M.D.
Department of Plastic and Reconstructive Surgery, Frenchay Hospital, Bristol, UK
e-mail: antonio.orlando@nbt.nhs.uk

Tips

Local Anesthetics

Otoplasty is frequently done in adult patients under local anesthesia, and in older children it may be an option. Unbuffered lidocaine 1 % with adrenaline 1: 200,000 (pH = 6.5) is commonly employed as a local anesthetic solution. The acidic nature of local anesthetic is at least partially responsible for the stinging or burning sensation at the injection site. A reduction in the pain associated with the infiltration of lidocaine has been reported by the use of alkalinized (buffered) local anesthetic solutions [1, 2]. This effect can be very easily achieved by adding 10 % of 8.4 % sodium bicarbonate into the local anesthetic solution. This will neutralize the acidic effect, resulting in less stinging and a more comfortable experience for the patient. If more than 10 % of sodium bicarbonate is added, then the excess will precipitate and appear as a cloudy solution.

Intrusion of Hair

To address the problem of hair intrusion into the operative field, we take various preemptive steps. In patients who have long hair, the hair is twisted into a single lock, and we tie this lock on top of the head with cotton gauze (Figs. 9.1 and 9.2). Even in patients with shorter hair, a copious amount of chlorhexidine scrubbing solution is applied to the hair around both ears. This not only

M.A. Shiffman (ed.), *Advanced Cosmetic Otoplasty*,
DOI 10.1007/978-3-642-35431-1_9, © Springer-Verlag Berlin Heidelberg 2013

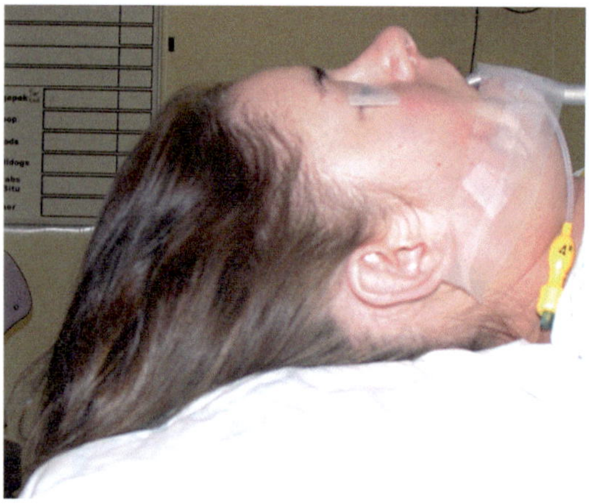

Fig. 9.1 Long hair placed together cranially

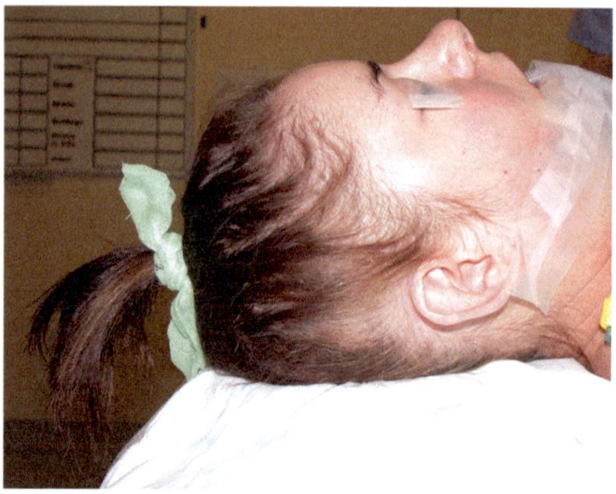

Fig. 9.2 Hair tied with cotton gauze

cleanses and decontaminates the scalp but also matts the hair, and as it dries it hardens to stick hair onto the scalp away from the surgical incision (Fig. 9.3).

Regardless of the length of hair and after the head drapes have been applied, a medium-sized clear adherent sheet dressing such as Tegaderm™ or Opsite™ is used. This adherent but transparent layer further isolates the ear from the rest of the face/scalp/neck. Cutting a longitudinal slit in the sheet or taking a 1–2-cm-wide ellipse out of the adherent dressing helps to facilitate application. The ear is passed through this fenestration, and the sticky portion of the dressings is placed over the hair (Figs. 9.4, 9.5, and 9.6). This maneuver will control even short hair on the dressing, resulting

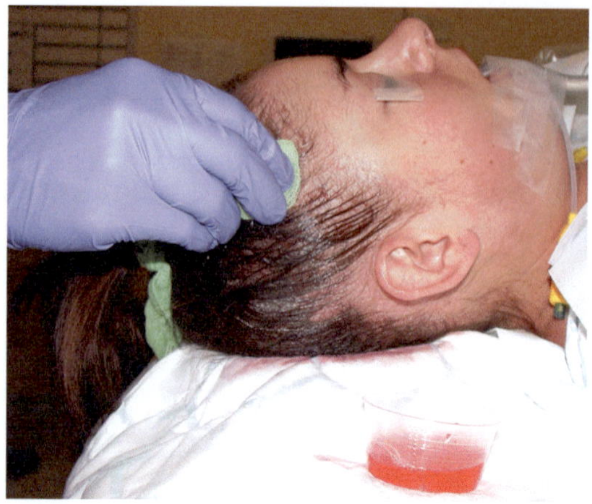

Fig. 9.3 Hair is being soaked with chlorhexidine scrubbing solution

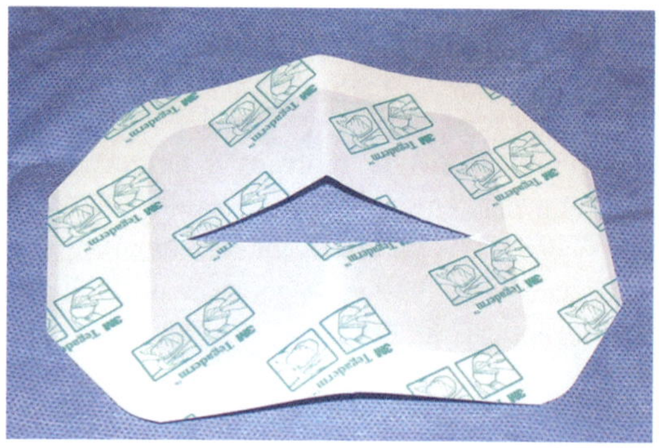

Fig. 9.4 Medium-sized Tegaderm™ with an ellipse cut out in the center

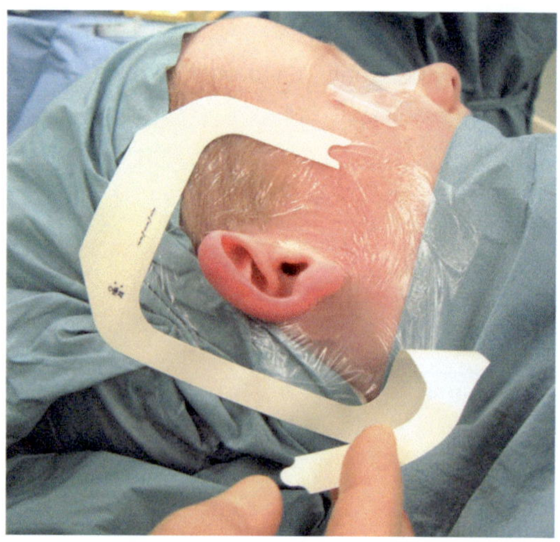

Fig. 9.5 Application of Tegaderm™ around the ear

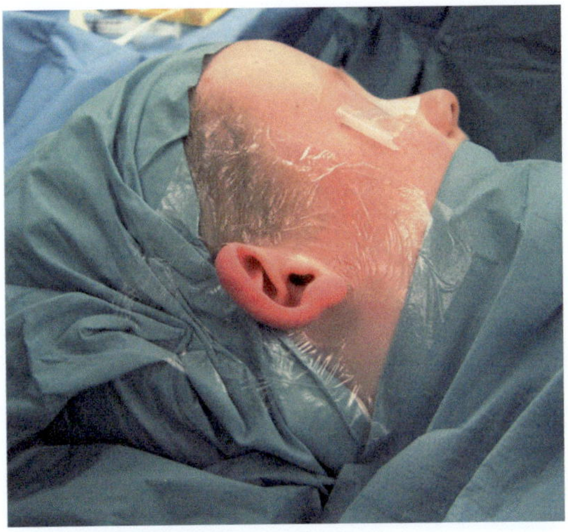

Fig. 9.6 Tegaderm™ in place

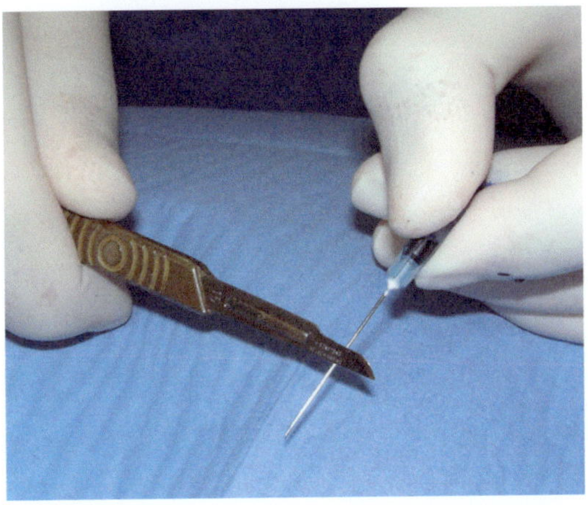

Fig. 9.7 Removing silicon coating from hypodermic needle

in no hair intruding into the operative field. Care must be taken to dry the whole of the operative field before application of the dressings, otherwise it will not stick properly.

Tattooing the Cartilage

For tattooing the cartilage, we use a hypodermic needle with its silicone surface roughened for better holding of ink. This can be achieved by running the back of a scalpel blade along its length (Fig. 9.7).

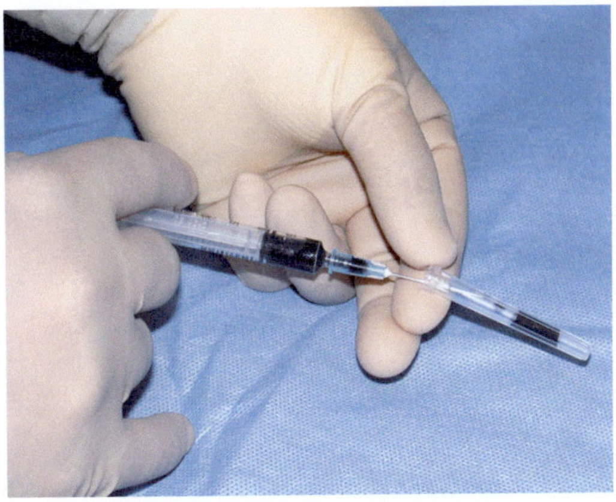

Fig. 9.8 Injecting ink into the needle sheath

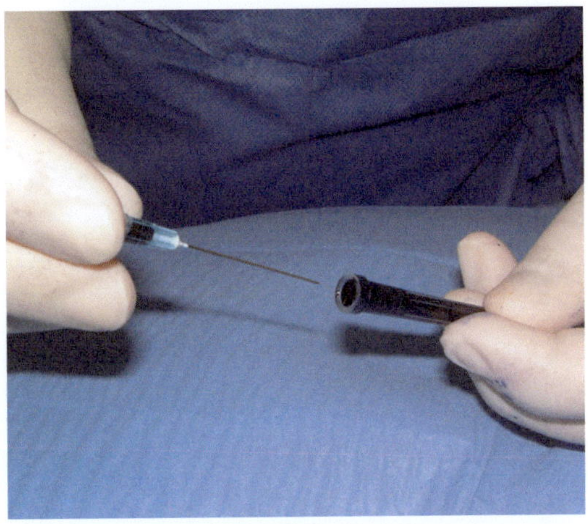

Fig. 9.9 Dipping needle into the ink container

The sheath of the needle itself can be used as an ink container. The usage of the sheath is superior to having ink in a pot. The sheath will allow ink to bath the whole length of needle as compared to only tip encounter with ink in a pot. This technique should result in more loading of ink to the surface of needle and better tattooing. The needle sheath can easily be filled by drawing ink into a 2-mL syringe and then injecting with the same needle into the sheath (Fig. 9.8).

The needle is dipped into the ink before puncture and again prior to its withdrawal through the cartilage. This has proven in our practice to be a reliable method of tattooing both sides of the cartilage (Figs. 9.9, 9.10, and 9.11). Care must be

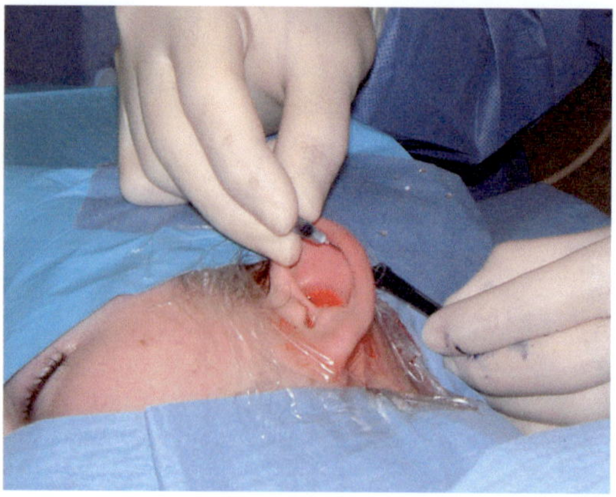

Fig. 9.10 Dipping needle into the ink container after its passage through the cartilage

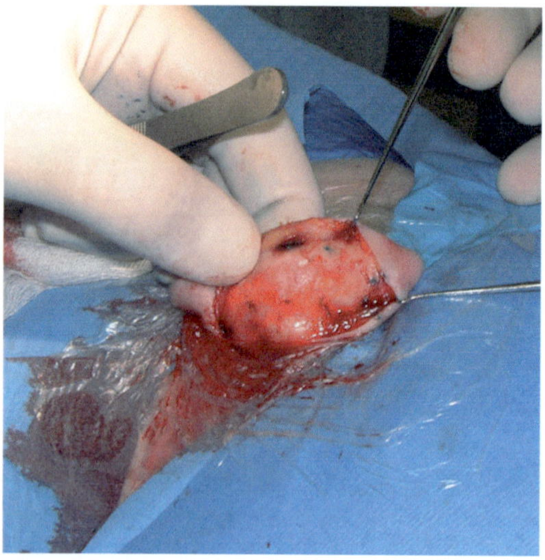

Fig. 9.11 Visible intraoperative cartilage marks

taken not to puncture your finger with the sharp needle tip before it is dipped into the sheath. Alternatively, the sheath can be held in a hemostat or forceps.

Ear Dressings

Application of dressings to the operated ear can also be challenging. A small length of a plain or proflavin-impregnated cotton is used and rolled into a 6–8 cm long strip. A small piece of Jelonet is further rolled over it to enhance its malleability

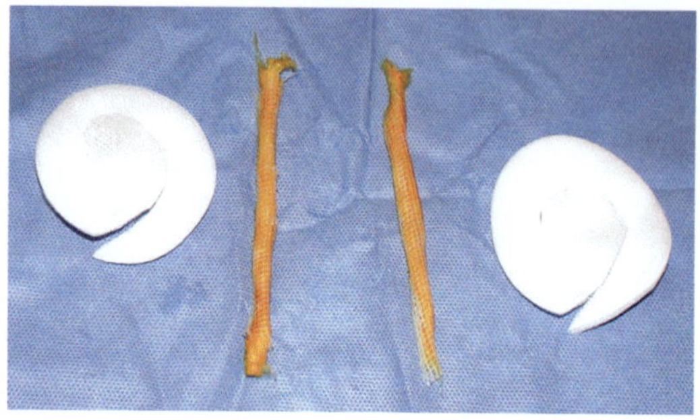

Fig. 9.12 Proflavin-soaked wool strings wrapped in Jelonet along with cutout eye pads

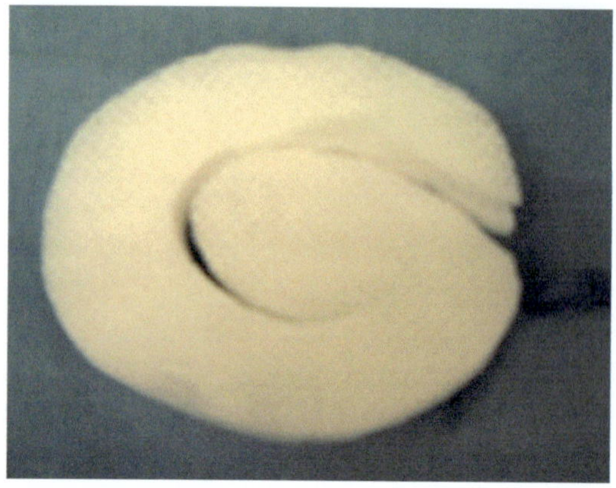

Fig. 9.13 Spiral cutting of an eye-pad dressing

and is placed from the newly formed scaphoid fossa to the concha of the ear (Figs. 9.12, 9.13, and 9.14). This placement will keep the gentle pressure over the dissected area to keep in shape and reduce any ooze from the deep surface of the ear skin.

An oval dressing pad is cut in a spiral manner and in a comma shape. An eye-pad dressing is ideal for this purpose. The central portion is applied on the conchal area, and the peripheral portion is hooked over the upper pole, and rest is placed behind the ear (Figs. 9.15 and 9.16). This maneuver is excellent for holding the dressing in position. Moreover, it provides a soft cushion to both outer and inner surfaces of the ear, dispersing any pressure and thus preventing necrosis. This can be reinforced further by placing small piece of cotton wool secured in position by a head dressing if required (Fig. 9.17).

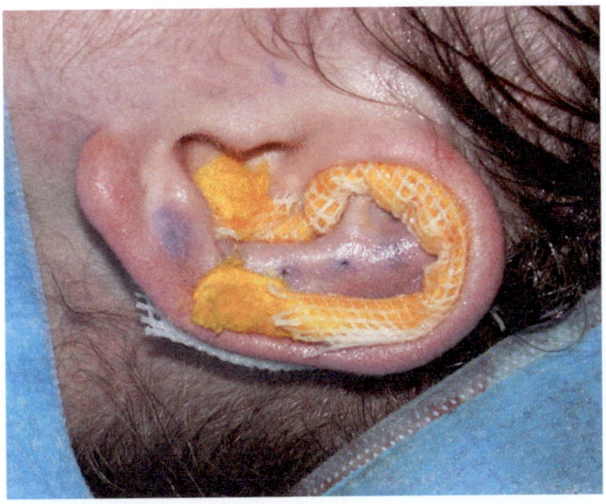

Fig. 9.14 Proflavin-impregnated wool strings wrapped in Jelonet placed at otoplasty site

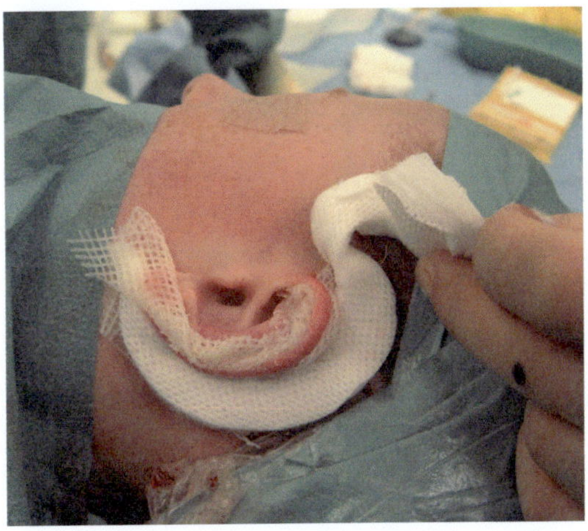

Fig. 9.15 Application of spiral dressing

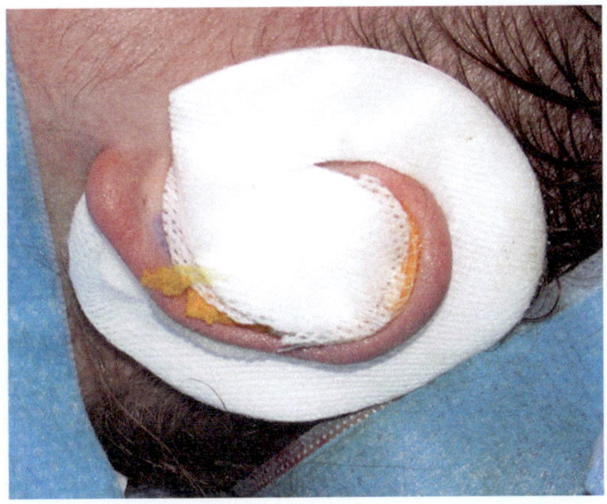

Fig. 9.16 Spiral dressing in place

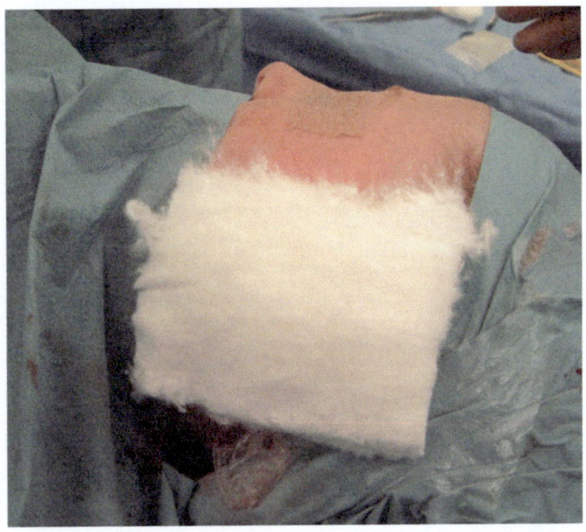

Fig. 9.17 Cotton wool in place

Application of Head Bandage

The challenge here is to apply a robust head bandage which stays in the position for a week postoperatively. To enable such a dressing, we use 4-inch-wide crepe bandage which is wrapped around the head at the position of the ears. This initially covers both eyes. It should be neither too tight nor too loose. Once the crepe bandage has been applied, the portion of the bandage covering the eyes is reflected onto the forehead and secured in the position with adhesive tape (Figs. 9.18, 9.19, and 9.20).

These simple measures have proven safe and useful adjuncts to this commonly performed procedure and reliably produce a satisfactory result.

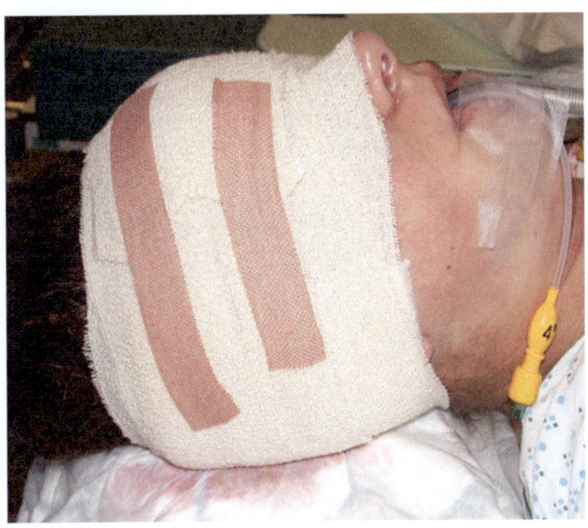

Fig. 9.18 Crepe bandage wrapped around head covering eyes

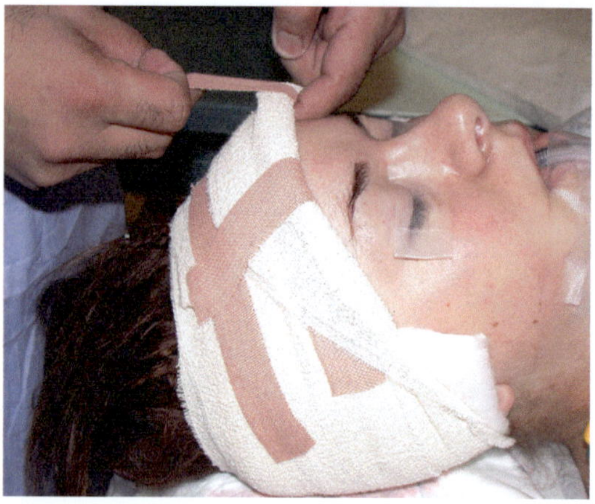

Fig. 9.19 Front portion of the bandage is reflected and secured in position by adhesive tape

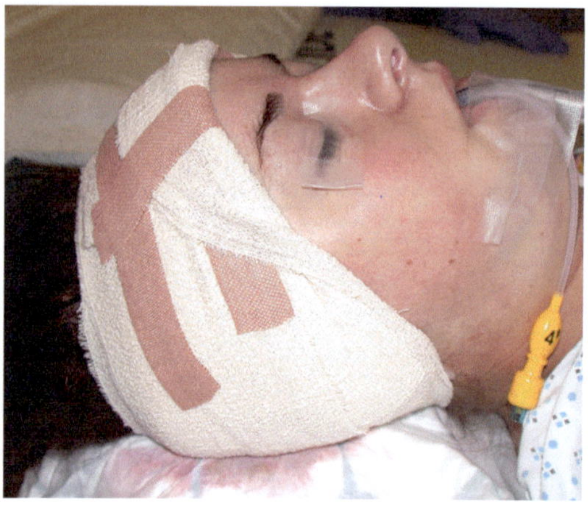

Fig. 9.20 Final appearance of head bandage

References

1. Barnett TA, Kapp DS. Reduction of pain and local complications when buffered lidocaine solution is used as a local anesthetic in conjunction with hyperthermia treatments: results of a randomized trial. Int J Radiat Oncol Biol Phys. 1992;23(3):585–91.
2. Masters JE. Randomised control trial of pH buffered lignocaine with adrenaline in outpatient operations. Br J Plast Surg. 1998;51(5):385–7.

Nuances of Otoplasty

10

Nathan T.N. Schreiber and Steven R. Mobley

Introduction

The ear is a complementary but integral part of one's appearance. Because the ear is more laterally located compared to other facial structures, it is often not the main focus when one examines the face. However, when prominent or otherwise abnormal, the ear can draw one's attention from the rest of the face, possibly resulting in social stigma or ridicule, especially in childhood. In 1881, Ely [1] performed the first truly cosmetic otoplasty on a 12-year-old boy for this very reason. Many variations of this operation have been described since, leaving today's practitioners with a number of techniques from which to choose.

In general, these techniques can be divided into two categories: cartilage cutting and cartilage shaping. Cartilage-cutting techniques involve scoring, incising, or excising cartilage to create the desired shape, while cartilage-shaping techniques involve suturing to bend cartilage into the desired shape. Cartilage-cutting techniques can result in unsightly irregularities, while cartilage-shaping techniques are at risk for suture failure and the ear springing back to its original position.

N.T.N. Schreiber, M.D. • S.R. Mobley, M.D. (✉)
Division of Otolaryngology-Head and Neck Surgery, Department of Surgery,
University of Utah School of Medicine,
50 North Medical Dr. 3C120, Salt Lake City,
UT 84132, USA
e-mail: ntschreiber@gmail.com;
mobley@mobleymd.com

The authors prefer a cartilage-shaping technique because the risk of cartilage irregularities is low, and in the case of suture failure, revision is relatively easily performed. Overall, however, excellent results can be achieved from the vast majority techniques that are available today as long as appropriate attention is given to each patient's anatomy.

Preoperative Workup

Patient Selection

As with any potential surgical candidate, a detailed history and physical exam is essential. Ear malformations may be associated with syndromes that include heart and kidney malformations or other craniofacial malformations that may complicate anesthesia, particularly airway management, and an anesthesiologist should be consulted preoperatively whenever appropriate. Although these concerns should always be kept in one's mind, it is still relatively uncommon to encounter such abnormalities in the otherwise healthy and anatomically normal appearing patient. As part of the exam, photographs should be taken for surgical planning. A series that includes full-face frontal, lateral, and posterior images as well as close-up frontal, lateral, oblique, and posterior images of each ear are helpful in the initial consultation (Fig. 10.1) [2]. These images assist in preoperative planning as well as the management of expectations and surgical goals.

M.A. Shiffman (ed.), *Advanced Cosmetic Otoplasty*,
DOI 10.1007/978-3-642-35431-1_10, © Springer-Verlag Berlin Heidelberg 2013

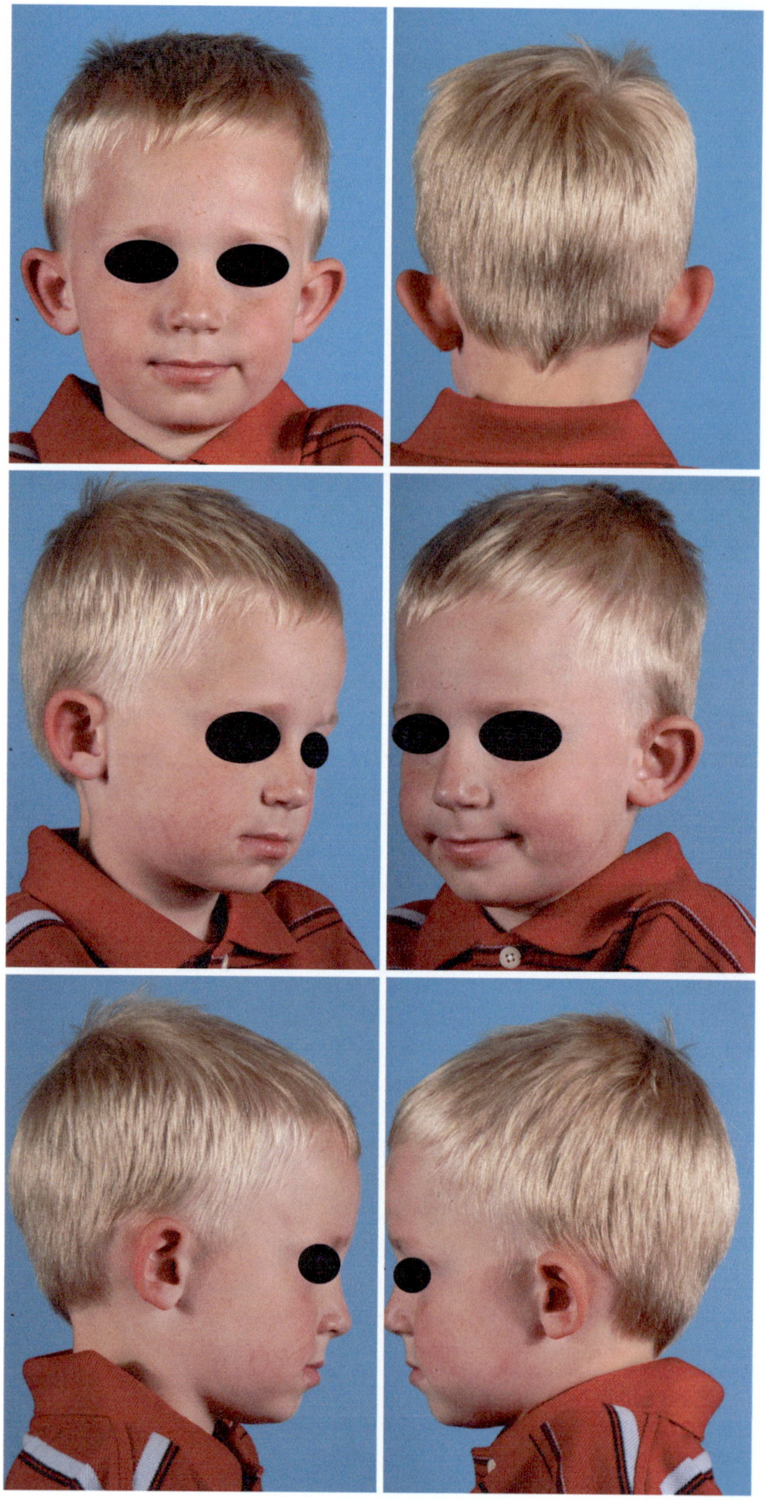

Fig. 10.1 Typical full-face images for otoplasty

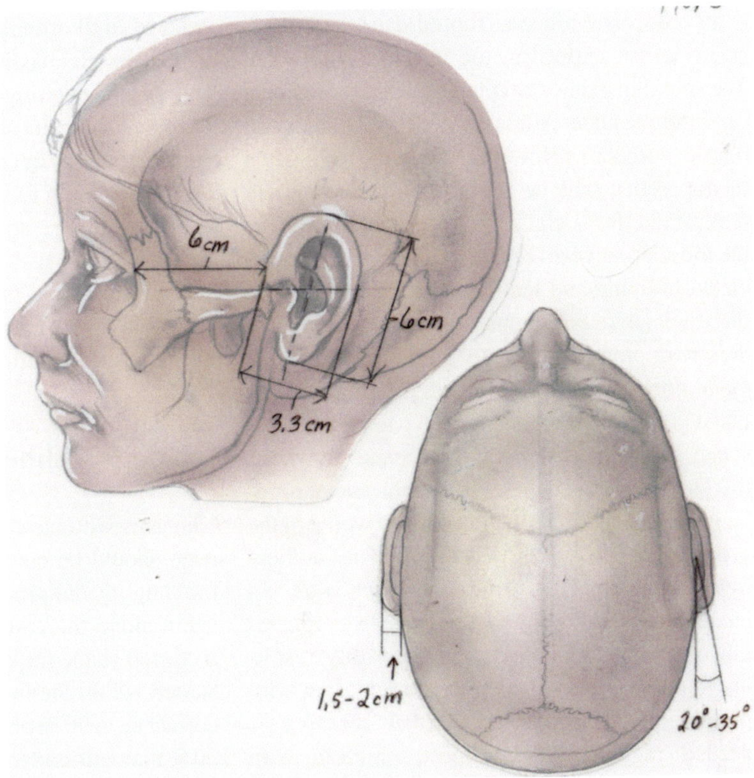

Fig. 10.2 Normal anatomic relationships of the ear (Image used with permission from [74])

Analysis of the patient's ears should be carefully documented so that any preexisting asymmetries and irregularities can be addressed. Measurements of the cephaloauricular angle, helix-to-scalp distance, as well as hypoplastic portions of the ear are often helpful in this regard. Prominent ears are often the result of a poorly formed antihelix and deep conchal bowl and have been defined alternatively as a cephaloauricular angle greater than 40° or a helix-to-scalp distance of 2 cm or greater (Fig. 10.2) [3, 4]. Regardless of published standards, patients with prominent ears will often present their own goals regarding ear appearance, especially when older. In the experience of the senior author, adult patients are much more likely to have contemplated otoplasty for many years and will often present with a well-defined idea of how close they desire their ears to be to their scalp. Individuals with longer hair, for example, may tolerate a greater degree of ear prominence compared to those with shorter hair, while men with shaved heads may request that their ears be quite close to the scalp, perhaps even closer than might be considered a cosmetic norm. As long as the request is reasonable, however, more extreme setbacks can still be accomplished with a high degree of patient satisfaction as long as goals and expectations are clear preoperatively. Younger patients, on the other hand, tend to have a much less specific idea of how close their ears should be to their scalp and an otoplasty should be performed with reasonable, standard goals in mind. One study noted a discrepancy between surgeon and patient identification of prominent ears, with surgeons labeling 10 % of patient ears as prominent but only 2 % of patients labeling their ears as prominent [5]. In other words, one may consider an ear prominent when a patient says it is. In this respect, goals regarding the ultimate appearance of one's ears are important to elicit.

Psychosocial concerns should also be acknowledged and discussed in the initial consultation. The social impact of having large protruding ears can often be underestimated by society and facial plastic surgeons. However, patients, and often their parents, will be the ones to most clearly understand this social stigma, particularly during the more cruel years of adolescence and its associated bullying and teasing. To further illustrate these social stresses, one study compared children with prominent ears to children with visible facial port-wine stains. One might initially think that a port-wine stain would prove to be a greater social handicap than prominent ears. However, this study suggested that self-esteem, social problems, and attention problems may be worse in the group with prominent ears [6]. The authors hypothesized that this difference may be due to a tendency to treat prominent ears as an exaggeration of normal rather than a true deformity, resulting in decreased social support for children with prominent ears. Although further research is needed regarding this subject, children with prominent ears may have a greater degree of psychosocial problems compared to children with other facial deformities. The potential psychosocial consequences of this condition are illustrated in heartbreaking detail by the following excerpt from a letter to the senior author written by the mother of a 9-year-old boy with prominent ears:

> …he recently had an incident on the school bus where an older boy punched him in the stomach and then mockingly asked, are you going to use your bat ears to fly away?… My son asks me on a regular basis, why people make fun of his ears?… It has gotten to the point where he is afraid to meet new people, is becoming increasingly shy, and is prone to hiding behind me or burying his face in my side when I introduce him to new people.

Stories similar to this are told by the majority of patients and families who are seen in consultation for an otoplasty and should be always be acknowledged so that appropriate family and social support can be encouraged.

Patient and family expectations regarding timing of surgery, potential complications, and ability to tolerate dressings and postoperative care should be addressed, particularly with younger patients. Traditionally, otoplasty in children is delayed until around 5–6 years of age, a time at which the ear has nearly reached its adult size and before entering grade school when teasing becomes a greater concern [7]. However, citing concerns about development of self-image with excessive family focus upon ear prominence prior to 5 years of age, some surgeons have performed otoplasty as early as 9 months without observing any disturbance in cartilage growth [8, 9]. Otoplasty much earlier than 5 years of age, however, remains controversial.

Molding Techniques

Neonates who have an auricular deformity, however, should be considered for ear molding. Ear molding techniques usually involve placing a splint along the contours of the ear to hold it in a desired shape for approximately 2–12 weeks. If started within the first week of life, molding may correct up to 90 % of auricular deformations, while 30 % may self-correct [10, 11]. Most authors advocate ear molding for neonates only. Yotsuyanagi [12, 13], however, suggested that ear molding can be performed in older children and even adults, reporting 72 % success in achieving adequate correction with a variety of auricular deformities after splinting from 2 weeks to 2 months depending on the deformity, cartilage elasticity, and response. Of these deformities, however, prominent ears were the most resistant to treatment, only responding 54 % of the time. The most significant barrier to ear molding, however, is tolerability of the splint. Younger children who are most likely to benefit from molding are less likely to tolerate prolonged, consistent use of the splint.

In 2011, however, Leclere [14] reported a 4-year experience of laser-assisted cartilage reshaping (LACR) for prominent ears. The Er:Glass laser used in this study has a wavelength of 1,540 nm, allowing penetration through the entire ear cartilage. Once treated, the cartilage is malleable and generates new cartilage that is thought to be the cause of long-term shape stability. In this study, 32 prominent ears of 17 patients with an average age of 34.5 years were treated with an Er:Glass laser, followed by placement of a silicone elastomer splint to hold the helix in the desired shape. The splint was worn at all times for 2 weeks and then only at night for an additional 4 weeks. Overall, 2 patients developed contact dermatitis thought to be related to the splint, 2 patients noticed ear asymmetry, and 1 patient rated the result as unsatisfactory but would have been willing to undergo the procedure again. This technique appears to have promise and may be more widely used in the future; however, at this time, larger studies are needed to further define indications and limitations for LACR.

Table 10.1 Goals of otoplasty [17]

1. Correct all upper third ear protrusion
2. The helix should be visible beyond the antihelix on frontal view
3. The helix should have a smooth, regular contour
4. The postauricular sulcus should not be excessively decreased or distorted
5. The helix-to-scalp distance should be: (a) 10–12 mm at the upper third (b) 16–18 mm at the middle third (c) 20–22 mm at the lower third
6. The helix-to-scalp distance should match the opposite side within 3 mm at any point

Operative Techniques

Positioning

Traditionally, the patient is placed in the supine position for otoplasty. If available, a Mayfield-type head rest can be helpful to allow easier access to the postauricular areas. Both ears should remain visible within the operative field, even if only one ear is to be operated upon so that ear-to-ear comparisons can be made during surgery. Alternatively, Manushakian et al. [15] reported performing otoplasty with the patient in the prone position, citing superior ability to compare each ear for symmetry without needing to turn the head from side to side. However, while symmetry can be appreciated from the prone position, it is clearly not the posterior view about which patients are usually concerned. Patients present to the office almost universally disturbed by how their ears look on frontal view. While operating on someone in the prone position may allow for an advantage visualizing posterior symmetry, this position makes it nearly impossible to assess the most important view to the patient, a seeming mismatch of intraoperative planning and technique with ultimate surgical goals. In addition, the prone position may expose the patient to an increased risk of serious complication, including accidental endotracheal extubation and corneal injury [16]. Although the overall risk for such complications may be low, any increased risk along these lines in an elective procedure may be unacceptable to the patient and surgeon. Regardless of positioning, symmetry is of the utmost importance, and for that reason the more challenging ear should be addressed first. It is often helpful to keep the goals of otoplasty in mind throughout surgery as a guide (Table 10.1).

Anesthesia

In general, conscious sedation with local anesthesia has become increasingly recommended in aesthetic surgery due to decreased postoperative morbidity as compared to general anesthesia. In one study of conscious sedation agents, remifentanil compared to propofol and midazolam was found to provide better perioperative pain control in patients undergoing otoplasty and blepharoplasty [18]. Another study of ambulatory surgery patients suggested significantly decreased postoperative pain and time to discharge when local anesthesia was injected intraoperatively [19]. For younger children, general anesthesia is still the safest and most practical option. For adults, these options should be discussed as a part of preoperative counseling. The senior author usually frames the discussion that general anesthesia will have a slightly higher incidence of postoperative nausea and possibly a sore throat, while conscious sedation has the advantage of a quicker wake-up and quicker discharge from the surgical facility. Overall, these are relatively minor decision points, and excellent patient experiences can usually be achieved with either general anesthesia or conscious sedation depending on each individual patient's desires and concerns. Whether conscious sedation or general anesthesia is used, local anesthesia infiltration is a must.

Local Anesthesia Injection

Many surgeons will inject standard concentrations of local anesthetic with epinephrine when performing otoplasty. The most common epinephrine concentration for this purpose is 1:100,000. One must keep in mind, however, that a hypertensive crisis may result from excessive epinephrine injection in patients who are taking vasoactive medications or who have cardiovascular disease, uncontrolled hypertension, pheochromocytoma, or hyperthyroidism [20, 21]. In patients with severe cardiovascular disease, some advocate maximum epinephrine doses of 0.04 mg (4 mL of anesthetic with 1:100,000 epinephrine) that can be administered up to every 30 min [22]. The majority of patients selected for elective otoplasty are in general healthy and without significant medical comorbidities. In our experience with such patients, epinephrine concentrations of 1:50,000 can be injected along the anterior and posterior ear without cardiovascular or ischemic complication. Under general anesthesia, 2–3 mL of a custom mixture of 0.25 % bupivacaine with 1:50,000 epinephrine will be injected along both sides of each ear. When using conscious sedation, a custom mixture of 1 % lidocaine with 0.25 % bupivacaine and 1:50,000 epinephrine will be injected. This dilution can be attained by combining 5 mL of 2 % lidocaine with 5 mL of 0.5 % bupivacaine and 0.2 mL of 1:1,000 epinephrine.

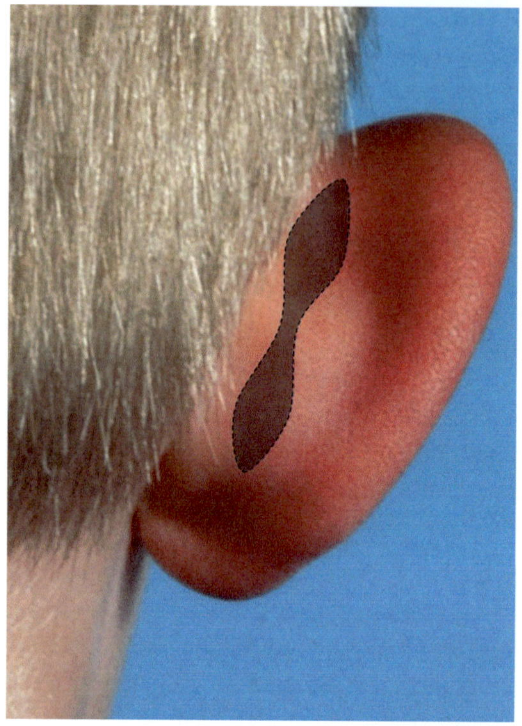

Fig. 10.3 Traditional dumbbell-shaped skin excision

Incision

Most otoplasty techniques involve a postauricular incision and skin excision in the shape of a dumbbell (Fig. 10.3). A skin excision of this shape will help to avoid creating a telephone ear deformity in which the upper and lower thirds of the ear are not adequately corrected and remain excessively prominent in the shape of a traditional telephone (Fig. 10.4). Some surgeons, on the other hand, advocate a simple postauricular skin incision without skin excision [23, 24]. In either case, the incision should be designed based upon the amount of correction that is needed as well as cartilage access. For example, the incision may be extended

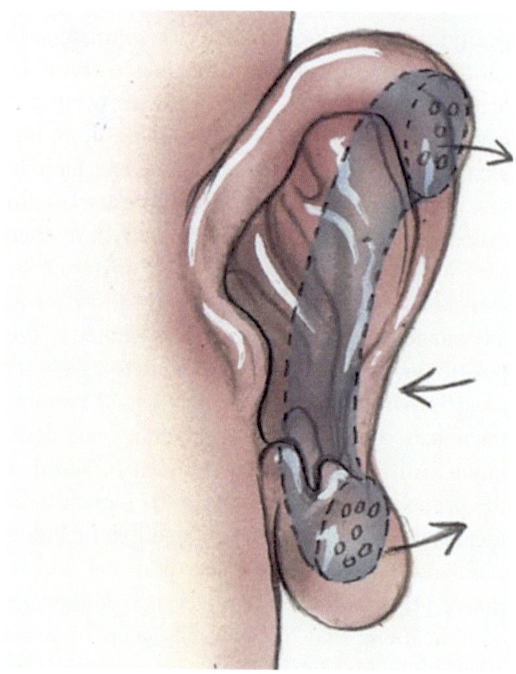

Fig. 10.4 Telephone ear (Image used with permission from [74])

superoanteriorly to the helical root and inferiorly to the lobule and should be used to access the planned antihelix and conchal cartilage.

Alternatively, some surgeons who prefer to recreate an antihelix by scoring the anterior cartilage surface advocate an anterior skin incision [25]. An anterior incision can allow easier access to the anterior surface of the cartilage, but does create a visible scar. Others have attempted to reduce incision size as much as possible to minimize risk of scar and keloid formation. One such technique, endoscopic-assisted otoplasty, trades a larger postauricular incision for a 2-cm temporal scalp incision for placement of an endoscope and a postauricular stab incision for placement of instruments [26]. Importantly, endoscopic-assisted otoplasty is not recommended for ears in which the lobule requires reduction independent to that of the helix or prominence is the result of a deep conchal bowl only. An additional technique called incisionless otoplasty avoids a traditional incision through percutaneous suture placement [27].

Conchal Bowl

Conchal setback involves securing the conchal cartilage closer to the mastoid periosteum and can be performed in either a cartilage-cutting or cartilage-shaping manner. Cartilage-shaping techniques will work for the majority of ears. Particularly deep conchal bowls or stiff cartilage, however, may be easier to address with a cartilage-cutting technique.

Cartilage-Cutting Techniques for the Conchal Bowl

The first cosmetic otoplasty as described by Ely involved a simple excision of skin and conchal cartilage [1]. In descriptions of their modified techniques, Converse and Farrior similarly excised strips of conchal cartilage, resuspending the cut edge of cartilage to the mastoid periosteum to decrease ear prominence [28, 29]. This technique was the preeminent practice of the early twentieth century and was noted to be long lasting but carried with it the risk of creating a noticeable cartilage irregularity.

Cartilage-Shaping Techniques for the Conchal Bowl

In 1968, Furnas [30] described placing three permanent sutures from the conchal cartilage to the mastoid periosteum to correct the excessively deep conchal bowl without incising the cartilage. This technique had been described previously, but with frequent deformity recurrence. Furnas achieved longer lasting results by emphasizing the importance of sutures penetrating entirely through the conchal cartilage as well as the mastoid periosteum. Ideal suture placement in this technique is identified prior to making any incisions by using a cotton-tipped applicator to press the conchal cartilage against the mastoid and marking the most aesthetically pleasing locations. Placing sutures too far posteriorly at the conchal cartilage or too far anteriorly at the mastoid periosteum can rotate the conchal bowl anteriorly, narrowing the entrance to the external auditory canal. It is recommended that one removes a disk of soft tissue above the mastoid periosteum to allow for adequate ear medialization (Fig. 10.5).

Fritsch [27] described incisionless otoplasty in 1992, in which he reduced conchal bowl prominence through a small incision up to a few millimeters in length directly in the postauricular sulcus. Electrocautery is used to ablate soft tissue above the mastoid periosteum, and a suture needle is passed subcutaneously through a portion of distal conchal bowl cartilage until it passes through the skin posteriorly. The suture needle is then passed back through the same opening through which it had just passed, through an adjacent portion of distal conchal bowl cartilage, and out through the small postauricular incision. The needle is then passed through mastoid periosteum and tied in place to achieve the desired correction.

In 2001, Horlock [31] described a modification of the conchal setback that involves creating a posteriorly based fascial flap from tissue that is initially left along the posterior surface of the auricular cartilage. This flap is elevated off of the mastoid to create adequate space for conchal medialization and attached above the newly created antihelix to provide additional coverage for the permanent sutures in this location. This modification is intended to provide additional

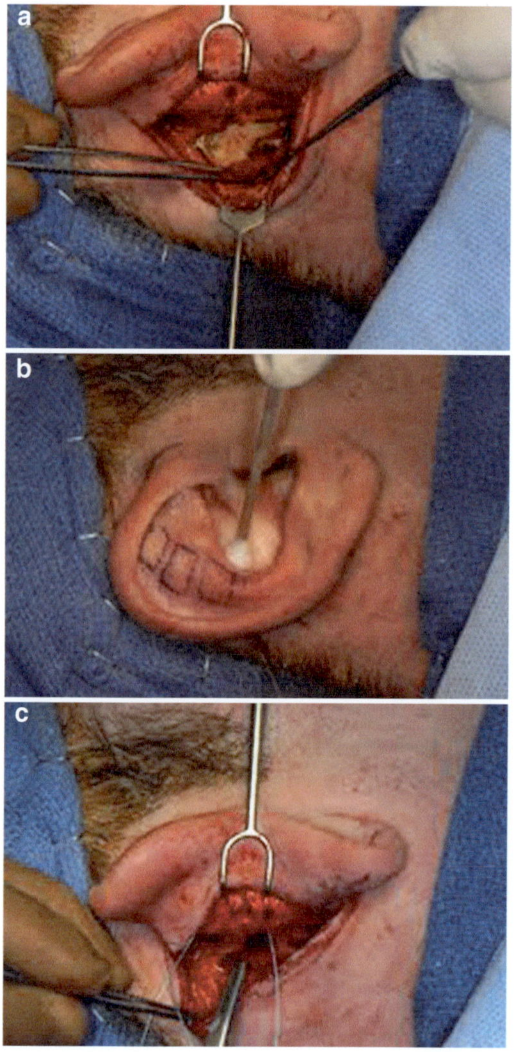

Fig. 10.5 Steps of conchal setback. Removing disk of soft tissue behind conchal cartilage (**a**), identifying ideal suture placement at posterior concha (**b**), and placing conchal setback suture (**c**)

stability and reduce postoperative ear lateralization as well as suture extrusion and discomfort.

Antihelix

On average, an unfolded antihelix accounts for 73 % of ear prominence [5]. For this reason, recreation of the antihelical fold is perhaps the most important single factor in otoplasty and may be performed without a conchal setback. The antihelix can also be recreated with either a cartilage-cutting or cartilage-shaping technique. Again, cartilage-shaping techniques will work for most ears, but cartilage-cutting techniques may be better suited for very stiff cartilage.

Cartilage-Cutting Techniques for the Antihelix

In 1910, Luckett [32] described a transcartilaginous incision at the antihelix in order to create a fold. This technique has also been described with excision of a cartilage strip [17, 33]. The resulting antihelix, however, may appear sharp and unnatural. Converse attempted to improve the appearance of the new antihelix by folding the cartilage upon itself after performing the transcartilaginous incision [28]. Other surgeons recognizing a persistent irregular appearance then began partial thickness cartilage incision or excision along the posterior surface. Farrior [29] excised a series of partial thickness cartilage wedges posteriorly at the planned antihelix and then made two transcartilaginous incisions at either side of the planned antihelix, allowing this strip of cartilage to be positioned anteriorly and curved slightly in a more natural shape. One such method involves using monopolar electrocautery in "cut" mode to create a "Y"-shaped partial thickness trough along the antihelix and superior and inferior crura after being marked with methylene blue [34]. This trough weakens the cartilage, allowing easier creation of an antihelix with horizontal mattress sutures. A similar technique of cartilage ablation to create troughs using the CO_2 laser was described by Ragab in 2010 [35], with the idea that cartilage remodeling may be induced to create a more stable cartilage shape.

Alternatively, some surgeons prefer to score the antihelical cartilage along its anterior surface, making use of cartilage's tendency to bend aware from a scored surface [36]. From a postauricular approach, Chongchet [37] described a transcartilaginous incision between the helix and antihelix to allow anterior cartilage access. Stenström and Heftner [38] described access to the antihelix from a postauricular incision, dissecting the entire auricular cartilage from the overlying skin to score the anterior cartilage surface. In variations of these techniques, the anterior cartilage surface is weakened with partial thickness incisions or scoring [23, 39]. These techniques, however, involve a greater degree of skin undermining and potentially a greater risk of hematoma if careful attention is not given to hemostasis or dressing application intraoperatively.

The anterior cartilage surface can be accessed from an anterior auricular incision along the posterior border of the conchal cartilage as well. From this incision, the anterior cartilage surface can be scored, abraded, or accessed endoscopically for greater scoring precision [25]. An anterior incision allows for decreased skin undermining, but does create a scar in a visible location.

An alternative technique described by Fritsch in 1992 [27] addresses both of these concerns. This technique, incisionless otoplasty, involves percutaneous scoring of the anterior cartilage along the planned antihelix with a 20-gauge phlebotomy needle followed by percutaneous placement of permanent horizontal mattress sutures.

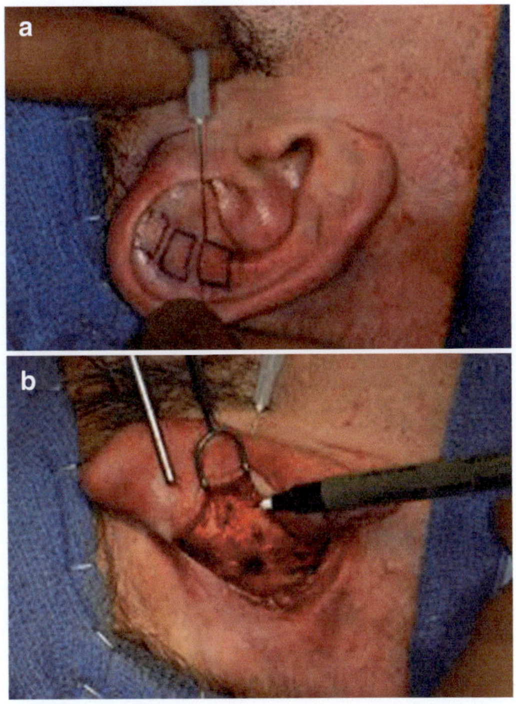

Fig. 10.6 Planning horizontal mattress sutures for antihelix using a 30 gauge needle to enter the cartilage through the skin at the anterior surface marking (**a**) and marking the posterior surface of the cartilage at the needle's exit (**b**)

Cartilage-Shaping Techniques for the Antihelix

In 1963, Mustarde [40] described placing a series of permanent horizontal mattress sutures through a postauricular incision without incising the cartilage to recreate the antihelix.

Some have noted that it can be difficult to place these sutures exactly from the posterior ear and have advocated the use of transcutaneous silk sutures placed intraoperatively as a guide for permanent suture placement [41]. In either case, it is often helpful to manually bend the antihelix to the desired natural shape and place markings where horizontal mattress sutures will be most effective (Fig. 10.6). Most surgeons will use 4-0 polyester sutures in this technique. Horlock's [31] postauricular fascial flap is designed to provide additional coverage of these permanent sutures and reduce the risk of suture extrusion and discomfort.

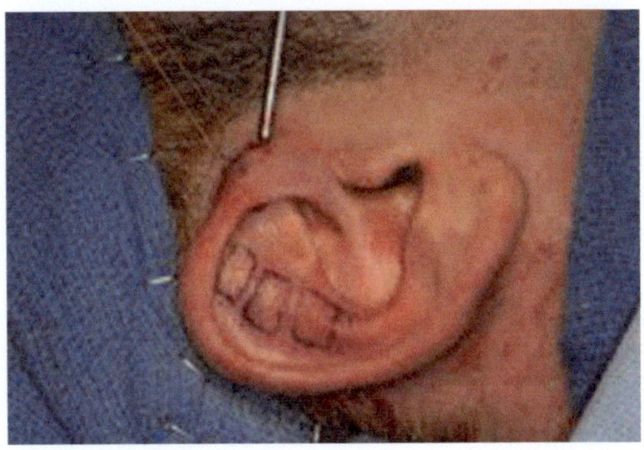

Fig. 10.7 Helical root suture and incision placement

Helical Root

Often, after performing a conchal setback and recreating the antihelix, the helical root will protrude laterally in a majority of cases. This problem was addressed by Hatch in 1958 [42], when he described securing the helical root to the temporalis fascia. This area can be accessed by extending the postauricular incision superiorly and anteriorly along a natural skin crease in front of the helical root or creating a separate 5–10-mm incision. A 4-0 polyester suture can then be placed securely, deep into the temporalis fascia and through the inferior-most helical root cartilage. When this stitch is tightened, the helical root should be brought into a more natural position (Fig. 10.7). This technique helps one avoid a telephone ear deformity [24].

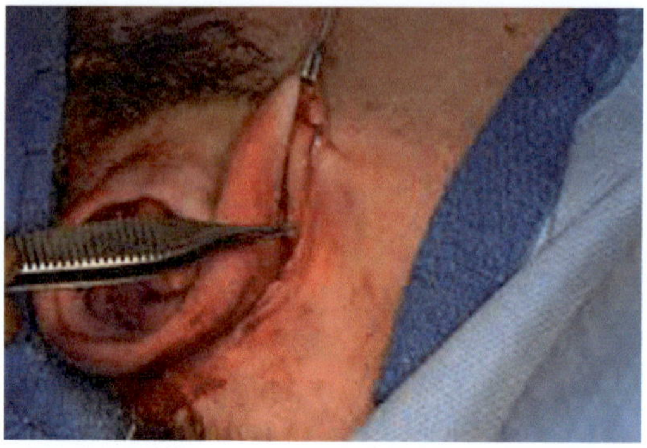

Fig. 10.8 Lobule reduction with posterior wedge excision

Lobule

Traditionally, the lobule is addressed by excising a vertical ellipse of skin along its posterior surface (Fig. 10.8) [7, 30]. In Fritsch's [27] incisionless otoplasty, however, lobule projection can be reduced by percutaneously dissecting the cauda helicis from the helix with a 20-gauge phlebotomy needle and securing the flail segment of cauda helicis cartilage to the posterior conchal bowl. The lobule is important to address if needed as it may also contribute to a postoperative telephone ear deformity.

Closing the Incision

In traditional otoplasty with a postauricular incision, it is important to close the incision meticulously to minimize the postoperative scar. Even though it is hidden behind the ear, a poorly closed incision may be bothersome to the patient. The authors prefer to close this incision using 5-0 fast-absorbing catgut suture, leaving three small, 3–4-mm gaps to allow egress of blood and decrease risk for hematoma. This modification of leaving small, purposeful 3–4-mm gaps in the closure has anecdotally reduced the senior author's rate of postoperative hematoma to zero without compromising final wound aesthetics or risk of infection.

Postoperative Care

Dressing

The majority of surgeons who perform otoplasty use some sort of compression dressing postoperatively to keep the ears in a fixed position during initial healing. Dressings used for this purpose range from fluffed gauze padding held in place by circumferential gauze or Silastic foam to a dust mask, a doorknob cover, or a wrestling headgear [43–47]. These dressings, however, may cause pressure necrosis of pinna and forehead or reduce the likelihood that a hematoma or infection will be recognized at an earlier time. In addition, dressings that require frequent replacement are coated with dried blood or have an odor may cause embarrassment and limit an earlier return to work or school [48, 49]. Because of these concerns, some surgeons have questioned the duration and even need for dressings after otoplasty, especially in cartilage-shaping techniques when permanent sutures are holding the newly positioned cartilage in position. Ramkumar et al. [50] randomized 80 children receiving otoplasty into 24-h versus 10-day dressing groups and found no difference between them. Orabi et al. [51] reviewed a series of 84 patients in which 23 did not receive a postoperative dressing and did not find any difference in complication rate. Overall, these studies suggest that postoperative dressings may be kept in place for shorter amount of time and may, perhaps, not even be necessary. Currently, however, there are no clear evidence-based recommendations, and, for this reason, the traditional approach of using a compression dressing is favored.

In our patients, a soft compression dressing is used in every case. Petrolatum gauze is cut into five 5-mm strips and packed along the newly shaped anterior and posterior ear surfaces. This dressing is covered by fluffed 4 × 4 in. gauze sponges and either size seven or eight elastic net bandage doubled over the face after twisting at the top of the head. A gap is cut over the eyes, nose, and mouth, while the inferior edge is pulled

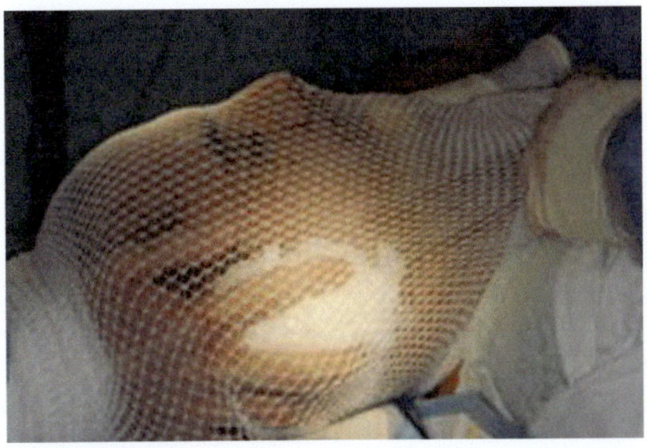

Fig. 10.9 Elastic net bandage placement

under the chin for patient comfort (Fig. 10.9). This dressing is left in place for 48 h and is removed when the patient returns to clinic on postoperative day 2.

Antibiotics

Many surgeons prescribe postoperative antibiotics after otoplasty, and unfortunately there are no studies specific to this topic. One study found no benefit for postoperative antibiotics in the setting of middle ear surgery and tympanoplasty [52]. Another study by Sylaidis et al. [53] suggests a 5 % wound infection rate for surgery near the ear mostly involving local flaps after oncologic resection. If antibiotics are to be used, one that covers typical skin flora, such as cephalexin, should be adequate.

Complications

Complications after otoplasty are uncommon, but can be severe when they occur. Therefore, any complications should be dealt with expeditiously. Early postoperative complications include bleeding, hematoma, skin necrosis, infection, and chondritis, while late complications include asymmetry inadequate correction, telephone ear deformity, abnormal ear contours, suture granulomas, extruded or broken sutures, and keloids. Complication rates are summarized in Table 10.2 [3, 23, 31, 37, 54–71]. Hematoma usually presents as sudden swelling at the surgical site and is often caused by inadequate hemostasis or postoperative trauma. Hematomas should be drained to prevent infection, calcification, and cartilage loss. Infection, on the other hand, will often present as ear swelling and drainage with worsening pain around postoperative day 3 or 4. In this situation, fluid collections should be drained, cultures should be obtained, and antibiotics should be initiated. Oral antibiotics may be given at first, but if infection persists at 48–72 h, broad-spectrum intravenous antibiotics that include pseudomonal coverage should be started. Excessive pain can be a sign of either of these complications but can also indicate a hypersensitivity reaction or excessive dressing tightness resulting in skin necrosis.

Overall, the most common complication of otoplasty is inadequate correction, a situation that may require revision surgery. The ear will often lateralize with time as well, possibly resulting in a late presentation. One type of inadequate correction is telephone ear deformity, a condition in which there are a residual laterally protruding helical root and lobule that give the ear the appearance of a traditional telephone. Telephone ear deformity can be prevented by performing a helical root setback and lobule reduction in the initial surgery. Overcorrection can also occur, although much less frequently. When this does occur, it can almost always be improved by placing a folded 2 × 2 in. gauze between the posterior surface of the ear and the scalp to push the ear laterally by 10–15°. This splint can be held in place with an athletic sweatband placed above and behind the ears and generally takes 2–6 weeks to achieve the desired amount of correction. This complication is very rare and has occurred in only a few of the senior author's patients, but each was adequately resolved using the aforementioned technique.

Abnormal ear contours can also result from otoplasty, most commonly from cartilage-cutting techniques in which sharp edges may cause an unnatural appearance. Cartilage-shaping techniques, however, are more susceptible to suture

Table 10.2 Complications of otoplasty

					Early complications		
Type of otoplasty	Author	Year	Study size	Method	Bleeding (%)	Hematoma (%)	Skin necrosis (%)
Cartilage-cutting	Chongchet	1962	21	Cartilage incising and scoring		5	
	Tan	1986	101	Cartilage incising and scoring	8		
	Calder and Naasan	1994	562	Cartilage incising and scoring	2		1.4
	Jeffery	1999	118	Cartilage incising and scoring		3.4	1.7
	Caouette-Laberge et al.	2000	500	Cartilage incising and scoring	2.1	0.4	0.6
	Peker et al.	2002	178	Cartilage incising and scoring	5.6	2.2	0
	Kompatscher et al.	2004	50	Cartilage incising and scoring		7.1	
	Kompatscher et al	2004	14	Anterior cartilage scoring and suturing		0	
	Panettier et al.	2004	33	Cartilage incising and scoring		0	0
	Panettier et al.	2004	30	Posterior cartilage scoring and suturing		0	0
	Bulstrode et al.	2003	114	Anterior cartilage scoring and suturing	0.9	0	0
	Di Mascio et al.	2003	40	Cartilage incising and scoring +/– suturing		7.5	
	Rubino et al.	2005	10	Cartilage incising and scoring	10	0	0
	Mandal et al.	2006	68	Anterior cartilage scoring and suturing	1.5		0.7
	Salgarello et al.	2007	135	Anterior cartilage scoring and suturing	6.6	0	1.5
	Olivier et al.	2009	104	Posterior cartilage scoring and suturing	1		
Cartilage-shaping	Rigg	1979	101	Cartilage suturing			
	Minderjahn et al.	1980	135	Cartilage suturing			
	Attwood and Evans	1985	52	Cartilage suturing	2.2		
	Tan	1986	45	Cartilage suturing	33		
	Adamson et al.	1991	55	Cartilage suturing	0.8		
	Foda	1999	39	Cartilage suturing	0	0	0
	Horlock et al.	2001	51	Cartilage suturing with fascial flap	2	0	0
	Mandal et al.	2006	94	Cartilage suturing	5.3		
	Mandal et al.	2006	41	Cartilage suturing with fascial flap	2.4		
	Schaverien et al.	2010	30	Cartilage suturing with fascial flap	3.3		
	Sinha	2012	227	Cartilage suturing with fascial flap		0	

[a]Recurrence and inadequate correction reported separately when possible as % + %
[b]Suture extrusion and granuloma reported separately when possible as % + %

	Late complications					
Infection (%)	Recurrence or inadequate correction (%)[a]	Asymmetry (%)	Suture extrusion or granuloma (%)[b]	Hypertrophic scar (%)	Keloid scar (%)	Dysaesthesia (%)
	10		0			
	9.9 + 4.4					
5.2	8		0			
3.3	12.7			0.8	0	4.1
0	4.4	5.6			1.6	9.6
	0		0			
	50					
	14					
	4		0			
	2		0			
	0.9 + 5.3		0			
	5					
	0		0			
1.5	11				1.4	
0	3			1.5	0.7	
	11.3	4.9	4.8	1	2.9	
	2		11			
	12.3	40				
	0		4.6			
	24.4		15			
	6.6		8.4	0.8	0.8	
	5.1		12.8			
	11.8		0			
1.1	8		1.1 + 2.1		2.1	
0	4.8		1.1			
	4.5		10			
0.4	3.7		2.6		1.3	

failure or extrusion and may require revision surgery. Asymmetry can also result from failure to adequately address preexisting differences between each ear as different techniques or degrees of medialization may be required from side to side. Suture granulomas can appear at any time postoperatively and are often noticed as a firm, subcutaneous irregularity that can be treated with skin incision and suture removal. Finally, scarring may occur at the skin incisions used in otoplasty. Keloid scars are often the most distressing but can be treated with triamcinolone injections, similar to keloid scar treatment at other body sites. With any postoperative complication, the patient is often distressed, and more frequent clinic visits can be very helpful in providing the reassurance necessary for long-term patient satisfaction.

Long-Term Results

Overall, the vast majority of patients undergoing otoplasty can expect to be satisfied with the result. Over time, however, the ear can be expected to lateralize to some degree. Schlegel-Wagner et al. [72] performed otoplasty using an anterior cartilage scoring technique with suture fixation and found that 2 mm of lost medialization could be expected at 6 years postoperatively, especially at the superior third of the ear. Because of this, excessive medialization is often performed initially, especially with cartilage-shaping techniques in which a greater degree of lateralization has been noted to occur. Messner and Crysdale [73] performed a retrospective review of 31 patients 3.7 years after cartilage-sparing otoplasty using the techniques described by Mustarde and Furnas and found that 29 % of ears returned to the original position, 28 % of ears stayed in the initial postoperative position, and the remaining 43 % of ears ended up somewhere in between. Overall, 0.9–5.8 mm of medialization was lost 1 year after surgery, with the majority of medialization loss at the superior rim. Despite loss of medialization, 90 % of families and patients in Schlegel-Wagner's [72] study reported "good" or "very good" results, while 85 % of families and patients in Messner and Crysdale's [73] study were happy with the results but only 73 % would choose to undergo otoplasty again.

Conclusions

Otoplasty is a rewarding procedure with low morbidity and high rates of surgical success and patient satisfaction. Patient and family satisfaction is also dependent on adequate preoperative counseling and the surgeon's understanding of patient expectations and psychosocial concerns. The psychosocial impact of having prominent ears, particularly in childhood and adolescence, should not be underestimated, and bullying and teasing should be addressed, particularly with younger patients, in the initial otoplasty consultation. In a newborn with an ear deformity, molding techniques should be considered. In the future, laser-assisted cartilage reshaping may be a useful technique in older individuals, but specific indications and limitations are yet to be defined. At this time, surgery is the primary modality for correction of prominent ears. A large number of otoplasty techniques and modifications have been described since the original report in 1881 and have been reviewed in this chapter. A thorough understanding of normal ear anatomy as well as a variety of the otoplasty techniques described in this chapter will allow one to tailor surgery to each individual ear and achieve excellent results.

References

1. Lam SM. Edward Talbot Ely: father of aesthetic otoplasty. Arch Facial Plast Surg. 2004;6(1):64.
2. Nuara MJ, Mobley SR. Nuances of otoplasty: a comprehensive review of the past 20 years. Facial Plast Surg Clin North Am. 2006;14(2):89–102.
3. Adamson PA, McGraw BL, Tropper GJ. Otoplasty: critical review of clinical results. Laryngoscope. 1991;101(8):883–8.
4. Richards SD, Jebreel A, Capper R. Otoplasty: a review of the surgical techniques. Clin Otolaryngol. 2005; 30(1):2–8.
5. Alexander KS, Stott DJ, Sivakumar B, Kang N. A morphometric study of the human ear. J Plast Reconstr Aesthet Surg. 2011;64(1):41–7.

6. Sheerin D, MacLeod M, Kusumakar V. Psychosocial adjustment in children with port-wine stains and prominent ears. J Am Acad Child Adolesc Psychiatry. 1995;34(12):1637–47.
7. Mobley SR, Vartanian AJ, Toriumi DM. Otoplasty: surgical correction of the protruding ear. Oper Tech Otolaryngol Head Neck Surg. 2002;13(1):29–35.
8. Songu M, Adibelli H. Otoplasty in children younger than 5 years of age. Int J Pediatr Otorhinolaryngol. 2010;74(3):292–6.
9. Gosain AK, Kumar A, Huang G. Prominent ears in children younger than 4 years of age: what is the appropriate timing for otoplasty? Plast Reconstr Surg. 2004;114(5):1042–54.
10. Byrd HS, Langevin CJ, Ghidoni LA. Ear molding in newborn infants with auricular deformities. Plast Reconstr Surg. 2010;126(4):1191–200.
11. Ullmann Y, Blazer S, Ramon Y, Blumenfeld I, Peled IJ. Early nonsurgical correction of congenital auricular deformities. Plast Reconstr Surg. 2002;109(3):907–13; discussion 914–5.
12. Yotsuyanagi T, Yokoi K, Urushidate S, Sawada Y. Nonsurgical correction of congenital auricular deformities in children older than early neonates. Plast Reconstr Surg. 1998;101(4):907–14.
13. Yotsuyanagi T. Nonsurgical correction of congenital auricular deformities in children older than early neonates. Plast Reconstr Surg. 2004;114(1):190–1.
14. Leclère FM, Trelles M, Mordon SR. Cartilage reshaping for protruding ears: a prospective long term follow-up of 32 procedures. Lasers Surg Med. 2011;43(9):875–80.
15. Manushakian HS, Wilson PA, De Souza BA, McGrouther DA. The prone position in otoplasty. Plast Reconstr Surg. 2005;115(3):963–4.
16. Mobley SR, Miller BT, Astor FC, Fine B, Halliday NJ. Prone positioning for head and neck reconstructive surgery. Head Neck. 2007;2911:1041–5.
17. McDowell AJ. Goals in otoplasty for protruding ears. Plast Reconstr Surg. 1968;41(1):17–27.
18. Ferraro GA, Corcione A, Nicoletti G, Rossano F, Perrotta A, D'Andrea F. Blepharoplasty and otoplasty: comparative sedation with remifentanil, propofol, and midazolam. Aesthetic Plast Surg. 2005;29(3):181–3.
19. Pavlin DJ, Chen C, Penaloza DA, Polissar NL, Buckley FP. Pain as a factor complicating recovery and discharge after ambulatory surgery. Anesth Analg. 2002;95:627–34.
20. Rizzi MD, Weil RJ, Lorenz RR. Severe transient hypertension after greater palatine foramen block in a patient taking midodrine. Am J Otolaryngol. 2010;31(1):67–9.
21. Berbaum MW, Bredle DL, Futamara W. Absence of significant adverse effects from low-dose subcutaneous epinephrine in dermatologic procedures. Arch Dermatol. 1997;133(10):1318–9.
22. Becker DE, Reed KL. Essentials of local anesthetic pharmacology. Anesth Prog. 2006;53(3):98–108.
23. Caouette-Laberge L, Guay N, Bortoluzzi P, Belleville C. Otoplasty: anterior scoring technique and results in 500 cases. Plast Reconstr Surg. 2000;105(2):504–15.
24. Spira M. Otoplasty: what I do now – a 30-year perspective. Plast Reconstr Surg. 1999;104(3):834–40.
25. Erol OO. New modification in otoplasty: anterior approach. Plast Reconstr Surg. 2001;107(1):193–202.
26. Graham KE, Gault DT. Endoscopic assisted otoplasty: a preliminary report. Br J Plast Surg. 1997;50(1):47–57.
27. Fritsch MH. Incisionless otoplasty. Otolaryngol Clin North Am. 2009;42(6):1199–208.
28. Converse JM, Nigro A, Wilson FA, Johnson N. A technique for surgical correction of lop ears. Plast Reconstr Surg. 1955;15(5):411–8.
29. Farrior RT. A method of otoplasty; normal contour of the antihelix and scaphoid fossa. AMA Arch Otolaryngol. 1959;69(4):400–8.
30. Furnas DW. Correction of prominent ears by concha mastoid sutures. Plast Reconstr Surg. 1968;42(3):189–93.
31. Horlock N, Misra A, Gault DT. The postauricular fascial flap as an adjunct to Mustardé and Furnas type otoplasty. Plast Reconstr Surg. 2001;108(6):1487–90.
32. Rogers BO. The classic reprint. A new operation for prominent ears based on the anatomy of the deformity by William H. Luckett, M.D. (reprinted from Surg Gynec. & Obst., 10: 635–7, 1910). Plast Reconstr Surg. 1969;43(1):83–6.
33. Cloutier AM. Correction of outstanding ears. Plast Reconstr Surg Transplant Bull. 1961;28:412–6.
34. Epstein JS, Kabaker SS, Swerdloff J. The 'electric' otoplasty. Arch Facial Plast Surg. 1999;1(3):204–7.
35. Ragab A. Carbon dioxide laser-assisted cartilage reshaping otoplasty: a new technique for prominent ears. Laryngoscope. 2010;120(7):1312–8.
36. Stenstroem SJ. A 'natural' technique for correction of congenitally prominent ears. Plast Reconstr Surg. 1963;32:509–18.
37. Chongchet V. A method of antihelix reconstruction. Br J Plast Surg. 1963;16:268–72.
38. Stenström SJ, Heftner J. The Stenström otoplasty. Clin Plast Surg. 1978;5(3):465–70.
39. Tolhurst DE. The correction of prominent ears. Br J Plast Surg. 1972;25(3):261–5.
40. Mustarde JC. The correction of prominent ears using simple mattress sutures. Br J Plast Surg. 1963;16:170–8.
41. de la Torre J, Tenenhaus M, Douglas BK, Swinburne JK. A simplified technique of otoplasty: the temporary Kaye suture. Ann Plast Surg. 1998;41(1):94–6.
42. Hatch MD. Common problems of otoplasty. J Int Coll Surg. 1958;30(2):171–8.
43. Converse JM, Wood-Smith D. Technical details in the surgical correction of the lop ear deformity. Plast Reconstr Surg. 1963;31:118–28.
44. Bandey SA, Atkins J, Neil WF. Silastic foam dressing in pinnaplasty. J Laryngol Otol. 1986;100(2):201–2.

45. Mitsukawa N. Auricular protection after ear surgery using a dust mask. J Craniofac Surg. 2008; 19(6):1639–40.
46. Mitsukawa N. Auricular protection after ear surgery using a door knob cover. J Craniofac Surg. 2007;18(6):1416–8.
47. McIntire MR, Morgan RF, Kenney JG, Edgerton MT. Postoperative protection for the external ear. Ann Plast Surg. 1983;11(3):261–2.
48. Bartley J. How long should ears be bandaged after otoplasty? J Laryngol Otol. 1998;112(6):531–2.
49. Bradbury ET, Hewison J, Timmons MJ. Psychological and social outcome of prominent ear correction in children. Br J Plast Surg. 1992;45(2):97–100.
50. Ramkumar S, Narayanan V, Laing JH. Twenty-four hours or 10 days? A prospective randomised controlled trial in children comparing head bandages following pinnaplasty. J Plast Reconstr Aesthet Surg. 2006;59(9):969–74.
51. Orabi AA, Chintamani BH, Timms MS. Is a head bandage useful after otoplasty? A quasi-randomized controlled study of complications and patient satisfaction. Ear Nose Throat J. 2009;88(10): E17–22.
52. Jackson CG. Antimicrobial prophylaxis in ear surgery. Laryngoscope. 1988;98(10):1116–23.
53. Sylaidis P, Wood S, Murray DS. Postoperative infection following clean facial surgery. Ann Plast Surg. 1997;39(4):342–6.
54. Tan KH. Long-term survey of prominent ear surgery: a comparison of two methods. Br J Plast Surg. 1986;39(2):270–3.
55. Calder JC, Naasan A. Morbidity of otoplasty: a review of 562 consecutive cases. Br J Plast Surg. 1994;47(3):170–4.
56. Jeffery SL. Complications following correction of prominent ears: an audit review of 122 cases. Br J Plast Surg. 1999;52(7):588–90.
57. Peker F, Celiköz B. Otoplasty: anterior scoring and posterior rolling technique in adults. Aesthetic Plast Surg. 2002;26(4):267–73.
58. Kompatscher P, Schuler CH, Clemens S, Seifert B, Beer GM. The cartilage-sparing versus the cartilage-cutting technique: a retrospective quality control comparison of the Francesconi and Converse otoplasties. Aesthetic Plast Surg. 2003;27(6):446–53.
59. Panettiere P, Marchetti L, Accorsi D, Del Gaudio GA. Otoplasty: a comparison of techniques for antihelical defects treatment. Aesthetic Plast Surg. 2003; 27(6):462–5.
60. Bulstrode NW, Huang S, Martin DL. Otoplasty by percutaneous anterior scoring. Another twist to the story: a long-term study of 114 patients. Br J Plast Surg. 2003;56(2):145–9.
61. Di Cio D, Castagnetti F, Baldassarre S. Otoplasty: anterior abrasion of ear cartilage with dermabrader. Aesthetic Plast Surg. 2003;27(6):466–71.
62. Rubino C, Farace F, Figus A, Masia DR. Anterior scoring of the upper helical cartilage as a refinement in aesthetic otoplasty. Aesthetic Plast Surg. 2005;29:88–93.
63. Mandal A, Bahia H, Ahmad T, Stewart KJ. Comparison of cartilage scoring and cartilage sparing otoplasty – a study of 203 cases. J Plast Reconstr Aesthet Surg. 2006;59(11):1170–6.
64. Salgarello M, Gasperoni C, Montagnese A, Farallo E. Otoplasty for prominent ears: a versatile combined technique to master the shape of the ear. Otolaryngol Head Neck Surg. 2007;137(2):224–7.
65. Olivier B, Mohammad H, Christian A, Akram R. Retrospective study of the long-term results of otoplasty using a modified Mustardé (cartilage-sparing) technique. J Otolaryngol Head Neck Surg. 2009;38(3):340–7.
66. Rigg BM. Suture materials in otoplasty. Plast Reconstr Surg. 1979;63(3):409–10.
67. Minderjahn A, Hüttl WR, Hildmann H. Mustardé's otoplasty – evaluation of correlation between clinical and statistical findings. J Maxillofac Surg. 1980; 8(3):241–50.
68. Attwood AI, Evans DM. Correction of prominent ears using Mustardé's technique: an out-patient procedure under local anaesthetic in children and adults. Br J Plast Surg. 1985;38(2):252–8.
69. Foda HM. Otoplasty: a graduated approach. Aesthetic Plast Surg. 1999;23(6):407–12.
70. Schaverien MV, Al-Busaidi S, Stewart KJ. Long-term results of posterior suturing with postauricular fascial flap otoplasty. J Plast Reconstr Aesthet Surg. 2010;63(9):1447–51.
71. Sinha M, Richard B. Postauricular fascial flap and suture otoplasty: a prospective outcome study of 227 patients. J Plast Reconstr Aesthet Surg. 2012; 65(3):367–71.
72. Schlegel-Wagner C, Pabst G, Müller W, Linder T. Otoplasty using a modified anterior scoring technique: standardized measurements of long-term results. Arch Facial Plast Surg. 2010;12(3):143–8.
73. Messner AH, Crysdale WS. Otoplasty. Clinical protocol and long-term results. Arch Otolaryngol Head Neck Surg. 1996;122(7):773–7.
74. Schreiber NTN, Mobley SR. Advanced Cosmetic Otoplasty. In: Johnson J. Head and Neck Surgery: Otolaryngology. 5th Ed. 2013. In press.

11 Anterior Versus Posterior Approach to Otoplasty

Rosa Maria Echarri, Mónica Hernando, and Guillermo Plaza

Introduction

Prominent ear (lop ear) is a common birth defect, occurring in 5 % of the white population [1]. This malformation is inherited in an autosomal dominant pattern with variable penetrance [2]. In most patients, two deformities usually coexist, determining the greatest separation of the auricles: an inadequate development of the antihelix fold and an overdevelopment of the concha [3].

More than 200 surgical techniques have been described for its correction, indicating the lack of an ideal technique [4]. These can be classified into two categories: with conservation of cartilage or with cartilage section. Section methods attempt to eliminate the inherent memory of the cartilage so that the shape of the auricle can be modified. These techniques may leave significant asymmetries. In contrast, methods designed to reshape the cartilage are based on the Mustardé technique, which consists of placing three or four horizontal mattress sutures with permanent suture material along the ridge of the helix, to create an antihelix fold. These techniques have higher rates of relapse and require surgical revisions more frequently due to failure of correction, compared with section techniques [5].

Moreover, it is still unclear which approach should be used. The posterior or retroauricular approach was described initially [1, 4, 5], but subsequently, anterior [6–9] or combined approaches were recommended or even those without any incision whatsoever, so-called incisionless otoplasty [10].

The aim of this chapter is to review the usefulness and advantages of the anterior approach, in comparison with the retroauricular approach, after review of our own experience on a consecutive series of suture-based otoplasties without cartilage section, which have been recently published [11].

Surgical Technique

An individual evaluation of the auricles of every patient should be our first step while planning surgery. Pictures should be obtained of every case to measure sizes and distances between the lateral helical rim and the mastoid surface and to discuss possible surgical procedures and results with the patients and their families.

The authors have been performing otoplasties for more than 15 years. The technique has evolved into one that is similar to the recently described Lucerne technique, which follows five basic surgical steps [12]:

R.M. Echarri, M.D. (✉) • M. Hernando, M.D.
G. Plaza, M.D., Ph.D.
Servicio de Otorrinolaringología,
Hospital Universitario de Fuenlabrada,
Universidad Rey Juan Carlos,
C° del Molino, 2, Fuenlabrada, Madrid 28942, Spain
e-mail: recharri.hflr@salud.madrid.org;
monica.hernando@salud.madrid.org;
gplaza.hflr@salud.madrid.org

M.A. Shiffman (ed.), *Advanced Cosmetic Otoplasty*,
DOI 10.1007/978-3-642-35431-1_11, © Springer-Verlag Berlin Heidelberg 2013

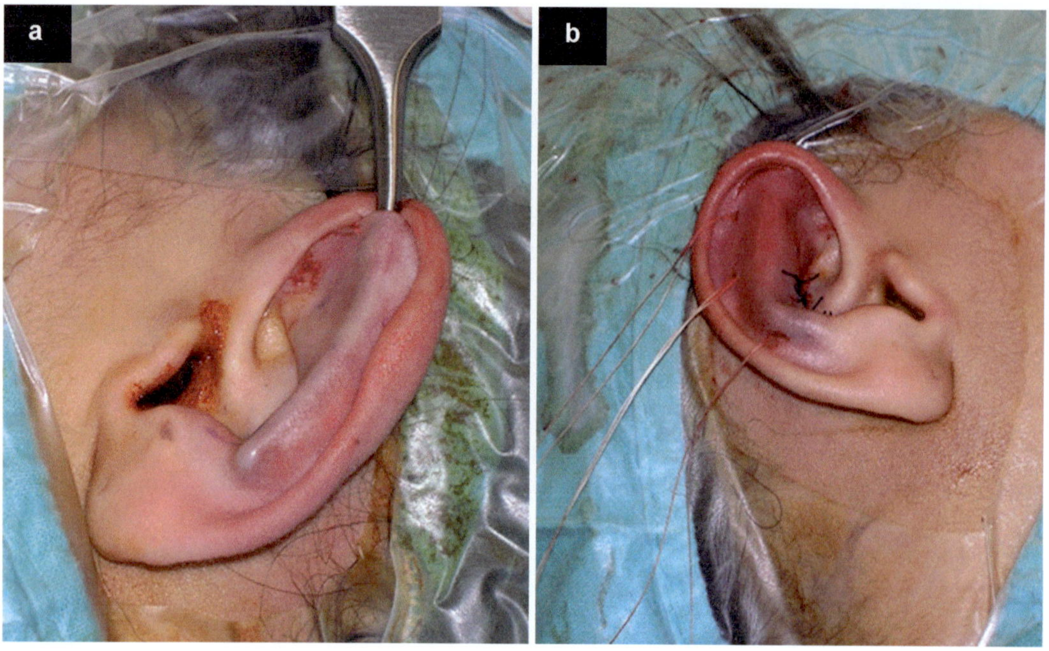

Fig. 11.1 Otoplasty by anterior approach. (**a**) Rasping the anterior perichondrium. (**b**) Nonabsorbable, ivory-colored stitches, through the incisions and passing through the posterior part of the auricular pavilion, to create the new antihelical fold

1. Skin incision, which may be anterior or retroauricular
2. Anterior scoring to reshape antihelical cartilage
3. Contouring of the antihelical fold by postauricular fixation sutures
4. Correction of auricular position, usually without cartilage excision
5. Refinements, specially lobuloplasty

Anterior Approach

Local infiltration of a combination of 1 % lidocaine and epinephrine 1:100,000 on both sides of the auricle is used. An incision of 1–2 cm is made, following the ridge of the helix, to prevent it being seen later. Using a Freer elevator, the skin is separated from the anterior cartilage, and the area is then scraped with a rasp (Fig. 11.1) to remove the anterior perichondrium. Three hypodermic needles are passed through the anterior skin and cartilage to serve as a guide for the creation of the new antihelical fold. Small incisions are made in the skin in the entry and exit areas of the needles. Nonabsorbable, ivory-colored sutures (Lorca-Marin®, Supramid, ref 65343, white polyamide, Tb-15, 3/0) are passed through these incisions and back through the posterior auricular part to create the new antihelical fold (Fig. 11.1). In case of prolapsed concha, an ellipse of skin and cartilage is removed in the area where the concha joins the antihelix, below the antitragus. This is completed with 4/0 silk suture of the incisions, which is removed after 7 days. Compression is done with cotton soaked in soap solution on the concha and the antihelical fold, covered with loose gauze and bandage for 1 week.

Posterior Approach

This approach also begins with infiltration of a combination of 1 % lidocaine and epinephrine 1:100,000 on both sides of the auricle. A posterior skin incision is carried out in an elliptical

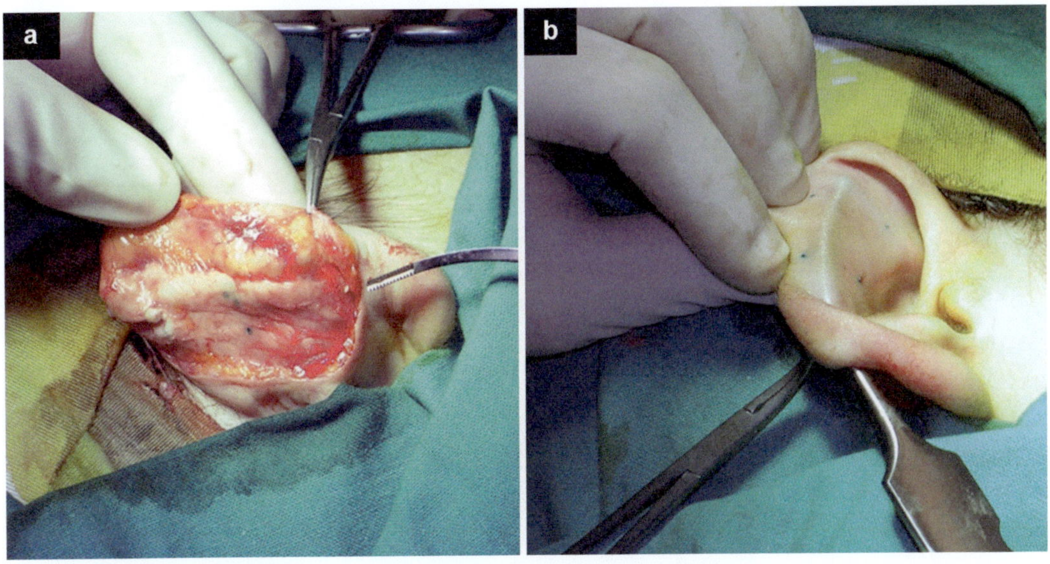

Fig. 11.2 Otoplasty by posterior approach. (**a**) Posterior elliptical skin incision, resection of a strip of skin to the level of the perichondrium. (**b**) Rasping from the retroauricular incision

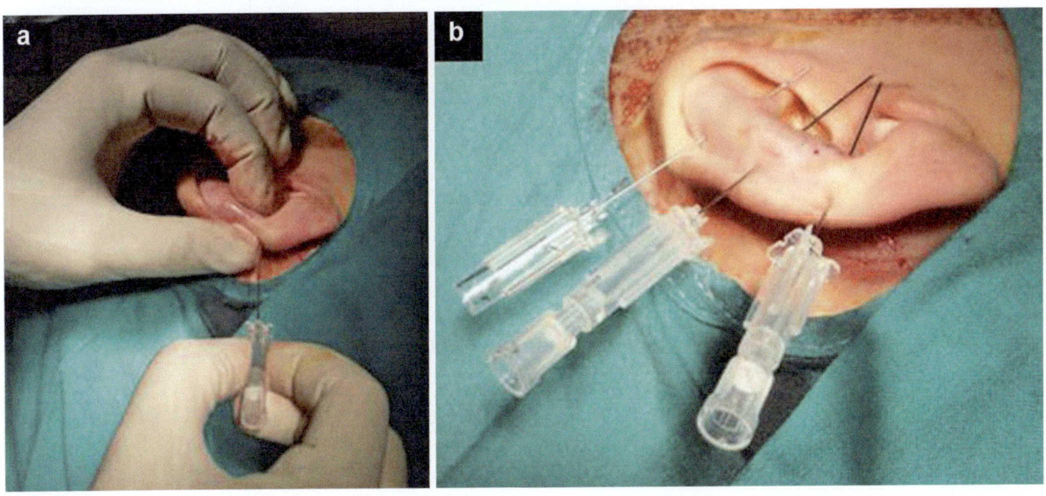

Fig. 11.3 Careful design of the new antihelical fold, passing needles several times until the desired result is achieved (**a**). Hypodermic needles are placed through the skin and cartilage to serve as a guide for the creation of a new antihelical fold (**b**)

shape, approximately 1 cm from the edge of the helix, and the skin is resected to the level of the perichondrium (Fig. 11.2). Dissection is performed up to the proximity of the retroauricular sulcus, and in a cranial direction, it should reach the proximity of the edge of the helix. Using the Freer elevator, the skin is separated from the anterior cartilage, and a rasp (Fig. 11.2) is then used to remove the anterior perichondrium. If it is necessary to reduce the height of the concha, a half-moon of cartilage of approximately 6 mm is resected at the junction of the antihelical fold and the root. Careful design of the new antihelical fold is planned, passing needles several times until the desired result is achieved (Fig. 11.3). Hypodermic needles are placed through the skin

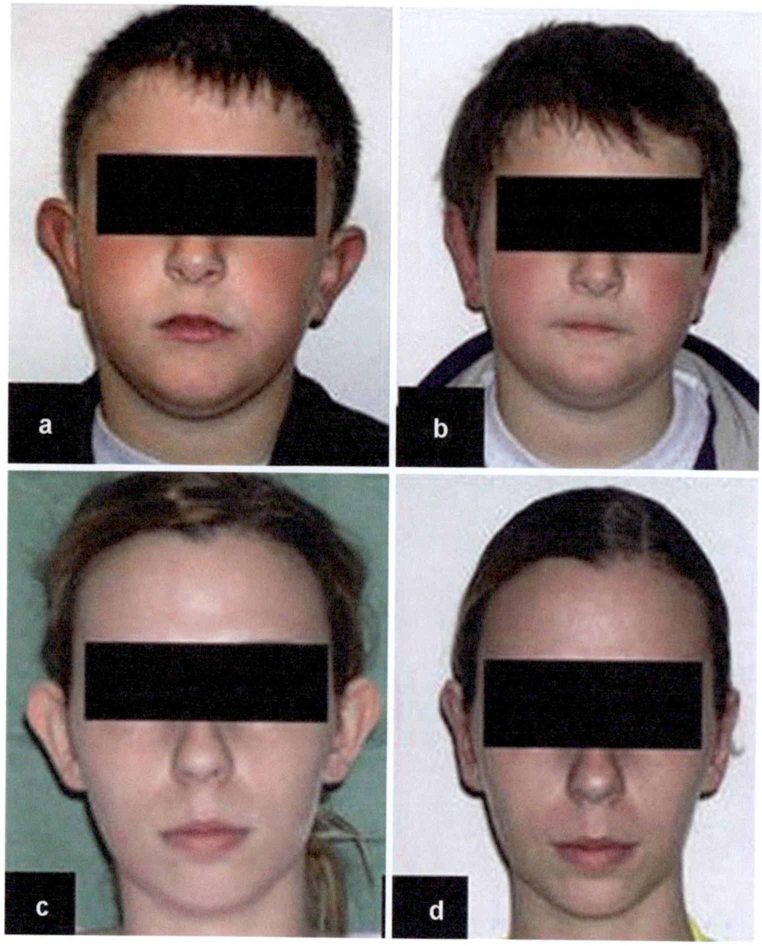

Fig. 11.4 Results after otoplasty. Anterior approach: (**a**) preoperative. (**b**) Control at 12 months. Posterior approach: (**c**) preoperative. (**d**) Control at 12 months

and cartilage to serve as a guide for the creation of a new antihelical fold (Fig. 11.3). Mattress sutures are applied, passing above and below the fold created through the anterior cartilage and perichondrium but not the skin, with three or four nonabsorbable ivory-colored sutures (identical to those used in the anterior approach). In adults with tough cartilage, before suturing, it is necessary to detach the anterior skin and thin the cartilage to facilitate the creation of the new fold. In patients with highly prolapsing conchas, a suture from the concha to the mastoid periosteum has to be done to approximate the concha to it. Lastly, the retroauricular skin is sutured with 4/0 silk. Swabs soaked in soap are used to model the new auricular shape, and dressing is maintained for 4–5 days.

Surgical Tips

The goal of surgery in the treatment of prominent ears is to obtain symmetrical and natural ears, with no signs of being operated on [13]. The variants of otoplasty can be classified into techniques which remodel the cartilage, as advocated by Mustardé [14], Furnas [15, 16], and Farrior et al. [17]; techniques which weaken it, as advocated by Stenstrom and Heftner [18, 19]; and techniques which section it, as advocated by Chongchet [20] and Converse et al. [21]. Some of these techniques also include the excision of an ellipse of retroauricular skin and other fixation of the cartilage to the mastoid.

Obtaining a good antihelical fold is crucial in every case [22], and this can be attempted with a

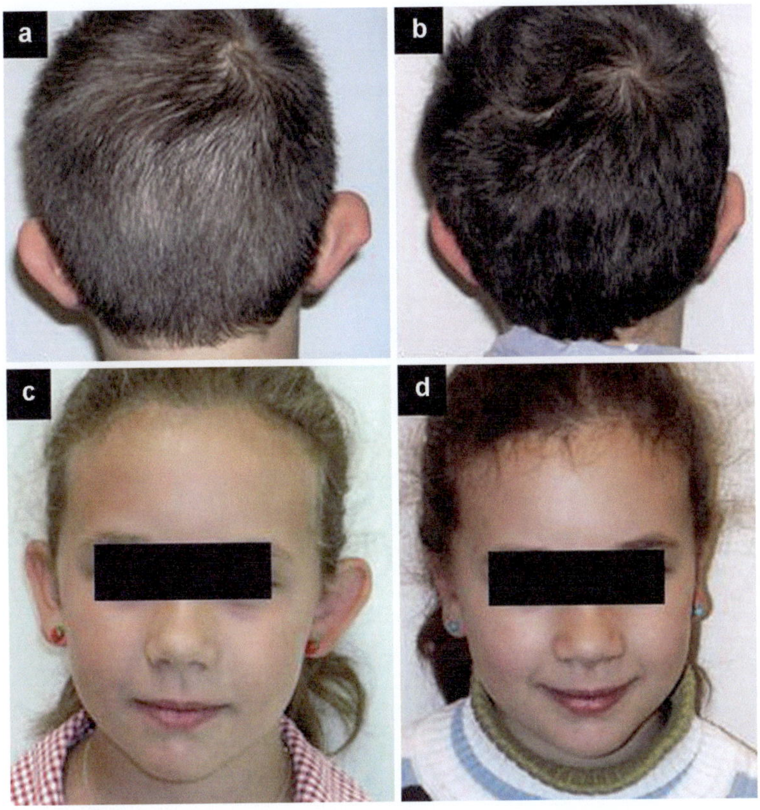

Fig. 11.5 Results after otoplasty. Anterior approach: (**a**) preoperative. (**b**) Control at 12 months. Posterior approach: (**c**) preoperative. (**d**) Control at 12 months

multitude of surgical techniques, such as horizontal sutures which fold the cartilage backward, through the weakening of the anterior side of the cartilage by filing, by multiple incisions in the back of antihelix to make the cartilage more flexible, etc.

The authors' technique includes a combination of these techniques through thinning of the anterior side of the antihelix to obtain a new antihelical fold which look harmonious and natural, as described by other authors [23, 24], and creating at least three Mustardé-type sutures that have to be correctly designed [25, 26]. The cosmetic results and patient satisfaction are good when using these techniques (Figs. 11.4, 11.5, and 11.6).

Regarding the approach, both the anterior and the posterior allow creating a new antihelical fold, without the need to make cuts through the cartilage. However, the use of sutures is related to the most common complication in our series, which was extrusion of the sutures. This occurred primarily when using an anterior approach (four times more frequently than in the posterior). It has been described by other authors in 10 % of patients [27], although it may be more frequent with some sutures that with others [28]. When suture extrusion appears, it is sometimes manifested as a continuous discharge at a particular point of the skin before the suture is exposed. Its early detection is important to avoid the possibility of triggering chondritis and because the tension effect of the stitches may disappear, favoring the recurrence of detachment of the operated ear, thus relapsing the prominent ear. In fact, in our series, this was the main cause of secondary operations, which were also more frequent in the anterior approach than in the posterior (28 % vs. 7 %).

The remaining complications described [29– 31] were less frequent; they did not represent major problems in our series. There may be infection of the skin, cartilage, or both. The importance of sequelae varies, with chondritis

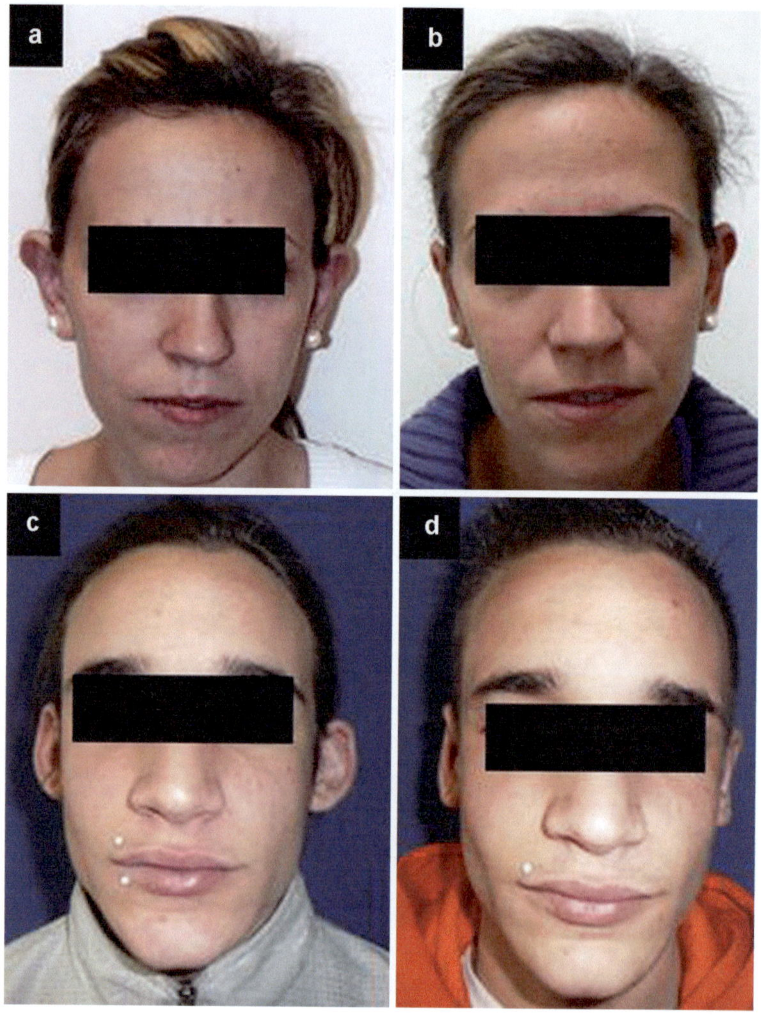

Fig. 11.6 Results after otoplasty. Anterior approach: (**a**) preoperative. (**b**) Control at 12 months. Posterior approach: (**c**) preoperative. (**d**) Control at 12 months

being one of the worst because it can make the pavilion disappear [32]. Treatment is carried out with broad-spectrum antibiotics to cover Staphylococcus and Pseudomonas, along with drainage of any collections that may appear.

Another important complication are hematomas. It is very important to monitor the possible formation of hematomas in the immediate postoperative period. Early symptoms include skin tightness, pain, and sensation of fullness. Patients should learn to recognize this rare complication, which has been described in 2 % of cases [33, 34].

As for aesthetic results (Figs. 11.3 and 11.4), there may be a late relapse in which the auricles become unstuck months after being operated on, which takes place in 2–13 % of cases according to the series, depending on the technique [33, 35, 36]. The authors observed more relapses with the anterior approach, probably due to the increased extrusion of sutures, decreasing tension.

Conclusions

Otoplasty allows for good cosmetic results in the treatment of protruding ears. The most common complication is the extrusion of stitches. The retroauricular approach to create a new antihelix without cartilage section allows achieving good results with fewer complications.

References

1. Mang WL. Otoplasty. In: Mang WL, editor. Manual of aesthetic surgery. Heidelberg: Georg Thieme Verlag; 2002. p. 191–223.
2. Weerda H. Classification and surgery of auricular defects. In: Weerda H, editor. Surgery of the auricle. Stuttgart: Georg Thieme Verlag; 2007. p. 43–233.
3. Barberan MT, Til G. Orejas en asa. In: Barberan MT, Sprekelsen MB, editors. Sociedad Española de Otorrinolaringología y Patología Cérvico-Facial. Girona: Gràfiques Alzamora; 2000. p. 151–6.
4. Adamson PA, Litner JA. Otoplasty technique. Otolaryngol Clin North Am. 2007;40(2):305–18.
5. Mandal A, Bahia H, Ahmad T, Stewart KJ. Comparison of cartilage scoring and cartilage sparing otoplasty – a study of 203 cases. J Plast Reconstr Aesthet Surg. 2006;59(11):1170–6.
6. Bassot DJ. The anterior approach to otoplasty. Plast Reconstr Surg. 2001;108(6):1823.
7. Burres S. The anterior-posterior otoplasty. Arch Otolaryngol Head Neck Surg. 1998;124(2):181–5.
8. Zambudio G, Ruiz JI, Guirao MJ, Sánchez JM, Girón O, Gutiérrez MA. Otoplastia por vía anterior para el tratamiento de las orejas prominentes. Una técnica mínimamente invasiva. Cir Pediatr. 2007;20(2): 119–21.
9. Erol OO. New modification in otoplasty: anterior approach. Plast Reconstr Surg. 2001;107(1):193–203.
10. Fritsch MH. Incisionless otoplasty. Otolaryngol Clin North Am. 2009;42(6):1199–208.
11. Echarri R, Hernando M, Montojo J, Plaza G. Otoplasty: results after anterior versus posterior approach. Acta Otorrinolaringol Esp. 2011;62:188–93.
12. Schlegel-Wagner C, Pabst G, Müller W, Linder T. Otoplasty using a modified anterior scoring technique: standardized measurements of long-term results. Arch Facial Plast Surg. 2010;12(3):143–8.
13. Petersson RS, Friedman O. Current trends in otoplasty. Curr Opin Otolaryngol Head Neck Surg. 2008;16(4):352–8.
14. Mustarde JC. The correction of prominent eras using simple mattress sutures. Br J Plast Surg. 1963;16:170–8.
15. Furnas DW. Correction of prominent ears by conchamastoid sutures. Plast Reconstr Surg. 1968; 42(3):189–93.
16. Janz BA, Cole P, Hollier Jr LH, Stal S. Treatment of prominent and constricted ear anomalies. Plast Reconstr Surg. 2009;124(1 Suppl):27e–37.
17. Scharer SA, Farrior EH, Farrior RT. Retrospective analysis of the Farrior technique for otoplasty. Arch Facial Plast Surg. 2007;9(3):167–73.
18. Stenstroem SJ. A "natural" technique for correction of congenitally prominent ears. Plast Reconstr Surg. 1963;32:509–18.
19. Stenstrom SJ, Heftner J. The stenstrom otoplasty. Clin Plast Surg. 1978;5(3):465–70.
20. Chongchet V. A method of antihelix reconstruction. Br J Plast Surg. 1963;16:268–72.
21. Converse JM, Nigro A, Wilson FA, Johnson N. A technique for surgical correction of lop ears. Plast Reconstr Surg. 1955;15(5):411–8.
22. Becker DG, Lai SS, Wise JB, Steiger JD. Analysis in otoplasty. Facial Plast Surg Clin North Am. 2006; 14(2):63–71.
23. Salgarello M, Gasperoni C, Montagnese A, Farallo E. Otoplasty for prominent ears: a versatile combined technique to master the shape of the ear. Otolaryngol Head Neck Surg. 2007;137(2):224–7.
24. Nolst Trenité GJ. Otoplasty: a modified anterior scoring technique. Facial Plast Surg. 2004;20(4):277–85.
25. Olivier B, Mohammad H, Christian A, Akram R. Retrospective study of the long-term results of otoplasty using a modified Mustardé (cartilage-sparing) technique. J Otolaryngol Head Neck Surg. 2009; 38(3):340–7.
26. Yugueros P, Friedland JA. Otoplasty: the experience of 100 consecutive patients. Plast Reconstr Surg. 2001;108(4):1045–51.
27. Barberán MT. Complicaciones en la otoplastia. In: Sprekelsen MB, Gomez JG, Ramos AM, Tomás MB, editors. Riesgos y Complicaciones en la Cirugía Oral y de Cabeza y Cuello. Kenilworth: Schering-Plough; 2008. p. 237–44.
28. Maslauskas K, Astrauskas T, Viksraitis S, Samsanavidius D. Comparison of otoplasty outcomes using different types of suture materials. Int Surg. 2010;95(1):88–93.
29. Limandjaja GC, Breugem CC, van der Mink Molen AB, Kon M. Complications of otoplasty: a literature review. J Plast Reconstr Aesthet Surg. 2009;62(1): 19–27.
30. Owsley TG, Biggerstaff TG. Otoplasty complications. Oral Maxillofac Surg Clin North Am. 2009;21(1): 105–18.
31. Bermúdez Polonio R. Acerca de ciertos fracasos estéticos menores en las otoplastias de las orejas en asa. An Otorrinolaringol Ibero Am. 1982;9(1):5–40.
32. Firmin F, Sanger C, O'Toole G. Ear reconstruction following severe complications of otoplasty. J Plast Reconstr Aesthet Surg. 2008;61(1 Suppl):S13–20.
33. Caouette-Laberge L, Guay N, Bortoluzzi P, Belleville C. Otoplasty: anterior scoring technique and results in 500 cases. Plast Reconstr Surg. 2000;105(2):504–15.
34. Messner AH, Crysdale WS. Otoplasty: clinical protocol and long-term results. Arch Otolaryngol Head Neck Surg. 1996;122(7):773–7.
35. Mompó L, Pastor G, Carrasco M, Cuesta MA, Dalmau J. Otoplasty without cartilage section using the Mustardé technique. Presentation of our experience. Acta Otorrinolaringol Esp. 2011;62(3):181–7.
36. de la Fuente A, Sordo G. Minimally invasive otoplasty: technical details and long-term results. Aesthetic Plast Surg. 2012;36(1):77–82.

Minimally Invasive Otoplasty: Technical Details and Long-Term Results

12

Antonio de la Fuente and Gustavo Sordo

Introduction

Correction of protruding ears remains a challenge. The literature describes a wide spectrum of techniques, ranging from incision-suture techniques [1], suture-only techniques [2], cartilage-scoring techniques [3–5], and others that combine some of the aforementioned procedures [6]. This wide variety of techniques suggests that no ideal method exists for the correction of protruding ears.

Pleasant results have been obtained with the aforementioned techniques. Nevertheless, they imply permanent buried sutures, extensive incisions, and ample dissections, which might increase the risk of complications such as bacterial contamination or intolerance of the sutures, visibility or palpability of foreign material, and skin and cartilage vascular compromise, to name a few.

Since 1992, the authors have been using a simplified and easily performed method for otoplasty that avoids the use of permanent sutures and wide dissection and addresses each aesthetic issue of the ear independently by separate incisions. This original technique was called "minimally invasive otoplasty," and a technical description of the procedure was published in 1998 [7].

A. de la Fuente, M.D., Ph.D.
Plastic, Aesthetic, and Reconstructive Surgery Unit, Hospital Rúber Internacional, Madrid, Spain
e-mail: secretaria@clinicadelafuente.es

G. Sordo, M.D. (✉)
Servicio de Cirugía Plástica, Hospital Central de la Cruz Roja/Private Practice, Madrid, Spain
e-mail: drgustavosordo@gmail.com

Preoperative Evaluation

Thorough analysis and diagnosis of each auricle was performed preoperatively, thus identifying every aesthetic deformity. Subsequently, surgical actions to be applied in each particular case were specified. The following algorithm was put into practice for each type of deformity:

1. Conchal cartilage hypertrophy: crescent-shaped conchal resection through a curved anterior incision
2. Lack of antihelical fold definition: anterior scoring with an ophthalmic knife through a stab wound at the root of the antihelical fold
3. Obtuse auriculomastoid angle: concho-mastoid sutures through a posterior incision over the auricular sulcus on separate tunnels
4. Hypertrophic scapha: crescent-shaped scaphal resection through an anterior curved incision
5. Hypertrophic lobule: wedge excision

Surgical Technique

Marking of the desired antihelical fold, excess conchal or scaphal cartilage, or lobule reduction is performed before surgery (Fig. 12.1).

With the patient under intravenous sedation and local anesthesia using 1 % lidocaine and

M.A. Shiffman (ed.), *Advanced Cosmetic Otoplasty*,
DOI 10.1007/978-3-642-35431-1_12, © Springer-Verlag Berlin Heidelberg 2013

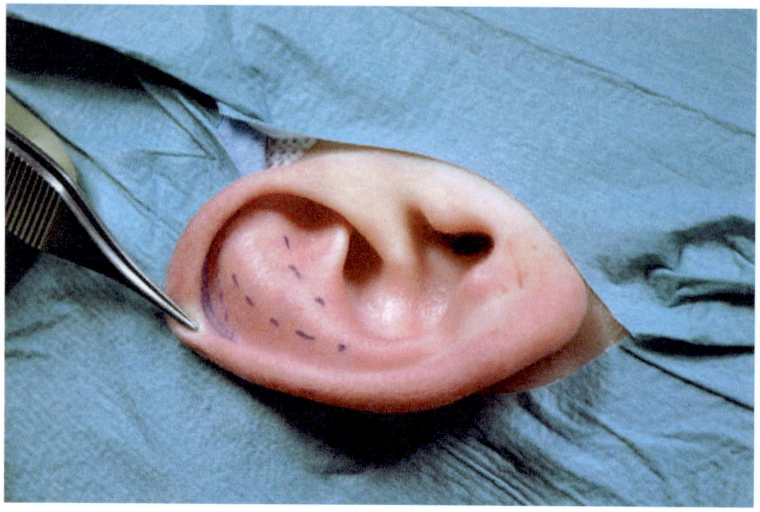

Fig. 12.1 Surgical markings including scaphal hypertrophy (crescent-shaped) and desired antihelical fold

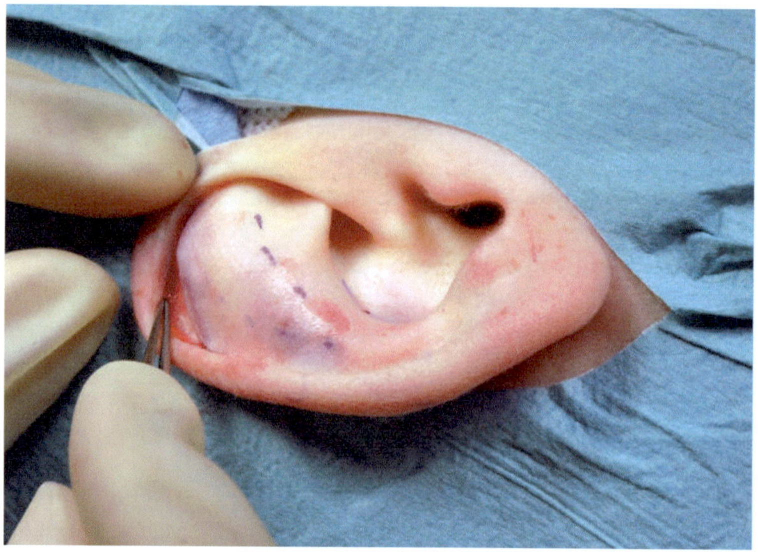

Fig. 12.2 Crescent-shaped excess scaphal cartilage

epinephrine 1:10,000, separate incisions are performed for independent treatment of the areas to be corrected.

Scaphal reduction is performed first. An incision is placed at the superior-most part of the anterior surface of the scapha where it meets the helix. Subperichondrial dissection is performed, releasing the soft tissues downward over the cartilage. This maneuver leaves a crescent-shaped scaphal cartilage exceeding the cutaneous border, which guides in calculating how much resection is needed (Fig. 12.2). Once this amount has been estimated, resection is performed, and skin is reapproximated with 6-0 absorbable sutures. No skin is removed.

Scaphal reduction has proved to be a powerful tool for solving the excess of cartilage height that conflicts with a short skin envelope at the upper pole. This type of deformity appears to be particularly frequent. It often is underestimated and may be the cause for an excessively projected upper pole of the auricle (Fig. 12.3).

Next, hypertrophic concha is addressed by a curved incision on the superior-most part of the concha's anterior aspect, where the scar will be hidden by the antihelical fold. A crescent-shaped

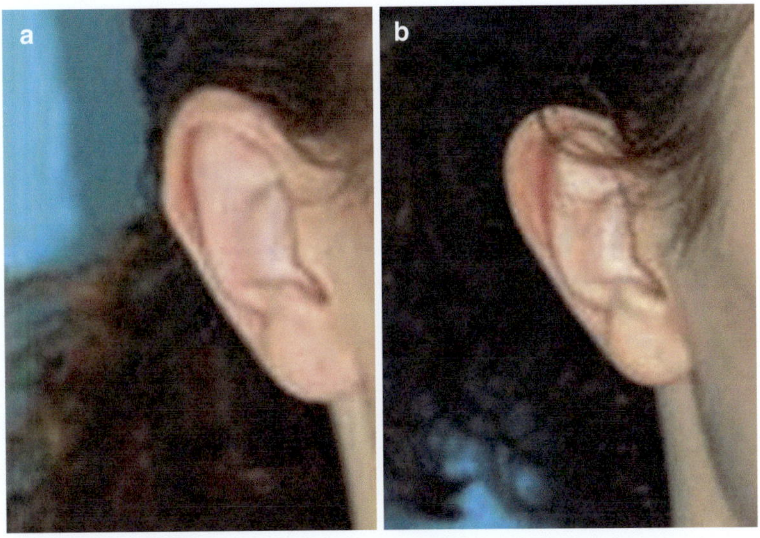

Fig. 12.3 (**a**) Preoperative. This patient was concerned about the height of her ears and requested to have her upper pole reduced. Hypertrophic scaphal cartilage is present. (**b**) One year postoperatively. Surgery included scaphal hypertrophy reduction and conchal-mastoid sutures. Note scaphal reduction and reduction of upper pole fullness. The antihelical fold was not modified by any means

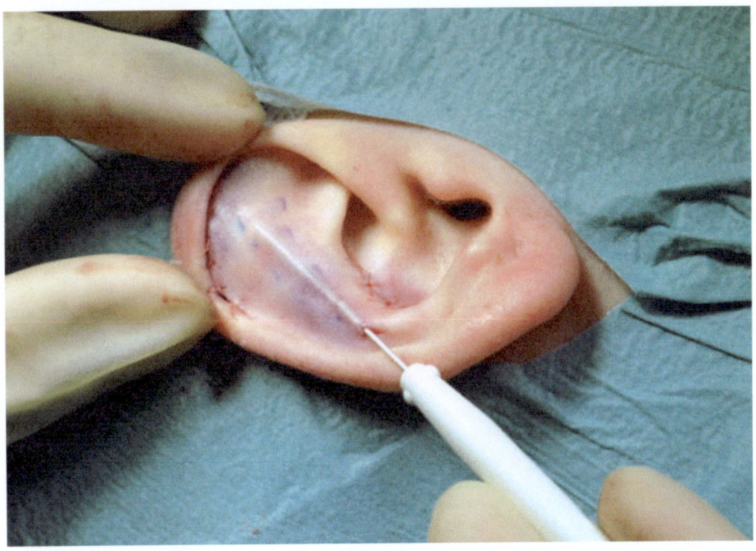

Fig. 12.4 Crescent-shaped excess conchal cartilage

portion of cartilage is subperichondrially dissected and then incised (Fig. 12.4). With the ear set back in its ideal position, conchal cartilage overlaps, and the amount of resection is estimated (Fig. 12.5). Skin is not resected to avoid undue tension and is approximated with 6-0 absorbable suture.

At this stage, the tendency to anteroposition of the ear is corrected, and deep sutures are used to set back and maintain the auricle. A narrow ellipse of skin (3–5 mm) is excised at the auriculomastoid sulcus, so the incision can be closed without undue tension. Two to three tunnels are bluntly dissected in the superior, medial, and inferior parts to expose the mastoid fascia, with no tissue removal (Fig. 12.6). The subcutaneous tissue and perichondrium of the ear's posterior surface is grasped with a 4-0 or 3-0 absorbable suture. The needle is passed all the way down through a tunnel, and a strong bite of mastoid fascia then is anchored (Fig. 12.7). The sutures are left untied, and the tension is estimated, especially at the central part of the ear, so as not to obliterate the postauricular sulcus.

Once the tension has been estimated, the sutures are tied at the same time to control the

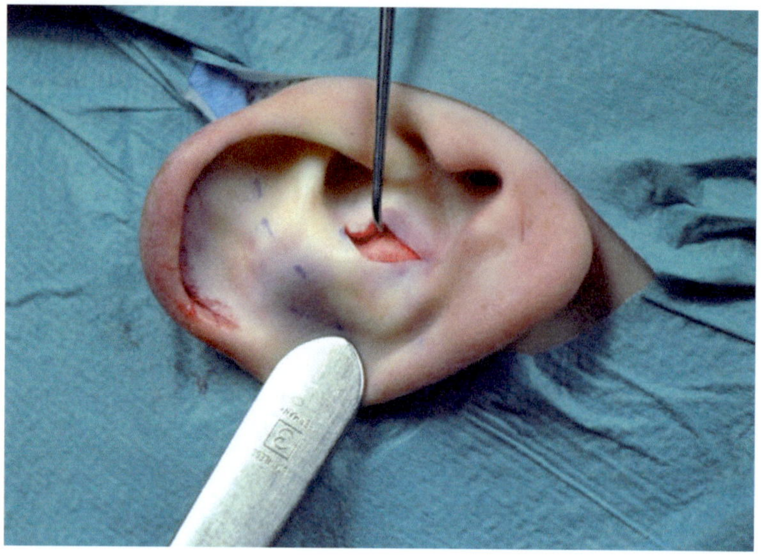

Fig. 12.5 Ophthalmic knife anteriorly scoring the antihelical fold

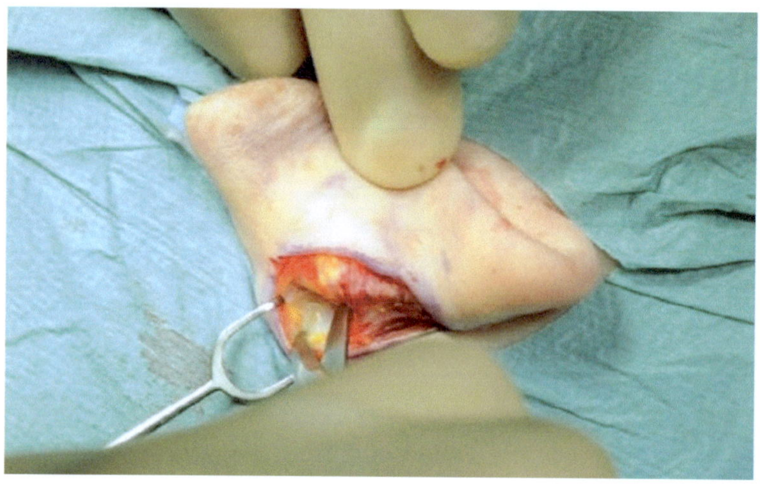

Fig. 12.6 Posterior tunnels exposing the mastoid fascia

tension and to produce a natural setback as well as a pleasant bending of the previously scored antihelix. A running 4-0 suture is used to close the posterior incision. If a hypertrophic lobule is found, reduction generally is performed by means of a wedge-shaped excision and direct closure.

Discussion

Minimally invasive otoplasty (96 bilateral and 4 unilateral) was performed for 100 patients (68 women and 32 men) with a mean age of 22.4 years. The respective surgical steps and their frequency are listed in Table 12.1. The complications are listed in Table 12.2.

All cases with mild discoloration or epidermolysis healed uneventfully. Partial recurrence took place in three cases, which was managed by reoperation 6 months postoperatively with very satisfactory results. One patient experienced partial upper pole necrosis, with tissue loss after application of undue tension to his bandage for 1 week. Scar revision and fat grafting were needed to improve the outcome.

Most of the patients were very satisfied (81 %) or satisfied (17 %) with the procedure. Two

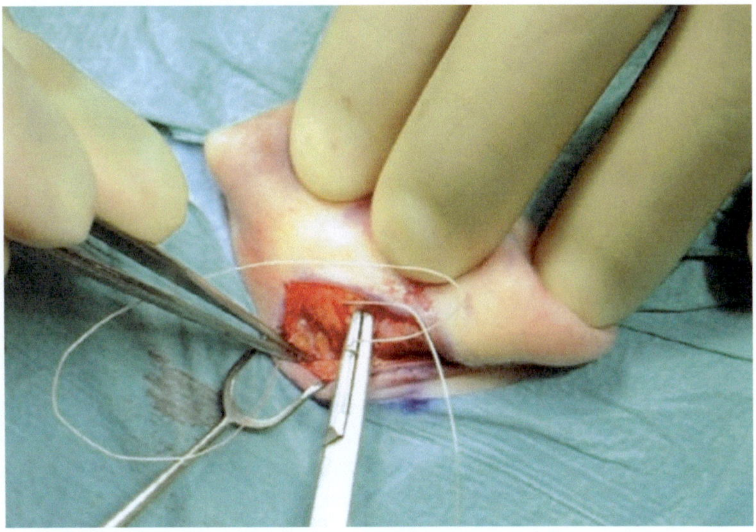

Fig. 12.7 A 3-0 absorbable suture passed all the way down the tunnel anchoring the ear to the mastoid fascia

Table 12.1 Techniques

Concho-mastoid sutures	81 %
Scaphal reduction	76 %
Antihelical folding	70 %
Conchal reduction	53 %
Earlobe reduction	19 %

Table 12.2 Complications

Discoloration/epidermolysis	5 %
Partial recurrence	2 %
Partial upper pole necrosis	1 %

patients were dissatisfied, but no patient reported great dissatisfaction with the outcome.

Like many techniques in otoplasty, the authors' procedure is based on the papers published by Stenstroem [3], Ju and Crikelair [4], and Chongchet [5], all of them inspired by Gibson and Davis's [8] interlocked stresses of cartilage. Following Stenström, we confine our dissection to a tunnel beneath the perichondrium, scoring blindly with an ophthalmic knife. This allows a natural, soft warping of the antihelix, with no permanent sutures (Fig. 12.8).

In addition to this, special attention is paid to the management of scaphal cartilage. Statistics show that a considerable number of patients seeking otoplasty (76 %) also would benefit from scaphal reduction. Thorough analysis of the upper pole shows a relatively constant combination of a lack of antihelical definition, with discrepancy between cartilage height and the skin envelope. Skin shortage produces a bending effect on a hypertrophic scapha, thus making the pinna look more separated from the head at the upper pole (Fig. 12.9).

Apart from defining the antihelix, we strongly recommend resizing the excess scaphal cartilage, adapting it to the amount of available skin. The anterior approach with downward release of skin leaves a crescent-shaped excess cartilage that eases the estimation of the resection. The posterior approach also is feasible but makes this maneuver more difficult due to the lack of guidance that the anterior skin release provides.

The size and overall appearance of the ear also can benefit from this action, especially in cases of patients concerned about excessive height of the ears (Fig. 12.3). Hypertrophic concha also is managed anteriorly. The principles of scaphal cartilage apply in such cases because anterior undermining leaves a crescent shape that guides the amount of resection needed in each case.

Three different incisions can be performed at the anterior surface, each aimed at solving a single problem. In addition to this, a posterior incision is performed when the ear must be set back.

Although other techniques advocate a single posterior incision for all the surgery, several objections could arise concerning the amount of

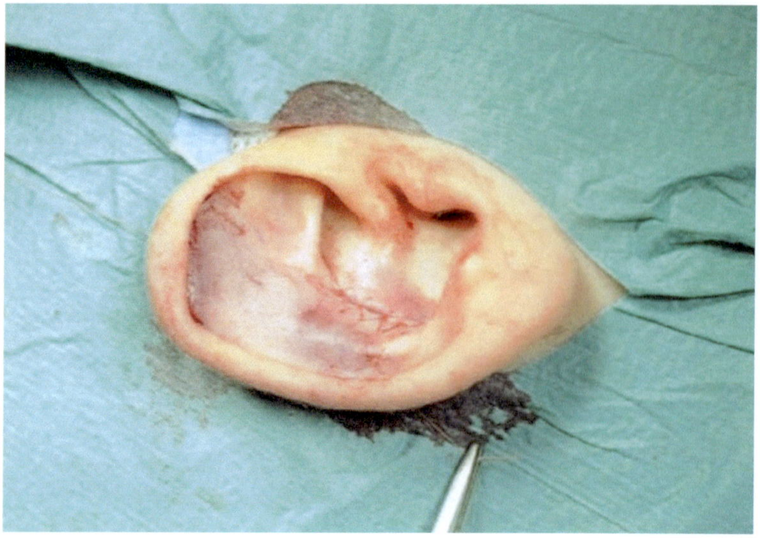

Fig. 12.8 Final aspect of the ear

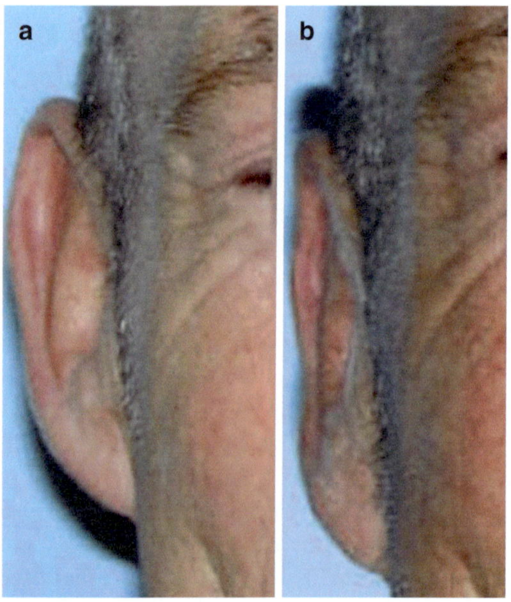

Fig. 12.9 (**a**) Preoperative. (**b**) One year postoperatively. Surgery included scaphal and conchal hypertrophy correction, anterior antihelical scoring, and conchal-mastoid sutures. Note the proper antihelical bending achieved

dissection needed to access the anterior aspect of the ear [5] or the need for permanent sutures to fold the antihelix [2]. In our experience, a combination of limited anterior and posterior approaches has proved to be safe in terms of tissue viability. All auricles have healed uneventfully. Patients with some mild discoloration and cyanosis (5 %) have been treated with topical antibiotic ointments and eventually have healed in 10–15 days.

Partial upper pole necrosis was found in one case that had continuous undue tension applied on the bandage for 1 week. Further corrections consisting of scar revisions, fat grafting, and the like were needed to achieve a satisfactory result.

Regarding incision visibility, inconspicuous scars on the anterior surface generally are obtained if the scars are hidden under the natural folds of the pinna. Careful manipulation of skin and perichondrium together with excellent skin edge approximation is mandatory.

Finally, concho-mastoid sutures are performed through two or three tunnels to minimize the amount of dissection needed. Absorbable sutures are preferred because we have observed that despite suture degradation, the ear maintains its position.

In conclusion, minimally invasive otoplasty provides long-term satisfactory results with an aesthetically pleasant pinna and a natural crease of the antihelical fold. The advantages of the technique are its simplicity, reliability, and safety. It avoids the use of permanent sutures and wide dissection and results in low complication, sequelae, and recurrence rates.

References

1. Converse JM, Nigro A, Wilson FA, Johnson N. A technique for surgical correction of lop ears. Plast Reconstr Surg. 1955;15(5):411–8.
2. Mustarde JC. The correction of prominent ears using simple mattress sutures. Br J Plast Surg. 1963;16:170–8.
3. Stenstroem SJ. A "natural" technique for correction of congenitally prominent ears. Plast Reconstr Surg. 1963;32:509–18.
4. Ju DM, Li C, Crikelair GF. The surgical correction of protruding ears. Plast Reconstr Surg. 1963;32:283–93.
5. Chongchet V. A method of antihelix reconstruction. Br J Plast Surg. 1963;16:268–72.
6. Schlegel-Wagner C, Pabst G, Müller W, Linder T. Otoplasty using a modified anterior scoring technique: standardized measurements of long-term results. Arch Facial Plast Surg. 2010;12(3):143–8.
7. de la Fuente A, Santamaría B. Minimally invasive otoplasty. Eur J Plast Surg. 1998;5:249–53.
8. Gibson T, Davis WB. The distortion of autogenous cartilage grafts: its cause and prevention. Br J Plast Surg. 1958;10:257–74.

13 Treatment of Prominent Ear Anomalies

Amy S. Xue, Edward I. Lee, Shayan Izaddoost, and Samuel Stal

Introduction

Prominent ear occurs in 5 % of the Caucasian population and is the most common congenital auricular deformity [1]. While it is a mild congenital defect within the spectrum of ear anomalies, its aesthetic and psychological impacts should not be neglected. Two-thirds of the prominent ear cases result from an underdeveloped antihelical fold, while one-third of the cases result from an excess of conchal bowl cartilage [2]. Associated secondary anomalies include excessive helical root protrusion, overprojected lobule, excessive antitragal protrusion, insufficient helical curling, cup ear deformity, and macrotia [3]. Studies have shown that prominent ear exhibits autosomal dominant inheritance [1].

The ultimate goal of surgery is to produce symmetrical, normal-appearing ears. Although quantitative measures to evaluate auricular dimensions serve as a useful guide when defining a deformity, prominence should be viewed in the context of the individual's face and patient's or family's perception. This chapter is intended to review the normal development and anatomy of the ear and the treatment options available for prominent ear otoplasty.

A.S. Xue, B.S. • E.I. Lee, M.D.
S. Izaddoost, M.D., Ph.D. (✉) • S. Stal, M.D.
Division of Plastic Surgery, Michael E. DeBakey Department of Surgery, Baylor College of Medicine, 6701 Fannin St, CC 610.00, Houston, TX 77030, USA
e-mail: xue@bcm.edu; eilee@bcm.edu; shayani@bcm.edu; sstal@bcm.edu

Development and Anatomy of the Ear

The external ear is composed of a tightly adherent skin over a cartilaginous framework. The posterior skin surface has a unique layer of adipose tissue. This layer extends anteroinferiorly to form the helical rim [4]. The average mature auricle is 6 cm in height and 3–4 cm in width (or 50–60 % of the height) [5]. The root of the helix is 6–7 cm posterior to the lateral canthus. The superior and inferior points align with the superior orbital rim and subnasales, respectively. The longitudinal axis is 15–20° off the sagittal plane, and the ear protrudes 1.5–2.0 cm from the postauricular skin [6] (Fig. 13.1).

The abnormal projection of the prominent ear results from variations in two basic anatomical structures: underdevelopment of the antihelix (Fig. 13.2) and/or overdevelopment of the conchal bowl. An obtuse conchoscaphal angle (>90°) is indicative of poor antihelical development leading to perception of prominence, while an enlarged or deepened conchal bowl (>1.5 cm) further lateralizes the ear, thereby exaggerating this prominence [3].

Embryologically, the ear arises from six hillocks of the first and second branchial arches during the second to fourth month of gestation [7]. Hillocks 1–3, from the first arch, form the anteromedial aspects of the auricle – tragus, helical crus, and helix, respectively. Hillocks 4–6, from the second arch, develop into the posterolateral aspects of the ear – the antihelix and antitragus, respectively [8]. Congenital ear deformities result

M.A. Shiffman (ed.), *Advanced Cosmetic Otoplasty*,
DOI 10.1007/978-3-642-35431-1_13, © Springer-Verlag Berlin Heidelberg 2013

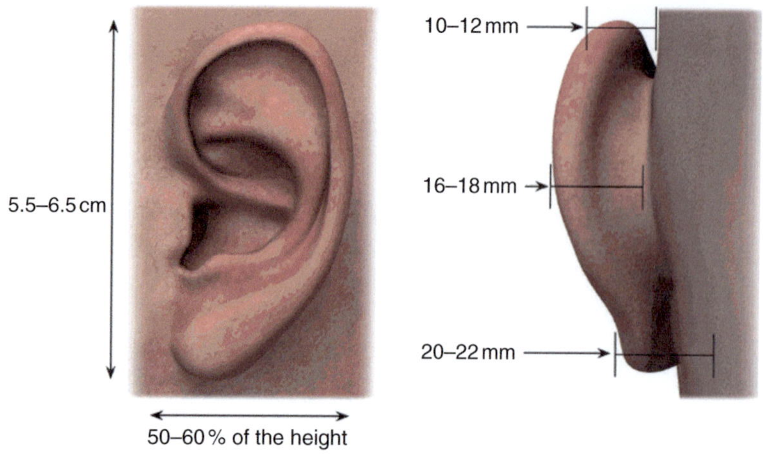

Fig. 13.1 Dimensions of the normal mature ear. The ears typically reach maturity by 10 years of age. Notice that the upper third of the helical rim typically projects 1.0–1.2 cm from the scalp, the middle third 1.6–1.8 cm, and the lobule 2.0–2.2 cm from the mastoid region. An underdeveloped antihelix leads to excessive projection of the upper third, while an overdeveloped conchal bowl results in lateralization of the middle third

from disruption of one or more of the auricular hillocks during embryogenesis.

Postnatally, the ear develops rapidly over the first decade of life. By age 10, the ear reaches 97–99 % of expected adult width and 93 % of adult length [3]. The fibrofatty lobule, however, continues to lengthen throughout adulthood. The auriculocephalic angle increases from 16 to 22° from age 1 to 10 years and retracts over the third decade before reaching an eventual plateau [9].

The ear is supplied by the branches from the superficial temporal artery anteriorly and the posterior auricular and occipital arteries posteriorly. The superficial temporal, posterior auricular, and retromandibular veins provide venous drainage. The lymphatic drainage of the anterior three hillocks is mainly to the anterior triangle of the neck while the posterior three hillocks ultimately drain into the posterior triangle of the neck. The ear is supplied by the great auricular nerve, lesser occipital nerve, and the auriculotemporal nerve. The concha is supplied by Arnold's nerve which is a branch of the vagus nerve.

Timing

Evaluation and treatment of auricular defects in children is similar to treating adults, with a few exceptions. First, the ear framework continues to grow during the first decade of life; therefore, any operative correction before this age must take into consideration its growth potential. Furthermore, children younger than 3 months old have very pliable ear cartilage due to maternal estrogen. For this reason, most ear deformities in young children can be treated with molding devices and do not require surgery. Expectedly, molding devices (using combination of tapes, glues, and stents) are most effective if implemented within 10 days of birth [10] and become less effective as the ear cartilage matures. For practical purposes, the ear is fully developed by 6–7 years of age, and correction can be performed at this time. Moreover, this age corresponds with age of school matriculation, which can have significant social ramifications for a child with prominent ears. Optimum results can be achieved only when both the parents and the child are motivated to undergo the procedure. Postoperative compliance with dressings is an integral part of prominent ear correction.

Surgical Principles

The primary goal of auricular reconstruction is to preserve function and restore form in the anterior and lateral views. Specifically, McDowell described the following reconstructive principles: (1) eliminate the protrusion in the superior third of the ear, (2) both helices should be visible lateral to the antihelix from the frontal view, (3) create a smooth and regular helical contour, (4) minimize distortion to the postauricular sulcus, (5) avoid placement of the

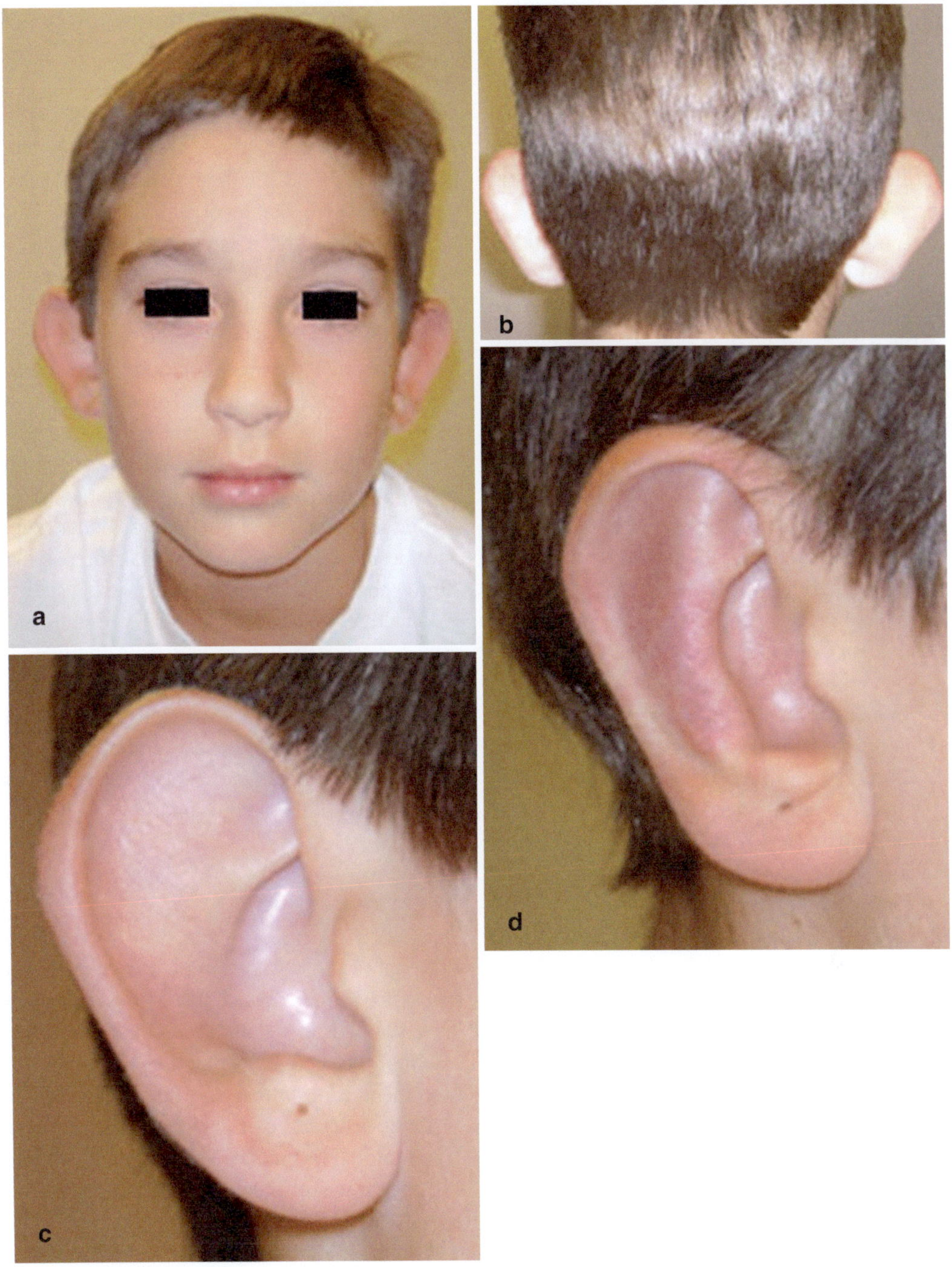

Fig. 13.2 (**a**, **b**) Anterior and posterior views of patient with bilateral prominent ears. Notice the underdeveloped antihelical fold and superior crus (**c**), leading to an obtuse conchoscaphal angle. (**d**) Twelve-month outcome after correction using Mustarde sutures

ear too close to the head, and (6) contours and positions of the two ears should be matched closely but not necessarily symmetric [11]. Since the lateral surface of the ear is rarely seen along with the contralateral ear, subtle variations can be tolerated. Therefore, corrective treatment should concentrate on the frontal view, which will allow for direct comparison of position, protrusion, and height.

Many techniques have been used to correct the underdeveloped antihelix. Initially, Ely described a technique where both skin and conchal cartilage were resected in two stages [12]. In 1910, Luckett described setback of the ear by excision of the postauricular skin, after realizing that the auricular prominence results from an underdeveloped antihelical fold. He also incised the ear cartilage leading to a sharp antihelix demonstrating a "surgically altered" ear [13]. In 1963, Mustarde [14] described a suture technique that creates a smooth and more natural fold. In his technique, permanent sutures are placed in the posterior surface of the ear cartilage and tied under enough tension to create the desired bend in the cartilage. While this allows great control in formation of the fold, suture failure can occur especially in adult males where the cartilage can be thick. These patients can benefit from Stenstroem's technique [15], where the fold is created by simply scoring the anterior surface of the auricular cartilage. Gibson and Davis [16] first noted this phenomenon in which the cartilage naturally curves away from the scored surface.

Several techniques have been described to address the conchal bowl hypertrophy. The Furnas technique [17] involves placement of conchal-mastoid sutures after removal of the posterior auricularis muscle and fibrofatty tissue from the postauricular groove. The Elliott technique [18] resects the excess cartilage through an anterior incision made at the conchal margin. Webster [19] described repositioning of the ear lobule using medial repositioning of the "tail" of the helix after posterior dissection. Current auricular reconstruction typically involves a combination of these techniques to optimize outcome. A thorough preoperative assessment, including history and physical, photography, and measurement, is necessary to determine the best surgical methods. In addition, it is particularly important to evaluate patient maturity and motivation for surgery, especially in the pediatric population.

Preferred Surgical Management

Preoperative

The first step in treatment of a prominent ear is preoperative assessment and creation of a surgical plan. Once the level of motivation of the patient and parents have been assessed and deemed to be appropriate for surgery, the helix, the concha, and the pliability of the cartilage need to be assessed. This will allow the surgeon to choose from the armamentarium of techniques described above. The patient should shower and shampoo his/her hair the night prior to surgery.

The surgery can be performed using a "Diamond Block" around the ear with 1 % Xylocaine with 1/100,000 epinephrine in adults or under general anesthesia in children. The patient is draped in the supine position such that both ears are visualized. Ophthalmic adhesive tape or 1010 drape can be used for sequestration of hair from the operative field. The ear should be prepped, including the external auditory canal, which should be occluded using a cotton plug. Lastly, digital pressure is exerted over the ear cartilage, thereby allowing visualization of the final results.

Operative

The goal of surgery is to produce perceptibly normal and symmetrical ears that are less noticeable. As discussed above, there is a large variety of existing corrective techniques available for prominent ears, which can be categorized into cartilage-scoring, cartilage-breaking, or cartilage-molding techniques [12, 17, 18, 20]. In general, a successful repair involves a combination of these techniques addressing the concha first, followed by the antihelix, and then, if needed, the lobule.

The conchal hypertrophy should be addressed first to minimize the risk of excessive Mustarde suture tightening [3]. For conchal depths of less than 2.5 cm, Furnas technique is sufficient whereby three to four conchomastoid sutures are placed to correct conchal excess (Fig. 13.3).

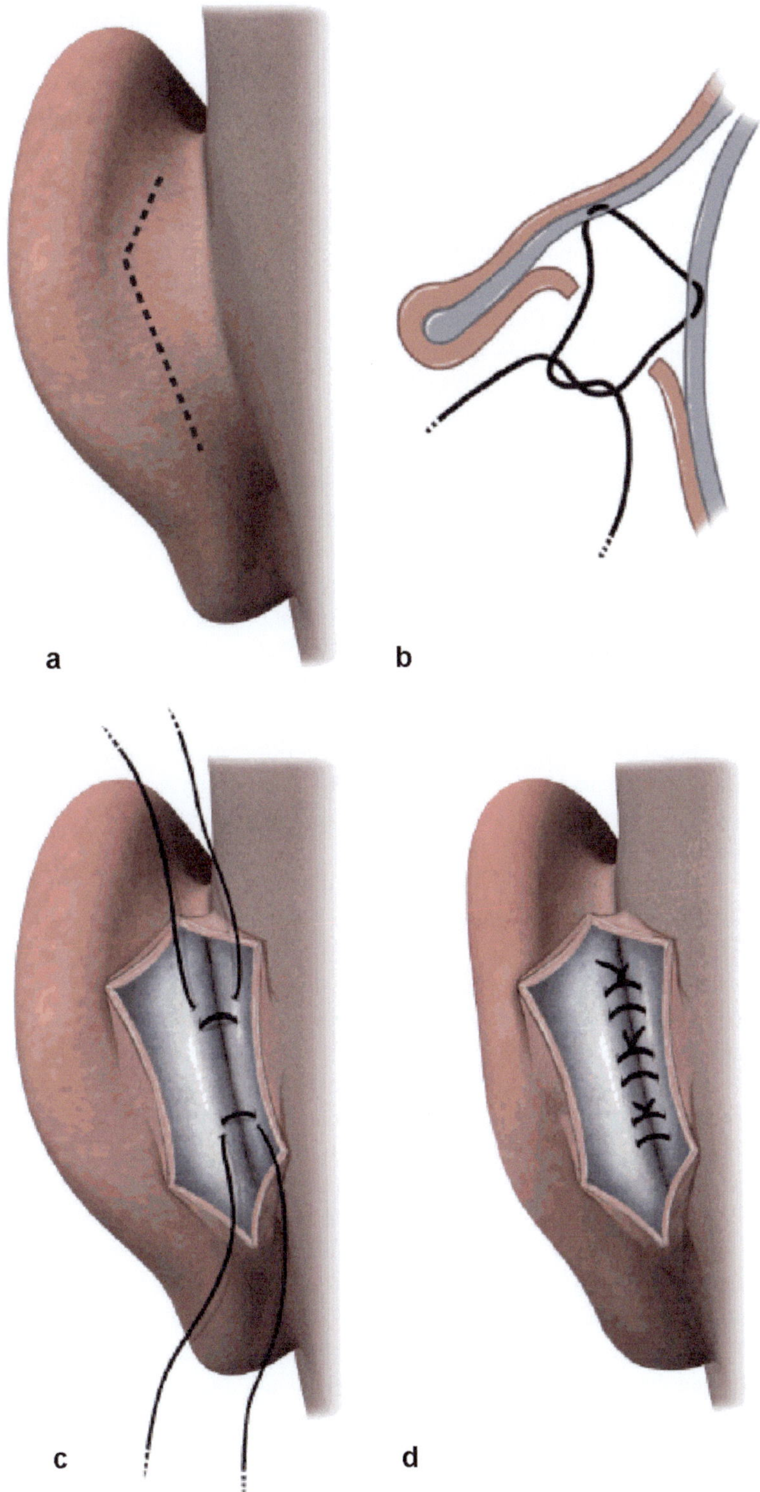

Fig. 13.3 Furnas conchomastoid sutures. (**a**) Access is established via a posterior skin incision. (**b**) The conchomastoid suture. (**c**, **d**) Horizontal mattress sutures are placed in a anteroposterior direction through the conchal and mastoid cartilages, respectively, to minimize narrowing of the external auditory canal

A vertical incision is made in the posterior conchal skin lateral to the sulcus. Anterior and posterior skin flaps are elevated to access the helical rim, scapha, and mastoid fascia. All skin flaps should be preserved, particularly the posterior flap, to maintain the posterior sulcus and decrease the incidence of suture granuloma formation [3]. The postauricular muscle and ligament are divided bluntly until the ponticulus is visualized and the soft tissue elevated. The ear is then drawn backward with nonabsorbable suture (4-0 Mersilene, Ethicon, Inc., Somerville, NJ) until desired shape is reached. The contact areas between the conchal cartilage and the mastoid fascia are marked and approximated with three to four mattress sutures (Fig. 13.4). The sutures must contain both the anterior and posterior perichondrium and must be placed in an anteroposterior direction to avoid forward rotation of the ear or narrowing of the external ear canal [3]. A Spira posterior conchal flap can be used to limit stenosis of the canal if narrowing is observed after Furnas sutures [21]. In the event of an overly deep concha, an anterior incision can be made over the shallow area of the concha, the cartilage incised, and excess cartilage resected, as described by Elliott [18].

The poorly defined antihelical fold is addressed next. The Mustarde technique (Fig. 13.5) places four to five scaphoconchal mattress sutures to reshape the ear and to decrease the perceived prominence [14]. A methylene-blue-dipped-25-gauge needle can be useful by marking the outline of suture placement on the concha and the outer aspect of the antihelix. Otherwise, temporary nylon sutures can be placed at 4-mm intervals to fold the scapha and create the neohelix prior to permanent suture placement (Fig. 13.4). When satisfactory antihelical definition is achieved, nonabsorbable mattress sutures (4-0 Mersilene) are placed incorporating the anterior and posterior perichondrium (Fig. 13.4). Sutures should be placed obliquely to maintain the anatomical curvature of the ear. The middle suture should be tied last to prevent telephone ear deformity (Fig. 13.6).

Anterior cartilage scoring is commonly required in case of rigid cartilage, such as in children older than 6 years of age [15]. Cartilage-scoring techniques are based on the observation that cartilage curls away from a cut surface, a phenomenon attributed to release of the interlocked stresses when the perichondrium is scored (Gibson's phenomenon) [16]. In this technique, a Dingman otoabrader is used to etch the anterior cartilage until the desired curvature is achieved. Access to the anterior ear can be achieved via a tunnel from the posterior incision or an anterior incision. A pocket is initially made between the skin and the cartilage to allow the introduction of the otoabrader (Fig. 13.7).

Prominent ear can also be associated with excessively large lobule. Moreover, excessive Mustarde sutures may inadvertently accentuate this finding, leading to telephone ear deformity (Fig. 13.7). Prominent lobule is addressed last with a simple full-thickness wedge excision or a modified fishtail excision [22]. A laterally positioned lobule is typically caused by a prominent cauda helicis that can be corrected by suturing it back to the concha, medial placement of the tail of the helix, or direct excision [2].

In more severe deformities or those involving stiffer cartilages, cartilage-breaking rather than cartilage-molding technique may be required [13, 22]. This is a powerful technique, the benefits of which must be weighed against the potential for secondary sharp ridging and contour irregularities.

Although cartilage-sparing techniques are preferred, cartilage-cutting ones may be useful in more severe prominent ear deformities. In cases of severe conchal hypertrophy, excision of the excess cartilage of the ascending conchal bowl may be necessary. In addition, excising the postauricular muscle and soft tissue can be useful to accentuate the setback [3]. Lastly, strict adherence to skin preservation cannot be overemphasized. None of the skin, even if appearing to be excessive after setback, should be excised.

A well-padded mastoid and auricular dressing is critical in the immediate postoperative period. Upon dressing removal, an elastic headband should be worn continuously for 3 weeks and at nighttime for 4–6 weeks.

Complications

The type of postoperative complication depends on the surgical technique. Hematoma is the most immediate and pressing postoperative

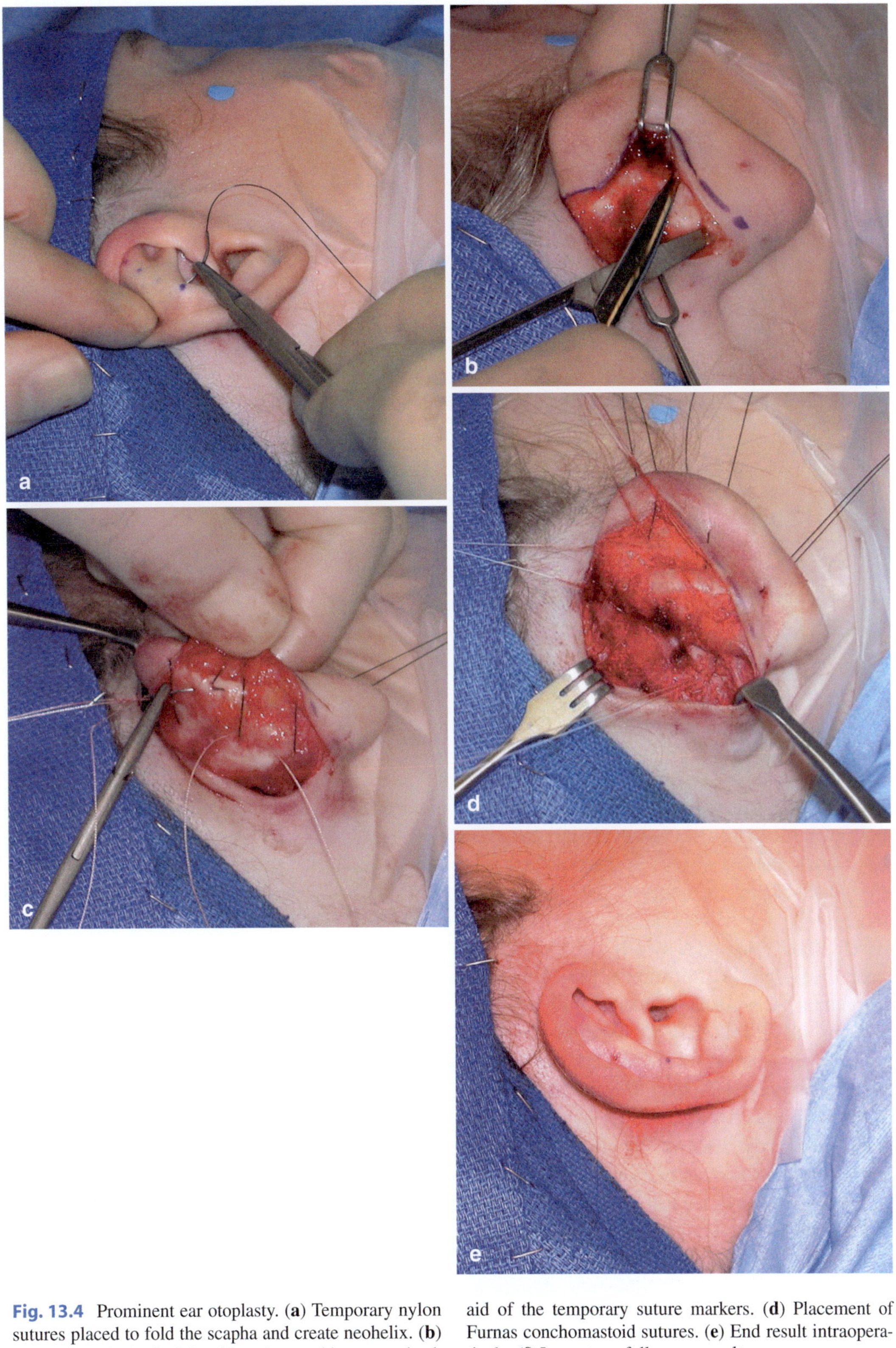

Fig. 13.4 Prominent ear otoplasty. (**a**) Temporary nylon sutures placed to fold the scapha and create neohelix. (**b**) Posterior auricular incision. Note that no skin was excised. (**c**) Placement of scaphaconchal mattress sutures with the aid of the temporary suture markers. (**d**) Placement of Furnas conchomastoid sutures. (**e**) End result intraoperatively. (**f**) Long-term follow-up results

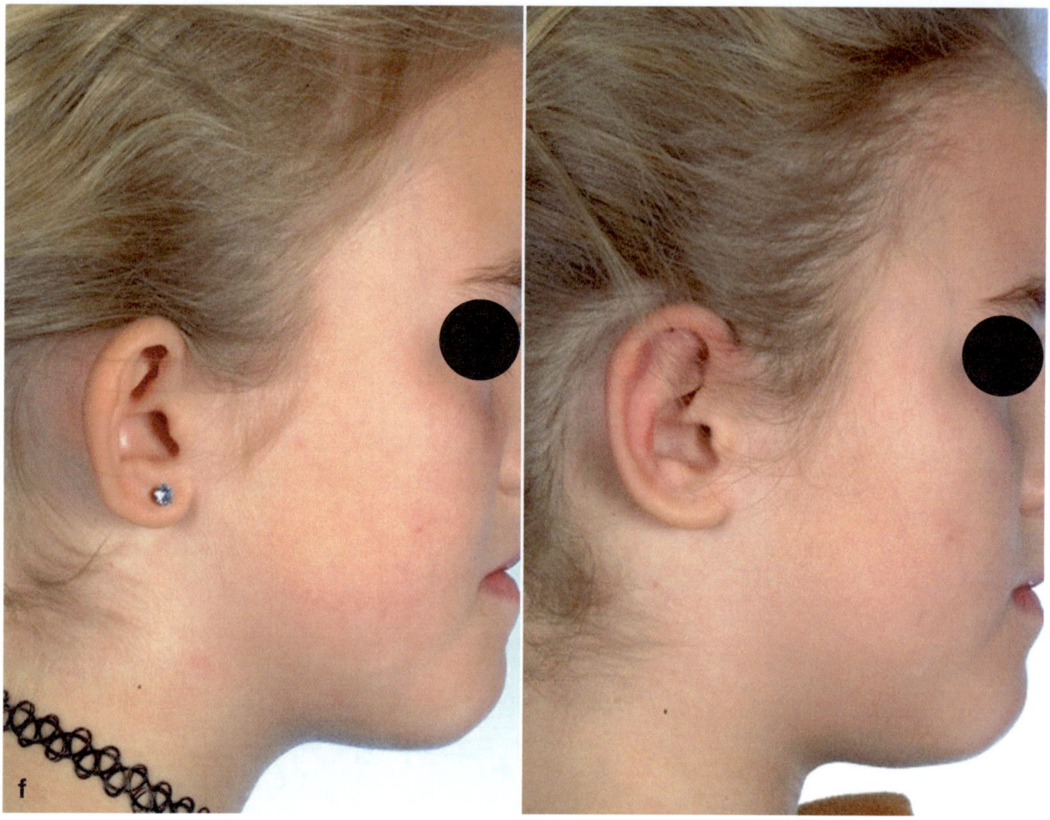

Fig. 13.4 (continued)

complication which may require reoperation if not amenable to local measures [23]. Insufficient hemostasis during surgery is the typical cause. Cartilage-scoring techniques are particularly more prone for hematoma formation [24]. Its development is heralded by disproportionate unilateral pain shortly after surgery [25]. Untreated hematomas can result in cauliflower deformities and elevate the risk of infection [25, 26]. Infection and chondritis are rare but may require re-exploration and removal of necrotic cartilage. A recent prospective study showed infection and cartilage necrosis rate at 0.44 % [24]. Suture protrusions on the other hand are quite common, particularly the nylon Mustarde sutures through the posterior skin. This complication may occur within the first few weeks postoperatively but usually years later [27]. Patients should be informed of this complication preoperatively and encouraged to return for follow-up. These sutures can usually be trimmed safely without endangering the reconstruction. If suture extrusion occurs several months postoperatively, the sutures can be removed.

The most common long-term complication is recurrence of the deformity, and patients need to be counseled preoperatively about this possibility. The surgical management discussed above minimizes the more serious complications, such as overcorrection, unnatural sharp contours, uneven setback, and telephone deformity. These typically manifest 6 months postoperatively and usually involve technical error. Telephone deformity results from uneven setback, leading to a C-shaped or telephone-shaped, helical contour with excessive protrusion of the lobule (Fig. 13.7). Fortunately, these more severe complications are preventable with

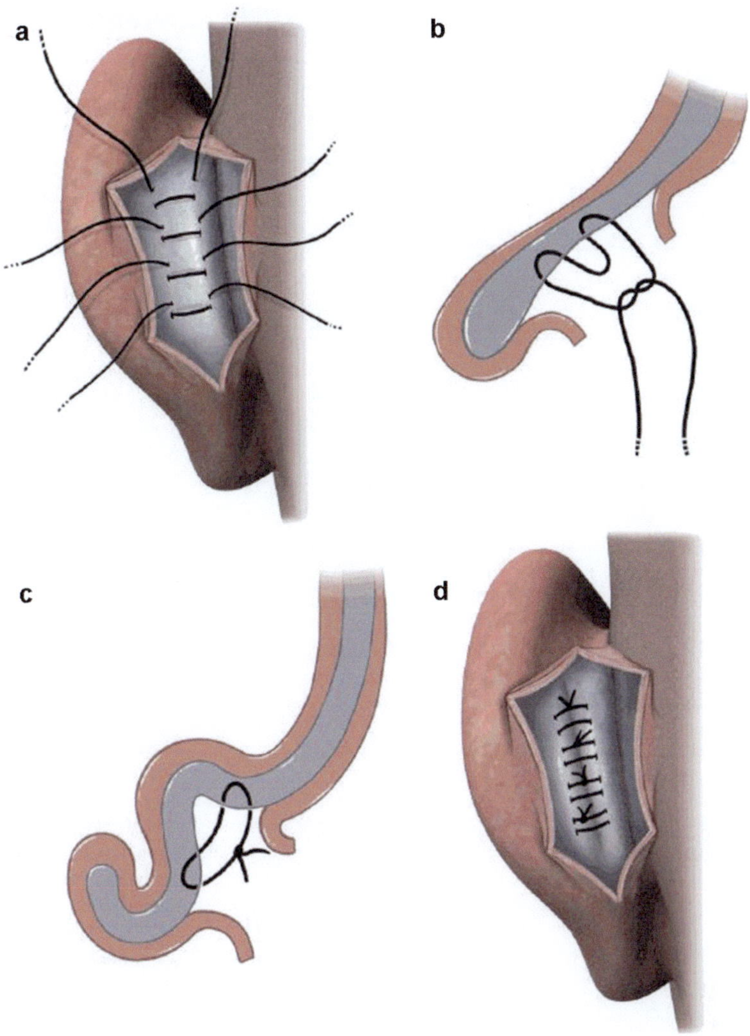

Fig. 13.5 Mustarde scaphoconchal sutures. (**a**–**d**) Five or six permanent, horizontal mattress sutures are typically needed to create the antihelix. The middle suture is tied last to prevent telephone ear deformity

good preoperative planning and careful technical execution.

Conclusions

Due to the large variety of available techniques, reconstruction of prominent ears is both highly versatile and also one of the more debated topics. Although the functional effects of the ear deformity are negligible, the psychological impact on a patient, particularly a child, can be profound and long lasting. The subjective nature of the perceived auricular projections makes "normalcy" difficult to define, despite quantitative measurements. Ultimately, the ears must be evaluated within the context of the face, while taking into consideration cultural and familial perceptions.

Prominence typically derives from varying degrees of antihelical hypoplasia or conchal bowl hyperplasia and is often associated with secondary auricular anomalies. A solid understanding of the anatomy of the ear is essential when choosing among the myriad of corrective techniques. A thoughtful and logical approach to reconstruction with careful surgical planning will provide consistent, optimized outcomes in form and symmetry.

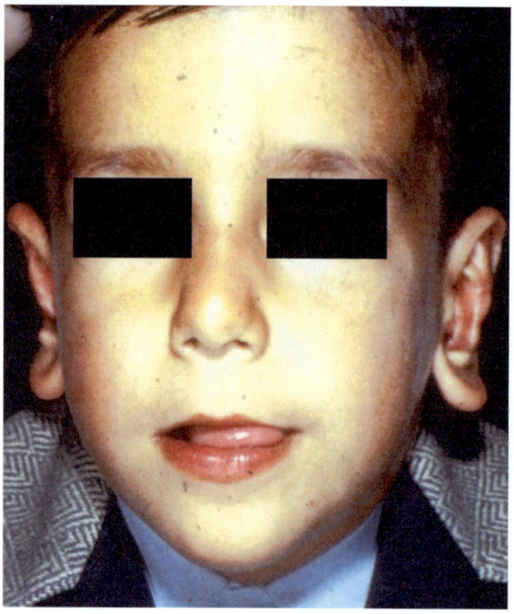

Fig. 13.6 Telephone ear deformity, marked by excessive projection of the lobule. The ear appears C-shaped from the lateral view. It can result from overtightening of Mustarde sutures

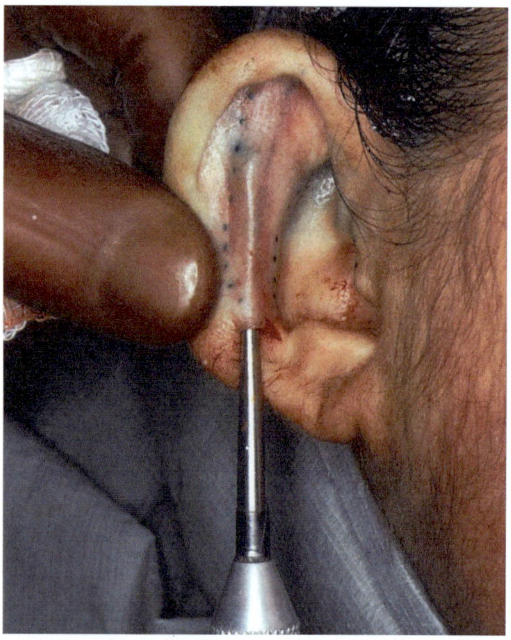

Fig. 13.7 Anterior cartilage scoring is necessary in more difficult cases with stiffer cartilage. A pocket is created to accommodate the otoabrader

References

1. Songu M, Adibelli H. Otoplasty in children younger than 5 years of age. Int J Pediatr Otorhinolaryngol. 2010;74(3):292–6.
2. Ambro BT, Lebeau J. Pediatric otoplasty. Oper Tech Otolaryngol Head Neck Surg. 2009;20:206–9.
3. Janz BA, Cole P, Hollier Jr LH, et al. Treatment of prominent and constricted ear anomalies. Plast Reconstr Surg. 2009;124(1 Suppl):27e–37.
4. Shonka Jr DC, Park SS. Ear defects. Facial Plast Surg Clin North Am. 2009;17(3):429–43.
5. Shaye D, Sykes JM. Reconstruction of acquired auricular deformity. Oper Tech Otolaryngol Head Neck Surg. 2011;22:47–52.
6. Tolleth H. Artistic anatomy, dimensions, and proportions of the external ear. Clin Plast Surg. 1978;5(3): 337–45.
7. Kösling S, Omenzetter M, Bartel-Friedrich S. Congenital malformations of the external and middle ear. Eur J Radiol. 2009;69(2):269–79.
8. Klockars T, Rautio J. Embryology and epidemiology of microtia. Facial Plast Surg. 2009;25(3):145–8.
9. Kelley P, Hollier L, Stal S. Otoplasty: evaluation, technique, and review. J Craniofac Surg. 2003;14(5): 643–53.
10. Byrd HS, Langevin CJ, Ghidoni LA. Ear molding in newborn infants with auricular deformities. Plast Reconstr Surg. 2010;126(4):1191–200.
11. McDowell AJ. Goals in otoplasty for protruding ears. Plast Reconstr Surg. 1968;41(1):17–27.
12. Ely ET. A classic reprint: an operation for prominence of the auricles (with two wood-cuts). Aesthetic Plast Surg. 1987;11(2):73–4.
13. Rogers BO. The classic reprint. A new operation for prominent ears based on the anatomy of the deformity by William H. Luckett, M.D. (reprinted from Surg Gynec Obst. 1910;10:635–7). Plast Reconstr Surg. 1969;43(1):83–6.
14. Mustardé JC. The correction of prominent ears using simple mattress sutures. Br J Plast Surg. 1963;16: 170–8.
15. Stenstroem SJ. A "natural" technique for correction of congenitally. Plast Reconstr Surg. 1963;32: 509–18.
16. Gibson T, Davis WB. The distortion of autogenous cartilage grafts: its cause and prevention. Br J Plast Surg. 1957;10:257–74.
17. Furnas DW. Correction of prominent ears by conchamastoid sutures. Plast Reconstr Surg. 1968;42(3): 189–93.
18. Elliott RA. Otoplasty: a combined approach. Clin Plast Surg. 1990;17(2):373–81.
19. Webster GV. The tail of the helix as a key to otoplasty. Plast Reconstr Surg. 1969;44(5):455–61.
20. Mustardé JC. The treatment of prominent ears by buried mattress sutures: a ten-year survey. Plast Reconstr Surg. 1967;39(4):382–6.

21. Spira M, Stal S. The conchal flap: an adjunct in otoplasty. Ann Plast Surg. 1983;11(4):291–8.
22. Wood-Smith D. Aesthetic plastic surgery. Philadelphia: Saunders; 1980.
23. Hoehn JG, Ashruf S. Otoplasty: sequencing the operation for improved results. Plast Reconstr Surg. 2005;115(1):5e–16.
24. Sinha M, Richard B. Postauricular fascial flap and suture otoplasty: a prospective outcome study of 227 patients. J Plast Reconstr Aesthet Surg. 2012;65(3):367–71.
25. Limandjaja GC, Breugem CC, van der Molen AB M, Kon M. Complications of otoplasty: a literature review. J Plast Reconstr Aesthet Surg. 2009;62:19–27.
26. Campbell AC. Otoplasty. Facial Plast Surg. 2005;21(4):310–6.
27. Thorne CH, Wilkes G. Ear deformities, otoplasty, and ear reconstruction. Plast Reconstr Surg. 2012;129(4):701e–16.

14 Precision and Suture Positioning in Otoplasty: Aspiring to the "Virgin" Ear

Kayvan Shokrollahi

Introduction

The ultimate goal in otoplasty is to achieve a natural result. While symmetry is important, the other crucial aspect is a natural shape to the ear. Many surgeons in the past have dismissed suture otoplasty as a technique that gives unnatural results. This is undoubtedly the case in the hands of an inexperienced surgeon or one whom has not understood the dynamics of the ear and its manipulation with sutures to create a natural result. However, the author believes that the most consistent and natural results are achieved with variations on suture techniques. My otoplasty practice has been based on the goal of a "virgin ear," whereby the ears have settled into a natural and symmetrical shape as soon as possible after surgery such that they do not look operated upon. This is very simple to achieve when following the recommendations below.

Suture Techniques Versus Anterior Scoring

Many surgeons routinely use anterior scoring methods that require degloving of the ear and get very good results. However, when complications do occur, these can be severe and potentially uncorrectable. Complications aside, a more holistic approach to surgery can be undertaken whereby patients have less bruising and are in less discomfort as their ear has not been degloved, they do not need head bandages, and they can shower the next day [1, 2]. These additional and important positive patient outcomes are difficult to achieve with cartilage scoring methods. The general techniques the author concentrates on are scar positioning, positioning and tying of Mustarde sutures, use of Furnas (concha-mastoid) sutures, and use of fascial flaps.

Preoperative Counseling and Managing Patient Expectations

Even more important than these surgical techniques is an in-depth discussion with the patient to realize their expectations. Some may not be happy unless they are slightly overcorrected, and others may have specific issues with parts of their ears that seem unusual to the surgeon. On many occasions the author has stood with a mirror with patients and bargained with them regarding their ear position. The author often suggests a position which is natural and that surgical colleagues would approve of, but the patient will adjust their ears to the position they want. In about 15 % of cases, this position will be slight overcorrection and 5 % very overcorrected. The author will slightly overcorrect both these groups, firstly because the patient will not be happy otherwise

K. Shokrollahi, M.D., BSc, MB, ChB, MSc, LLM, MRCS(Eng), FRCS(Plast)
Mersey Regional Burns and Plastic Surgery Unit, Ward 4D, Whiston Hospital, Warrington Rd, Liverpool L35 5DR, UK
e-mail: kshokrollahi@hotmail.com

M.A. Shiffman (ed.), *Advanced Cosmetic Otoplasty*,
DOI 10.1007/978-3-642-35431-1_14, © Springer-Verlag Berlin Heidelberg 2013

and secondly because what we perceive to be "overcorrected ears" actually occur naturally in many individuals if one cares to observe passersby. Nevertheless, the majority of patients will agree with my recommendation of a natural corrected position for their ears.

Scar Position

Where to position a skin incision or excision? Using the posterior approach is undoubtedly superior as it is hidden both as a scar and as a potential keloid scar complication. The general principles of scar positioning relate to visibility and surgical access. There is no question that placing the skin incision anterior/lateral to that described "traditionally" is of great benefit. The incision is best placed in the posterior groove of the helix and where the helix casts a shadow over the posterior of the ear. This scar is less visible when stood behind a patient, whereas scars in the center of the posterior ear or in the auriculocephalic sulcus are more visible. Secondly, access to the superior pole of the ear and the outer aspect of the ear is simpler. This allows for very accurate suture positioning to create specific and gentle corrections of parts of the ear, especially the tip. A "lop" ear is often encountered when using suture correction. When the tip of the ear droops downward, good access to the tip of the helical cartilage and positioning of a specific trajectory of suture downward will correct this problem very easily with a gentle and subtle suture tie. Raising a substantial fascial flap based on the helix is facilitated that can be used for a number of purposes.

Positioning and Tying of Mustarde Sutures

The most crucial element to a good result in suture otoplasty is the positioning of the Mustarde sutures. This will be the difference between an unnatural angulated and overcorrected appearance and an ear that is natural and appropriately corrected. I now undertake these suture positions by eye intraoperatively, but one technique that can be used is to create and then skewer the correct antihelical fold using a fine gauge syringe needle (Fig. 14.1) [3]. These can be left in or subsequently marked with ink as per the surgeons' preference. Three Mustarde sutures are usually sufficient, but if required, there should be no hesitation to using additional ones.

To achieve the most natural correction, the author recommends positioning and then tying the Mustarde sutures from inferior to superior. The reason is that the crucial superior pole of the ear should be a subtle and gentle "final correction" after all other sutures are positioned and tied. The sharp angular and overcorrected look is in my opinion most commonly seen because the superior pole was tied first. In addition to angularity, this means that the superior pole is always overcorrected because when both the central and inferior sutures are tied, they will cause further posterior movement of the superior pole, even if slight. By tying the inferior suture first, which gives only a very slight correction initially, and then the central suture, the final correction

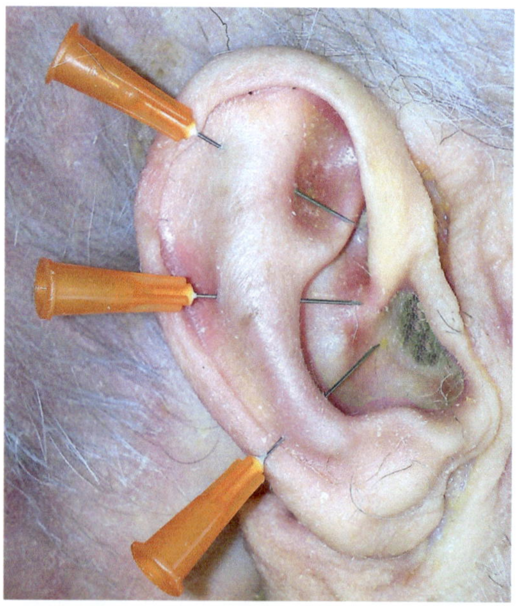

Fig. 14.1 Orange needles used to create and maintain antihelix, providing accurate localization for positioning of Mustarde sutures

required at the superior pole is much milder, without angularity, and can be judged with millimeter precision in comparison to the scalp.

4/0 Ticron or 4/0 Ethibond sutures are recommended. These can be found on suitably curved semicircular needles that are less easily lost in the tissues. These braided sutures anecdotally appear to form less rigid/crystalline knots that are less likely to extrude and are more resistant to fracture if weakened by stray needle damage. An anteriorly based fascial flap sutured to the mastoid combined with skin glue as postoperative splint will ensure almost no tension remains on these suture knots by the end of surgery [1, 2].

Furnas/Concha-Mastoid Sutures

Since using a fascial flap, which itself rotates the ear when sutured to the mastoid, there is reduced need for these sutures. However, their use to rotate the ear before positioning and tying Mustarde sutures is important for those ears with large and deep conchal bowls. When used to give gentle rotation, it ensures that the effect of subsequent Mustarde sutures is more reserved and gentle, ensuring a more natural contour with less angularity. Only in the most severe cases is the excision of cartilage ellipse required from the conchal bowl. I avoid this technique.

Fascial Flap

The author would encourage any surgeon undertaking suture otoplasty to raise a fascial flap [2]. This is simple and does not impact on differing techniques. However, raising and manipulating the flap when based on the helix allow the surgeon to experiment without changing their usual operative strategy.

References

1. Shokrollahi K, Cooper MA, Hiew LY. A new strategy for otoplasty. J Plast Reconstr Aesthet Surg. 2009;62(6):774–81.
2. Shokrollahi K, Tanner B. "Glue Ear": beginning of the end for head bandages after prominent ear correction? J Plast Reconstr Aesthet Surg. 2008;61(9):1077.
3. Mathur BS, Shokrollahi K. Precision and suture positioning in otoplasty. Experience with 380 cases. J Plast Reconstr Aesthet Surg. 2010;63(3):571–2.

Otoplasty with Mustarde Suture Cartilage Scratching and Rasping

15

Kutlu Sevin and Asuman Sevin

Introduction

Otoplasty is performed by different surgical specialities including otorhinolaryngology, plastic surgery, and maxillofacial surgery. As a result many papers have been published describing different techniques. However, the best technique may be the one that is flexible, simple, and versatile. Correction of prominent ears was first successfully conducted by Dieffenbach [1] to correct a post-traumatic prominent auricle in a patient. He excised retroauricular skin and used a conchomastoidal suture for the fixation of the ear. In 1910, Luckett [2] combined a skin-cartilage excision along the antihelical fold with horizontal mattress sutures to achieve a better formation of the scapha. Since then more than 200 surgical techniques have been described for this condition indicating that no single ideal technique has been universally adopted. Modern otoplasty techniques are based on two main surgical categories, cartilage sparing and cartilage cutting, along with many nuances. The anterior scoring methods, as described by Stenstrom [3] and Chongchet [4], are the most commonly performed cartilage-scoring procedures. However, these methods have been criticized for their complications, such as hematoma, anterior skin necrosis, chondritis, and irreparable cartilage damage [5]. Conchoscaphoid suturing to create the antihelical fold [6] and conchomastoid suturing to rotate the conchal angle [7] are commonly described cartilage sparing methods.

Renewed interest in suture-based techniques evolved through advances led by Horlock et al. [6] whom introduced the idea of using a proximally based fascial flap beneath which permanent sutures could be buried to prevent extrusion. Schaverien [8] stated good results using a proximally based fascial flap to cover the internal permanent sutures and reduce the risk of suture extrusion. Shokrollahi et al. [9] went further using a distally based fascial flap successfully.

Conchal reduction has been performed using various techniques. However, the use of conchomastoidal suturing was popularized by Furnas [10] and later modified by Spira et al. [11]. Becker [12] introduced the method involving a combination of cartilage incisions and suture techniques to soften the contour of the corrected prominent ear. This technique was refined later by Converse and Wood-Smith [13] in 1963. Mustarde' s [14] approach to the creation of antihelical tubing was to use permanent conchoscaphal mattress sutures.

K. Sevin, M.D. (✉)
Plastic Reconstructive and Aesthetic Surgery Department, Faculty of Medicine, Ankara University, 435. Cadde 72/53, Cankaya, Ankara 06550, Turkey
e-mail: ksevin@gmail.com

A. Sevin, M.D.
Plastic Reconstructive and Aesthetic Surgery Department,
Ankara Numune Training and Research Hospital, 435. Cadde 72/53, Cankaya, Ankara 06550, Turkey
e-mail: basevin@gmail.com

M.A. Shiffman (ed.), *Advanced Cosmetic Otoplasty*,
DOI 10.1007/978-3-642-35431-1_15, © Springer-Verlag Berlin Heidelberg 2013

Technique

The patient is prepared and draped. Subcutaneous injection of 1 % lidocaine with 1 in 100,000 epinephrine is used for local anesthesia along the posterior portion of the pinna. Using a no. 15 blade scalpel, an ellipse of postauricular skin is excised in the subdermal plane to optimize exposure. The amount of skin removed is determined by folding the pinna back and marking the superior and inferior fixation points needed to hold the antihelical roll. A vertical postauricular skin ellipse is excised 2–2.5 cm lateral to the sulcus. Skin flaps are elevated for access to the helical rim, scapha, and mastoid fascia. The perichondrium is cut along the antihelix line carefully sparing the cartilage, and then the perichondrium is first elevated by eye scissors and then by an elevator. After hemostasis, the antihelix line is softened with rasping and scratching. The cartilage is thinned to about 30 % of its thickness by the use of a surgical blade. Three Mustarde sutures are placed, superior, middle, and inferior, using 4-0 white polyester material. Two conchomastoidal sutures are placed superior and inferior. The sutures must contain both the anterior and posterior perichondrium, although great care must be taken to avoid inclusion of the anterior auricular skin. The inferior sutures are tied first, leaving the superior suture until last, to provide the best correction because the upper-pole suture should be tied to position the ear finally at appropriate distance from the side of the head. This distance cannot be correctly defined if the uppermost suture is tied first, as the distance will change when the lower sutures are tied. In case of protruding earlobe, a single lobule deep dermis-to-scalp periosteum suture is placed without wedge excision. The skin is closed with 4-0 absorbable sutures in continuous fashion. Following skin closure, the auricle is packed with moist cotton to maintain skin flexibility and the shape of the new auricle. A bolster of cotton is applied to prevent pressure ischemia or necrosis, followed by an external bandage. On the first postoperative day, the dressing is removed for evaluation and replaced again with a light dressing. The auricle is packed anteriorly and posteriorly to avoid maceration. A protective bandage is worn for 4 days, and patients are advised to continue wearing it at night for another 2 weeks. Prophylactic oral antibiotics are routinely continued for 1 week postoperatively.

Results

The authors performed a retrospective study of patients who underwent otoplasty from 2002 to 2009, using Mustarde suturing and cartilage softening by scalpel scratching and rasping. All of the patients have undergone the same procedure under local anesthesia. Only bilaterally affected patients were included. Of the 132 patients (264 primary otoplasties), 83 (63 %) were female and 49 (37 %) were male (Fig. 15.1). For nine patients, a secondary revision was performed for recurrence (Table 15.1). Postauricular keloid was found around the scar area after 1 year in two cases. The lesions were excised and treated with intralesional injection of triamcinolone acetonide successfully. Wound infection occurred in one patient. Suture extrusion was found in five cases. The remaining patients were satisfied with the outcome.

Discussion

The goals of otoplasty as described by McDowell [15] include (1) the helix should be just visible beyond the antihelix when the patient is viewed from the front, (2) protrusion of the upper one-third of the ear must be corrected, (3) the helix should have a smooth and regular line throughout, (4) the postauricular sulcus should not be markedly decreased or distorted, (5) the ear should not be inset too close to the head, and (6) the ear position should be within 3 mm between both ears. Modern otoplasty techniques are mainly based on two surgical categories, cartilage sparing and cartilage cutting along with different variations. The common aim of these methods is to create an ear that appears normal with acceptable protrusion, symmetry, and form. A good understanding of the anatomic features allows the surgeon to treat the patients effectively. Techniques that are based on scoring can be subdivided further into those that only superficially score the cartilage and those that score deeply enough to cut through the newly created antihelix. The scoring can be accomplished on either the anterior or posterior surface of the ear cartilage. In general, however, full-thickness penetration of the cartilage usually results in a sharper antihelical fold, which is not desirable [11, 16].

Scoring techniques are mainly based on the studies of Gibson and Davis [17] that the cartilage tends to warp away from an injured surface. Stenstrom [3] and Chongchet [4] applied this theory to otoplasty. Stenstrom's initial technique scored the anterior scapha to produce an antihelical fold and later modified his technique by adding a posterior approach [18]. Fry [19] studied human nasal septal cartilage and proposed that interlocked stresses released by partial-thickness incisions on one side of in vitro septal cartilage strips result in bending away from the side incised due to unopposed tensile stresses on the intact side. Later, however, in vitro studies in 1982 by Murakami et al. [20] on human septal cartilage strips found inconsistent results with partial-thickness cuts. Today, the exact mechanism for the observed warping behavior of cartilage is still a matter of debate.

Many different instruments have been used within different centers to warp the cartilage. Stenstrom and Heftner [18] scratched the cartilage surface anteriorly with razor blades. Later, devices reported for cartilage scoring include rasps, hypodermic needles [21], and dermabrasion tool [22]. Qureshi et al. [23] studied the use of bipolar

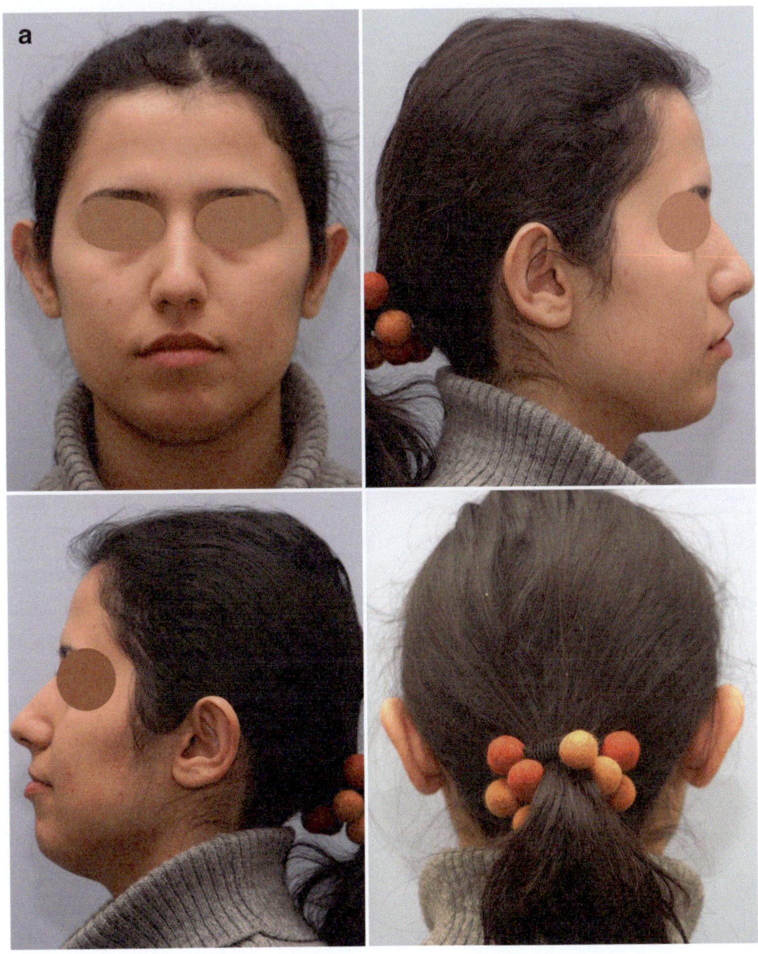

Fig. 15.1 (**a**) Preoperative view of 23-year-old female. (**b**) Six months postoperative view after otoplasty with Mustarde suture cartilage scratching and rasping

Fig 15.1 (continued)

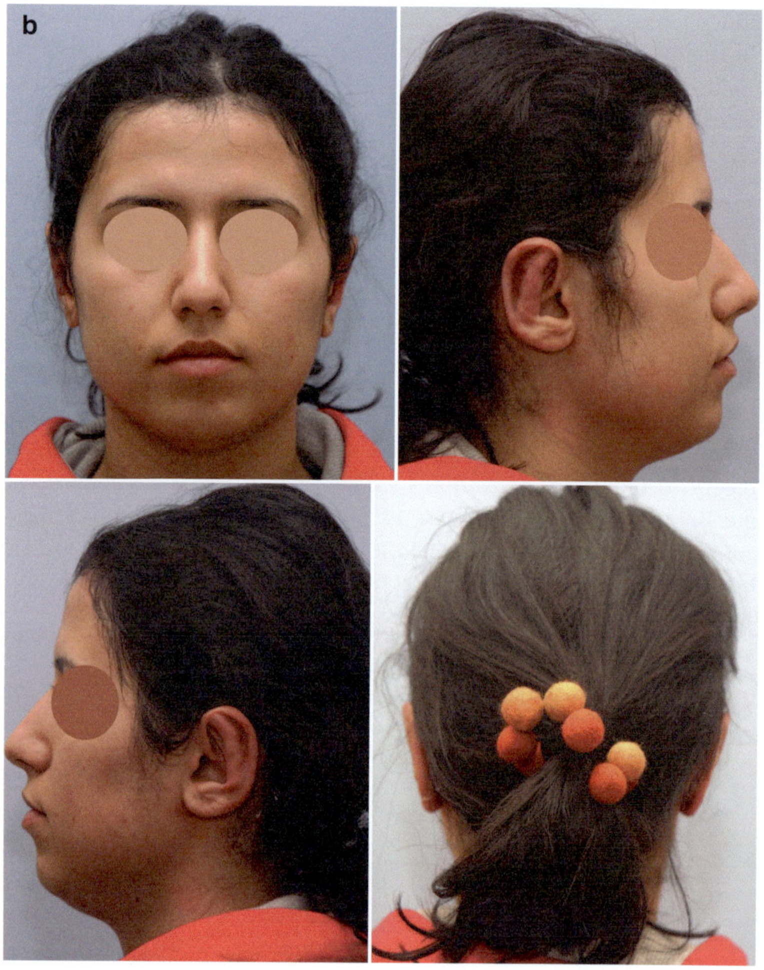

Table 15.1 Complications of otoplasty with Mustarde suture in a study of 132 cases

Complication	Number of cases	Percentage
Bleeding	2	1.5
Infection	1	0.7
Suture extrusion	5	3.8
Recurrence	9	6.8
Keloid	2	1.5

cautery to achieve a similar effect in an ex vivo pig ear model. No statistical difference was found in the degree of warping caused by either scalpel scoring or bipolar cautery. We should note that the desired amount of cartilage warping can be adjusted by the extent of the scratching and rasping. In our clinical practice, a scalpel blade is the usual and preferred method to scratch and rasp the cartilage. Contrary to a general belief that the cartilage tends to warp away from an injured surface, we were able to achieve an adequate antihelical fold by warping and rasping the posterior surface of the ear cartilage to produce a thin cartilage. Thus, no anterior approach for the cartilage was necessary, also eliminating the risk of anterior hematoma or bruising.

Excision techniques used to reduce conchal hypertrophy can be grouped into those that excise cartilage alone and those that excise both skin and cartilage [24]. Luckett's [2] procedure to create a new antihelical fold involved excising a crescent segment of cartilage from the posterior and reapproximating the remaining edges to each other. However, this creates a sharp fold with an unnatural appearance. The cartilage-only techniques are usually performed through a posterior approach, whereas the skin and cartilage techniques generally are performed using an anterior approach. Neither of the approaches has a proven advantage, and the choice is a matter of personal preference.

The Converse technique is an example of a classic, yet complicated, cartilage-cutting technique [13, 25]. Parallel, full-thickness cartilaginous incisions are made along the conchal rim and the desired antihelical fold to form an island of cartilage, which is then tubed and secured with sutures to create the new antihelical fold. Pitanguy [26] described a simpler technique which involves the formation of a smaller cartilage island by parallel incisions in the region of the desired antihelical fold; this island is then projected forward to create an antihelical fold by approximating the cartilage with mattress sutures. In 2011, Maricevich [27] reviewed their results of the Pitanguy island technique and stated that it is a simple and reliable method for carefully selected case since it is not appropriate for patients who have a normal antihelix.

Pilz et al. [22] modified the technique originally described by Stark and Saunders [28] by combining the posterior skin excision with controlled dermabrasion of the posterior cartilage surface. However, we believe that there is no need for cartilage abrasion, as it is possible to obtain the same result simply by scratching and rasping with a blade.

Reports in the literature on complication rates and especially long-term results have been few. Complications after otoplasty can be divided into early and late stage, with the former occurring up to 14 days postoperatively and the latter occurring after the initial 14-day period [29]. In the early phase, bleeding, hematoma, and infection are most seen complications [30]. Insufficient hemostasis during surgery or other errors in surgical technique are the usual reasons leading to hematoma formation. In our study, bleeding was seen in two cases and infection in one case (Table 15.1). Late complications include suture extrusion, scarring, asymmetry, and unsatisfactory results. Suture extrusion may be the result of either incorrectly placed sutures too close to the skin, tension on cartilage, or infection [31]. Abnormal scar formation includes hypertrophic scarring or keloid formation. Unsatisfactory results include overcorrection, undercorrection, recurrence, telephone deformities or reverse telephone deformities, and cartilage irregularities. Recurrence of prominent ear may be the result of postoperative trauma, insufficient cartilage weakening, and suture failure or insufficiency. Late complications especially recurrence can require revision surgery.

Mustarde suture and cartilage softening has been our preferred method for correcting the protruding ear. Cartilage softening with scratching provides a softer and narrower antihelix fold. With the use of this technique, the anterior skin overlying the concha is left undisturbed. The authors do not excise cartilage because it is believed the edges of the excised cartilage form a sharp unnatural antihelix. The authors also believe that the use of braided polyester suture prevents loosening of the knots. Polyester is more pliable than nylon, and the color of the suture material is very important because the sutures are close to the skin; they may become visible in time.

References

1. Dieffenbach JF. Die operative Chirurgie. Leipzig: F.A. Brockhaus; 1845.
2. Luckett WH. A new operation for prominent ears based on the anatomy of the deformity. Surg Gynecol Obstet. 1910;10:635–7.
3. Stenstroem SJ. A natural technique for correction of congenitally prominent ears. Plast Reconstr Surg. 1963;32:509–18.
4. Chongchet V. A method of antihelix reconstruction. Br J Plast Surg. 1963;16:268–72.
5. Calder JC, Naasan A. Morbidity of otoplasty: a review of 562 consecutive cases. Br J Plast Surg. 1994; 47(3):170–4.
6. Horlock N, Misra A, Gault DT. The post auricular fascial flap as an adjunct to Mustarde and Furnas type otoplasty. Plast Reconstr Surg. 2001;108(6):1487–90.
7. Mustarde JC. Correction of prominent ears with multiple sutures. Clin Plast Surg. 1978;5(3):459–64.
8. Schaverien MV, Al-Busaidi S, Stewart KJ. Long-term results of posterior suturing with postauricular fascial flap otoplasty. J Plast Reconstr Aesthet Surg. 2010; 63(9):1447–51.
9. Shokrollahi K, Cooper MA, Hiew LY. A new strategy for otoplasty. J Plast Reconstr Aesthet Surg. 2009;62(6):774–81.

10. Furnas DW. Correction of prominent ears by conchamastoid sutures. Plast Reconstr Surg. 1968; 42(3):189–93.
11. Spira M, McCrea R, Gerow FJ, Hardy SB. Correction of the principal deformities causing protruding ears. Plast Reconstr Surg. 1969;44(2):150–4.
12. Becker OJ. Correction of protruding deformed ear. Br J Plast Surg. 1952;5(3):187–96.
13. Converse JM, Wood-Smith D. Technical details in the surgical correction of the lop ear deformity. Plast Reconstr Surg. 1963;31:118–28.
14. Mustarde JC. The correction of prominent ears using simple mattress sutures. Br J Plast Surg. 1963;16:170–8.
15. McDowell AJ. Goals in otoplasty for protruding ears. Plast Reconstr Surg. 1968;41(1):17–27.
16. Elliott Jr RA. Complications in the treatment of prominent ears. Clin Plast Surg. 1978;5(3):479–90.
17. Gibson T, Davis W. The distortion of autogenous cartilage grafts: its cause and prevention. Br J Plast Surg. 1958;10:257–74.
18. Stenstrom SJ, Heftner J. The Stenstrom otoplasty. Clin Plast Surg. 1978;5(3):465–70.
19. Fry HJ. Interlocked stresses in human nasal septal cartilage. Br J Plast Surg. 1966;19(3):276–8.
20. Murakami WT, Wong LW, Davidson TM. Applications of the biomechanical behaviour of cartilage to nasal septoplastic surgery. Laryngoscope. 1982;92(3):300–9.
21. Mahler D. The correction of the prominent ear. Aesthetic Plast Surg. 1986;10(1):29–33.
22. Pilz S, Hintringer T, Bauer M. Otoplasty using a spherical metal head dermabrador to form a retroauricular furrow: five-year results. Aesthetic Plast Surg. 1995;19(1):83–91.
23. Qureshi TR, Hurren JS, Gourlay T. The effectiveness of scoring and bipolar diathermy on ear cartilage behavior: ex vivo study. Ann Plast Surg. 2007;58(3): 321–7.
24. Janis JE, Rohrich RJ, Gutowski KA. Otoplasty. Plast Reconstr Surg. 2005;115(4):60e–72.
25. Converse JM, Nigro A, Wilson FA, Johnson N. A technique for surgical correction of lop ears. Plast Reconstr Surg. 1955;15(5):411–8.
26. Pitanguy I, Müller P, Piccolo N, Ramalho E, Solinas R. The treatment of prominent ears: a 25-year survey of the island technique. Aesthetic Plast Surg. 1987; 11(2):87–93.
27. Maricevich P, de Gontijo Amorim NF, Duprat R, Freitas F, Pitanguy I. Island technique for prominent ears: an update of the Ivo Pitanguy clinic experience. Aesthet Surg J. 2011;31(6):623–33.
28. Stark RB, Saunders DE. Natural appearance restored to the unduly prominent ear. Br J Plast Surg. 1962;15: 385–97.
29. Weerda H, Siegert R. Complications in otoplastic surgery and their treatment. Facial Plast Surg. 1994;10(3): 287–97.
30. Limandjaja GC, Breugem CC, van der Mink Molen AB, Kon M. Complications of otoplasty: a literature review. J Plast Reconstr Aesthet Surg. 2009;62(1): 19–27.
31. Campbell AC. Otoplasty. Facial Plast Surg. 2005; 21(4):310–6.

The Négrevergne Otoplasty Technique

16

Murat Songu

Introduction

Otoplasty is a century-old procedure that has undergone many modifications over the years. Over 200 different procedures have been described in the literature that excise, bend, suture, scratch, or reposition the auricular cartilage. This plenty of surgical techniques show that no simple "best" technique exists.

The Négrevergne otoplasty technique is a simple method of cartilage weakening mainly preferred in young children in our practice [1]. This technique was developed by Michel Négrevergne and adopted in the Georges Portmann Institute in France [2]. In Négrevergne otoplasty technique, a surgical instrument (monopolar diathermy) which is already present in the surgical field is used. Since this technique is suture-free, low-complication rates can be obtained. Common complications such as suture failures and extrusions, suture material-induced foreign-body granulomas, and wound breakdown are never observed. In this chapter, preoperative issues are discussed; perioperative routine and the surgical technique are described in step-by-step detail.

M. Songu, M.D.
Department of Otorhinolaryngology,
Izmir Ataturk Research and Training Hospital,
Izmir 35360, Turkey

Department of Otorhinolaryngology,
Dr. Behçet Uz Children's Hospital,
Izmir, Turkey
e-mail: songumurat@yahoo.com

Preoperative Issues

The most common indication for performing otoplasty is the prominent ear (Fig. 16.1). Other indications for otoplasty include trauma, cupped ear deformity, or to correct a previous poor result. Anatomic norms for human ears have been established; thus, it is possible to more objectively quantify patients who have irregular, prominent ears. Janis and Rohrich summarized the proportions that are common in the normal, aesthetic ear (Table 16.1) [3–9].

While the measurements and proportions of a "normal" ear have been well documented, the position of anatomical landmarks and relation to one another at the end of the otoplasty procedure are far more important. The ears must look proportional to the facial features and have a natural appearance. Prominent ear occurs as a result of one or more anatomic variants. Most often there is a lack of an adequate antihelix; the ear is less furled back on itself and thus protrudes from the skull. Another common anatomic finding in patients with prominent ears is a relative excess of conchal bowl cartilage. A third component can be an ear lobule that is excessive in size or positioned laterally. The basic goals of otoplasty were summarized by McDowell in 1968 and are listed in Table 16.2 [3].

The appropriate time for the correction of prominent ears should depend on a rational approach based on auricular growth and age of school matriculation. Although the concern for ridicule and its effect on social development has been clearly

M.A. Shiffman (ed.), *Advanced Cosmetic Otoplasty*,
DOI 10.1007/978-3-642-35431-1_16, © Springer-Verlag Berlin Heidelberg 2013

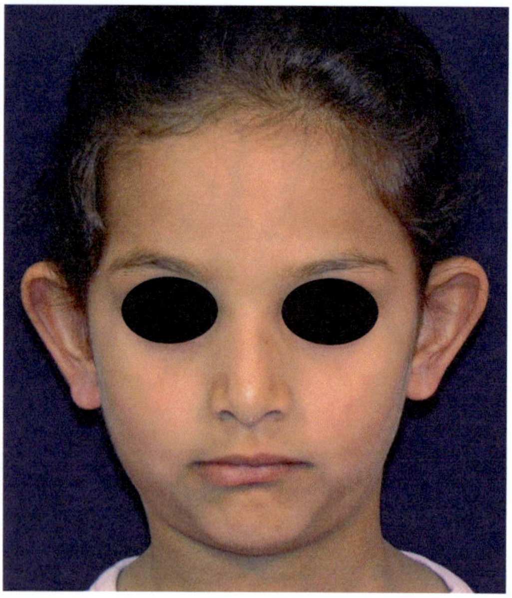

Fig. 16.1 Prominent ears showing increased helix-mastoid angle, antihelical hypoplasia, cavum hyperplasia, and protruding lobule

Table 16.1 Proportions of the aesthetic ear

The long axis of the ear inclines posteriorly at approximately a 20° angle from the vertical
The ear axis does not normally parallel the bridge of the nose (the angle differential is approximately 15°)
The ear is positioned at approximately one ear length (5.5–7 cm) posterior to the lateral orbital rim between horizontal planes that intersect the eyebrow and columella
The width is approximately 50–60 % of the length (width, 3–4.5 cm; length, 5.5–7 cm)
The anterolateral aspect of the helix protrudes at a 21–30° angle from the scalp
The anterolateral aspect of the helix measures approximately 1.5–2 cm from the scalp (although there is a large amount of racial and gender variation)
The lobule and antihelical fold lie in a parallel plane at an acute angle to the mastoid process
The helix should project 2–5 mm more laterally than the antihelix on frontal view

illustrated, many children are not referred for otoplasty until teasing becomes an issue [10, 11]. Otoplasty procedure in children is recommended to be performed prior to the start of schooling [12]. The hope is to correct the malformation before the time of socialization in order to minimize ridicule by peers. However, substantial psychological pressure exposed to children with protruding ears among the peers at the preschool period or in kindergarten is usually underestimated. Changing socioeconomic trends have increased the proportion of families in which both parents work outside of the home. As a result, children have been increasingly exposed to peers through daycare centers well before age 4 or 5 years. This intense early exposure to peers and caretakers outside of the family may significantly affect development of self-esteem. We observed that these children can provide information about their psychological strain or possible problems with other children associated with their protruding ears. Furthermore, these children can also express concern about the abnormal appearance of their ears before age five [13].

Table 16.2 McDowell's basic goals of otoplasty

All upper third ear protrusion must be corrected
The helix of both ears should be seen beyond the antihelix from the front view
The helix should have a smooth and regular line throughout
The postauricular sulcus should not be markedly decreased or distorted
The helix to mastoid distance should fall in the normal range of 10–12 mm in the upper third, 16–18 mm in the middle third, and 20–22 mm in the lower third
The position of the lateral ear border to the head should match within 3 mm at any point between the two ears

Like many procedures involving the child's face, there is a concern about how the operative site will respond to pressures of normal growth. Until recently, very few surgeons felt comfortable operating on the ear of a young child due to concerns about longevity and altered growth. Adamson et al. studied the growth patterns of the external ear of 2,300 ears and showed that the ear reaches 85 % of its adult size by 3 years of age [14]. On the other hand, Farkas differed some in his measurements stating that the ears reach 85 % of full size by age 6, 90 % by age 9, and 95 % by age 14 [15]. Balogh and Millesi were the only authors to objectively study growth alterations following otoplasty and concluded that growth of the ear is not arrested following otoplasty [16]. Recently, Gosain and colleagues reported that otoplasty can be safely performed under age 4

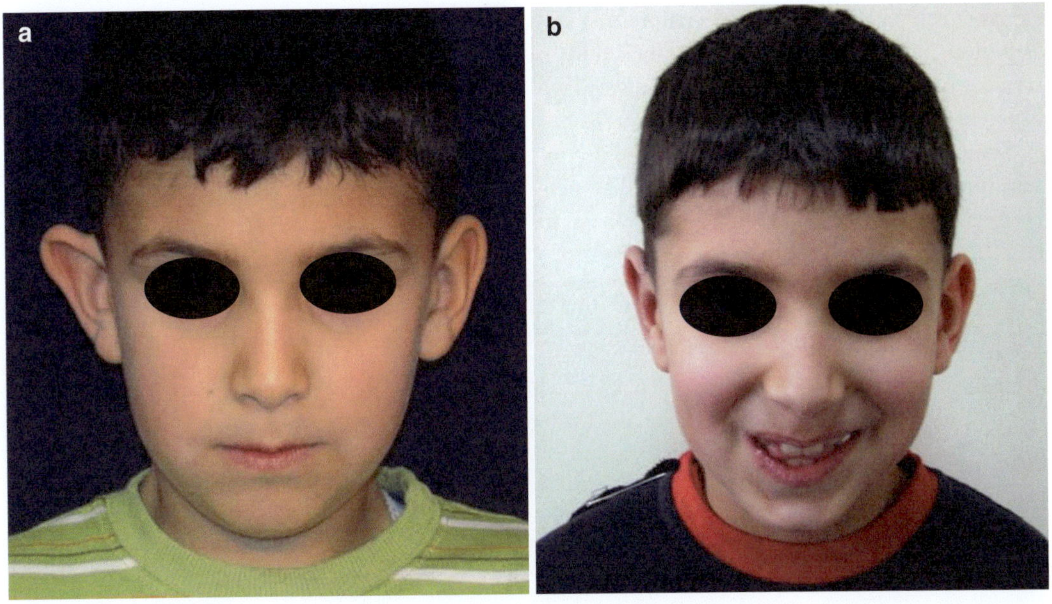

Fig. 16.2 (**a**) Preoperative. (**b**) Postoperative after undergoing right unilateral otoplasty and adenoidectomy that demonstrates the normal growth of the ear that had been operated on relative to the unaffected ear

and as young as 9 months without significant effect on ear growth in a cohort of 12 patients with prominent ears [17, 18]. Due to our experience, in unilateral "Jumbo" ears, we observed that the protruding ear is usually bigger than the unaffected ear in all dimensions. Growth alteration should be a desired consequence among these patients, and this desire is another rationale for the early surgical intervention. Nevertheless, we did not observe any visible disturbance or growth restriction in our patients, even in the unilateral operated group (Fig. 16.2).

An important advantage of performing otoplasty at these younger ages is the increased malleability of the auricular cartilage, decreasing the need to use cartilage-cutting techniques. At this age, the auricular cartilage is characteristically pliable; however, elasticity decreases with advancing age, often demanding more aggressive treatment. The softer the auricular cartilage, the easier it is to shape the cartilage or auricle into the appropriate form and pin it back, using gentle surgical techniques. The Négrevergne otoplasty technique was popularized in the Georges Portmann Institute in France. The technique includes partial-thickness posterior scoring of the auricular cartilage using monopolar cutting diathermy. Because the ear cartilage is weak under age five, cartilage scoring can be conservative, sufficient to release the cartilage spring only.

The main disadvantage of the surgery before age five is postoperative difficulties dealing with the dressing. The procedure is best performed when the auricle has reached maturation and the child is old enough to cooperate with the postoperative care. It must be kept in mind that correction before age five may complicate the postoperative course when the child, even if not intentionally, pulls apart the bandage and potentially disrupts the repair. Our practice has shown that all of the study patients were followed by multiple extra visits for redressings and their fingers were constantly inside the bandage which resulted in more swelling and certainly greater risk of postoperative complications. Nevertheless, at the end of the follow-up period, no serious complications occurred, and the patient showed full recovery in our series (Fig. 16.3) [13].

Another aspect with significant impact on procedure planning is the analysis of the cartilage consistency and, in particular, the stiffness and thickness of the cartilage. The consistency of the cartilage is typically evaluated by palpitation and cautious, controlled bending. It is important in surgical planning to remember that the cartilage becomes more calcified and brittle with age.

Standard preoperative photographs and consent form for the procedure are taken. The purpose of the photographic documentation is to document the preoperative situation. A basic series should include full facial frontals and laterals of both ears. Frontal close-ups, obliques, and posterior images of each ear are also helpful (Fig. 16.4).

Taking postoperative photos at intervals of 6 and 12 months helps to monitor postoperative

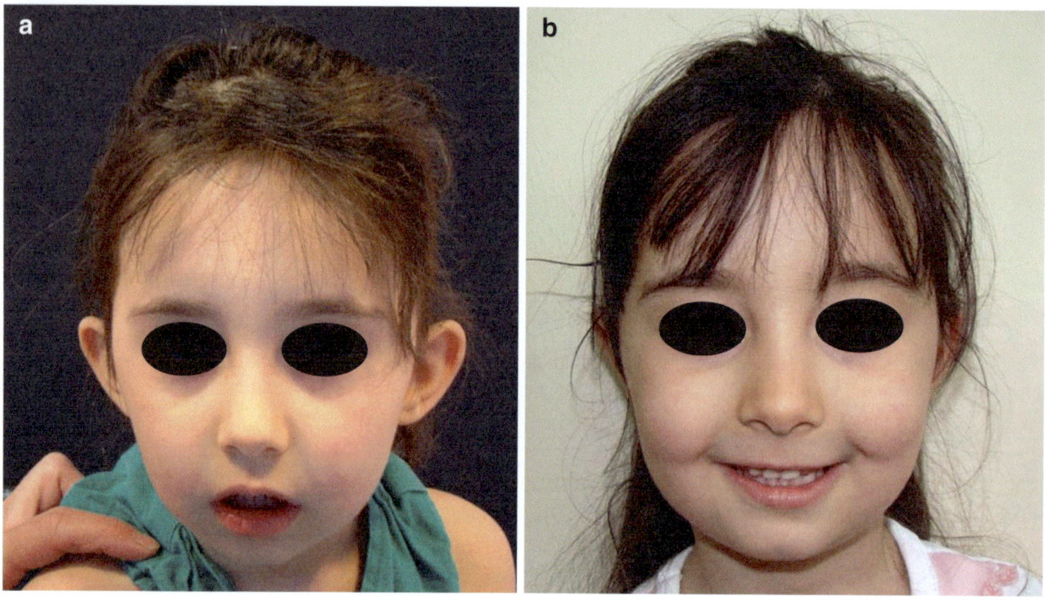

Fig. 16.3 (**a**) Preoperative. (**b**) Postoperative following bilateral otoplasty and adenoidectomy in combination with tonsillectomy. The ears remain relatively symmetrical postoperatively

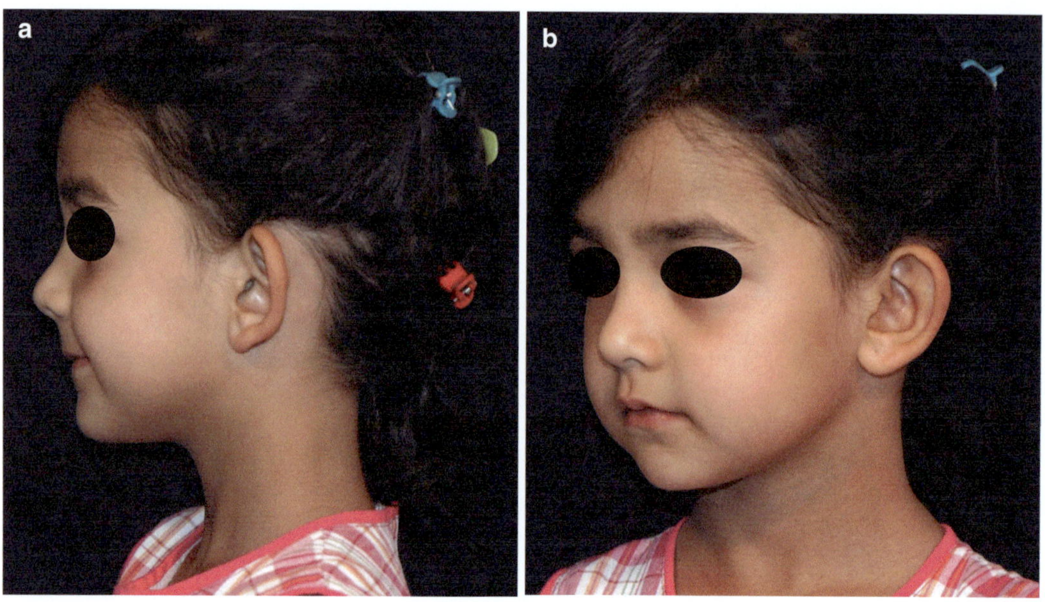

Fig. 16.4 Documentation showing left lateral (**a**), left oblique (**b**), frontal (**c**), right oblique (**d**), right lateral (**e**), and posterior (**f**) images

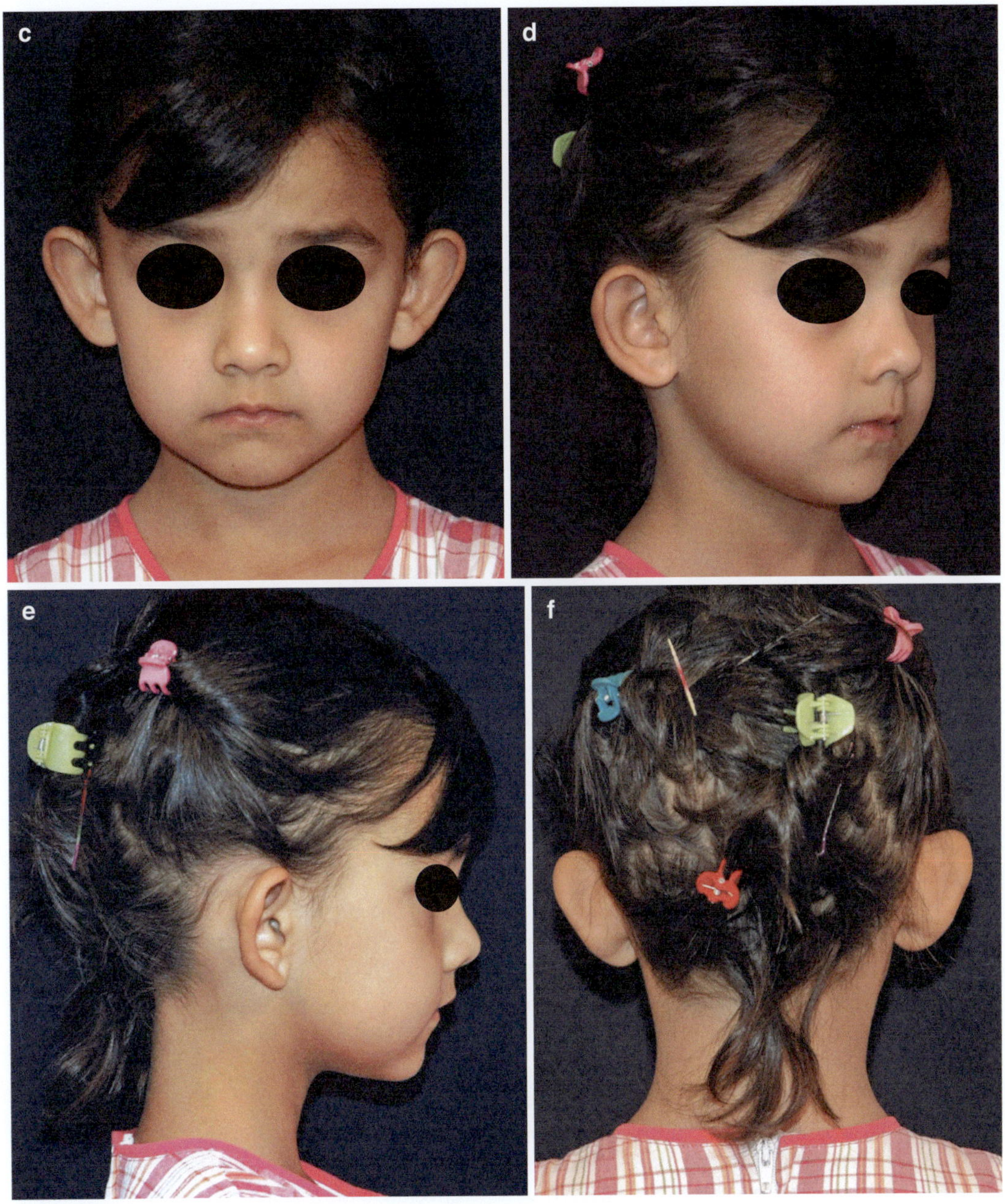

Fig. 16.4 (continued)

success and is also recommended for medical legal reasons (Fig. 16.5) [19, 20]. Prophylactic antibiotics are recommended for the majority of aesthetic and reconstructive procedures on the ear. The risk of chondritis is a sufficient indication to use an intraoperative dose of a broad-spectrum antibiotic and to prescribe a few postoperative days dosage of the similar agent.

Just as important as the anatomic irregularities of the auricle are the expectations of the patient and family. It is important to discuss the potential outcomes and complications and to ensure the patient has realistic expectations. The patients or the parents of the child are informed about the potential risks and unwanted complications, including hematoma

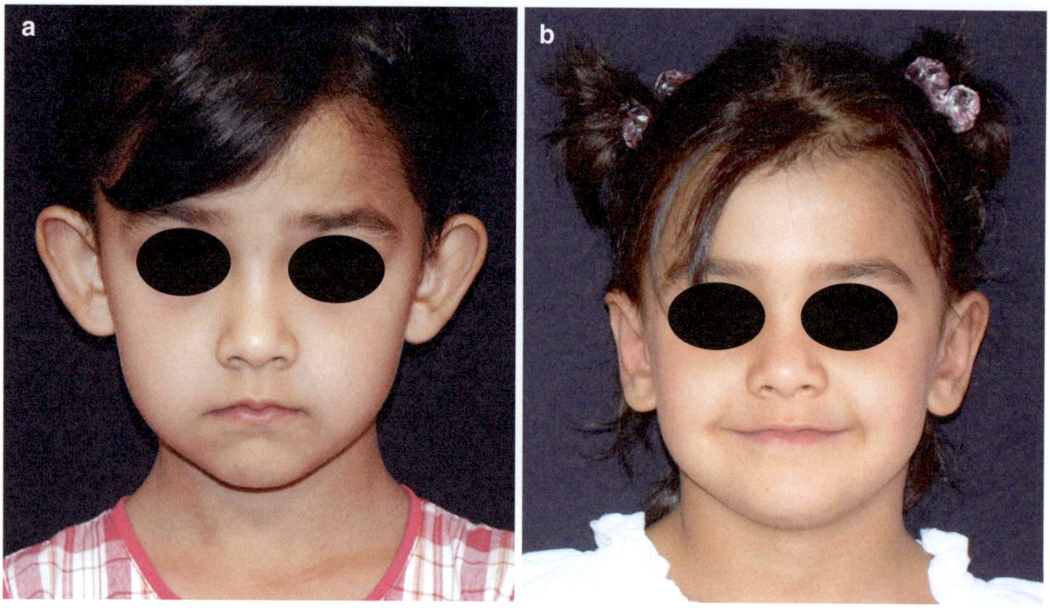

Fig. 16.5 (**a**) Preoperative. (**b**) Postoperative after bilateral otoplasty. The ears are symmetrical postoperatively and rising self-confidence is apparent even in the photograph

and infections of skin or cartilage, and also regarding the possibility of an unsatisfactory cosmetic result.

Anesthetic Considerations

In an effort to reduce the potential surgical morbidity related to general anesthesia, current trends in aesthetic surgery have moved toward local anesthesia combined with sedation, as opposed to general anesthesia [21]. Regardless of whether general anesthesia or monitored sedation is used, the use of local anesthesia results in decreased postoperative narcotic use and decreased pain scores [22]. Local anesthesia can be delivered in a number of ways. A peripheral nerve block can provide broad-range analgesia with one injection, as opposed to local infiltration, which must be precisely placed to have the appropriate effects. Local infiltration, however, has the added benefit of hemostasis when low-dose epinephrine is included. There are multiple choices of substances available as local anesthetics, including prilocaine, lidocaine, mepivacaine, bupivacaine, and ropivacaine.

Surgical Technique

In considering the proper surgical technique, there is room for surgeon preference and vision. The surgeon should develop a complete surgical plan that is a conglomerate of the individual techniques necessary to correct each observed anatomic irregularity. Surgical techniques for the correction of the prominent ear can be grouped into maneuvers used to create the antihelical fold, to correct the conchal defect, and to affect lobule positioning.

1. Perioperative Routine: There are as many variations in perioperative routine as there are in surgical technique for otoplasty. The hair is covered with a standard head bandage along the hairline. A small sterile cotton ball is placed in the external auditory canal to prevent blood from accumulating on the tympanic membrane (Fig. 16.6).

   The cleansing of the external ear is performed with povidone-iodine solution. Surgical draping with Tegaderm (3M Health Care, St. Paul, MN) or other clear sticky drape keeps the hair out of the surgical field. Drapes are placed so that both ears are simultaneously on view

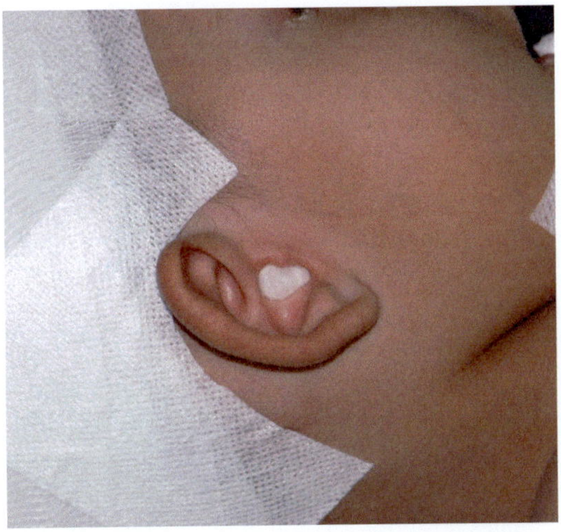

Fig. 16.6 Small sterile cotton ball placed in the external auditory canal

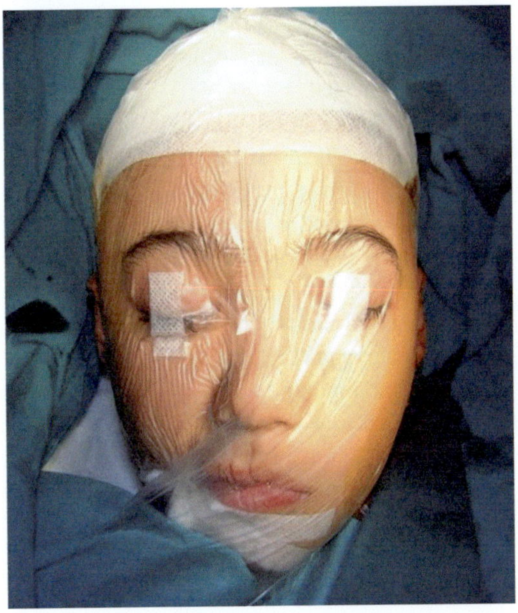

Fig. 16.7 Surgical draping with clear sticky drape

providing intraoperative comparison to obtain optimal symmetry (Fig. 16.7).

2. Skin Incision: As symmetry is the key, it is recommended to begin with the more severely affected side. Before local infiltration and associated tissue distortion, the area of redundant postauricular skin to be excised is estimated by gentle manipulation of the ear and traction in the desired position. The postauricular skin excision is then marked based on the estimation. Although most investigators have advocated an excision of skin, some have described a simple incision [19, 23]. The desired ear contours are simulated by exerting gentle digital pressure on the helix, and newly formed antihelical fold is marked on the skin (Fig. 16.8). The posterior auricular skin and mastoid soft tissues are infiltrated subcutaneously with 1 % Lidocaine HCl and 1:100,000 epinephrine solution. Local anesthesia enhances hemostasis and demarcates the plain of dissection.

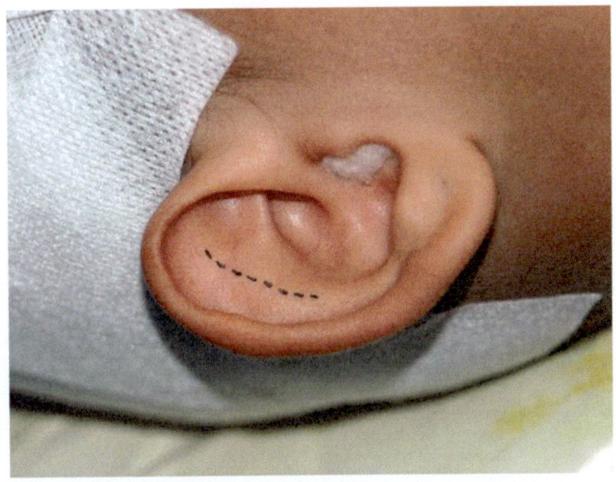

Fig. 16.8 Ear contours are simulated by exerting gentle digital pressure on the helix. Newly formed antihelical fold and planned mattress sutures are marked on the skin

The estimated skin excision on the posterior surface of the ear can be done safely with the narrowest width at the middle third to avoid "telephone ear" deformity. This occurs when the middle portion is reduced to a relatively greater degree than the superior helix and lobule. This overcorrection in the middle breaks the straight line of the caudal helix and leaves a relatively over-projected superior helix and lobule, giving the ear a convexity similar to the shape of a traditional telephone (Fig. 16.9). The reverse phenomenon can also occur if relatively less mid-portion correction is performed. This is termed a reverse telephone deformity.

If a lobule prominence accompanies, the skin excision is finished with a diamond-shaped inferior end to correct the lower pole prominence. The maximal width of the diamond-shaped excision is designed to rest at the point of maximal lobule prominence (Fig. 16.10). Others describe creating a medial-based skin flap that is redraped over the posterior auricle at the end of the case and excising the distal portion of the skin flap as needed to precisely fill the defect without tension or excess [10]. The main advantage of this approach is tension-free closures, which may reduce the incidence of hypertrophic scars.

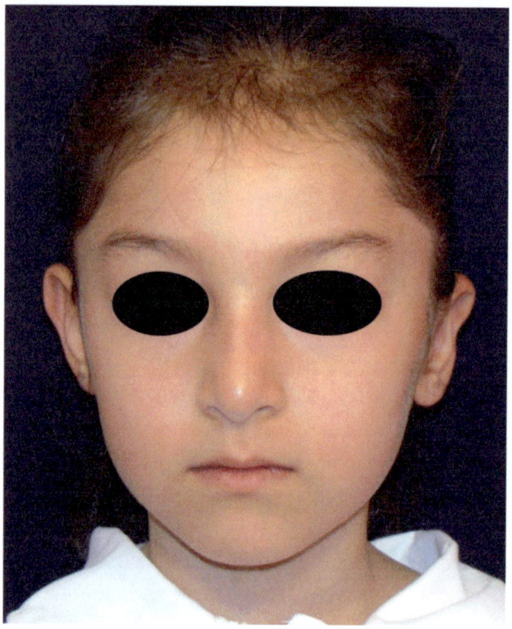

Fig. 16.9 "Telephone ear" deformity evident on the sixth month control

The previously marked postauricular skin is widely undermined exposing the perichondrium. Hemostasis is meticulously maintained, and dissection is developed peripherally to the free edge of the helix and posteriorly to the level of the mastoid bone. The bulky postauricular soft tissue, auricularis posterior muscle fibers, and fibrofatty tissues cleanly excised off the perichondrium and mastoid fascia with preservation of the periosteum (Figs. 16.11 and 16.12).

Creation of a deep, mastoid pocket accommodates the repositioned conchal cup, facilitates posterior rotation of the concha, removes the postauricular tissues that may act as a lever producing excessive prominence, and enhances the setback by effectively reducing conchal height. Utilization of the mastoid pocket also serves to reduce distortion of the external auditory meatus.

3. Reshaping the Antihelix and Repositioning the Concha: The proposed position of the antihelical fold was previously marked on the skin. The cartilage under the desired fold is marked by inserting dental needles at two or three points from anterior to posterior fashion. The inserted needles mark the lines of cartilage weakening (Fig. 16.13).

The monopolar diathermy in cutting mode is adjusted to a setting sufficient to create a partial-thickness trough through the cartilage. Three passes are made to form the antihelical

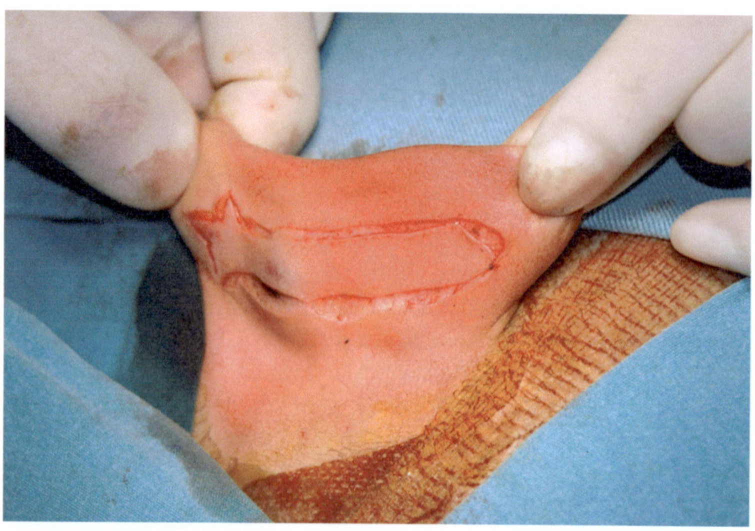

Fig. 16.10 The estimated skin excision with a diamond-shaped inferior end

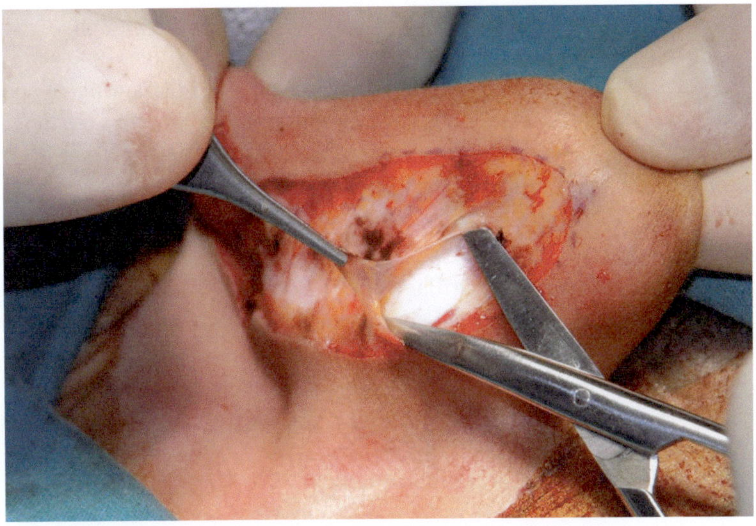

Fig. 16.11 The subcutaneous tissue over the mastoid surface of the cartilage is dissected

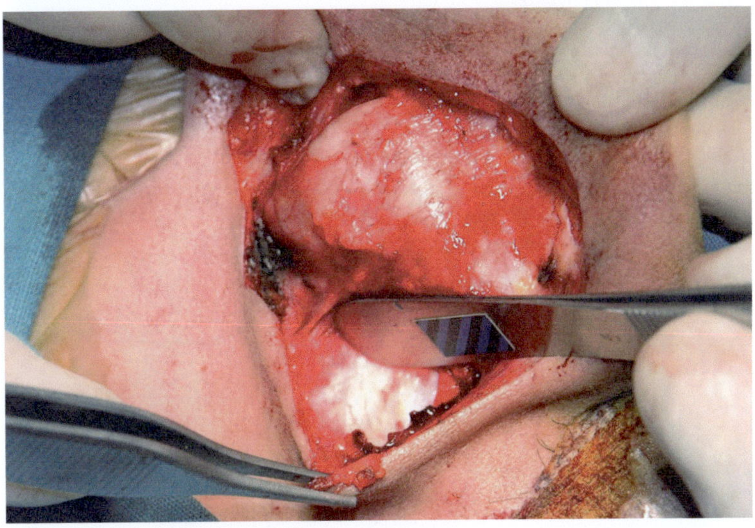

Fig. 16.12 The bulky postauricular soft tissue, auricularis posterior muscle fibers, and fibrofatty tissues excised

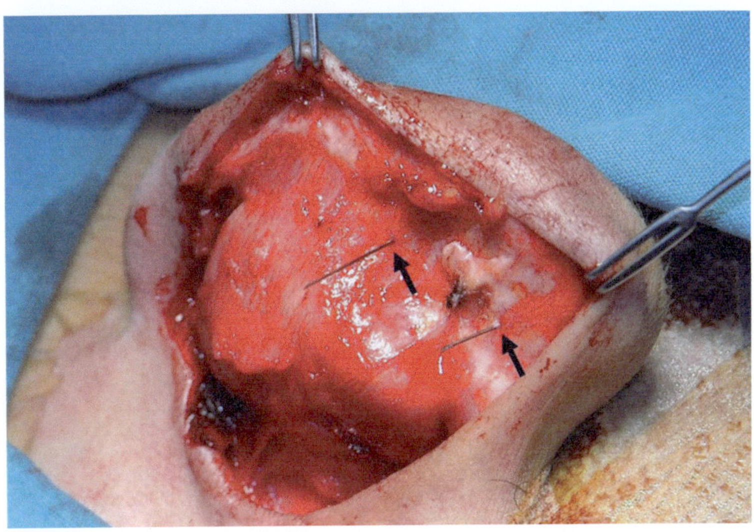

Fig. 16.13 Dental needles (*black arrows*) marking the lines of cartilage weakening

fold while maintaining sufficient flexibility to prevent a sharp angle at the fold (Figs. 16.14 and 16.15). Next, the conchal hypertrophy component is addressed. The conchal-mastoid groove has been cleared of the fibrofatty tissue and the postauricularis muscle previously as described. The ear is drawn backward into the desired position, and the site of contact between the conchal cartilage and mastoid fascia is checked. The marked conchal limits are used to mark proposed conchal scoring incisions, which are parallel the long axis of the ear. Two or three incisions are made with a monopolar diathermy in cutting mode (Figs. 16.14 and 16.15). This maneuver breaks the spring of the conchal bowl and lead the fibrosis to the mastoid fascia. Any excess conchal cartilage along the free edge of the external auditory meatus is excised, avoiding protrusion into the external auditory canal.

4. Lobule and Helical Rim Positioning: The lobule can be an overlooked component of the prominent ear and appears accentuated after the auricle is repositioned. Wood-Smith suggested a "fish taillike" retrolobular skin excision with a subsequent V-Y plasty [24].

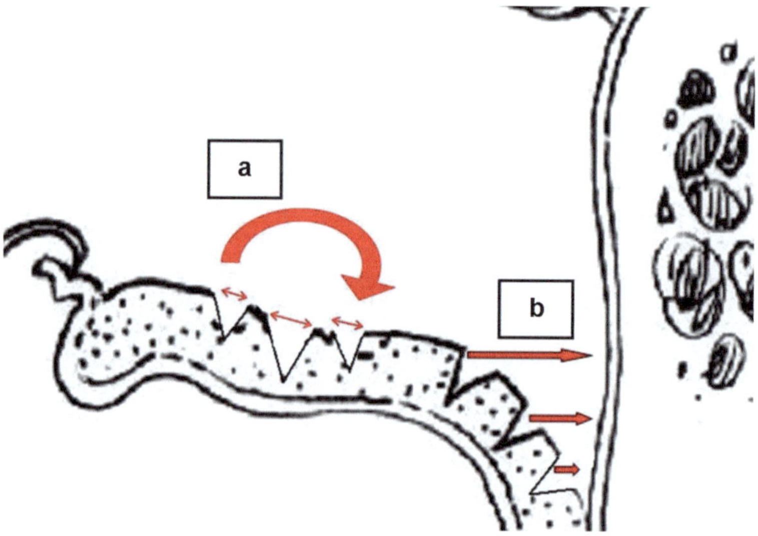

Fig. 16.14 Axial view demonstrates the sequential effects of surgical maneuvers on ear protrusion. (**a**) Partial-thickness scoring of scapha to create antihelical fold. (**b**) Partial-thickness scoring of concha to break the spring of the cartilage

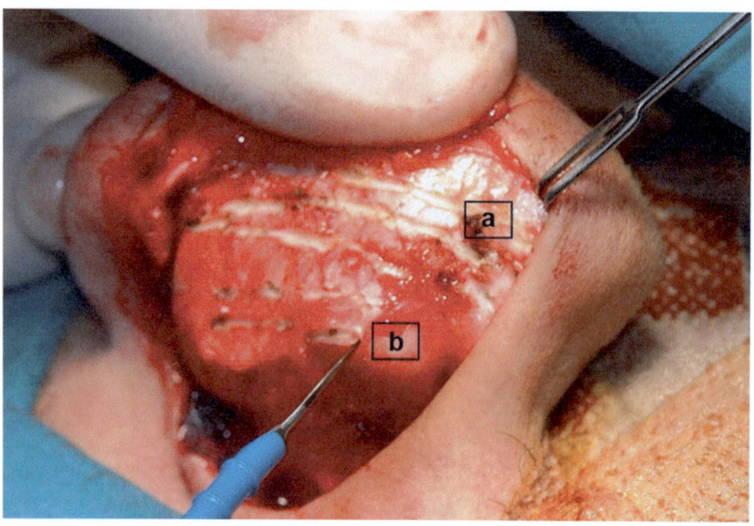

Fig. 16.15 (**a**) Partial-thickness scoring of scapha to create antihelical fold. (**b**) Partial-thickness scoring of concha to break the spring of the cartilage

Posterior lobule skin and fibrofatty tissue can be also excised in V-shaped, heart-shaped, and eccentric elliptical patterns with suture approximation producing the desired setback. Additionally, a Z plasty can be fashioned at the most inferior aspect of the postauricular incision, producing a similar effect. Gosain advocated a single stitch approach in which the lobule is secured to the mastoid region [25]. The excess skin is then excised, and the incision is closed. Spira et al. treat the protruding lobule by wedge excision and a periosteum suture between the dermis and the scalp [26]. Another method involves a curvilinear, fusiform excision from the anterior to posterior lobe margin with a central V excision to effect easy closure [27]. One further consideration in the prominent ear, not mentioned elsewhere, is the helical curl itself. Often this can be flattened and floppy, further contributing to the overly abnormal appearance. Few investigators have focused on this particular aspect. One study does describe a simple wedge excision along the helix alone without extending into the scaphae [28]. This shortens the outermost edge of the helix, enhancing its curl inward. This is used as an adjunct when the helix itself is noticeably flattened. In majority of our cases, we prefer a diamond-shaped posterior skin excision behind the lobule and suture the opposing points of the diamond in the closure using a running, locked, 4–0 long-term absorbable suture. It obviates the discomfort of suture removal, especially in children (Fig. 16.12).

5. Dressing and Postoperative Care: The appropriate dressing for the ear is a critical aspect of the procedure. At the completion of the procedure, the wounds are carefully cleansed and dressed with greasy gauzes soaked in Bepanthen Plus® (50-mg Dexpanthenol, 5-mg klorheksidin HCl). It is extremely important that the greasy gauze be carefully molded to fit the new folds and contours of the ear and to gently pad the postauricular surface (Fig. 16.16).

   All patients are placed on a 5-day regimen of antibiotics and acetaminophen as needed for pain. Aygit reported a custom-made mold for 2 weeks postoperative [29]. Azuara used a moldable porous polyester splint in a similar fashion for 72 h with a compression dressing full time for the first week postoperatively followed by 1 month of nighttime compression (Fig. 16.17) [30].

   In our practice, the dressing is removed on the first postoperative day to inspect the ears.

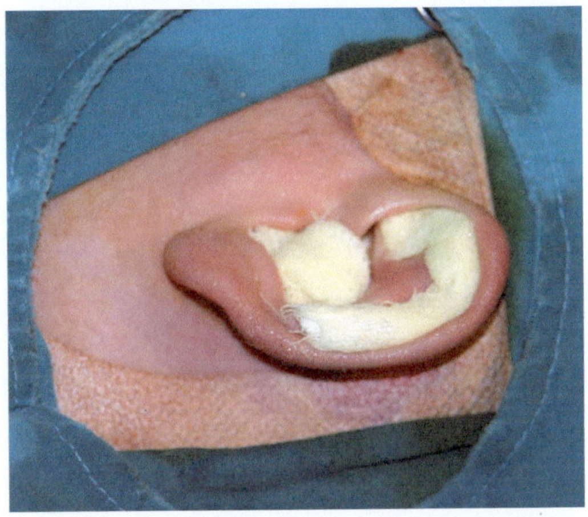

Fig. 16.16 Molded greasy gauze placed to fit the new folds and contours of the reconstructed ear

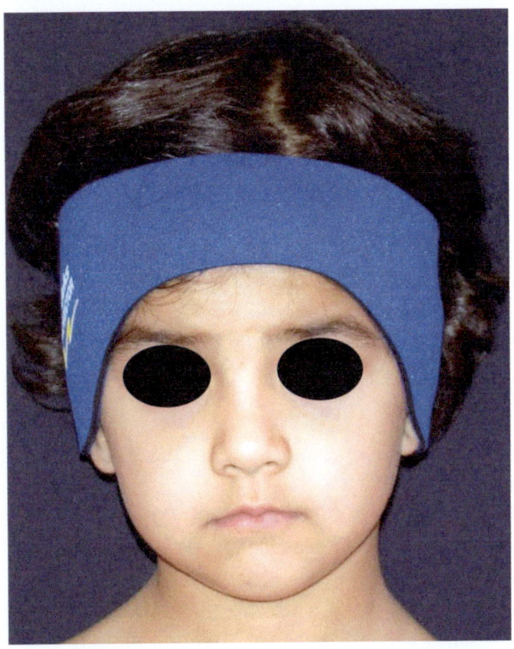

Fig. 16.17 Headband to prevent inadvertent nocturnal trauma

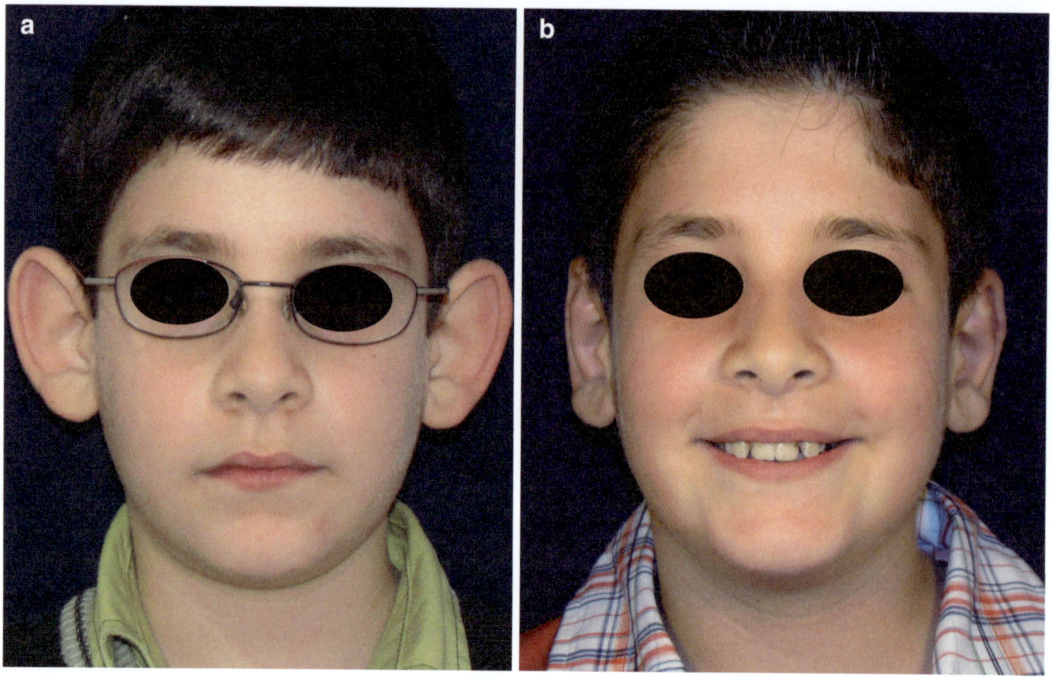

Fig. 16.18 (**a**) Preoperative 14 year-old boy. (**b**) Three months postoperative

This facilitates early identification of complications such as hematoma formation or skin ischemia. A slightly lighter dressing is replaced and is changed every other day for a further 7 days. After removal of the dressings, patients are instructed to wear a headband nightly for 1 month to prevent inadvertent nocturnal trauma. Patients are discouraged from any rough play or circumstances that might lead to accidental trauma, as a history of external trauma has been associated with about half of the cases of loss of correction requiring revision surgery [31]. Patients are then typically seen at 3–6 months postoperatively and 1 year postoperatively to document results (Fig. 16.18).

Conclusions

Although otoplasty is a century-old procedure that has undergone many modifications over the years, we are still unearthing the many advantages and disadvantages of a great variety of techniques. We herein described our effective and rapid procedure which maintains the natural contours of the auricle by addressing the poorly developed or absent antihelical fold, an abnormally large concha, and a prominent lobule.

Our controllable and intrinsically safe technique is relatively simple, can be applied to a wide variety of prominent ear deformities, and reproducible in the hands of other surgeons. We also believe that further investigations are required to characterize the physiological mechanisms involved in warping behavior of cartilage.

References

1. Songu M, Négrevergne M, Portmann D. The Négrevergne otoplasty technique. Ann Otol Rhinol Laryngol. 2010;119(1):27–31.
2. Mayaleh HA, Khalil HS, Portmann D, Négrevergne M. Otoplasty for prominent ears in children. The technique adopted in the Portmann Institute. Rev Laryngol Otol Rhinol (Bord). 2003;124(2):13513–6.
3. McDowell AJ. Goals in otoplasty for protruding ears. Plast Reconstr Surg. 1968;41(1):17–27.
4. Skiles MS, Randall P. The anesthetics of ear placement: an experimental study. Plast Reconstr Surg. 1983;72(2):133–40.

5. Farkas LG. Anthropometry of normal and anomalous ears. Clin Plast Surg. 1978;5(3):401–12.
6. Farkas LG. Anthropometry of the normal and defective ear. Clin Plast Surg. 1990;17(2):213–21.
7. Tolleth H. A hierarchy of values in the design and construction of the ear. Clin Plast Surg. 1990;17(2):193–207.
8. Smith HW. Calibrated otoplasty. Laryngoscope. 1979;89(4):657–65.
9. Janis JE, Rohrich RJ, Gutowski KA. Otoplasty. Plast Reconstr Surg. 2005;115(4):60e–72.
10. Horlock N, Vogelin E, Bradbury ET, Grobbelaar AO, Gault DT. Psychosocial outcome of patients after ear reconstruction: a retrospective study of 62 patients. Ann Plast Surg. 2005;54(5):517–24.
11. Keery H, Boutelle K, van den Berg P, Thompson JK. The impact of appearance-related teasing by family members. J Adolesc Health. 2005;37(2):120–7.
12. Kelley P, Hollier L, Stal S. Otoplasty: evaluation, technique, and review. J Craniofac Surg. 2003;14(5):643–53.
13. Songu M, Adibelli H. Otoplasty in children younger than 5 years of age. Int J Pediatr Otorhinolaryngol. 2010;74(3):292–6.
14. Adamson JE, Horton CE, Crawford HH. The growth pattern of the external ear. Plast Reconstr Surg. 1965;36(4):466–70.
15. Farkas LG. Growth of normal and re-constructed auricles. In: Tanzer RC, Edgerton MT, editors. Symposium on reconstruction of the auricle. Mosby: St. Louis; 1974. p. 24–31.
16. Balogh B, Millesi H. Are growth alterations a consequence of surgery for prominent ears? Plast Reconstr Surg. 1992;90(2):192–9.
17. Gosain AK, Recinos RF. Otoplasty in children less than four years of age: surgical technique. J Craniofac Surg. 2002;13(4):505–9.
18. Gosain AK, Kumar A, Huang G. Prominent ears in children younger than 4 years of age: what is the appropriate timing for otoplasty? Plast Reconstr Surg. 2004;114(5):1042–54.
19. Spira M. Otoplasty: what I do now – a 30-year perspective. Plast Reconstr Surg. 1999;104(3):834–41.
20. Becker W, Deutsch E, Knappen FJ, Nussgens K. Panel discussion: problems of the specialist's duty to inform the patient. HNO. 1976;24(6):181–96.
21. Cregg N, Conway F, Casey W. Analgesia after otoplasty: regional nerve blockade vs local anaesthetic infiltration of the ear. Can J Anaesth. 1996;43(2):141–7.
22. Pavlin DJ, Chen C, Penaloza DA, Polissar NL, Buckley FP. Pain as a factor complicating recovery and discharge after ambulatory surgery (table of contents). Anesth Analg. 2002;95(3):627–34.
23. Caouette-Laberge L, Guay N, Bortoluzzi P, Belleville C. Otoplasty: anterior scoring technique and results in 500 cases (review). Plast Reconstr Surg. 2000;105(2):504–15.
24. Wood-Smith D. Otoplasty. In: Rees T, editor. Aesthetic plastic surgery. Philadelphia: Saunders; 1980. p. 833.
25. Gosain AK, Recinos RF. A novel approach to correction of the prominent lobule during otoplasty. Plast Reconstr Surg. 2003;112(2):575–83.
26. Spira M, McCrea R, Gerow FJ, Hardy SB. Correction of the principal deformities causing protruding ears. Plast Reconstr Surg. 1969;44(2):150–4.
27. Adamson PA, Strecker HD. Otoplasty techniques. Facial Plast Surg. 1995;11(4):284–300.
28. Maurice PF, Eisbach KJ. Aesthetic otoplasty: wedge excision of a flattened helix to create a helical curl. Arch Facial Plast Surg. 2005;7(3):195–7.
29. Aygit AC. Molding the ears after anterior scoring and concha repositioning: a combined approach for protruding ear correction. Aesthetic Plast Surg. 2003;27(1):77–81.
30. Stenstroem SJ. A "natural" technique for correction of congenitally prominent ears. Plast Reconstr Surg. 1963;32:509.
31. Adamson PA, McGraw BL, Tropper GJ. Otoplasty: critical review of clinical results. Laryngoscope. 1991;101(8):883–8.

Island Technique for Prominent Ears 17

Ivo Pitanguy and Henrique N. Radwanski

Introduction

Prominent ears are commonly caused by overdevelopment of the concha, underdeveloped antihelical folds, and protruding earlobes [1, 2]. These may occur alone or in combination.

Otoplasty should be performed to correct the deformity early, usually around the age of 7 years when the child becomes exposed to social attention [3–6]. General anesthesia is usually required for patients under the age of 10 years. After 10 years, local anesthesia, with sedation under the supervision of an anesthesiology team, may be tolerated.

The surgeon should comprehend the final position of the ear; the angle of the ear and the mastoid is normally around 30°, the concha and scaphoid forming an angle of about 90° (conchascaphoid angle) and the angle between the head and the concha of about 90° (cephaloconchal angle) so that the scaphoid fossa lies parallel to the head. The goal of otoplasty is to reposition the ears so that the contours appear soft and natural. The helical rim should be visible from the frontal view protruding beyond the antihelix. Lateral view should show contours as smooth and round. From the posterior view, the contour of the helical rim should be straight [1, 6, 7].

There is no single ideal procedure to correct prominent ears, as can be attested by the various techniques [3, 6, 7]. Each surgeon should be versed in the different approaches and should adopt a procedure that aims to correct the presenting signs of this deformity. Conceptually, the "island technique" aims at creating an "island" of cartilage, which is fashioned and projected, thus mimicking the antihelix fold. This approach was originally devised by Pitanguy and Flemming [8] as an effective, simple, and reliable procedure to correct prominent ears. Since then, other publications have confirmed these principles [9–11].

Technique

The island of cartilage is marked as the surgeon holds the auricle with the thumb and index finger (Fig. 17.1) [8–10]. An ellipse of skin is excised from the posterior surface of the ear to give optimum visualization with the width of skin determined by the extent of auricle protrusion and by bending the auricle backwards. The demarcation of the island that will form the antihelical fold (Fig. 17.2) is transferred to the posterior surface of the auricle with needles stained with methylene blue (Fig. 17.3). After incision of the cartilage, edges are undermined to minimize tension in the suture line (Fig. 17.4). The carti-

I. Pitanguy, M.D.
Ivo Pitanguy Clinic,
Rua Dona Mariana, 65,
Rio de Janeiro 22280-020, Brazil
e-mail: pitanguy@pitanguy.com.br

H.N. Radwanski, M.D. (✉)
Department of Plastic Surgery,
Pontifical Catholic University of Rio de Janeiro and the
Carlos Chagas Post-Graduate Medical Institute,
Rio de Janeiro, Brazil
e-mail: dr.henrique@pilos.com.br

M.A. Shiffman (ed.), *Advanced Cosmetic Otoplasty*,
DOI 10.1007/978-3-642-35431-1_17, © Springer-Verlag Berlin Heidelberg 2013

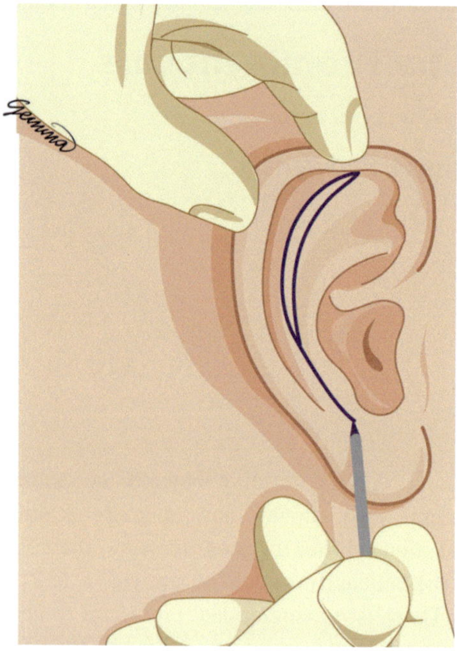

Fig. 17.1 The island of cartilage is marked as the surgeon holds the auricle with the thumb and index finger

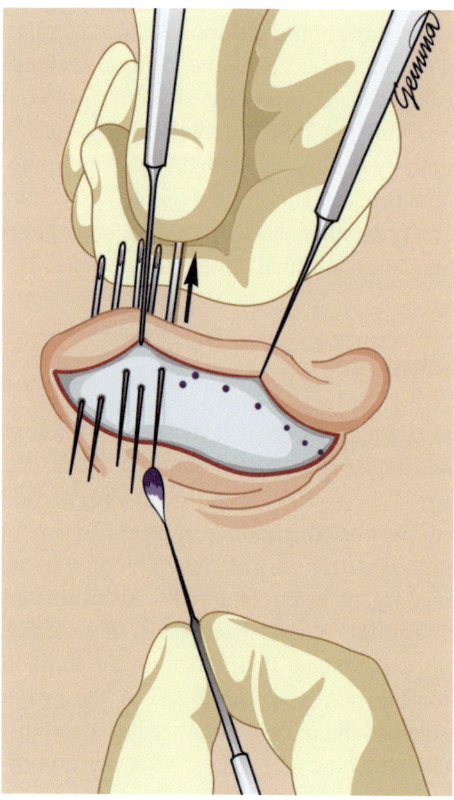

Fig. 17.2 Transferred to the posterior surface of the auricle with needles stained with methylene blue

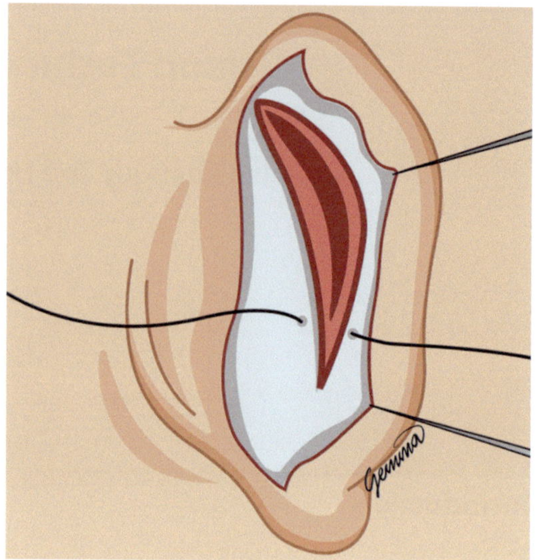

Fig. 17.3 The incised ellipse

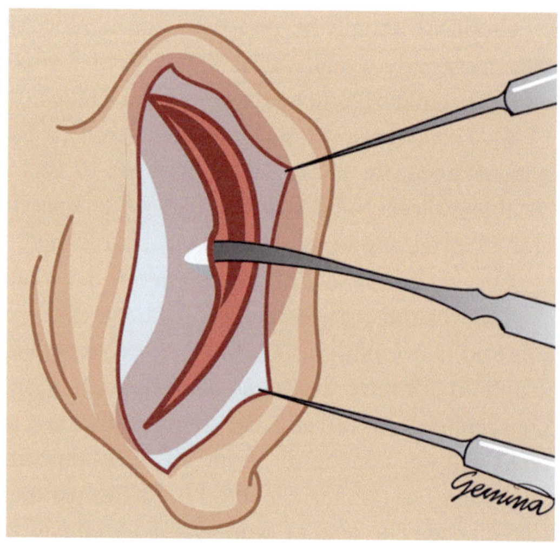

Fig. 17.4 The cartilaginous edges are undermined to minimize tension in the suture line

laginous edges are approximated without tension, projecting the island forwards, using 4-0 PDS, and one or two sutures passed through the perichondrium to unite the mobilized portion of the cartilage (Fig. 17.5). This projects the cartilaginous island anteriorly to simulate the antihelical fold (Fig. 17.6). The concha is repositioned by rotation and fixation to the periosteum of the mastoid bone. If necessary, excess concha can be excised, but skin folds must be avoided when suturing the incision. The concha is undermined from the medial edge of the postauricular skin incision to the external auditory meatus. The degree of rotation of the concha is limited because excess rotation can narrow the entrance to the external auditory meatus. The earlobe protrusion is brought into the same plane as the remainder of the auricle using a triangular or bow-shaped excision of skin between the earlobe and concha.

Dressing consists of packing the auricle with moist cotton, carefully inserting the cotton in all the crevices so as to maintain the shape of the new auricle. A bolster of cotton is applied to prevent pressure necrosis. External bandage wrapping is used. Oral antibiotics are routinely used for 5 days postoperatively.

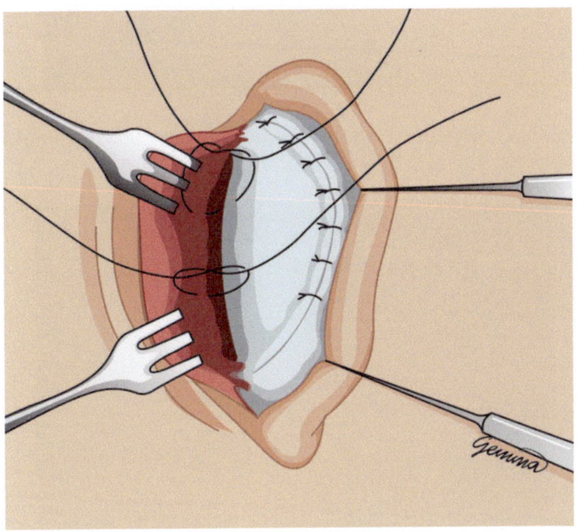

Fig. 17.5 The cartilage edges are approximated with 4-0 PDS, with no tension

The dressing is removed on the first postoperative day for evaluation and then replaced. On the 10th postoperative day, the sutures are removed. The child should use a protective bandage to cover the ears, and to ensure constant gentle pressure, for the first week. This bandage should also be used for the next 3 weeks at night.

Complications

Out of 111 patients there was one hematoma that required surgical evacuation. There was no evidence of chondritis, infection, necrosis, hypertrophic scars, granulomas, suture extrusion, or loss of sensibility. Five patients had residual deformity, 3 patients had asymmetry, 3 patients had under-correction, and 1 patient had both asymmetry and marked antihelical fold. There were no recurrences of the deformity.

Discussion

The island technique is indicated for patients who have any degree of underdevelopment of the antihelix, even if the main etiology is an overdeveloped concha (Figs. 17.7, 17.8, 17.9, and 17.10). The procedure is relatively simple and has few complications. There are some complications that are inherent in any otoplasty technique [12, 13] such as asymmetry and under-correction that are due primarily to intraoperative misjudgment. Some surgeons criticize the cartilaginous island as appearing too artificial; this is due to poor execution, where

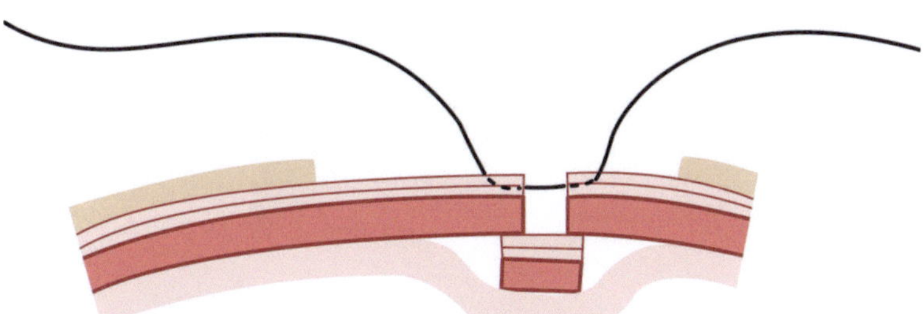

Fig. 17.6 This projects the cartilaginous island anteriorly to simulate the antihelical fold

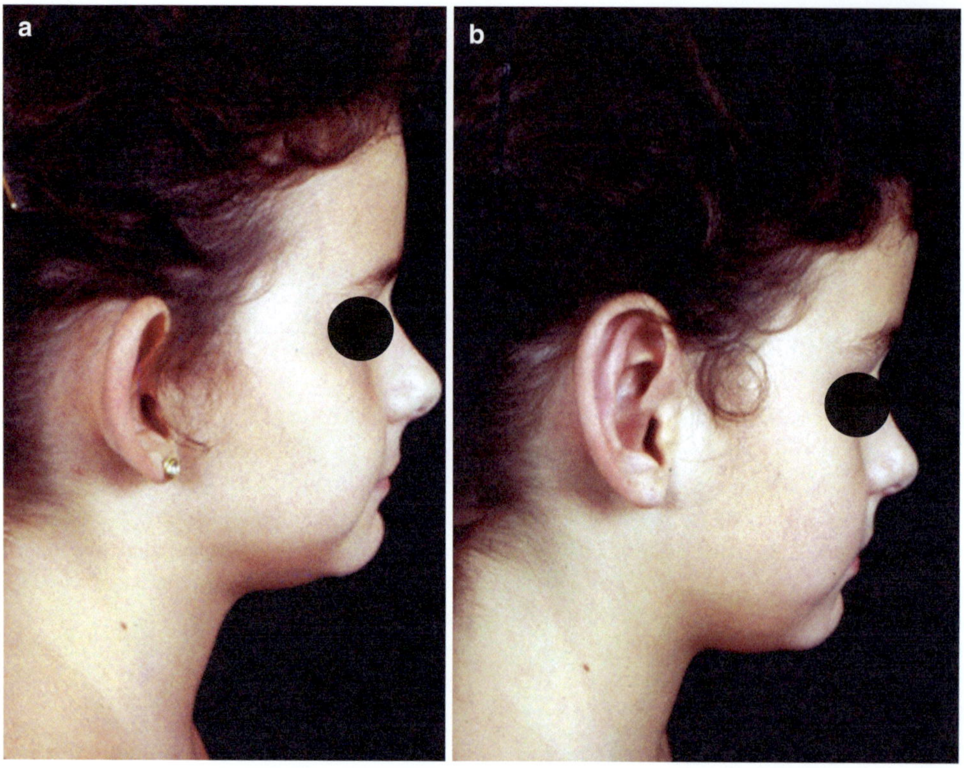

Fig. 17.7 (**a**) Preoperative 7-year-old girl with prominent ears. (**b**) Postoperative after correction by the island technique

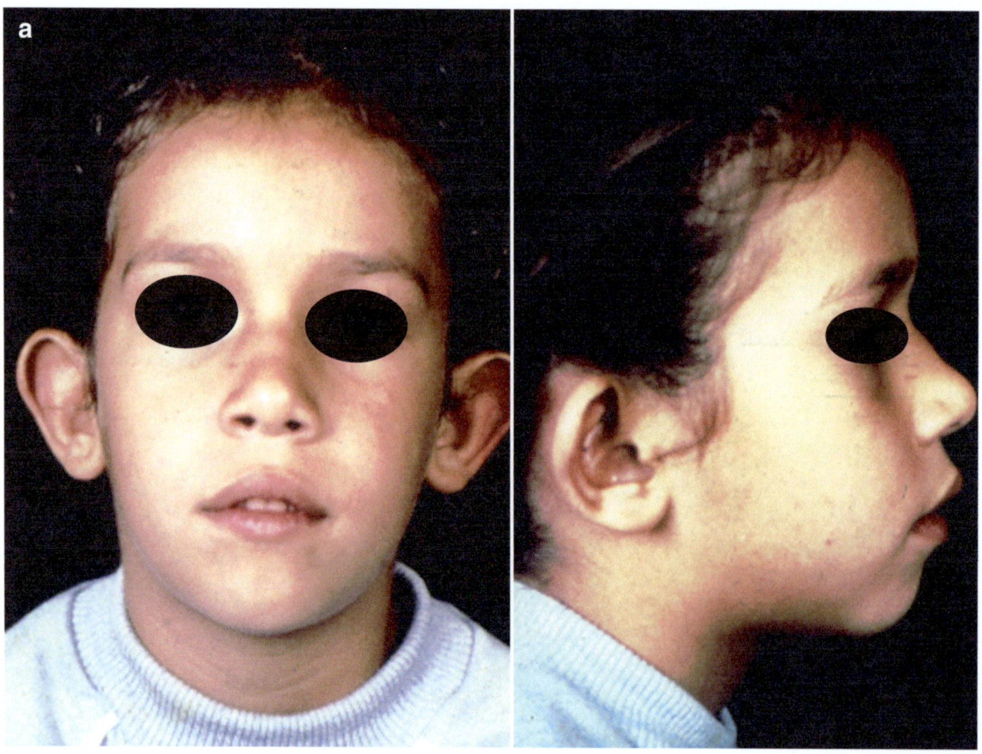

Fig. 17.8 (**a**) Preoperative 6-year-old girl with prominent ears. (**b**) Postoperative following correction by the island technique

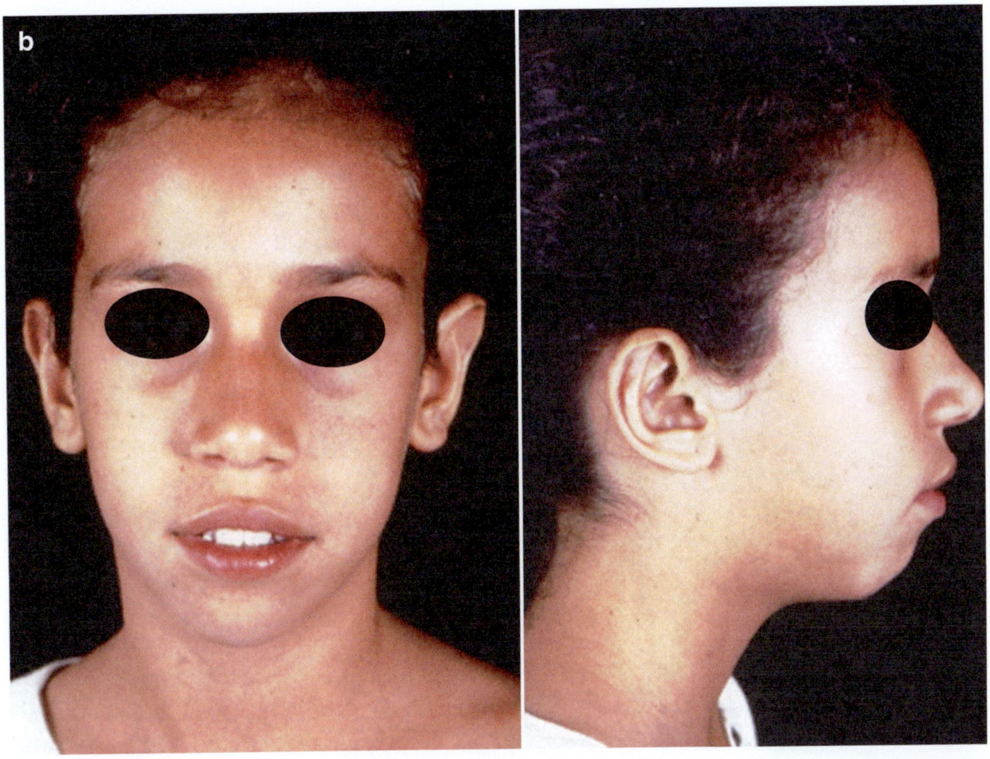

Fig 17.8 (continued)

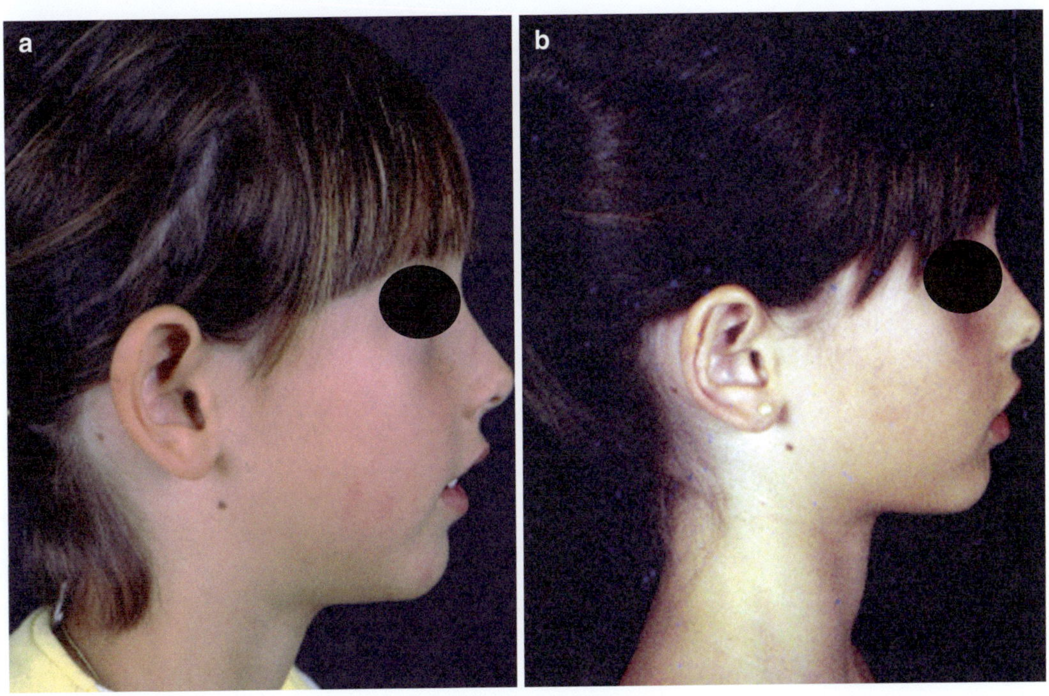

Fig. 17.9 (**a**) Preoperative 6-year-old girl with prominent ear. (**b**) Postoperative after use of the cartilage island

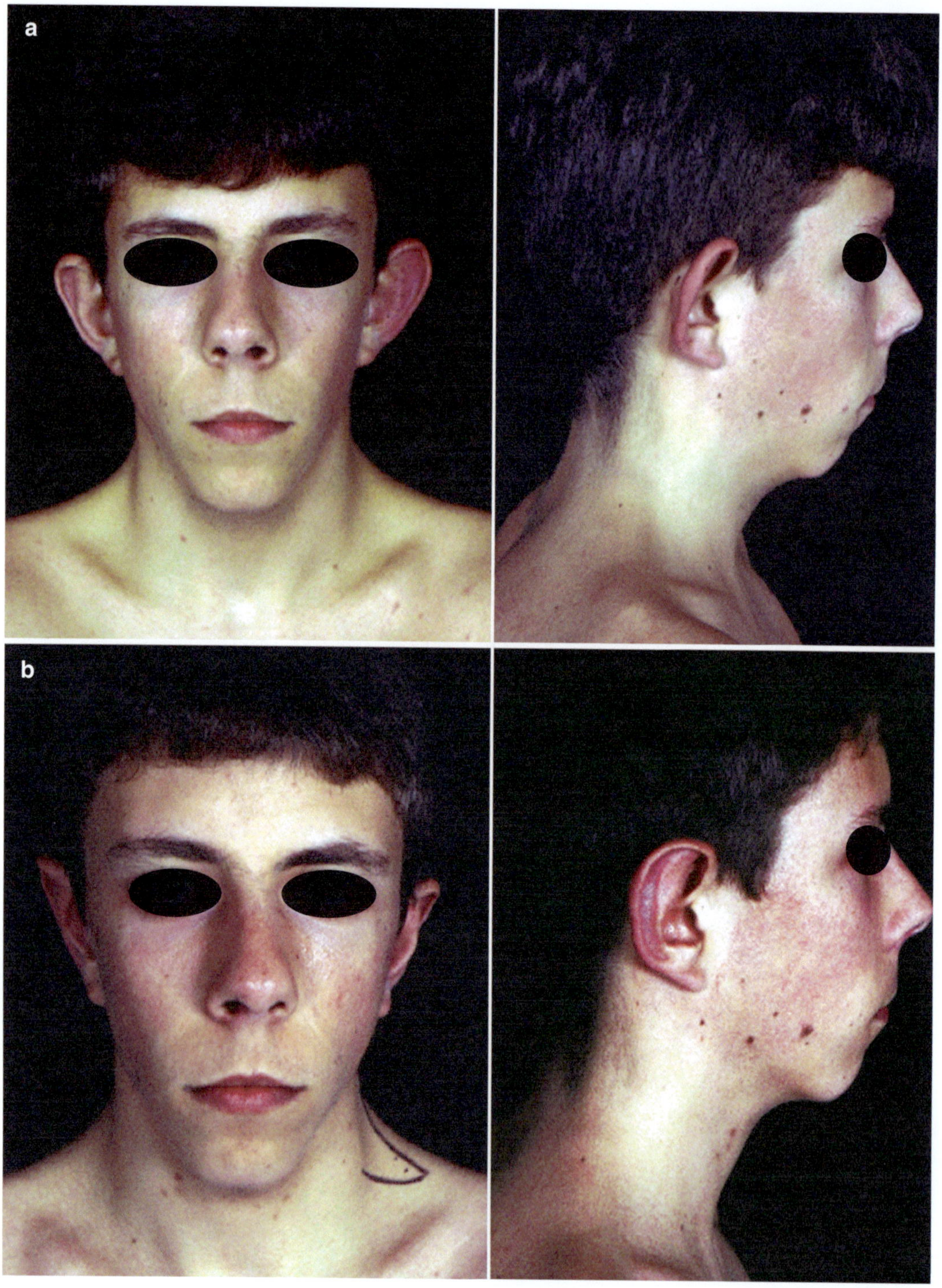

Fig. 17.10 (**a**) Preoperative 12-year-old boy with prominent ears. (**b**) Postoperative following correction by the island technique

sharp limits of the island produce a very prominent shape of the new antihelix, and can be avoided by carefully softening the edges.

Conclusions

The island technique, as originally described by the senior author, is an effective, simple, and reliable method of otoplasty to correct prominent ears. The procedure is reproducible and has had low recurrence and complication rates.

References

1. Macgregor FC. Ear deformities: social and psychological implications. Clin Plast Surg. 1978;5(3):347–50.
2. Bradbury ET, Hewison J, Timmons MJ. Psychological and social outcome of prominent ear correction in children. Br J Plast Surg. 1992;45(2):97–100.
3. Mustarde JC. The correction of prominent ears using simple mattress sutures. Br J Plast Surg. 1963;16:170–8.
4. Mustarde JC. The treatment of prominent ears by buried mattress sutures: a ten-year survey. Plast Reconstr Surg. 1967;39(4):382–6.
5. Stenstroem SJ. A "natural" technique for correction of congenitally prominent ears. Plast Reconstr Surg. 1963;32:509–18.
6. Stenstrom SJ, Heftner J. The stenstrom otoplasty. Clin Plast Surg. 1978;5(3):465–70.
7. Furnas DW. Correction of prominent ears with multiple sutures. Clin Plast Surg. 1978;5(3):491–5.
8. Pitanguy I, Flemming I. Plastiche Eingriffe an der Ohrmuschel. Stuttgart: Georg Thieme Verlag; 1976. p. 69.
9. Pitanguy I. Aesthetic plastic surgery of head and body. Berlin: Springer; 1981. p. 306–14.
10. Pitanguy I, Muller P, Piccolo N, Ramalho E, Solinas R. The treatment of prominent ears: a 25-year survey of the island technique. Aesthetic Plast Surg. 1987;11(2):87–93.
11. Bartkowski SB, Szuta M, Zapata J. Pitanguy's method of protruding ear correction from our own experience: review of 80 cases. Aesthetic Plast Surg. 2001;25(2):103–10.
12. Calder JC, Naasan A. Morbidity of otoplasty: a review of 562 consecutive cases. Br J Plast Surg. 1994;47(3):170–4.
13. Jeffery SL. Complications following correction of prominent ears: an audit review of 122 cases. Br J Plast Surg. 1999;52(7):588–90.

Otoplasty and Earlobe Repair

18

David J. Archibald and Edward H. Farrior

Introduction

Otoplasty is the reshaping of the ears, typically the correction of protruding ears or lop-ear deformities. Reshaping of the ears also occurs in the form of microtia repair on a more grand scale and earlobe reduction or repair of iatrogenic deformities to a more minor degree, but this is not typically considered otoplasty.

Otoplasty most commonly refers to the reduction of protruding ears. This usually involves recreating normal cartilaginous contours on the anterior surface of the ear and reducing the depth of the conchal bowl. Contour recreation and depth reduction of the bowl may be done independently; however, they are most often done together, to varying degrees. This affects the protrusion of the ear away from the side of the head and creation of the ideal postauricular angle or cephaloauricular angle of less than 45° [1]. The goal of this chapter is to summarize the abnormalities that produce the protruding ear, to describe how to correct them, and to offer relatively simple solutions for the aging lobule and postsurgical lobular deformities.

History

Otoplasty has an extensive history. Auricular reconstruction was described as early as the seventh century by Sushruta in ancient India [2]. In Die Operative Chirurgie (Operational Surgery, 1845), Dieffenbach (1794–1847) reported the first surgical approach for the correction of prominent ears. In his treatise, he described a pinna setback technique of excising postauricular skin and then suturing the auricular cartilage to the mastoid periosteum [3]. Almost 40 years later, in the Archives of Otology, Ely [4] advocated excising both skin and cartilage on the anterior as well as posterior surface. He reported a case of a 12-year-old boy who presented with a complaint of being ridiculed due to the prominence of his ears. A few years later, Keen [5] described an improved approach to the deformity, advocating the excision of only posterior skin and cartilage. In 1910, Luckett [6] acknowledged the importance of the antihelical fold and noted the deficiency of this structure in children with protruding ears. He described a procedure to create the antihelix by excising a crescent-shaped piece of cartilage and closing the defect with buried mattress sutures. In his original description, he also envisioned the possibility of reconstructing the antihelix without excising cartilage, but rather

D.J. Archibald, M.D.
Department of Plastic & Reconstructive Surgery, Rockwood Clinic, 801 West 5th Avenue, Suite 504, Spokane, WA 99204, USA
e-mail: david@drarchibald.com

E.H. Farrior, M.D. (✉)
Farrior Facial Plastic Reconstructive and Cosmetic Surgery Center, 2908 West Azeele Street, Tampa, FL 33609, USA
e-mail: ed@drfarrior.com; farrior@tampabay.rr.com; efarrior@tampabay.rr.com

M.A. Shiffman (ed.), *Advanced Cosmetic Otoplasty*,
DOI 10.1007/978-3-642-35431-1_18, © Springer-Verlag Berlin Heidelberg 2013

folding the cartilage in patients with thin, flexible cartilage. Many other surgeons subsequently reported on various methods of making relaxing cartilage incisions, excisions, and shavings, facilitating posterior plication to decrease projection of the concha and create the antihelix [7–13].

Modern otoplasty techniques have evolved to less invasive therapies, as surgeons have recognized the underlying anatomic defects. Though described previously, Mustarde [14] refined and popularized the technique of reestablishing the antihelical fold by using suture plication at three points without incision of the cartilage. Shortly thereafter, Furnas [15] published his method of addressing conchal excess by suturing the concha to the mastoid.

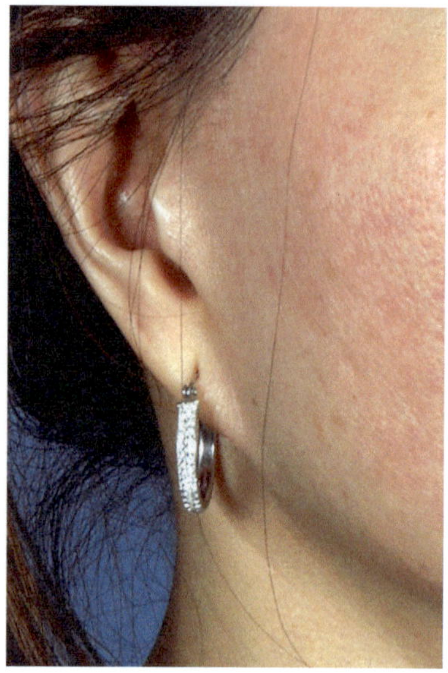

Fig. 18.1 The pixie deformity describes an elongated, downward displaced earlobe that may be caused by improper incision placement around the lobule, aggressive skin removal, or excessive tension at the time of closure

Embryology, Anatomy, and Malformations

During the sixth week of fetal life, the ear arises from the first and second branchial arch in the form of six auricular hillocks of condensed ectoderm and mesoderm that form within the first and second branchial arches. The first three hillocks (1 through 3) are attributed to the first branchial arch, and the second three hillocks (4 through 6) are attributed to the second branchial arch. It is the general consensus that the bulk of the ear is formed from the third through fifth hillocks and that the sixth hillock contributes to the lobule and antitragus with the tragus and helical crus originating from the first and second hillocks [16]. Development of the pinna primarily occurs during the first trimester of pregnancy; therefore, the majority of auricular deformities develop during this phase of embryological maturation.

Malformations of the external ear occur on a wide spectrum and may result in microtia, the absence of most external anatomy including the external auditory canal, and are frequently associated with underdevelopment of the middle and inner ear. This is considered a third-degree dysplasia (Weerda's classification) of the ear [17]. The cupped ear deformity, second degree, is most often represented by an undersized ear with reduced components, most frequently affecting the superior helical margin, superior crus of the antihelix, and scaphoid fossa. First-degree deformities of the ear are deformities of excess rather than absence and are manifested by the protruding or overly large ear. Lop-ear deformity, or protruding ears, is inherited as an autosomal dominant trait with variable penetrance, 59 % of patients having a positive family history [18]. Protruding ears affect 5 % of the Caucasian race, most commonly secondary to lack of development of the antihelical fold [19].

Abnormalities of the ear can also be caused by iatrogenic and traumatic sources. One of the most frequently occurring iatrogenic abnormalities is the pixie deformity that can be the sequelae of a facelift (Fig. 18.1). The pixie deformity describes an elongated, downward displaced earlobe that may be caused by improper incision placement around the lobule, aggressive skin removal, or excessive tension at the time of closure. There is a similar congenital variation in the degree of attachment of the lobule to the neck that can be released, if so desired, in the same fashion as the repair of the postsurgical pixie-ear deformity.

Abnormalities that are the consequence of aging may also affect the lobule, resulting in elongation and thinning. If these are not addressed at the time of a facelift, there will be a severe lack of harmony after completion of the facial rejuvenation, and this may distract from an otherwise satisfactory result.

In performing otoplasty, it is imperative to realize that for each eminence, there is a fossa and that by recreating the normal convexities and concavities of the auricular cartilage, it is possible to create an ear that looks normal, with long-lasting results.

Patient Selection

The ear continues to grow after birth and reaches approximately 85 % of its adult size by age three. Slower growth of the ear proceeds until 6 years of age, at which time the ear has reached adult size, approximately 6 by 3 cm. Ears that protruded often become the source of ridicule and can be corrected as early as 5 or 6 years of age. There is evidence to suggest that teasing and harassment will begin when the patient enters elementary school [20]. This of course may depend upon the degree of protrusion, the gender of the patient, and the hairstyle. The parents of male children are more likely to seek correction at a younger age than those of females. There is an upper limit on the age at which an otoplasty can be performed. In elderly patients, the cartilage becomes more rigid and may require more aggressive surgical techniques.

Surgical Management

Lop-Ear Deformity

Correction of the lop-ear deformity takes many forms and has been covered extensively in the past [10, 14, 15, 21]. Regardless of technique, surgery must be customized to address the deformities that exist to prevent over- or undertreatment.

In the senior author's (EHF) practice, there is a 93 % occurrence of absent or underdeveloped superior crus of the antihelix in patients with protruding ears. This may present in isolation, resulting in the protrusion of the superior pinna or in conjunction with the absence or underdevelopment of the antihelix along its entire length, which occurs in 75 % of the patients and results in the protrusion of the entire helical margin. Protrusion of the entire helical margin in the absence or underdevelopment of the antihelix is almost universally associated with a prominent cauda helicis, contributing to protrusion of the lobule. A deep conchal bowl, which further exacerbates the protrusion, occurs in approximately 45 % of patients.

Absence of the superior crus is the most straightforward and most consistently encountered deformity. It is addressed through the excision of an ellipse of skin on the posterior surface of the ear over the desired fossa of the superior crus of the antihelix. This is determined by folding the ear to recreate the superior crus and identifying the corresponding position on the posterior surface. This can be accomplished by the placement of Keith needles through the ear from the anterior surface. Needles are placed at the junction of the superior and inferior crus of the antihelix in the fossa triangularis, the lateral conchal bowl at the junction of the superior and inferior crus, and the anterior margin of the scaphoid fossa (Fig. 18.2). These are used guide posts for the scoring of the posterior surface of the ear in the antihelical fossa while avoiding incisions that would cross the inferior crus, a devastating error. After scoring, horizontal mattress sutures are placed from the scaphoid eminence to the eminence triangularis and the lateral conchal bowl sequentially. These sutures are performed with a 4-0 Mersilene and then tightened to the desired projection, positioning the helical margin 1.5–2 cm off the mastoid at the junction of the superior and inferior crus [22, 23].

When the antihelix is entirely absent, the posterior skin excision is extended as an elliptical dumbbell inferiorly until the beginning of the lobule (Fig. 18.3). After the skin incision is complete, the skin is dissected off the posterior surface of the cauda helices, and the lateral margin of the distal 5–7 mm is resected obliquely (Fig. 18.4).

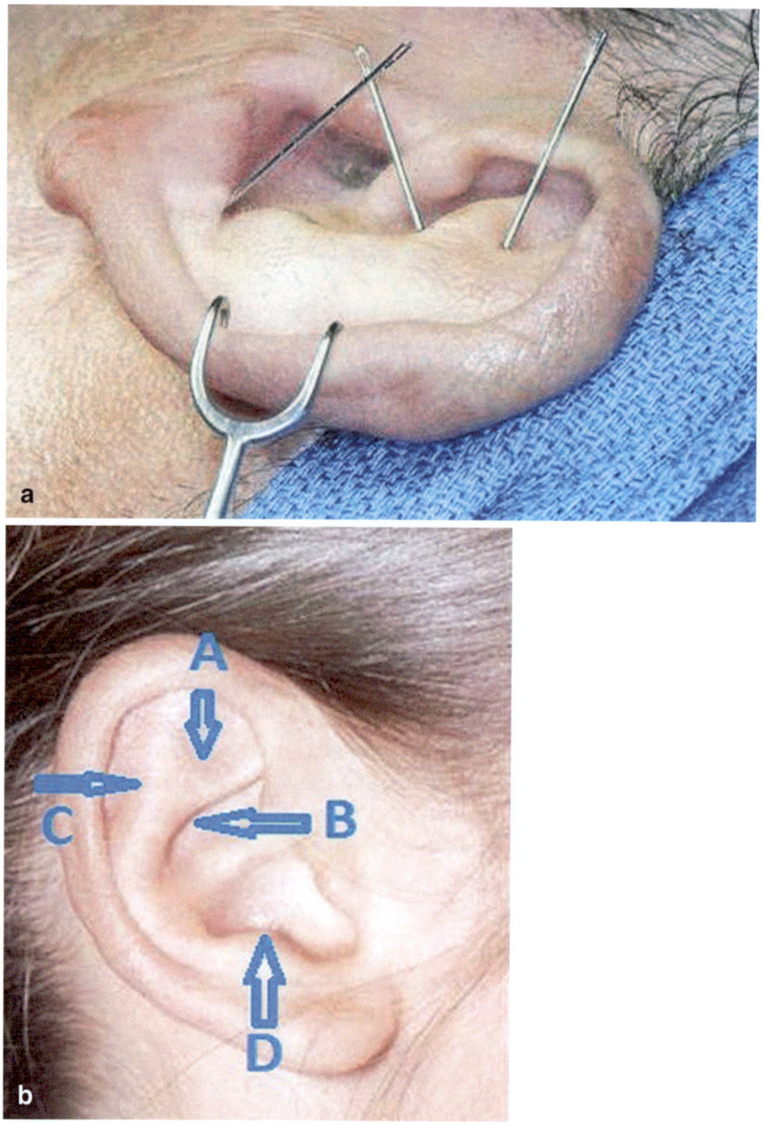

Fig. 18.2 (**a**) Recreation of the superior crus and identifying the corresponding position on the posterior surface can be accomplished by the placement of Keith needles through the ear from the anterior surface. (**b**) Needles are placed at the junction of the superior and inferior crus of the antihelix in the fossa triangularis, the lateral conchal bowl at the junction of the superior and inferior crus, and the anterior margin of the scaphoid fossa

The scoring is then performed, extending down the entire length of the antihelix (Fig. 18.5). Horizontal mattress suture of 4-0 Mersilene is placed from the scaphoid eminence to the lateral conchal bowl (Fig. 18.6). The sutures all radiate from the external auditory canal. When placing the sutures, care is taken to avoid the skin on the anterior surface.

In the presence of a deep conchal bowl, conchal reduction or conchal setback needs to be performed. Conchal reduction is more reliable and results in much less postoperative pain and discomfort. With conchal setback alone, there is no recreation of the antihelix in its absence. To perform conchal reduction, the posterior surface of the cartilage is marked with trans-auricular Keith needles, corresponding to the previously described locations, in addition to the placement of a needle at the lateral conchal bowl even with the antitragus (Fig. 18.2a, b). The index or middle finger is placed in the conchal bowl to palpate the deep surface of the conchal incision, and an ellipse of lateral bowl cartilage is resected with the width dependent on need (Fig. 18.7). This defect is then incorporated into the posterior suturing. The additional sutures are placed from the scaphoid eminence in a horizontal fashion to the lateral and subsequently medial

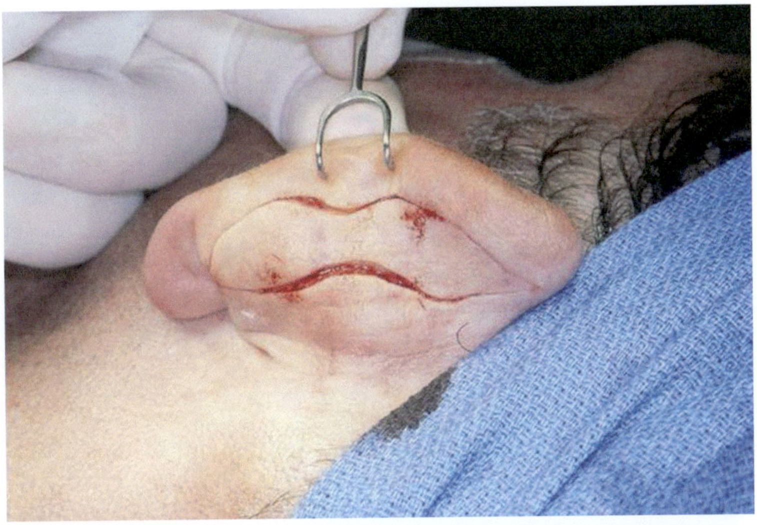

Fig. 18.3 When the antihelix is entirely absent, the posterior skin excision is extended as an elliptical dumbbell inferiorly until the beginning of the lobule

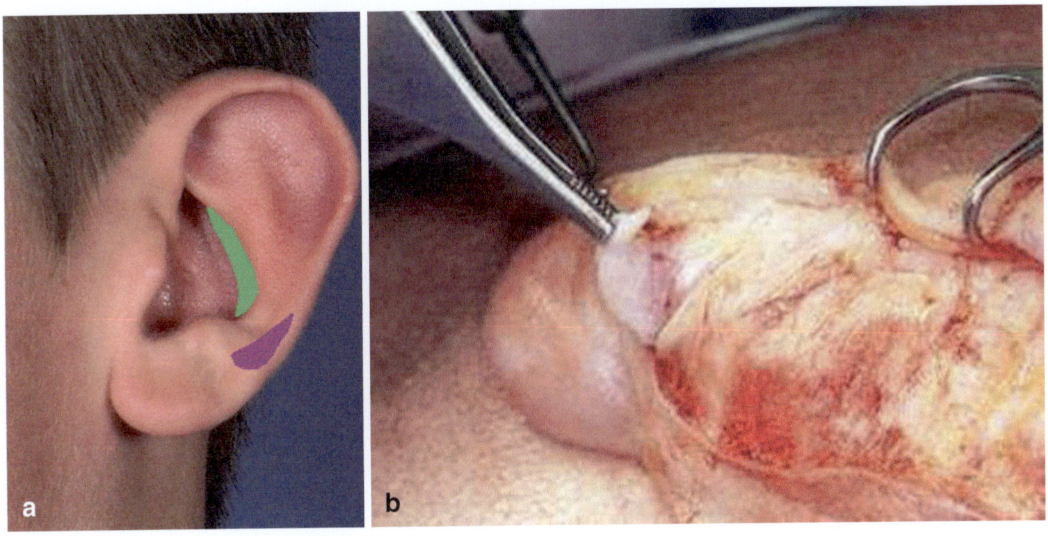

Fig. 18.4 (**a**) Green is the ellipse of lateral bowl of concha to be excised, purple is leteral margin of the distal 5–7 mm to be resected obliquely. (**b**) After the skin incision is complete, the skin is dissected off the posterior surface of the cauda helicis.

margin of the conchal bowl, as a vertical suture (Fig. 18.6).

The postauricular incision is closed with a running, locked, 5-0 plane gut suture. Antibiotic ointment is applied to the incision, and mineral-oil-impregnated cotton is placed in the postauricular sulcus, fossa triangularis, scaphoid fossa, concha cavum, and concha cymba (Fig. 18.8). Fluffed cotton 4 × 4 gauze is secured over the ears with a circumferential dressing encompassing both ears.

When the elliptical dumbbell excision of posterior auricular skin, trimming of the cauda helicis, and a combination of conchal reduction, posterior scoring, and mattress suture are applied appropriately, anatomically correct-appearing ears can be created with little to no evidence of surgical correction (Figs. 18.9 and 18.10).

Earlobe Abnormalities

Earlobe abnormalities may take many forms. They may be postsurgical in nature, the result of a congenital variation, or part of the aging process. The most common variation is the congenital

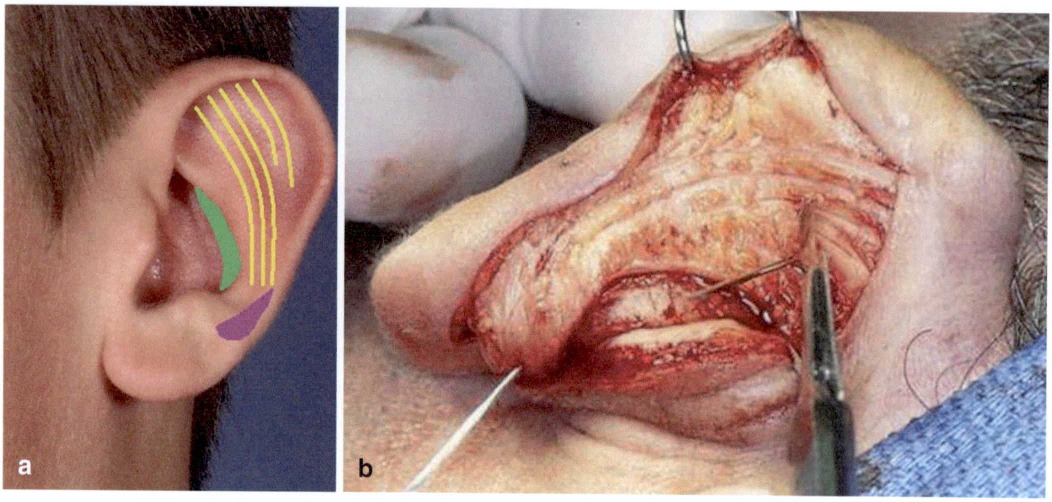

Fig. 18.5 (**a**, **b**) Cartilage scoring (*yellow lines*) is performed extending down the entire length of the antihelix

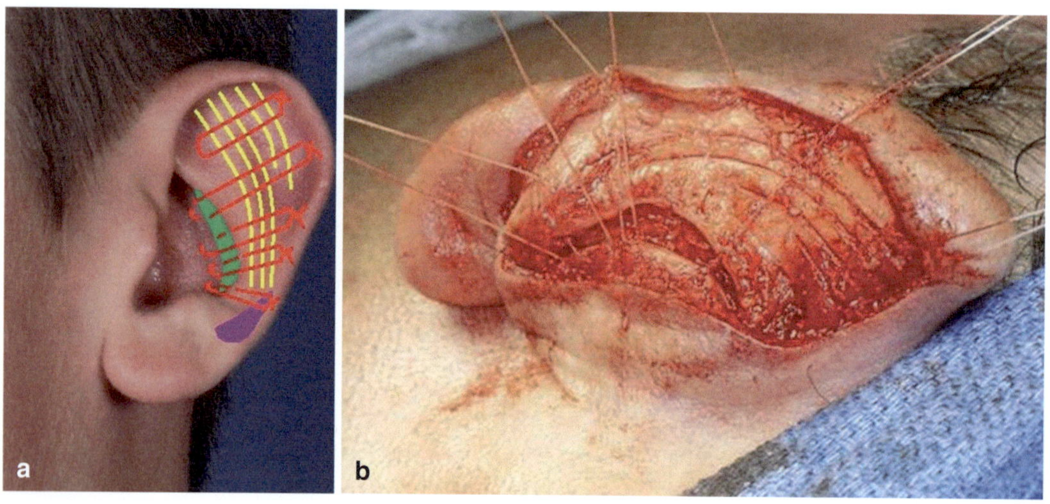

Fig. 18.6 (**a**, **b**) Horizontal mattress sutures of 4-0 Mersilene (*red lines*) are placed from the scaphoid eminence to the lateral conchal bowl. The sutures all radiate from the external auditory canal. When placing the sutures, care is taken to avoid the skin on the anterior surface

attached lobule. The management of the congenital attached lobule is similar to the technique for correcting the postsurgical pixie deformity. The technique for correction of the senile and large lobule will depend upon the vertical and horizontal dimensions of the earlobe and the nature of the attachment of the lobule to the posterior face, as well as the patient's desire or lack thereof to change that attachment. With the large lobule, simple marginal excision, as described by Adamson, can be performed [22].

With the normal-sized attached lobule, whether congenital or iatrogenic, the goal is achieving a more acute angle of attachment without a scar extending vertically into the neck. This is best achieved with a simple transposition flap created from the skin of the inferior margin of the lobule (Fig. 18.11). This flap is repositioned into a postauricular recipient incision, maintaining all visible incisions in the postauricular sulcus and mastoid.

When the attached lobule is enlarged, and overall size reduction as well as release is desired,

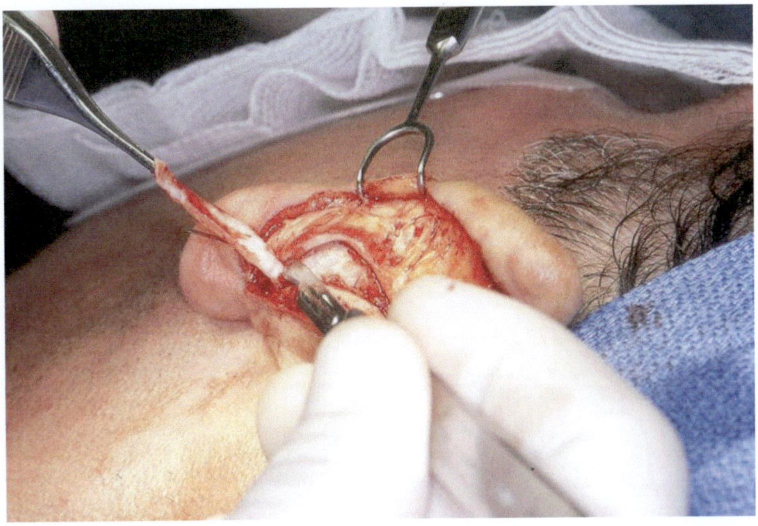

Fig. 18.7 An ellipse of lateral bowl cartilage is resected with the width dependent on need. This defect is then incorporated into the posterior suturing

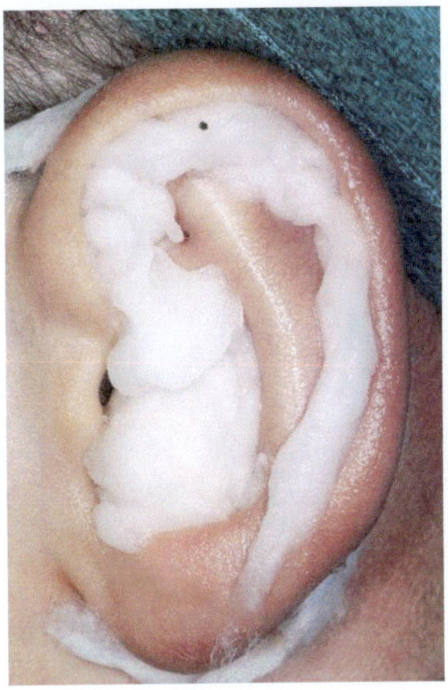

Fig. 18.8 Antibiotic ointment is applied to the incision, and mineral-oil-impregnated cotton is placed in the postauricular sulcus, fossa triangularis, scaphoid fossa, concha cavum, and concha cymba

creativity is the key to a successful release and camouflaged scar. If this is being performed in conjunction with a facelift, it is easy to avoid a vertical cervical incision when lobular reduction is performed first and the facelift flap trimming is executed. This accommodates the repositioning of the earlobe, i.e., eliminating infra-lobular tension with minimal flap resection.

Attached lobule size reduction is achieved through a hemi-crescentic resection of the lobule, with the wider portion anterior at the lobular facial junction (Fig. 18.12). The incision can be blended into the soft tissue furrow of the inferior extent of the scaphoid fossa. If the desired result is to reduce the overall size and release the lobule from its attachments to the posterior face and neck, it is then necessary to butterfly the inferior segment, creating a transposition flap as in the release of the attached lobule prior to creating the hemi-crescentic excision.

For the lobule that is detached and of increased horizontal and vertical dimension, stellate excision is performed. This is planned to include any preexisting rhytids and will more than likely necessitate the repiercing of the ear after completion. With both the stellate and pie-shaped excision, the pattern is offset at the inferior margin of the lobule to prevent a circumferential scar and contracture between the anterior and posterior surface (Fig. 18.13).

Postoperative Care

The otoplasty dressing remains in place for 5 days, but is removed for any complaints of discomfort, pain, or bleeding. After the dressing is removed, the patient is instructed to secure the ears while asleep for 6 weeks postoperatively.

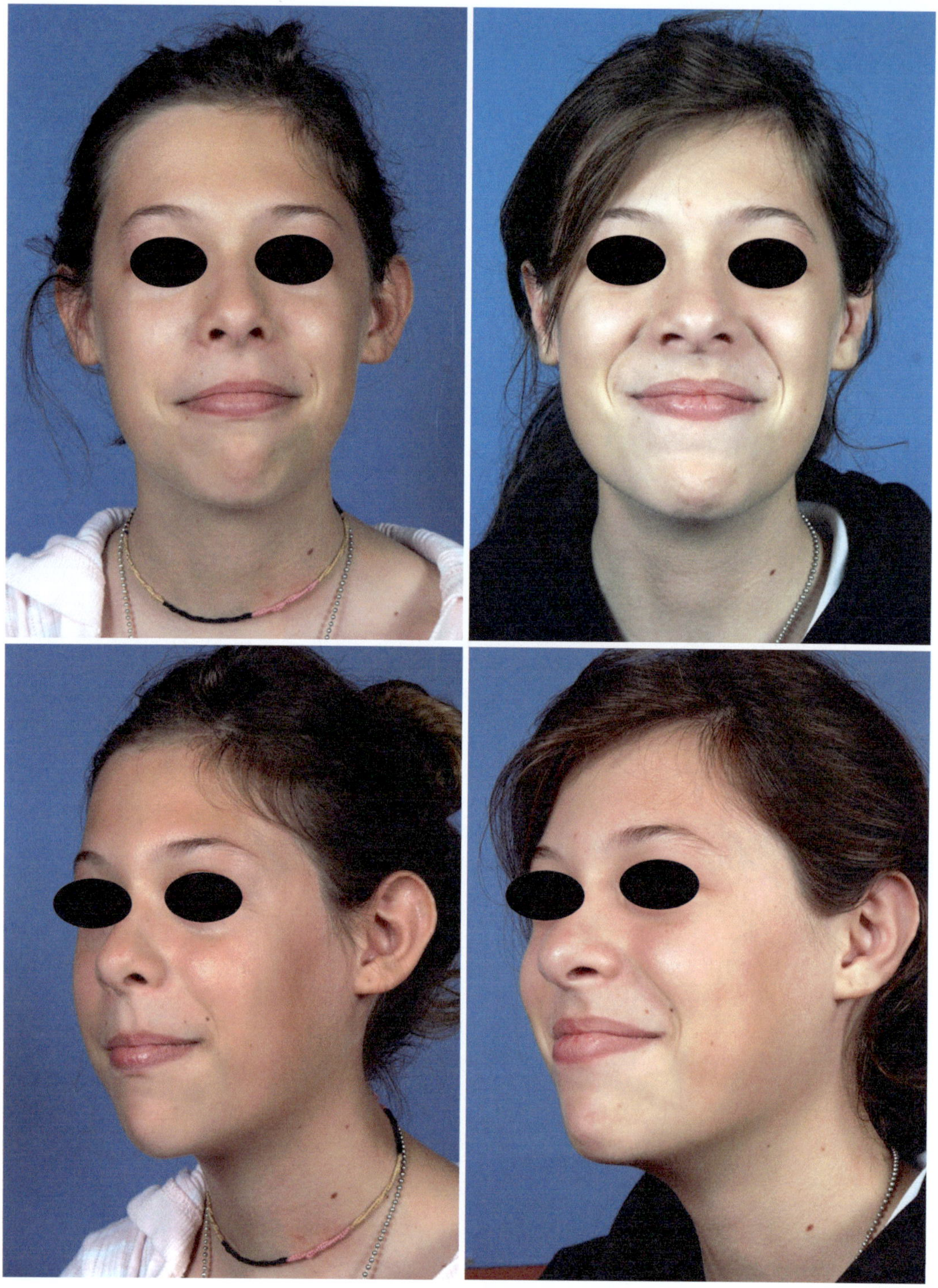

Fig. 18.9 (*Left*) Preoperative. (*Right*) Postoperative following otoplasty

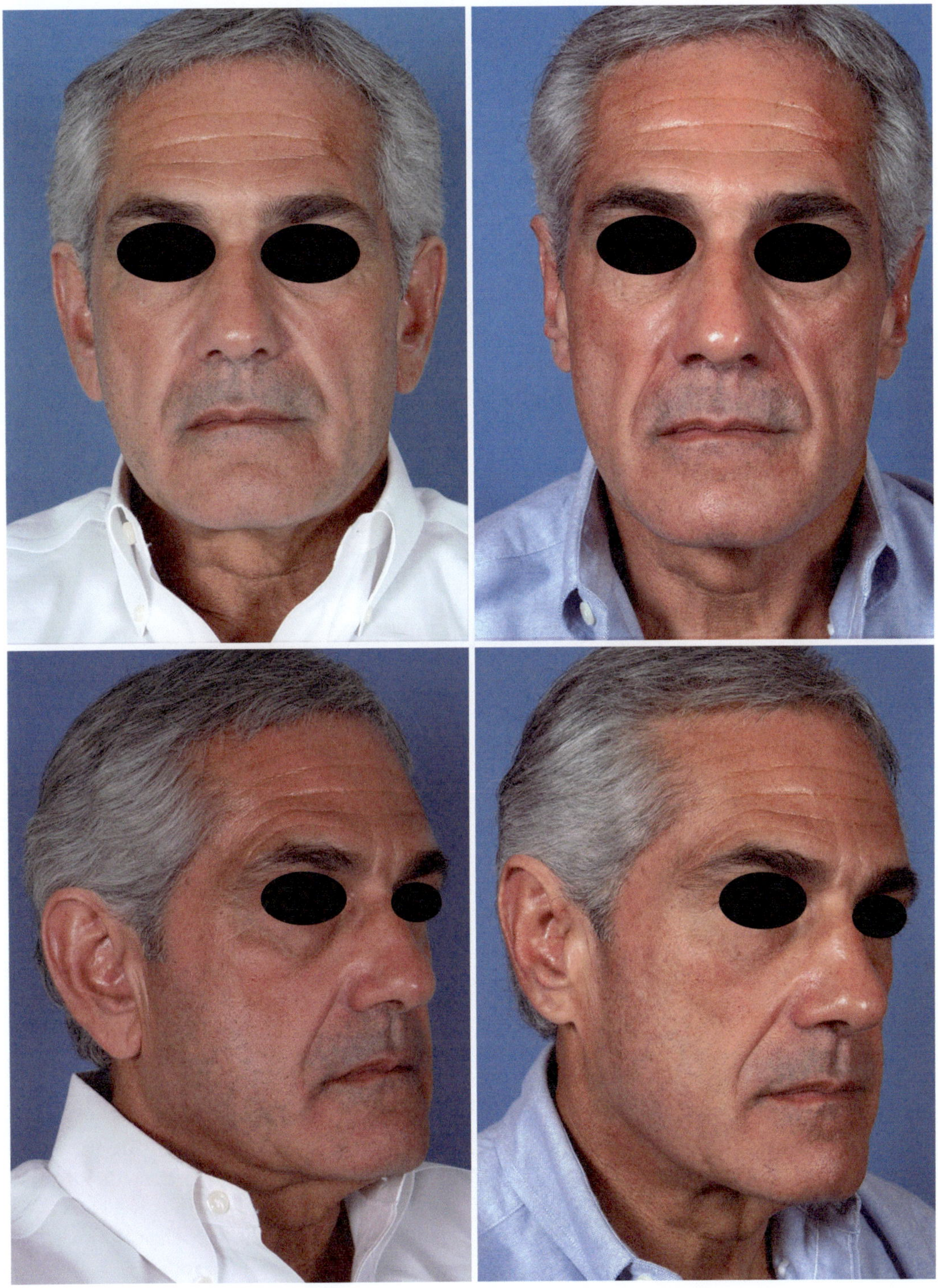

Fig. 18.10 (*Left*) Preoperative. (*Right*) Postoperative following otoplasty with earlobe reduction

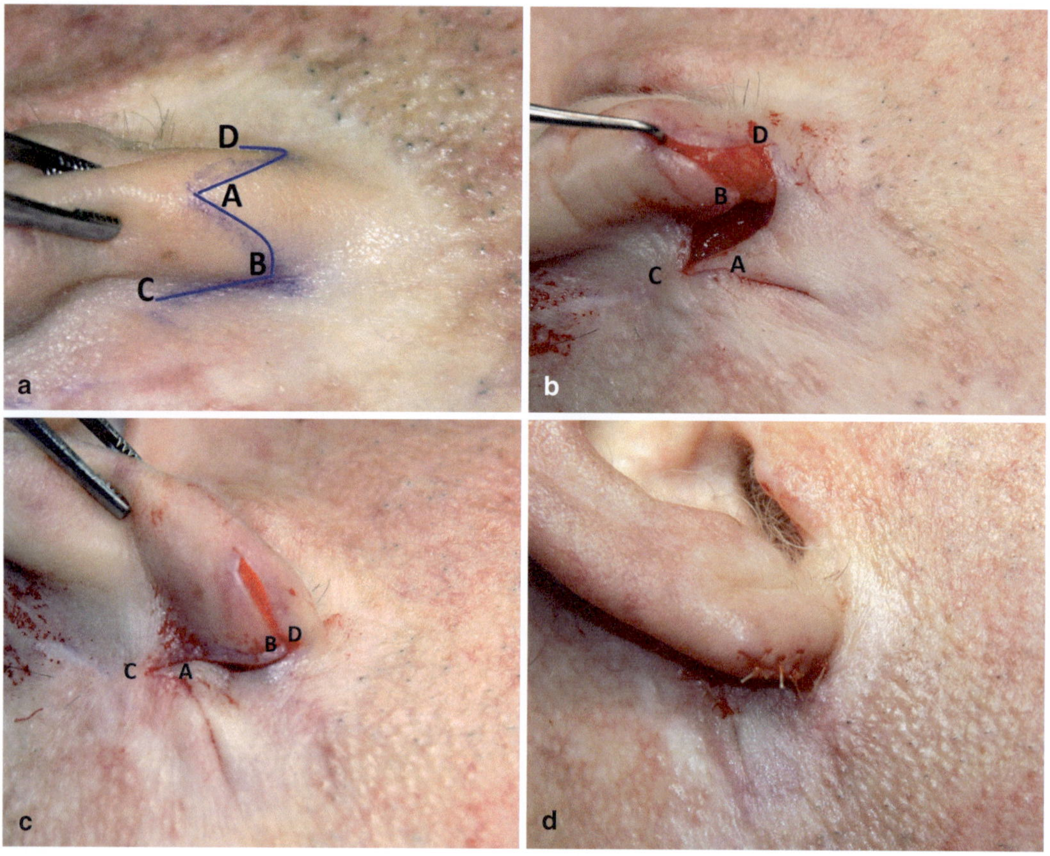

Fig. 18.11 (**a–d**) Correction of the normal-sized attached lobule is best achieved with a simple transposition flap created from the skin of the inferior margin of the lobule. This flap is repositioned into a postauricular recipient incision, maintaining all visible incisions in the postauricular sulcus and mastoid

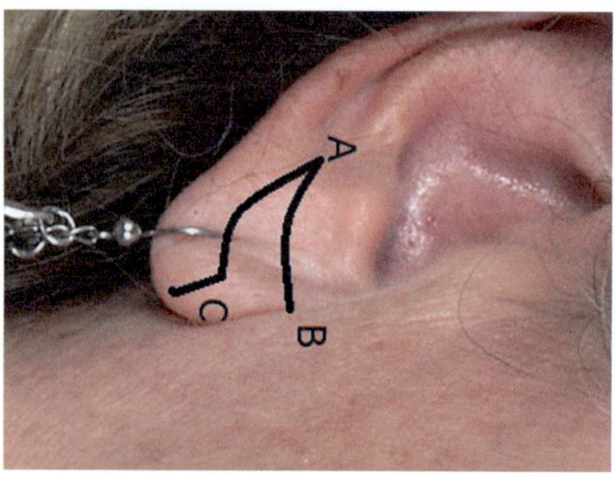

Fig. 18.12 Attached lobule size reduction is achieved thought a hemi-crescent resection of the lobule (C to A to B) with the wider portion anterior at the lobular facial junction

This can be accomplished with an athletic headband. The postauricular incision is cleaned with hydroperoxide and dressed with antibiotic ointment until the fast-absorbing sutures have resorbed. Swimming is allowed immediately after the head dressing is removed, but diving is prohibited for 6 weeks postoperative. Patients are also forbidden from wearing athletic or recreational headgear for 6 weeks.

With earlobe reduction, it is virtually impossible to dress the lobule. Patients are instructed to clean the surgical incisions with peroxide and apply antibiotic ointment twice a day. If the ear is pierced at the time of the procedure, the 14-karat-gold post remains in place for 6 weeks to allow epithelialization and is then changed under the supervision of a nurse in the office.

Complications

As is the case with most elective cosmetic surgical procedures, the rate of complications or adverse incidents is minimal. The most common

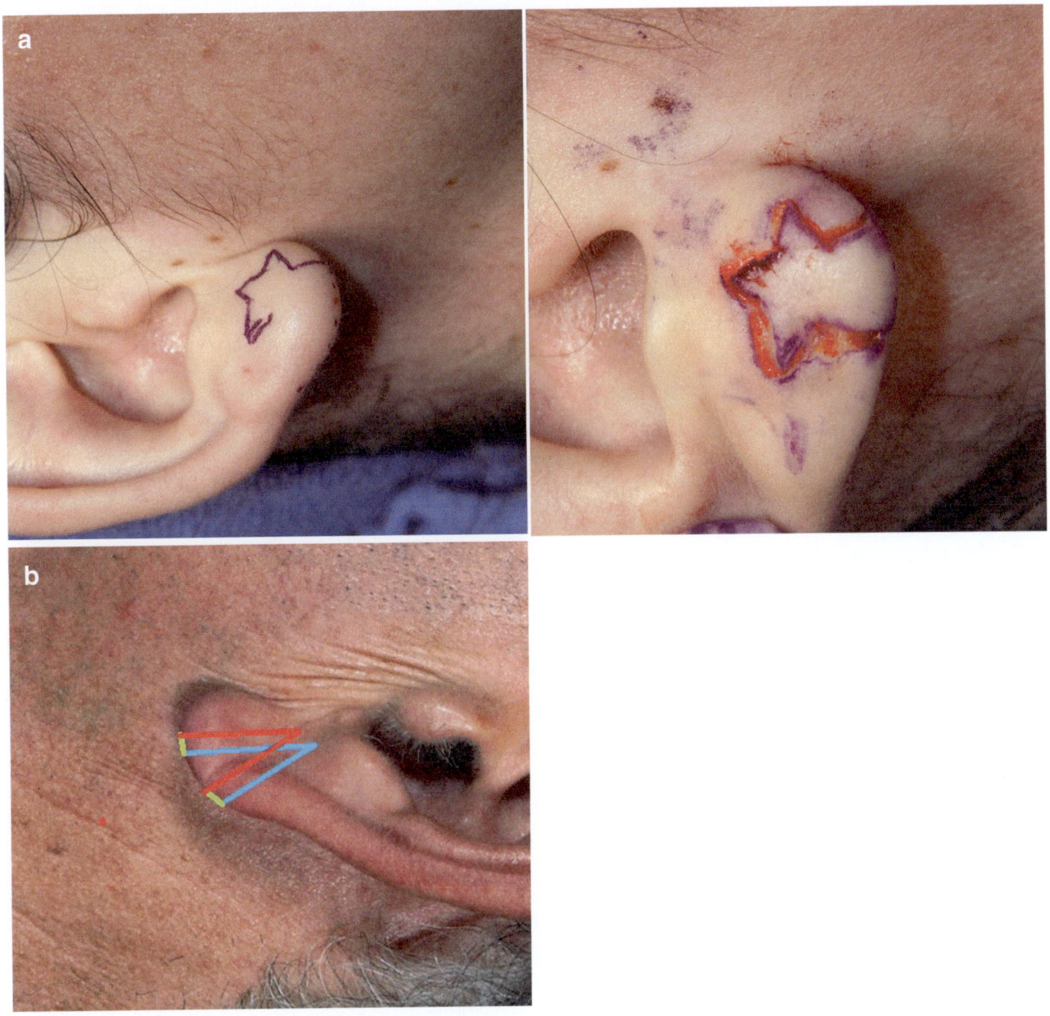

Fig. 18.13 (**a**, **b**) Correction of the enlarged attached lobule is by either stellate or pie-shaped excision and is offset at the inferior margin of the lobule to prevent a circumferential scar and contracture between the anterior and posterior surface (*red line* anterior incision, *blue line* posterior incision)

complication of otoplasty may in fact be the previously unidentified preoperative asymmetry. It is therefore imperative to point out any preoperative differences prior to surgery. These preoperative asymmetries may or may not have been identified by the parents or patient before surgery, but will assuredly be noticed postoperatively. If a postoperative asymmetry exists, this can be addressed with local anesthesia as an outpatient. Most patients are initially counseled to avoid intervention for at least 12 months after surgery. Cartilaginous irregularities may occur on the anterior surface of the ear where cartilaginous incisions were made. When performing a conchal setback, careful posterior suture placement must be performed to avoid anterior displacement of the posterior border of the external auditory canal.

The second most common complication is the extrusion of one of the contouring sutures. This may happen years after the original procedure. In most cases, the cartilage will have recontoured and the protruding suture can be removed without consequence. Hypertrophic and keloid scar formation in the postauricular incision can occur and will more than likely require excision and scar repair, but should initially be treated with intralesional steroid injections.

Postoperative hematoma can develop and necessitate evacuation. If left untreated, the likelihood of developing a wound infection is increased and this may lead to perichondritis and the possible loss of the affected ear.

Conclusions

The graduated technique for otoplasty incorporates the reduction of conchal depth and recreating the antihelix. The most consistent combination of surgical techniques is reducing conchal depth through conchal reduction and recreating the antihelix with scoring in the antihelical fossa on the posterior surface of the ear, followed by the placement of vertical mattress sutures from the scaphoid fossa to approximate the lateral conchal bowl and medial antihelix.

Modifications of lobular size, position, and attachment may be performed as stand-alone procedures or as adjunct to facial rejuvenation or otoplasty for the protruding ear. Their use in facial rejuvenation patients can sometimes be essential to overall facial harmony. Ignoring an enlarged earlobe at the time of a facelift will create an inconsistent appearance postoperatively. These procedures are a safe and simple approach to enhancing outcomes from otoplasty and rhytidectomy, as well as simply reducing an enlarged lobule.

References

1. Richards SD, Jebreel A, Capper R. Otoplasty: a review of the surgical techniques. Clin Otolaryngol. 2005;30(1):2–8.
2. Hauben DJ. Sushruta Samhita (Sushruta'a collection) (800–600 B.C.?). Pioneers of plastic surgery. Acta Chir Plast. 1984;26(2):65–8.
3. Tanzer RC, Converse JM, Brent B. Deformities of the auricle. In: Converse JM, editor. Reconstructive plastic surgery. Philadelphia: WB Saunders Co.; 1977.
4. Ely E. An operation for the prominence of the auricles. Arch Otolaryngol. 1881;10:97–9.
5. Keen WW. New method of operating for relief of deformity from prominent ears. Ann Surg. 1890;11(1): 49–51.
6. Luckett WH. A new operation for prominent ears based on the anatomy of the deformity. Surg Gynecol Obstet. 1910;10:635–7.
7. Becker OJ. Surgical correction of the abnormally protruding ear. Arch Otolaryngol. 1949;50(5):541–60.
8. Converse J, Nigro A, Wilson FA. A technique for surgical correction of lop ear. Plast Reconstr Surg. 1955;15:411.
9. Davis JS, Kitlowski EA. Abnormal prominence of the ears: a method of readjustment surgery. Surgery. 1937;2:835–47.
10. Farrior RT. A method of otoplasty; normal contour of the antihelix and scaphoid fossa. AMA Arch Otolaryngol. 1959;69(4):400–8.
11. Gibson T, Davis WB. The distortion of autogenous cartilage grafts, its cause and prevention. Br J Plast Surg. 1958;10:257–74.
12. Stenstrom SJ. A natural technique for correction of congenital ear deformities. Br J Plast Surg. 1963;99:562.
13. Kaye BL. A simplified method for correcting the prominent ear. Plast Reconstr Surg. 1967;40(1):44–8.
14. Mustarde JC. The correction of prominent ears using simple mattress sutures. Br J Plast Surg. 1963;16: 170–8.
15. Furnas DW. Correction of prominent ears by conchamastoid sutures. Plast Reconstr Surg. 1968;42(3): 189–93.
16. Rogers BO. Microtic, lop, cup and protruding ears: four directly inheritable deformities? Plast Reconstr Surg. 1968;41(3):208–31.
17. Weerda H. Classification of congenital deformities of the auricle. Facial Plast Surg. 1988;5(5):385–8.
18. Potter EL. A hereditary ear malformation transmitted through five generations. J Hered. 1937;28:255–8.
19. Bardach J. Congenital ear deformities. Surgery for congenital and acquired malformations of the auricle. In: Cummings FJ, Fredrickson JM, Harker LA, Krause CJ, Schuler DE, editors. Otolaryngology-head and neck surgery. St. Louis: Mosby; 1986.
20. Nachlas NE, Duncan D, Trail M. Otoplasty. Arch Otolaryngol. 1970;91(1):44–9.
21. Farrior RT. Modified cartilage incisions in otoplasty. Facial Plast Surg. 1985;2(2):109–18.
22. Adamson PA, Litner JA. Otoplasty technique. Facial Plast Surg Clin North Am. 2006;14(2):79–87.
23. Larrabee WF, Adams JB. Otoplasty. In: Smith BR, editor. Pediatric facial plastic and reconstructive surgery. New York: Raven; 1993. p. 78–98.

The Bauer Otoplasty Technique

19

Ahmed M.S. Ibrahim, Samuel J. Lin,
and Bruce S. Bauer

Introduction

The ear pinna in humans adds very little to auditory function; besides helping to collect sound, some have stated that its main purpose is to "appear normal" [1]. Naturally, the term "normal" is subjective and based on what any specific society in general deems as "acceptable." Prominent ears are sometimes referred to as "cup ears" or "lop ears." These prominent ears are often portrayed in cartoon characters depicting an oddball or a less intelligent individual [1]. The prominent ear is a congenital anatomic finding found in approximately 5 % of the population and is characterized by deformities of various auricular structures such as concha valga, hypertrophy of the concha, change in the auricular-cranium angle, and absence of antihelix modeling [2, 3]. An ear is termed prominent if the ear projects more than 15–20 mm or more than 21–30° from the temporomastoid plane of the skull. In boys, the mean length of the ear is 55 mm at 6 years, 60 mm at 12 years, and 62 mm at 18 years; in girls, the mean length of the ear is 54 mm, 58 mm, and 58 mm at 6, 12, and 18 years, respectively. The mean width of the ear in boys is 34, 35, and 36 mm at 6, 12, and 18 years while in girls, the mean width of the era is 33, 34, and 34 mm, respectively [1]. If an ear is 2 or more standard deviations from the mean (2.0–2.5 for width, 3.0–3.5 for length), it is considered abnormally large (macrotia).

Children with prominent ears are often the target of abuse resulting in long-term psychological complications [4–6]. Studies have shown that following corrective surgery, there is a marked improvement in the quality of life experienced by these individuals [6–9]. Even with known standards for ideal anthropomorphic measurements and facial proportions, societal standards

A.M.S. Ibrahim, M.D. • S.J. Lin, M.D.
Divisions of Plastic Surgery
and Otolaryngology-Head and Neck Surgery,
Beth Israel Deaconess Medical Center,
Harvard Medical School,
110 Francis Street, Suite 5A, Boston, MA 02215, USA

Division of Plastic Surgery,
Beth Israel Deaconess Medical Center,
Harvard Medical School,
Boston, MA, USA
e-mail: aibrahim@bidmc.harvard.edu;
sjlin@bidmc.harvard.edu

B.S. Bauer, M.D. (✉)
Pediatric Plastic Surgery, NorthShore University
HealthSystem, Northbrook, IL, USA

Department of Surgery, University of Chicago, Pritzker
School of Medicine, Chicago, IL, USA

Section of Pediatric Plastic Surgery,
Division of Plastic and Reconstructive Surgery,
NorthShore University Health System,
University of Chicago Medical School,
501 Skokie Blvd, Northbrook, IL 60062 USA
email: bbauer@northshore.org

M.A. Shiffman (ed.), *Advanced Cosmetic Otoplasty*,
DOI 10.1007/978-3-642-35431-1_19, © Springer-Verlag Berlin Heidelberg 2013

continue to change. Naturally, humans understand how a "normal" face should appear, and any deviation from that (such as prominent ears) may elicit a negative response [1].

Many authors have contributed to the evolution of otoplasty [3, 10–53]. In essence, a majority of otoplasty procedures are effective in reducing the prominence of the ear; however, one approach may be better suited for a particular problem than another, and each is characterized by variations based on the nature or the shape of the auricle.

History of the Procedure

Sushruta is credited with the development of the first otoplasty in ancient India in the fifth century BC. His otoplastic principles, slightly modified, are still being applied nearly two millenniums later. Johann Friedrich Dieffenbach (1794–1847) reported the first surgical approach for correction of prominent ears which combined excision of excess cartilage from the posterior sulcus of the ear with suturing of the corrected pinna to the mastoid periosteum. In 1881, Ely [54] is reported as having performed the first otoplasty in medical literature. Ely's technique was then expanded upon by Hippolyte Morestin in 1903 where he described the use of concha-mastoid (C-M) sutures, antihelix (Mustarde) sutures, an antihelix incision, and thinning of the posterior surface of the cartilage. In addressing the flat antihelix, in 1910, Luckett reported incising the cartilage and creating a crest by joining the cut edges with mattress sutures. In 1920, Harold D. Gillies was able to reproduce the pinna by burying an external-ear support framework constructed with autologous rib cartilage under the skin of the mastoid region followed by separation of the reconstructed pinna from the skin of the mastoid area using a cervical flap. GW Pierce in 1930 was able to weaken the line of the crest of the antihelix and hence facilitate formation of the fold by scoring the posterior surface of the cartilage. In 1958, Gibson showed that disrupting a balanced cross section of costal cartilage could cause warping distal to the site of disruption. While working with Pierce, Stenstrom and Heftner [55] noted that cartilage would curl away from a scored surface, and therefore, anterior scoring replaced posterior scoring of the antihelix. A tubelike crest was formed by making parallel cartilage incisions, and mattress sutures were later employed to create the fold of the antihelix [56–58]. To reduce the deep concha, Furnas [59] expanded on Morestin's original C-M sutures; this technique was later modified by Gault et al. [60] and Elliott [33].

Kaye [15] and Davis [61] later described anterior approaches for altering the antihelix which were recently modified by Nordzell [62] and Erol [10]. More recently, the importance of conchal enlargement on overall ear structure and prominence has been emphasized. The senior author (BSB) presents an approach in which chondrocutaneous resection rather than being an adjunctive procedure became the cornerstone of otoplasty recognizing that release of the conchal support to the antihelical body allowed gentle reshaping of the antihelix avoiding many of the drawbacks of prior approaches. Additionally, with more experience, the anterior approach to the concha allows for precise correction of more subtle aspects of the challenging prominent ear patient as well as a means of preventing and correcting secondary deformities; this technique may decrease the revision rate following correction of the prominent ear.

Indications

In assessing a patient for otoplasty, one needs to consider the anatomic causes for protrusion of the ear. Prominence is typically a result of three variants: (1) underdevelopment of the antihelical fold, (2) overdevelopment of the conchal bowl and wall, and (3) a scaphoconchal angle greater than 90°. Additionally, contributing factors may include (1) protrusion of the lower auricular pole, (2) prominence of the mastoid process, and (3) a prominent-tipped upper auricular pole. Protrusion of the auricle may also be one component of a more complex deformity such as constricted ear, Stahl ear (third crus), macrotia, or syndromic facial deformity [63].

A majority of the patients who present for otoplasty have visibly prominent ears; however, not all patients have a desire to change their appearance. Generally, the parents of children with prominent ears will bring them in for correction in an effort to spare their child embarrassment and teasing [64]. Children under the age of 5 years are rarely perceptive enough about their appearance to feel that surgery is necessary; this dynamic may occasionally result in difficulty cooperating with postoperative care. Regardless, ear surgery is best addressed at a younger age as the ear becomes firmer, less malleable, and calcified with age. At infancy, the prominent ear can even be addressed with nonsurgical molding. More subtle cases of ear prominence, distortion of ear shape, or ear asymmetry may not necessitate the need for correction until a child is older and oriented with his or her appearance. Ultimately, a decision regarding surgery needs to be made on a case-by-case basis.

Adults seeking otoplasty must be able to adequately provide substantial reasoning for seeking a change, demonstrate an understanding of the realistic expectations of a postoperative result, and understand postoperative management. It is vital that cases be meticulously selected especially when the deformity is a minimal or a subtle finding.

Contraindications

Contraindications may exist with each patient. In children, potential contraindications include (1) a strong resistance by the child to undergo surgery which may be hidden in the form of misbehavior or becoming extremely nervous about going to the doctor or to the hospital and (2) a history of chronic ear infections and ear drainage that have not been thoroughly treated. Conditions such as scalp infections or acne must also be treated well in advance of surgery. A simple surgical wound infection can lead to an ear-threatening chondritis.

There are various ethnic and cultural considerations that the operating surgeon should take into consideration in preoperative planning. In Japanese culture, prominent ears denote intelligence while in Celtic communities they are very common. Most children quickly conform to the cultural values of their adopted country.

Preoperative Preparation

A thorough history and physical examination should be obtained. Sufficient time for adequate preoperative planning is paramount. Proper assessment of the auricular deformity is key. The specifics of the deformity are discussed, and the procedure is described in detail; preoperative discussion includes anesthesia type and postoperative routine. Possible risks such as hematoma, chondritis, and infection are reviewed. It is important to carefully listen to what the patient (and parent) is expressing and attempt to adequately answer their questions. The patient (and parent) should express an understanding of the expectations and possible complications of the procedure. Dealing with any concerns that the patient might have in the preoperative period increases the likelihood that a technically excellent otoplasty will be viewed with satisfaction and gratitude. It is not necessary to worry the patient, but full disclosure dictates that patients understand the risks and benefits of otoplasty. All patients should be told that there is a risk that a revision may be necessary.

Anesthesia

Local Anesthesia

A potential ideal candidate for local anesthesia without premedication is a suitably mature child aged at least 10 years with uncomplicated prominent ears. A eutectic mixture of local anesthetics (EMLA) cream is applied to the postauricular area 2–3 h before surgery. An oral antibiotic is administered an hour prior to surgery. A 27- or 30-gauge needle is used to infiltrate the retroauricular and posterior surfaces of the ear with buffered 1 % lidocaine (Xylocaine) with epinephrine 1:100,000. Bupivacaine (0.25 %) with epinephrine 1:100,000 is then administered, and lidocaine or bupivacaine (Marcaine) is reinforced during the procedure. All throughout the procedure, a parent may read a favorite story or play a favorite audio tape for the child.

General Anesthesia

General anesthesia is recommended in younger patients. Following induction, an endotracheal tube is placed in the midline and secured with a circum-mandibular or transalveolar suture of 0 or #1 Prolene. The table is then turned 180° with the anesthesiologist at the foot of the table. A broad-spectrum antibiotic is then administered intravenously. After all markings have been placed, the anterior and posterior surfaces of both ears are injected with 0.5 % lidocaine with 1:200,000 epinephrine solution. The patient is also injected with 0.25 % bupivacaine to provide bilateral great auricular nerve blocks for postoperative analgesia.

Position/Markings

The patient is placed in the supine position, prepped and draped in the usual sterile fashion with both ears and the retroauricular skin exposed. Skin prepping solution is used to sterilize the face and both ears. These areas are then draped with a standard head drape with both ears exposed. A Tegaderm or other clear sterile drape is used to secure any stray hairs. Surgical soap is then used to shampoo the hair, and Betadine is applied to prep the face, neck, ears, and adjacent ventilating tube. Mastisol adhesive solution is applied to the face, and a series of 1-in. Steri-Strips are placed to hold the head towels securely to the face and neck. Steri-Strips are also placed over the eyes. A body sheet is used that is made of clear plastic and thereby provides visibility of the entire ventilating system. The patient's head may be placed on a doughnut.

The incision is marked along the retroauricular sulcus and less frequently on the posterior surface of the concha if a conchal excision is planned. If a lobular setback is planned, a triangular area of the skin is marked for incision at the most medial area of retrolobular skin. The intended region of antihelical fold creation is marked.

Technique

The procedure begins with incisional injection of local vasoconstrictive/anesthetic agents. This local solution not only helps with hemostasis but also aids in soft tissue dissection from cartilage. In addition, bipolar cautery is used throughout the procedure. The incision is made with a #15 blade on the anterior surface of the concha; it is placed at the junction of the floor of the concha and the posterior conchal wall. It starts in the cymba concha and continues along the cavum concha to a point below the antitragus but does not extend as far as the external auditory meatus. It is important to avoid placing the incision too high in the concha which will reduce control of the antihelical fold leading to disfigurement of the antihelix. The incision continues through both the anterior skin and conchal cartilage and is stopped just before the posterior conchal skin. Using sharp dissection in the loose areolar plane behind the concha, the incision is then deepened through the subcutaneous tissues to expose soft tissue and skin from the posterior surface of the conchal bowl. A crescent-shaped chondrocutaneous segment is then excised. To ensure a tension-free closure, it is fundamental that more cartilage than skin be resected especially along the inferior concha deep to the antitragus. The amount of cartilage and skin resection needed to create an aesthetically pleasing position for the ear and to address conchal hypertrophy can be accurately assessed with by applying finger pressure to produce a gentle setback of the antihelix. Three or four interrupted 5-0 clear nylons are used to suture the edges of the conchal cartilage. The most inferior suture should be placed at the junction of cavum concha and antitragus to aid the cartilage in supporting the lobule. A slight overlapping of cartilage (antitragal segment over conchal segment) will cause the lobule to tip posteriorly.

Next, using a combination of 5-0 chromic gut with horizontal mattress sutures and a running

6-0 mild chromic gut, the anterior skin is closed. Initially, the ear and helical rim may appear prominent; this is easily corrected by gently applying pressure to the antihelix which will cause relaxation of the tension required in order to bend the antihelix. To correct prominence of the lobule and the effaced antihelix, a dumbbell-shaped ellipse of skin with the inferior end widened to a diamond shape (positioned with its maximal width at the point of maximal lobule prominence) is excised down to the perichondrium. This maneuver will help to correct lower pole prominence by providing access to the posterior surface of the scapha and helical sulcus for the placement of sutures. When exposing the posterior surface of the conchal bowl and scapha, it is important to preserve the perichondrium to reduce the chances of subsequent sutures pulling through the cartilage. Care is also taken to properly identify and free the helical tail. Cartilage of the tail from the skin overlying its anterior surface must not be freed as this may diminish the effectiveness of correcting prominence of the lobule. Finally, dissection proceeds onto the mastoid surface, where soft tissues are freed ensuring that sutures placed later can be securely fastened into the mastoid fascia.

Before proceeding with the placement of sutures to further correct the ear prominence, it is important to assess the spring or resistance of the cartilage to further shaping by putting pressure on the helical rim and antihelix. Even a limited amount of conchal resection results in lessening of this spring and increased ease of shaping the antihelix. At this stage, any additional sutures needed to complete an accurate closure of the conchal defect are placed. To correct prominence of the upper and middle thirds of the ear, two or three 4-0 clear nylon sutures are placed from the scaphal cartilage and helical sulcus cartilage to the mastoid fascia. The most superior suture is placed from the region of the triangular fossa to the temporal fascia. To ensure proper placement of these sutures, a straight Keith needle is used to apply pressure to the preferred points on the anterior surface of the ear. The point of the needle is then passed through the selected spot and visualized on the posterior surface of the cartilage. A nylon suture is then placed at each specific point, and the needle is withdrawn; sutures are passed through either the temporal or mastoid fascia. When all the sutures are placed, they are carefully tied beginning with the scaphal suture (one should be meticulous of the relationship of the helical rim and the reshaped antihelix so that the helical rim remains visible from the frontal view). It is imperative that the sutures be tied at the proper tension to create a smooth antihelical fold. If there is a need to approximate the helical root and head, an additional suture is placed from the triangular fossa to the temporal fascia. In adult patients, the cartilage of the antihelix may be less flexible, and therefore, extra sutures may be needed to shape and round the antihelix (placed prior to the ones described previously to preshape the antihelix before further correcting the prominence). These sutures are placed from the helical sulcus to the cut edge of concha at right angles to the antihelix and from the scapha to the cut edge of the concha and deep to the inferior crus.

Following correction of the upper and mid auricular prominence, position of the lobule is addressed. Lobule position is determined by the closure of the squid-shaped ellipse using 5-0 chromic gut. The optimum shape, contour, and projection of the lobule is obtained by altering the initial position of the suture; the remaining closure is continued with a running 5-0 chromic suture. Correcting the more prominent side first provides a symmetrical setback; guiding the placement of sutures defines the antihelix and lobule prominence.

Correction of irregularities of the helical rim in the area of Darwin's tubercle and reduction of prominence of the antitragus are the most common adjunctive procedures. A small incision is created parallel to the border of the prominence; excess cartilage is exposed and resected. This is then closed with an interrupted and running 6–0 mild chromic suture. Enlargement of the lobule can be addressed by a large resection at the junction of the lobule and middle third where the splice can be stair stepped at the splice point or small wedge resection within the lobule itself for smaller degrees of lobule enlargement.

Postoperative Period

The ends of the subcuticular sutures are taped with Steri-Strips. Petroleum jelly gauze is molded into the lateral contours of the ear and in the postauricular sulcus. The ears are covered with soft gauze pads. Kerlix strips are placed over each eye, and the head is wrapped with a roll of Kerlix gauze. Each of the vertical gauze strips is tied, compressing the head wrap to clear the visual fields. To minimize shifting, the wrap is taped to the skin at several points.

Follow-Up

Dressings are removed on postoperative day one to check for shifts in position, pressure points, and hematomas. Skin sutures are removed on postoperative day 5–7 (the subcuticular suture in the postauricular sulcus is removed on postoperative day 10 or later). Patients are asked to look in the mirror daily to familiarize themselves with the features of their newly positioned ears and to report any changes that are noticed.

Discussion

A thorough understanding of the anatomy of the prominent ear and meticulous analysis of the complex deformity that comprises the prominent ear are required to perform the best possible otoplasty procedure [65, 66]. The ultimate goal is to achieve an aesthetically pleasing result that conforms to the patient's appearance in accordance with the patient's body image [1].

The prominent ear has numerous etiologies, but the common denominator has always been hypertrophy of the concha [67]. Understanding this fact is imperative; even with minor resection and resuturing of the cut concha, posterior placement of sutures will cause the antihelix to yield with a soft, smooth, rounded shape unmarred by any sharp irregular surfaces [67].

Attainment of perfect symmetry is highly unlikely in every single patient undergoing this procedure; however, the application of adjunctive procedures (see technique) at the initial procedure has helped to evade this concern. To date, all revision procedures, even in younger children, have been accomplished with a single procedure under local anesthesia in the office setting [1].

In the senior author's (BSB) experience with this technique, there have been no major or minor complications. In a series of 292 patients, Baker and Converse [32] reported a 3 % incidence of telephone deformity, 1.2 % localized cellulitis, 0.7 % chondritis, and 0.8 % hematoma. Keloids developed in 11 % of black patients (one bilateral) and 2.1 % of white patients. Despite other authors criticizing this approach as a potential source of keloid formation [39, 68, 69], Bauer has not reported keloids in any cases including a larger series of conchal donor sites for composite grafts used for ear reconstruction [70]. Limandjaja et al. [71] found that the incidence of early complications (hematoma, bleeding, infection, skin necrosis, and wound dehiscence) associated with otoplasty was low (0–8.4 %) while late complications (suture extrusion, scarring, hypersensitivity, asymmetry) occurred more frequently (up to 47.3 % of the time). Occasionally, patients develop tenderness in the postauricular area which decreases over time.

Recurrence of prominence of the ear is quite rare. Should that scenario present itself, a repeat procedure is selected, taking into account the causes of the relapse. The patient is asked to wear an elastic headband in the postoperative period for anywhere from 6 to 12 months. Bauer has reported a higher incidence of recurrence in younger children with a constriction component to the prominence. To avoid this occurrence, an additional scaphal suture to the cut edge of the concha is placed to resist the forward spring of the upper pole of the ear. Following this approach, no recurrence has been noted [65]. It is also important to note that it is not uncommon for an otoplasty that appears pleasing at the end of a surgery to curl, buckle, or shift as a result of external pressures such as gravitational pressure when sleeping. These phenomena can easily be dealt with in the early postoperative period using molding material. They key to a favorable response is early recognition and rapid treatment.

To achieve the best outcomes, it is important to remember that correct analysis of each ear deformity is the most important step. A failure to appreciate all the elements causing distortion of ear position will result in a poor aesthetic outcome. One must remember to avoid placing the incision for conchal resection too high in the concha, assure a tension-free closure of the concha, stay away from excessive resection of skin or cartilage, and attempt to preserve the perichondrium on both surfaces of the cartilage. Additionally, when designing the dumbbell-shaped excision, it is imperative that the skin excision be tapered at its midportion to prevent the development of postoperative telephone ear deformity. This approach has been consistent and durable and can serve as viable option when considering otoplasty for the correction of prominent ears.

Conclusions

Various otoplasty techniques exist that have been modified over time. Many of these procedures are useful in addressing prominence of the ear. Depending on the shape and nature of the auricle in addition to patient expectations, one approach may be better suited than another. A myriad of techniques exist for otoplasty suggesting that there is not one definitive approach, and each surgery must be tailored to the individual patient. The Bauer Otoplasty Technique offers an alternative option and can be applied to a multitude of ear deformities requiring reconstruction. To yield the best possible aesthetic outcomes not only is a proper understanding of the normal anatomy essential, it is paramount that the operating surgeon comprehend the principles of this procedure and have an appreciation of the minor details that this approach entails (Figs. 19.1, 19.2, 19.3, 19.4, 19.5, 19.6, 19.7, and 19.8).

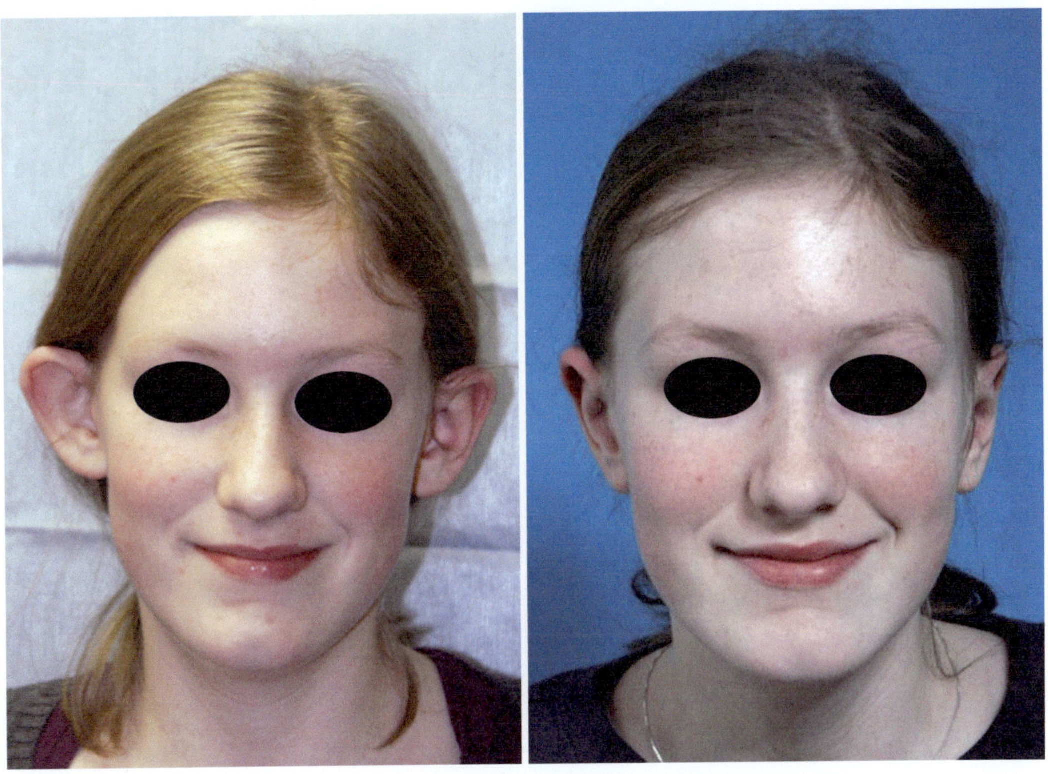

Fig. 19.1 Preoperative image of patient with prominent ears (*left*). Postoperative image following correction (*right*)

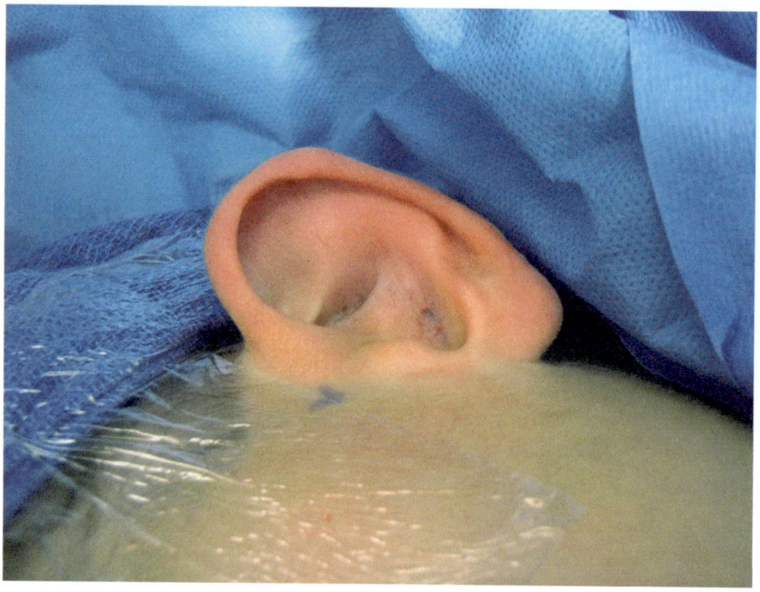

Fig. 19.2 Intraoperative view of the patient's left ear

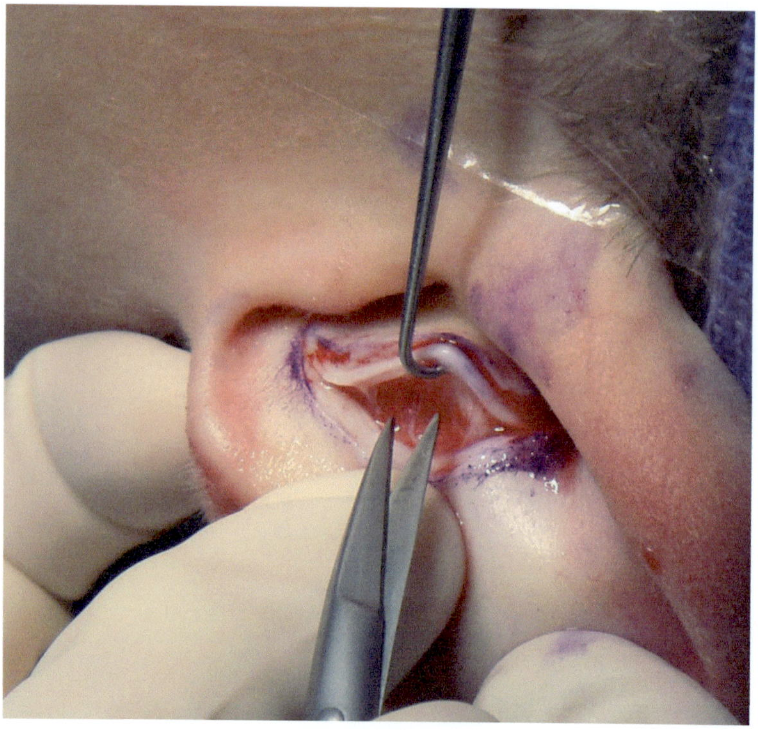

Fig. 19.3 Beginning of cartilage dissection using an anterior approach

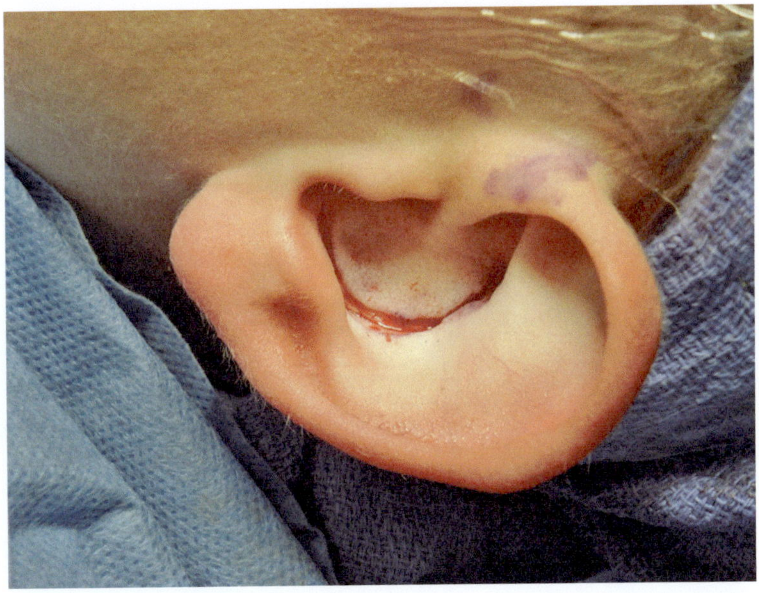

Fig. 19.4 Dissection of concha by an anterior approach

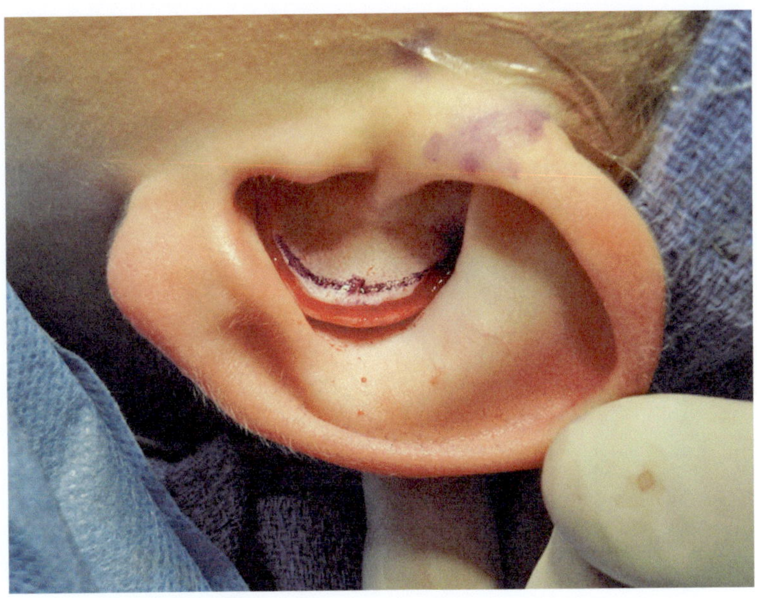

Fig. 19.5 Planned resection of a chondrocutaneous section of the concha from an anterior approach

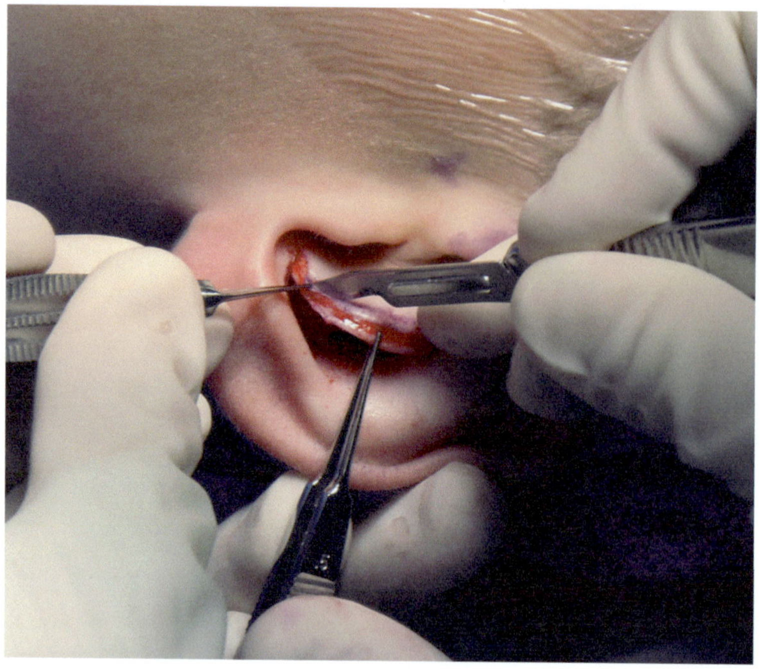

Fig. 19.6 Dissection of the chondrocutaneous portion of the concha

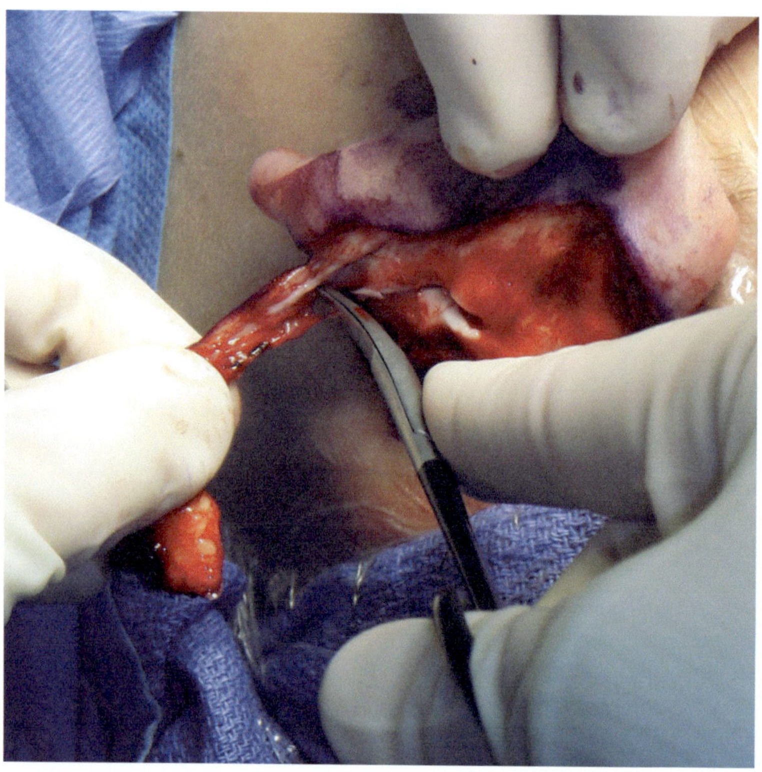

Fig. 19.7 Resection of the chondrocutaneous portion of the concha

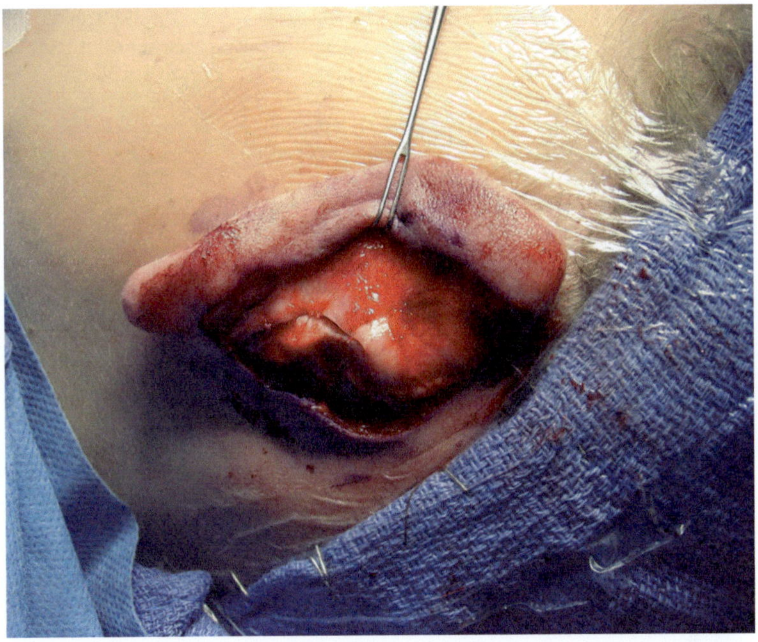

Fig. 19.8 Placement of sutures and closure

References

1. Lin SJ, Furnas D. Prominent ear. In: Narayan D, editor. emedicine.medscape.com/article/1290275-overview; 2009.
2. Amaro JWF. Aspectos psicolo'gicos e psicossociais da cirurgia reparadora. In: Sucena RC, editor. Cirurgia Plastica. Sao Paulo: Roca; 1981. p. 95–169.
3. Guyuron B, DeLuca L. Ear projection and the posterior auricular muscle insertion. Plast Reconstr Surg. 1997;100(2):457–60.
4. Bradbury E. The psychology of aesthetic plastic surgery. Aesthetic Plast Surg. 1994;18(3):301–5.
5. Bradbury ET, Hewison J, Timmons MJ. Psychological and social outcome of prominent ear correction in children. Br J Plast Surg. 1992;45(2):97–100.
6. Klassen A, Jenkinson C, Fitzpatrick R, Goodacre T. Patients' health related quality of life before and after aesthetic surgery. Br J Plast Surg. 1996;49(7):433–8.
7. Sarwer DB, Wadden TA, Pertschuk MJ, Whitaker LA. The psychology of cosmetic surgery: a review and reconceptualization. Clin Psychol Rev. 1998;18(1):1–22.
8. Hasan JS. Psychological issues in cosmetic surgery: a functional overview. Ann Plast Surg. 2000;44(1):89–96.
9. Gasques JA, de Godoy JM P, Cruz EM. Psychosocial effects of otoplasty in children with prominent ears. Aesthetic Plast Surg. 2008;32(6):910–4.
10. Erol OO. New modification in otoplasty: anterior approach. Plast Reconstr Surg. 2001;107(1):193–202; discussion 203–5.
11. Stenstroem SJ. A "natural" technique for correction of congenitally prominent ears. Plast Reconstr Surg. 1963;32:509–18.
12. Spira M, Stal S. The conchal flap: an adjunct in otoplasty. Ann Plast Surg. 1983;11(4):291–8.
13. Furnas DW. Correction of prominent ears by conchamastoid sutures. Plast Reconstr Surg. 1968;42(3):189–93.
14. Connolly A, Bartley J. 'External' Mustarde suture technique in otoplasty. Clin Otolaryngol Allied Sci. 1998;23(2):97–9.
15. Kaye BL. A simplified method for correcting the prominent ear. Plast Reconstr Surg. 1967;40(1):44–8.
16. Gay Jr EC. Auricular repositioning otoplasty. Laryngoscope. 1974;84(3):468–84.
17. Yarchuk NI, Limberg AA, Nekachalov VV. Clinical and histological characteristics of late results of otoplasty using diced cadaver cartilage. Acta Chir Plast. 1975;17(4):188–97.
18. Smith R, Dickinson JT, Teachey WS. Medial conchal excision in otoplasty. Laryngoscope. 1975;85(4):738–50.
19. Stucker FJ, Christiansen TA. Otoplasty techniques. Trans Pa Acad Ophthalmol Otolaryngol. 1976;29(1):52–4.
20. Maniglia AJ, Maniglia JJ, Witten BR. Otoplasty – an eclectic technique. Laryngoscope. 1977;87(8):1359–68.
21. Elliott Jr RA. Complications in the treatment of prominent ears. Clin Plast Surg. 1978;5(3):479–90.
22. Dingman RO, Peled I. Corrective cosmetic otoplasty: a simple and accurate technique. Ann Plast Surg. 1979;3(3):250–2.

23. Minderjahn A, Huttl WR, Hildmann H. Mustarde's otoplasty – evaluation of correlation between clinical and statistical findings. J Maxillofac Surg. 1980; 8(3):241–50.
24. Senechal B, Chauffete JP, Senechal G. Complications and failures of otoplasty. Ann Otolaryngol Chir Cervicofac. 1983;100(7):493–8.
25. Hebisch A. Prominent ears: a simple surgical method of otoplasty using the Kaye and Stenstrom technic. Bull Soc Sci Med Grand Duche Luxemb. 1983;120(1): 37–41.
26. Campbell G. Otoplasty: something old, something new. Reconstruction of the external ear using fresh cadaver homograft ear cartilage and a sternomastoid myocutaneous flap. Br J Plast Surg. 1983;36(2): 262–6.
27. Hinderer UT, del Rio JL, Fregenal FJ. Otoplasty for prominent ears. Aesthetic Plast Surg. 1987;11(2): 63–9.
28. Adamson PA, McShane DP, Feldman RI. Otoplasty: an update. J Otolaryngol. 1987;16(4):258–62.
29. Oneal RM, Dodenhoff RJ, McClatchey KD. The role of perichondrium in modifying curved cartilage: an experimental study. Ann Plast Surg. 1987;19(4): 343–8.
30. Matsuo K, Hayashi R, Kiyono M, Hirose T, Netsu Y. Nonsurgical correction of congenital auricular deformities. Clin Plast Surg. 1990;17(2):383–95.
31. Allison GR. Anatomy of the auricle. Clin Plast Surg. 1990;17(2):209–12.
32. Baker DC, Converse JM. Correction of protruding ears: a 20-year retrospective. Aesthetic Plast Surg. 1979;3:29–39.
33. Elliott Jr RA. Otoplasty: a combined approach. Clin Plast Surg. 1990;17(2):373–81.
34. Furnas DW. Complications of surgery of the external ear. Clin Plast Surg. 1990;17(2):305–18.
35. Koch A, Andes C, Federspil P. Otoplasty: results of a modified form of Mustarde's method. Rev Laryngol Otol Rhinol (Bord). 1991;112(3):249–53.
36. Van de Heyning-Meier J. Controversies in otoplasty. Acta Otorhinolaryngol Belg. 1991;45(3):297–304.
37. Botta SA. A technique for otoplasty. Aesthetic Plast Surg. 1991;15(4):339–42.
38. Adamson PA, McGraw BL, Tropper GJ. Otoplasty: critical review of clinical results. Laryngoscope. 1991; 101(8):883–8.
39. Buchwald C, Nielsen LH, Rosborg J. Keloids of the external ear. ORL J Otorhinolaryngol Relat Spec. 1992;54(2):108–12.
40. Johnson PE. Otoplasty: shaping the antihelix. Aesthetic Plast Surg. 1994;18(1):71–4.
41. Romo 3rd T, Sclafani AP, Shapiro AL. Otoplasty using the postauricular skin flap technique. Arch Otolaryngol Head Neck Surg. 1994;120(10):1146–50.
42. Rohrich RJ, Friedman RM, Liland DL. Comparison of otoplasty techniques in the rabbit model. Ann Plast Surg. 1995;34(1):43–7.
43. Pilz S, Hintringer T, Bauer M. Otoplasty using a spherical metal head dermabrader to form a retroauricular furrow: five-year results. Aesthetic Plast Surg. 1995;19(1):83–91.
44. Brenda E, Marques A, Pereira MD, Zantut PE. Otoplasty and its origins for the correction of prominent ears. J Craniomaxillofac Surg. 1995;23(2):99–104.
45. Peled IJ. Knifeless otoplasty: how simple can it be? Aesthetic Plast Surg. 1995;19(3):253–5.
46. Adamson PA, Strecker HD. Otoplasty techniques. Facial Plast Surg. 1995;11(4):284–300.
47. Dudley WH, Peet AL, Flaggert 3rd JJ. Otoplasty for correction of the prominent ear. J Oral Maxillofac Surg. 1995;53(12):1386–91.
48. Messner AH, Crysdale WS. Otoplasty. Clinical protocol and long-term results. Arch Otolaryngol Head Neck Surg. 1996;122(7):773–7.
49. Beasley NJ, Jones NS. Otoplasty: the problem of the deep conchal bowl. J Laryngol Otol. 1996;110(9): 864–8.
50. Okajima H, Suzuki K, Takeichi Y, Umeda K, Baba S. Long-term results of otoplasty for microtia. Acta Otolaryngol Suppl. 1996;525:25–9.
51. Hell B, Garbea D, Heissler E, Klein M, Gath H, Langford A. Otoplasty: a combined approach to different structures of the auricle. Int J Oral Maxillofac Surg. 1997;26(6):408–13.
52. Lazaridis N, Tilaveridis I, Dimitrakopoulos I, Karakasis D. Correction of the protruding ear with a modified anterior scoring technique. J Oral Maxillofac Surg. 1998;56(3):307–13.
53. Hagerty TA, Barone EJ, Cohen IK. Endoscopic otoplasty in the rabbit model: effect of mechanical abrasion on ear cartilage deformation. Plast Reconstr Surg. 1998;101(2):487–93.
54. Lam SM. Edward Talbot Ely: father of aesthetic otoplasty. Arch Facial Plast Surg. 2004;6(1):64.
55. Stenstrom SJ, Heftner J. The Stenstrom otoplasty. Clin Plast Surg. 1978;5(3):465–70.
56. Tanzer R. Congenital deformities. In: Converse J, editor. Reconstructive plastic surgery. 2nd ed. Philadelphia: Saunders; 1977. p. 1705–10.
57. Mustarde JC. Correction of prominent ears using buried mattress sutures. Clin Plast Surg. 1978;5(3):459–64.
58. Mustarde JC. The correction of prominent ears using simple mattress sutures. Br J Plast Surg. 1963;16: 170–8.
59. Furnas DW. Correction of prominent ears with multiple sutures. Clin Plast Surg. 1978;5(3):491–5.
60. Gault DT, Grippaudo FR, Tyler M. Ear reduction. Br J Plast Surg. 1995;48(1):30–4.
61. Davis J. Prominent ears. Clin Plast Surg. 1978;5(3): 471–7.
62. Nordzell B. Open otoplasty. Plast Reconstr Surg. 2000;106(7):1466–72.
63. McDowell AJ. Goals in otoplasty for protruding ears. Plast Reconstr Surg. 1968;41(1):17–27.
64. Macgregor FC. Ear deformities: social and psychological implications. Clin Plast Surg. 1978;5(3):347–50.

65. Bauer BS, Song DH, Aitken ME. Combined otoplasty technique: chondrocutaneous conchal resection as the cornerstone to correction of the prominent ear. Plast Reconstr Surg. 2002;110(4):1033–40; discussion 1041.
66. Lentz AK, Plikaitis CM, Bauer BS. Understanding the unfavorable result after otoplasty: an integrated approach to correction. Plast Reconstr Surg. 2011;128(2):536–44.
67. Bauer BS, Margulis A, Song DH. The importance of conchal resection in correcting the prominent ear. Aesthet Surg J. 2005;25(1):72–9.
68. Burres S. The anterior-posterior otoplasty. Arch Otolaryngol Head Neck Surg. 1998;124(2):181–5.
69. Kim DY, Kim ES, Eo SR, Kim KS, Lee SY, Cho BH. A surgical approach for earlobe keloid: keloid fillet flap. Plast Reconstr Surg. 2004;113(6):1668–74.
70. Bauer BS. Reconstruction of microtia. Plast Reconstr Surg. 2009;124(1 Suppl):14e–26.
71. Limandjaja GC, Breugem CC, van der Molen AB M, Kon M. Complications of otoplasty: a literature review. J Plast Reconstr Aesthet Surg. 2009;62(1):19–27.

Use of Multiple Techniques for Otoplasty (Stenstrom, Mustarde, Furnas)

20

Jack A. Friedland and Renata Souza Maricevich

Introduction

Prominent ears are the most common congenital deformity in the head and neck region, with an incidence described for Caucasians of about 5 % [4]. Prominent ears are usually not associated with other abnormalities or syndromes, but may be considered an aesthetic handicap [45]. The forces governing the development of this deformity are unknown, and only 8 % of patients with this condition have some family history [3]. In approximately 61 % of children with this condition, the deformity can be diagnosed at birth [42], and there is no apparent sex predilection. Since Luckett's original description [22], a number of anatomical features associated with prominent ears have been described. These have been summarized as (1) absence of an adequate antihelical fold; (2) presence of a large, deep conchal bowl; (3) inadequate definition of the helical rim; and (4) abnormalities of the lobule [20]. Patients usually present with a combination of all these features.

J.A. Friedland, M.D., FACS (✉)
Clinical Professor of Surgery (Plastic),
University of Arizona Medical School,
Phoenix, Arizona, AZ, USA

Associate Professor of Plastic Surgery,
Mayo Medical School,
Rochester, Minnesota, USA
e-mail: jaf@jackafriedlandmd.com

R.S. Maricevich, M.D.
Division of Plastic Surgery, Department of Surgery,
Mayo Clinic, 200 First Street SW,
Rochester, MN 55901, USA
e-mail: maricevich.renata@mayo.edu

Although Sushruta and Tagliacozzi described otoplasty techniques, the modern era of otoplasty can be traced to 1848, when the term "otoplastick" was first used by Dieffenbach in his description of the repair of microtia [12]. In 1881, Ely removed a complete-thickness strip of the auricle from the cephaloauricular angle, but this left a visible scar in front of and behind the ear [14].

Keen modified the same technique by leaving the anterior skin bridge intact to prevent a noticeable scar [19]. After the turn of the century, many attempts were made to correct the protruding ear by using various antihelical and conchal cartilage excisions through a postauricular approach [5, 6, 11, 20, 26, 28, 34, 46]. Later, in the late 1940s, attempts were made to weaken the cartilage by mechanically thinning or placing partial-thickness incisions in it. Initially, parallel incisions were made on the posterior surface of the auricle with or without cartilage excision, allowing the antihelical fold to form [24, 32]. Abrasive brushes were then used to weaken the antihelix [39]. In the 1960s, Mustarde used permanent retention mattress sutures in a combined technique with a fusiform skin excision to recreate the antihelical fold [29]. The simplicity and good results obtained have gained this procedure widespread application, especially with regard to the delicate form of the antihelix. In 1963, Stenstrom [40] and Chongchet [10] scored the anterior part of the antihelix through a posterior incision, allowing the elastic forces to bend the cartilage along the antihelical fold, a maneuver that offers a more normal, rounded shape. In 1968, Furnas [17] described a procedure based on Miller's technique (further

M.A. Shiffman (ed.), *Advanced Cosmetic Otoplasty*,
DOI 10.1007/978-3-642-35431-1_20, © Springer-Verlag Berlin Heidelberg 2013

developed by Owens and Delgado [30]), which consisted of securing the concha to the mastoid periosteum posteriorly, thereby decreasing the concha-scaphoid angle.

In 1981, Pitanguy described the island technique, which consisted of dissecting a cartilaginous island to reconstruct the antihelix and form the triangular fossa, in addition to correcting the conchascaphal angle. This technique is not indicated for patients with a normal antihelix [23].

Anterior and posterior approaches have been described. Incisionless techniques were initially reported in 1995 by Fritsch, and multiple versions have been created since then [15, 16]. Ragad and Leclere published the use of laser-assisted cartilage reshaping with and without additional surgical intervention [21, 33]. There is lack of long-term results for these techniques.

Early splinting of the newborn ear may correct a degree of prominence and may obviate the need for surgery in later life [41], but most patients will require an operation. And when it becomes necessary, the surgeon should be able to select the best features of the most useful techniques to create the ideal procedure for correction of the deformity. Overall, more than 200 techniques have been described for the correction of prominent ears [1, 2, 7–9, 13, 18, 25, 27, 31, 35–38, 43, 44], and the procedures have become increasingly complex because of the aesthetic requirements of patients and the efforts by surgeons to achieve the fine and harmonious shape typical of the normal human auricle.

The goal of surgery for prominent ears is to produce symmetrical, natural-looking ears, with no obvious signs of surgery having been performed. Therefore, a combination technique of the most beneficial features of three previously described techniques, without cartilage resection, which has been tested over time and which provides excellent cosmetic results, a high level of patient satisfaction, and minimal complications, is presented in this chapter [47].

Preoperative Evaluation

First and foremost, patients should be asked to describe the bothersome aspects of their deformities, their motivation to have the deformities corrected, and their expectations for the procedure. The abnormalities and asymmetries have to be discussed with the patient and his or her family.

A complete preoperative work-up should include assessment of medical, personal, and family histories, including a tendency for bleeding and any previous occurrences of hypertrophic scars or keloids.

Preoperative photographic documentation consists of frontal, posterior, right and left lateral, and oblique views. No specific measurements are taken.

Technique

Local anesthesia with 1 % lidocaine and 1:100,000 epinephrine and intravenous sedation is used in most cases, but pediatric procedures are always performed under general anesthesia.

The surgical technique (Figs. 20.1, 20.2, 20.3, 20.4, 20.5, 20.6, 20.7, 20.8, and 20.9) includes excision of a small ellipse of posterior auricular skin, scoring of the antihelical cartilage on its anterior surface in a subcutaneous position (as described by Stenstrom), suturing to recreate the fold of the antihelix (in the fashion of Mustarde), and concha-mastoid suturing applied to the back of the ear to decrease the concha-scaphoid angle (in the manner of Furnas).

Postoperative dressings consist of antibiotic ointment and Xeroform gauze (Sherwood Medical, St. Louis, MO) placed over the postauricular incisions, saline-soaked cotton placed in all anterior crevices of the ears, gauze fluffs covered by circumferential Kerlix (Kendall Healthcare Products, Mansfield, MA), and an elastic bandage held in place by a woven net dressing. Drains are not used.

Results and Complications

The combined technique presented is safe, easy to perform, and has few complications. Excellent symmetry, as perceived both by the surgeon and the patient, is achieved resulting in high patient satisfaction (Fig. 20.10).

Undercorrection that requires intervention is rare with this combination of techniques, noted in

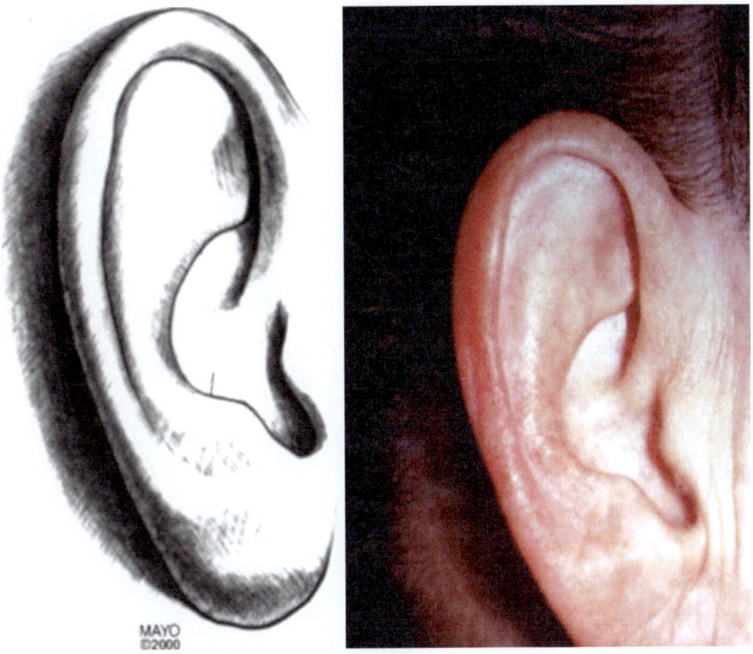

Fig. 20.1 Preoperatively, there is unfurling of the antihelix and increase of concha-scaphoid angle

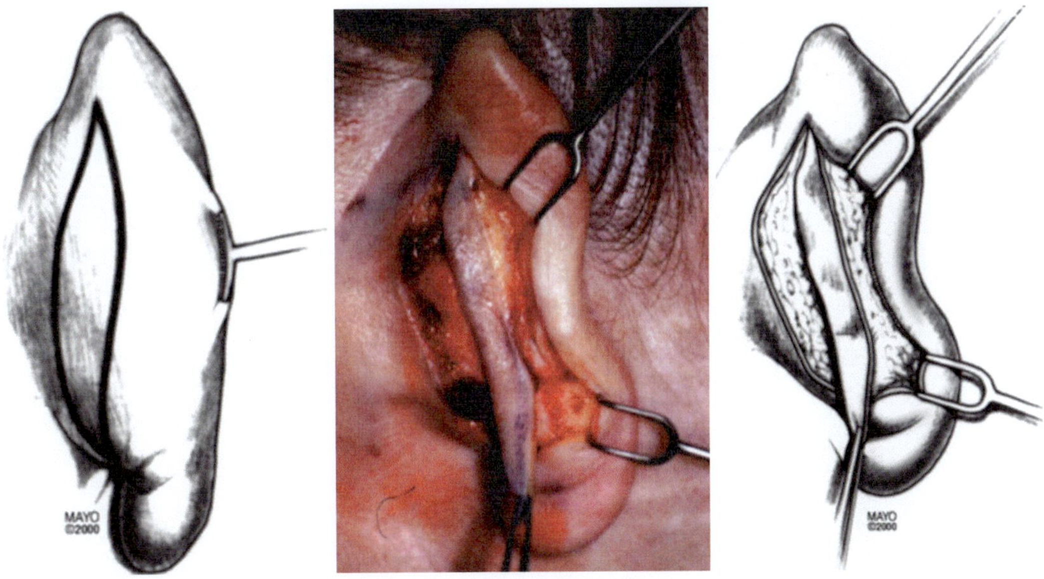

Fig. 20.2 A small ellipse of skin is usually excised from the back of the ear to assist with exposure and closure

less than 5 % of patients [47]. A few patients may experience a Mustarde suture extrusion, which can be easily dealt with under local anesthetic in an outpatient setting in the office.

The authors have not experienced any cases of hemorrhage, hematoma formation, skin breakdown, hypoesthesia, or perichondritis using this technique. In case of loss of initial correction, which has not been observed with this previously published technique, revision operation is relatively easy to perform on intact cartilage (Fig. 20.11).

There are usually no cases of postoperative lobule prominence since any lobule deformity is addressed during the initial operation, with a wedge excision being performed on the posterior surface, if necessary.

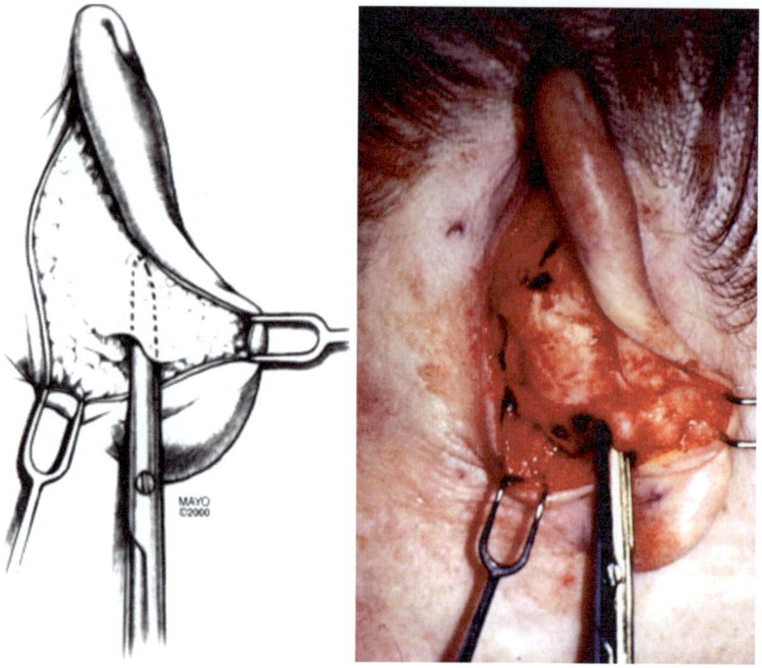

Fig. 20.3 The skin is elevated from the anterior surface of the antihelix through a posterior approach below the tail of the antihelix

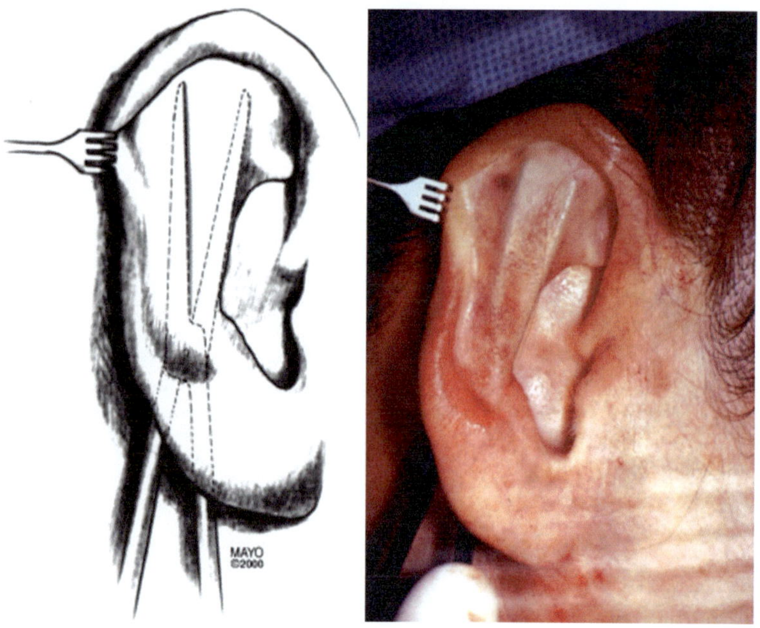

Fig. 20.4 Elevation of the skin is performed with a small Stevens scissors from the anterior aspect of the cartilage before otobrasion

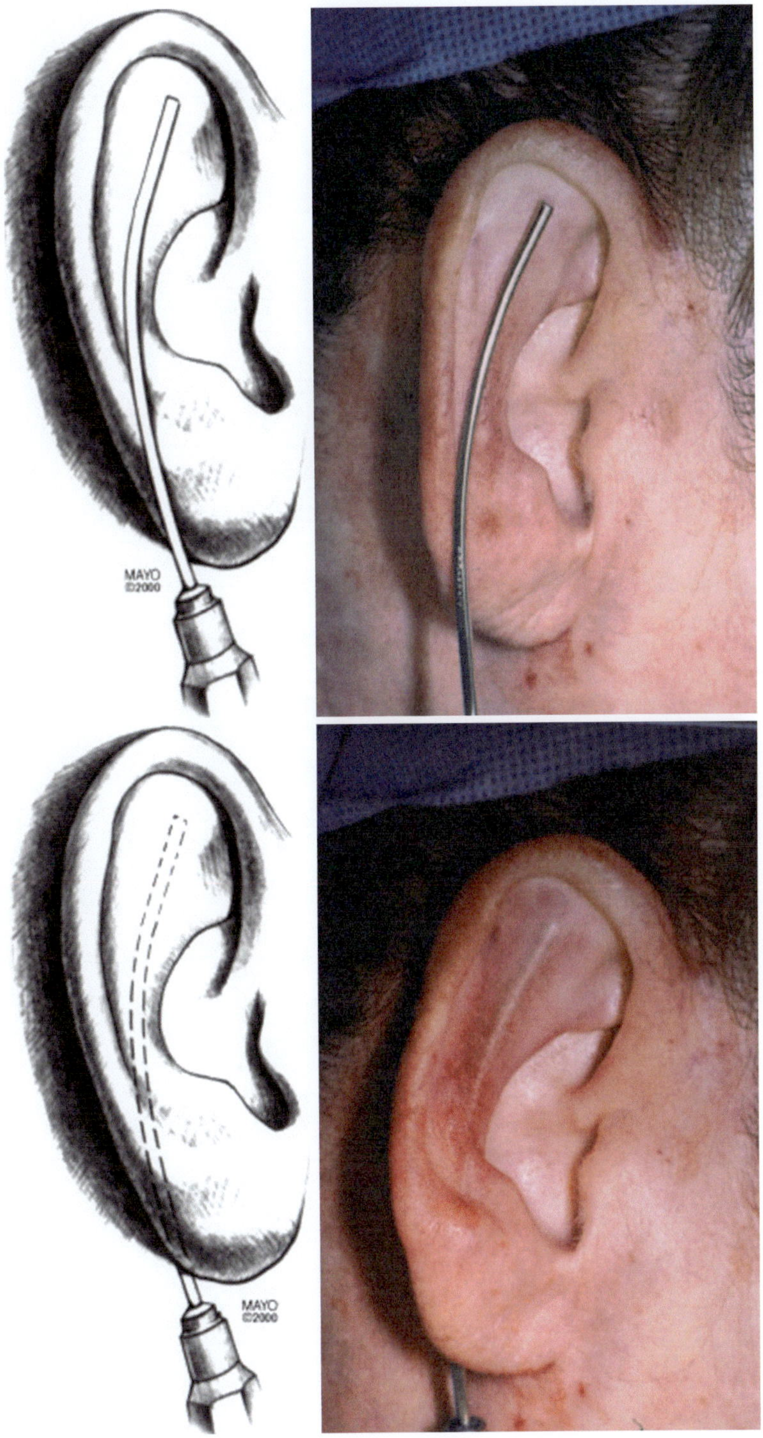

Fig. 20.5 A Dingman otoabrader is inserted posteriorly to subcutaneously abrade the anterior aspect of the antihelical cartilage (Stenstrom)

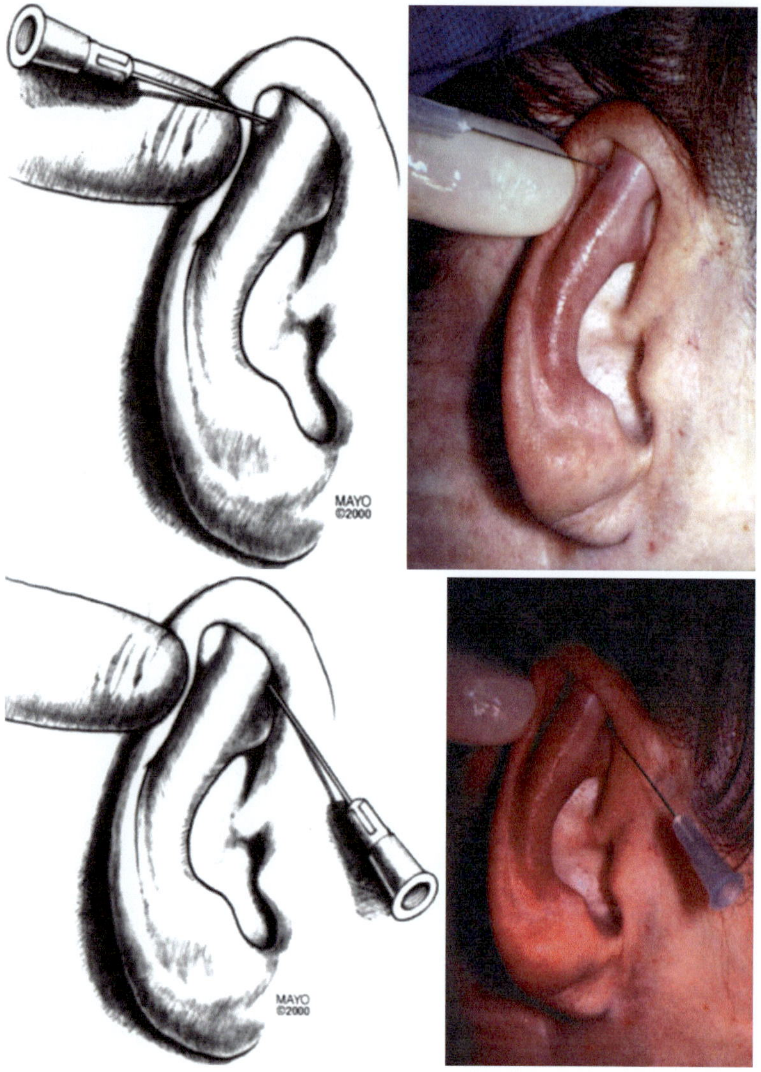

Fig. 20.6 A 27-gauge needle is inserted anteriorly on each side of the antihelix to assist in placement of 4-0 clear nylon monofilament horizontal mattress sutures tied posteriorly to create the fold of the antihelix

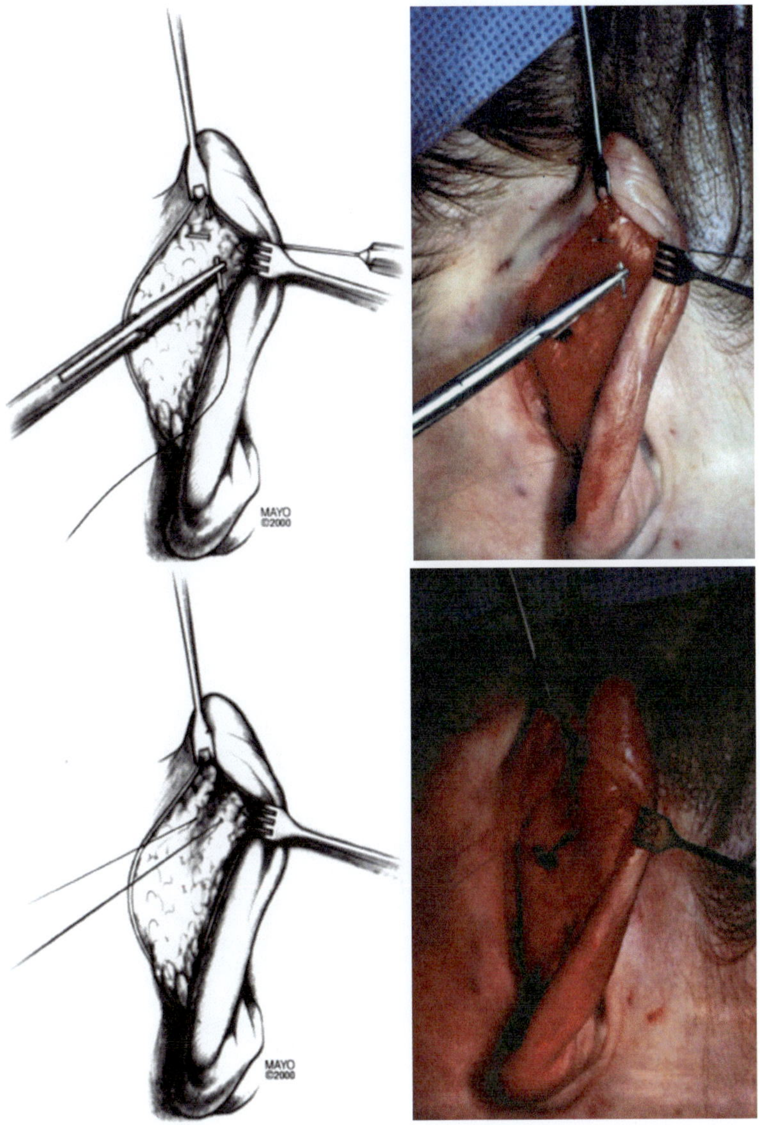

Fig. 20.7 At least three horizontal mattresses sutures (Mustarde) are placed to create the antihelical fold

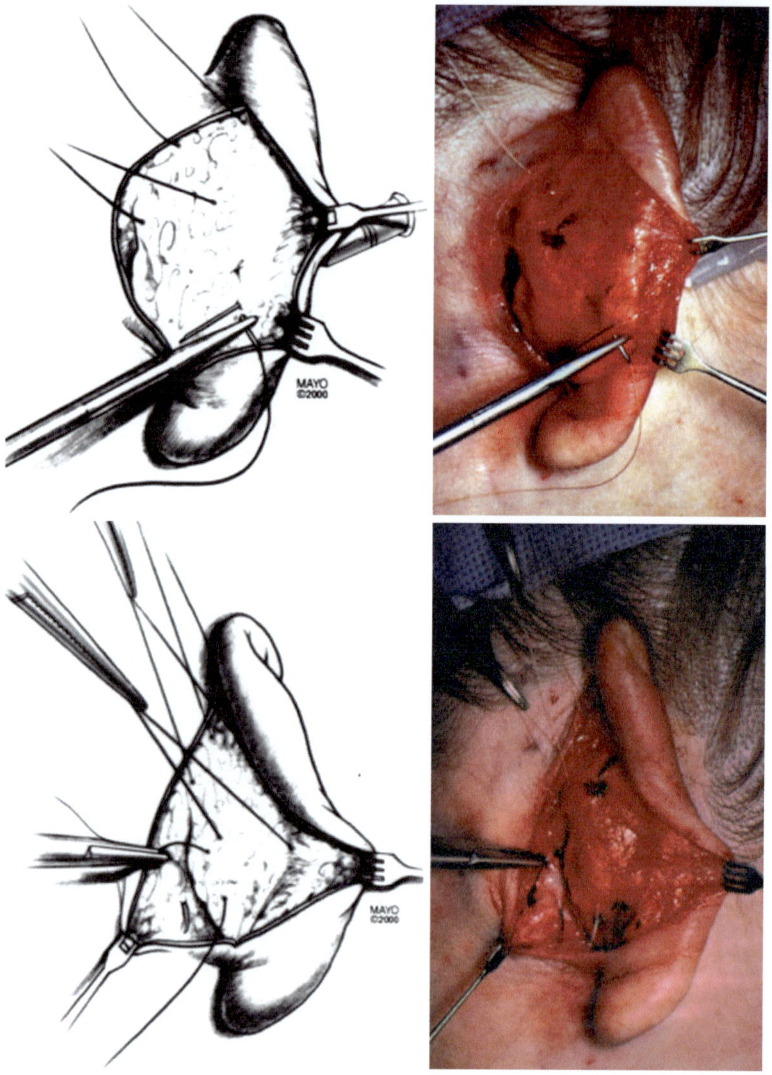

Fig. 20.8 One or two concha-mastoid sutures are placed (Furnas) to decrease the concha-scaphoid angle

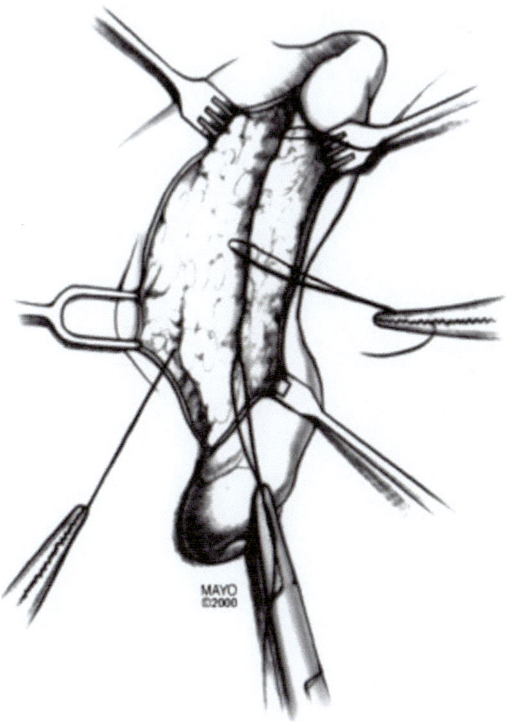

Fig. 20.9 After sutures are tied, the skin incision is closed with an intracuticular 4.0 Monocryl suture

Conclusions

Controlling the degree and position of the fold of the antihelix is a basic requisite for good results. This is the reason why cartilage-sparing techniques offer the surgeon the ability to achieve this goal without disrupting the structural integrity of the ear. Cutting techniques irreversibly subject the antihelix to unpredictable distortion by wound contraction forces, and for this reason no conchal resections are performed.

The combination of techniques allows for a more delicate approach, and the aesthetic improvement becomes evident even in the immediate postoperative period. The final outcome of this combined technique is reproducible and long-lasting. It can be considered a standard technique to be used for treating patients of any age and with any magnitude of defect.

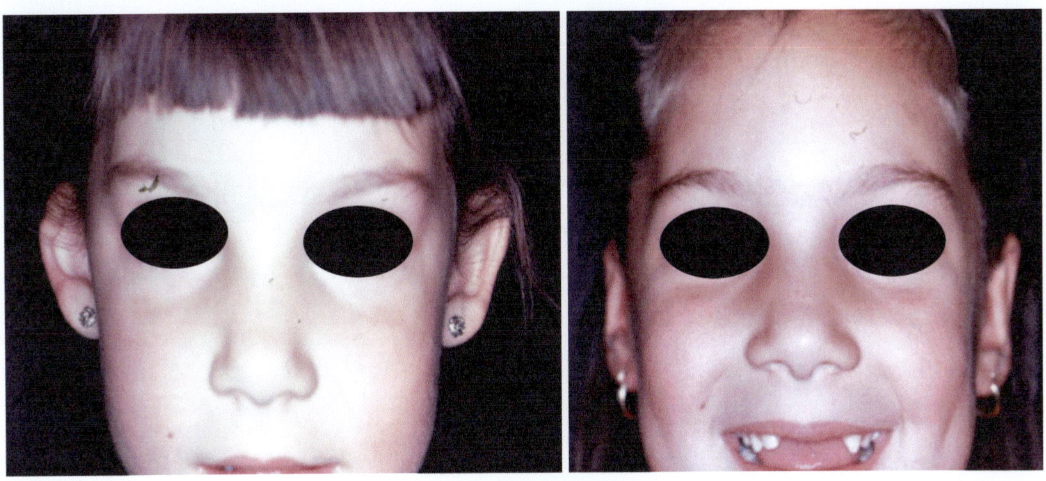

Fig. 20.10 (*Left*) Preoperative. (*Right*) Postoperative using combined technique

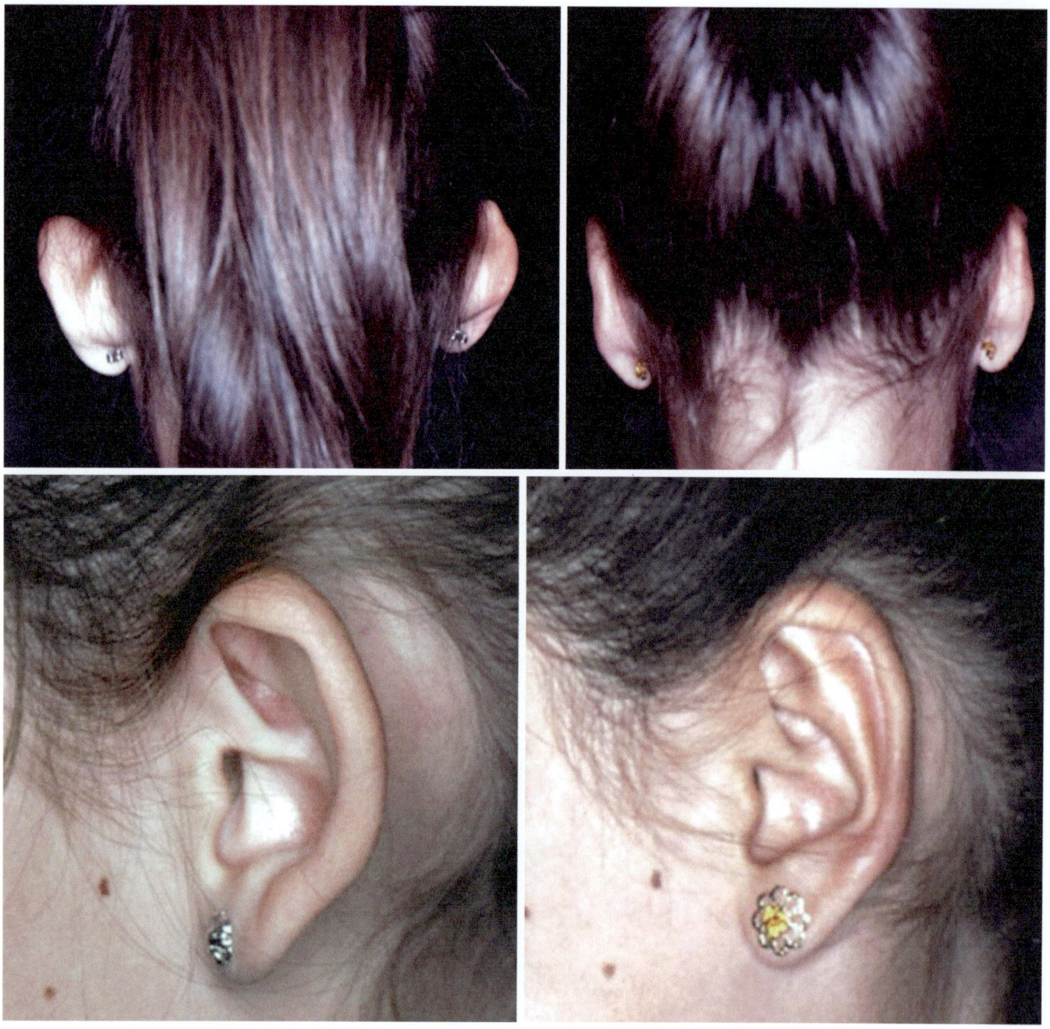

Fig. 20.10 (continued)

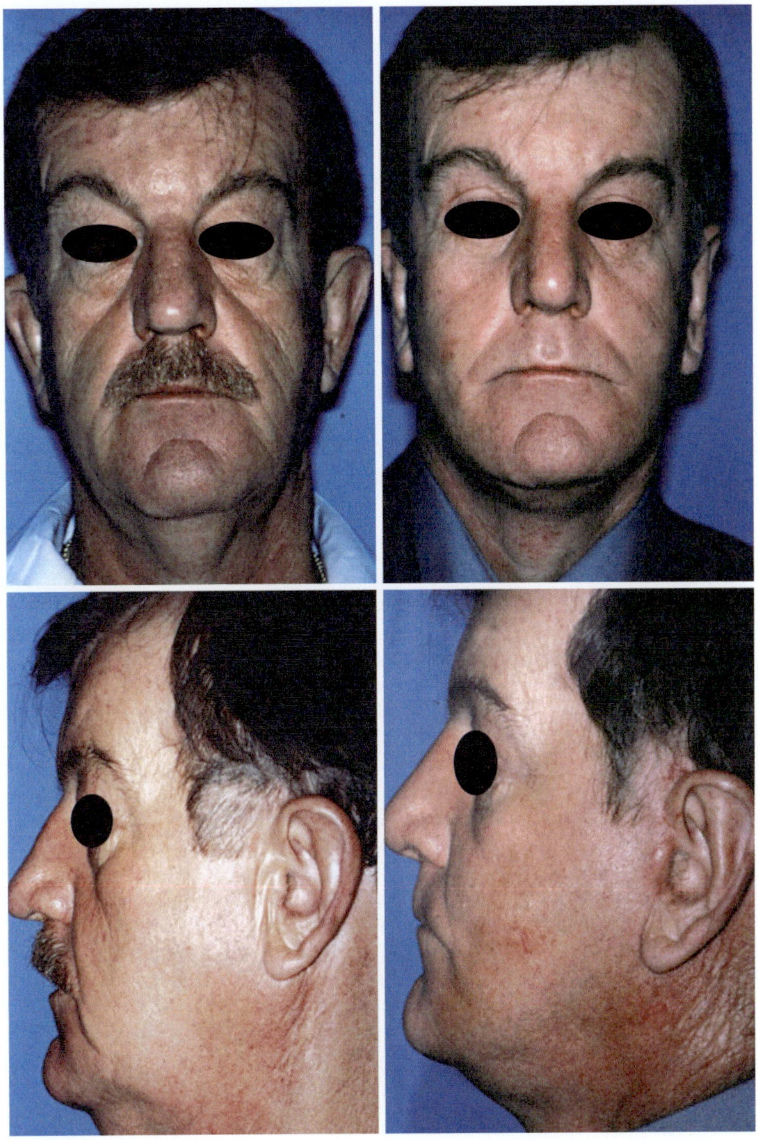

Fig. 20.11 (*Left*) Preoperative. (*Right*) Postoperative using combined technique

References

1. Adamson PA, Litner JA. Otoplasty technique. Facial Plast Surg Clin North Am. 2006;14(2): 79–87.
2. Adamson PA, McGraw BL, Tropper GJ. Otoplasty: critical review of clinical results. Laryngoscope. 1991; 101(8):883–8.
3. Baker DC, Converse JM. Correction of protruding ears: a 20-year retrospective. Aesthetic Plast Surg. 1979; 3:29–39.
4. Bardach J. Surgery for congenital and acquired malformation of the auricle. In: Cummings CW, Fredrickson JM, Harker LA, Krause CJ, Schuller DE, editors. Otolaryngology: head and neck surgery. St. Louis: Mosby; 1986. p. 2861.
5. Barsky AJ. Plastic surgery. Philadelphia: Saunders; 1938. p. 178–80.
6. Baxter H. Plastic correction of protruding ears in children. Can Med Assoc J. 1941;45(3):217–20.
7. Burstein FD. Cartilage-sparing complete otoplasty technique: a 10-year experience in 100 patients. J Craniofac Surg. 2003;14(4):521–5.

8. Calder JC, Naasan A. Morbidity of otoplasty: a review of 562 consecutive cases. Br J Plast Surg. 1994;47(3): 170–4.
9. Caouette-Laberge L, Guay N, Bortoluzzi P, et al. Otoplasty: anterior scoring technique and results in 500 cases. Plast Reconstr Surg. 2000;105(2):504–15.
10. Chongchet V. A method of antihelix reconstruction. Br J Plast Surg. 1963;16:268–72.
11. Davids JS, Kitlowski EA. Abnormal prominence of the ears: a method of readjustment. Surgery. 1937;2: 835–8.
12. Dieffenbach JE. Die ohrbildung otoplastik. In: Die operative Chirurgie. Leipzig: Brockhaus; 1848. p. 395–7.
13. Echarri SMR, Cunado HM, Woodeson MJ, Mayor PG. Otoplasty: results after anterior versus posterior approach. Acta Otorrinolaringol Esp. 2011;62(3): 188–93.
14. Ely ET. An operation for prominence of the auricles. Arch Otolaryngol. 1881;10:97–9.
15. Fritsch MH. Incisionless otoplasty. Laryngoscope. 1995;105:1–11.
16. Fritsch MH. Incisionless otoplasty. Otolaryngol Clin North Am. 2009;42:1199–208.
17. Furnas DW. Correction of prominent ears by conchamastoid sutures. Plast Reconstr Surg. 1968;42(6): 189–93.
18. Graham KE, Gault DT. Endoscopic assisted otoplasty: a preliminary report. Br J Plast Surg. 1997;50(1): 47–57.
19. Keen WW. New method of operating for relief of deformity from prominent ears. Ann Surg. 1890;11(1): 49–51.
20. Lavy J, Stearns M. Otoplasty: techniques, results and complications – a review. Clin Otolaryngol Allied Sci. 1997;22(5):390–3.
21. Leclere FM, Trelles M, Mordon SR. Cartilage reshaping for protruding ears: a prospective long term follow-up of 32 procedures. Lasers Surg Med. 2011;43(9): 875–80.
22. Luckett WH. A new operation for prominent ears based on the anatomy of the deformity. Surg Gynecol Obstet. 1910;10:635–7.
23. Maricevich P, de Amorim NF G, Duprat R, Pitanguy I. Island technique for prominent ears: an update of the Ivo Pitanguy clinic experience. Aesthet Surg J. 2011;31(6):623–33.
24. McEvitt WG. The problem of the protruding ear. Plast Reconstr Surg (1946). 1947;2(5):481–96.
25. Messner AH, Crysdale WS. Otoplasty. Clinical protocol and long-term results. Arch Otolaryngol Head Neck Surg. 1996;122(7):773–7.
26. Miller C. Operations for corrections of outstanding ears. In: Miller CC, editor. Cosmetic surgery: the correction of featural imperfections. Philadelphia: Davis; 1925. p. 201–11.
27. Mompo L, Pastor G, Carrasco M. Otoplasty without cartilage section using the Mustarde technique. Presentation of our experience. Acta Otorrinolaringol Esp. 2011;62(3):181–7.
28. Morestin MH. De la reposition et du plissement cosmetiques du pavillon de l'oreille. Rev Orthop. 1903;4:289–303.
29. Mustarde JC. The treatment of prominent ears by buried mattress sutures: a ten-year survey. Plast Reconstr Surg. 1967;39(4):382–6.
30. Owens N, Delgado DD. The management of outstanding ears. South Med J. 1965;58:32–3.
31. Peker F, Celikoz B. Otoplasty: anterior scoring and posterior rolling technique in adults. Aesthetic Plast Surg. 2002;26(4):267–73.
32. Pierce GW, Klabunde EH, Bergeron VL. Useful procedures in plastic surgery. Plast Reconstr Surg (1946). 1947;2(4):358–61.
33. Ragab A. Carbon dioxide laser-assisted cartilage reshaping otoplasty: a new technique for prominent ears. Laryngoscope. 2010;120(7):1312–8.
34. Ruttin E. Eine Methode zur Korrektur abstehender Ohren und zum Verschluss retroaurikulaerer Oeffnungen. Monatsschr Ohrenheilkd. 1910;44:196.
35. Salgarello M, Gasperoni C, Montagnese A, Farallo E. Otoplasty for prominent ears: a versatile combined technique to master the shape of the ear. Otolaryngol Head Neck Surg. 2007;137(2):224–7.
36. Scharer SA, Farrior EH, Farrior RT. Retrospective analysis of the Farrior technique for otoplasty. Arch Facial Plast Surg. 2007;9(3):167–73.
37. Schlegel-Wagner C, Pabst G, Muller W, Linder T. Otoplasty using a modified anterior scoring technique: standardized measurements of long-term results. Arch Facial Plast Surg. 2010;12(3):143–8.
38. Sinha M, Richard B. Postauricular fascial flap and suture otoplasty: a prospective outcome study of 227 patients. J Plast Reconstr Aesthet Surg. 2012;65(3): 367–71.
39. Stark RB, Saunders DE. Natural appearance restored to the unduly prominent ear. Br J Plast Surg. 1962; 15:385–97.
40. Stenstrom WJ. An aid to accurate fixation during fundus photography. Arch Ophthalmol. 1963;70: 389–90.
41. Tan ST, Shibu M, Gault DT. A splint for correction of congenital ear deformities. Br J Plast Surg. 1994;47(8): 575–8.
42. Tan ST, Gault DT. When do ears become prominent? Br J Plast Surg. 1994;47(8):573–4.
43. Valente AS. Separating the helix from the antihelix: a new concept in prominent ear correction. Aesthet Surg J. 2010;30(2):139–53.
44. Vital V, Printza A. Cartilage-sparing otoplasty: our experience. J Laryngol Otol. 2002;116(9): 682–5.
45. Vuyk HD. Cartilage-sparing otoplasty: a review with long-term results. J Laryngol Otol. 1997;111(5): 424–30.
46. Young F. The correction of abnormally prominent ears. Surg Gynecol Obstet. 1944;78:541.
47. Yugueros P, Friedland JA. Otoplasty: the experience of 100 consecutive patients. Plast Reconstr Surg. 2001;108(4):1045–51; discussion 1052–3.

Combined Technique in Aesthetic Otoplasty

21

Marzia Salgarello and Giuseppe Visconti

Introduction

Dieffenbach [1] is credited with the first otoplasty report (1845) describing the correction of a posttraumatic protruding ear by simple postauricular sulcus skin excision, with suture affixing the auricle to the mastoid periosteum. However, the first report of a purely aesthetic otoplasty is accredited to Ely (1881) [2], who performed a full-thickness vertical wedge crescent excision of the antihelix for the correction of a protruding ear.

Since these first reports, throughout the 20th century, there has been an increasing volume of publications in the plastic surgery and otolaryngology literature on different operative techniques for the correction of ear deformities, each of them with their own advantages and limits.

M. Salgarello, M.D. (✉)
Department of Plastic and Reconstructive Surgery, Università Cattolica del "Sacro Cuore", Largo A. Gemelli 8, 00168 Rome, Italy

Department of Plastic and Reconstructive Surgery, Università Cattolica del "Sacro Cuore" – University Hospital "A. Gemelli", Largo A. Gemelli 8, 00168 Rome, Italy
e-mail: m.salgarello@mclink.it

G. Visconti, M.D.
Department of Plastic and Reconstructive Surgery, Università Cattolica del "Sacro Cuore" – University Hospital "A. Gemelli", Largo A. Gemelli 8, 00168 Rome, Italy
e-mail: joevisconti@hotmail.com

This chapter describes the combined otoplasty technique of the senior author (MS), demonstrating the reliability and flexibility of this technique in treating a wide variety of deformities, from simple protruding ears to those with accompanying moderate degrees of constriction, lobule protrusion, and deformities of the helical rim [3]. Besides the description of the surgical technique, a comprehensive analysis of the relevant applied external ear anatomy along with the associated pathological conditions and a brief summary of basic otoplasty techniques is provided.

Relevant Applied Anatomy of the External Ear

Embryology

Embryologically, the external ear develops from six mesenchymal prominences that align themselves superiorly on the first (mandibular) brachial arch and inferiorly on the second (hyoid) brachial arch. The auricular portion of the mandibular arch is responsible for the development of the tragus and the helical crus. The auricular portion of the hyoid arch, the main contributor to ear formation. It leads to the development of the helix, scapha, antihelix, concha, antitragus, and lobule. The superiorly located mandibular arch slides inferiorly and the inferiorly located hyoid arch moves superiorly, thus defining the ear draft.

M.A. Shiffman (ed.), *Advanced Cosmetic Otoplasty*,
DOI 10.1007/978-3-642-35431-1_21, © Springer-Verlag Berlin Heidelberg 2013

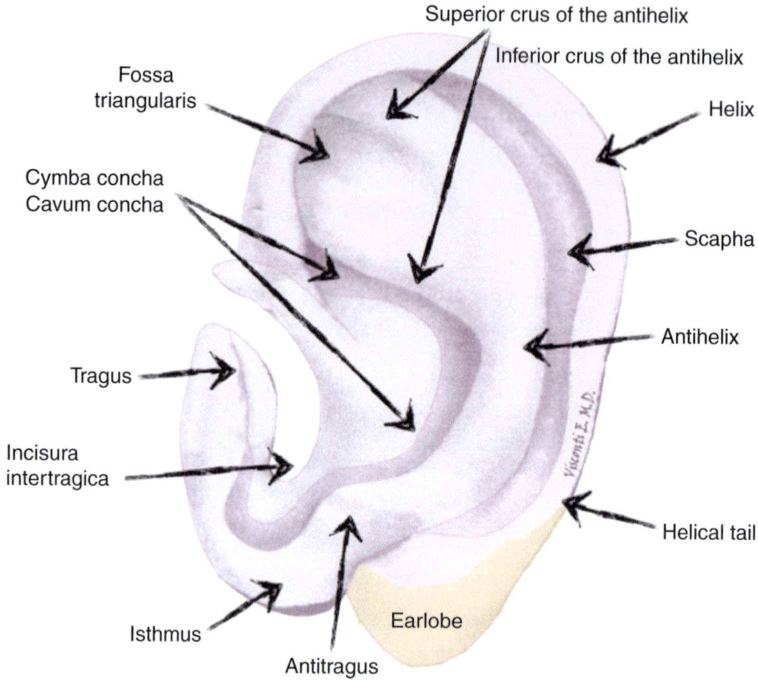

Fig. 21.1 The cartilaginous ear framework is shown with all its involutions, protuberances, and folds. In *yellow*, the fibrofatty earlobe

The ear normally develops between the fifth and the ninth weeks of gestation. At the age of 3 years, the ear is approximately 85 % of its adult size. The ear width becomes mature at 6 years in females and at 7 years in males; the ear length reaches its mature size at 12 years in females and at 13 years in males. As time goes on, the mature ear acquires the features of the aged ear, which is characterized by a stiffer and more calcified cartilage along with the sequelae of skin aging and elastosis, such as lobule ptosis.

Applied Anatomy of the External Ear

The Chondrocutaneous Portion

The external ears are paired organs mounted on the bony base of the underlying temporal bone. These organs are a complex chondrocutaneous composite and are endowed with many intricate involutions, protuberances, and folds. These complex and unique structures serve to capture and guide sounds through the external auditory canal since humans have lost the ability to move the ear appropriately to direct different sounds. With the presence of intrinsic and extrinsic auricular muscles, human ears are relatively fixed compared with the mobile ears of many animals.

The surface anatomy of the external ear is defined by a complex chondrocutaneous structure in the superior and middle third and a dermoadipose appendix in the inferior third, forming the lobule. The chondrocutaneous structure is defined by five main components: the helix, antihelix, scapha, concha, and tragus. Other defining elements are Darwin's tubercle, the antitragus, and the intertragic incisure (Fig. 21.1). The fine relationships among all these elements define the "normal" ear.

The Auricle Muscles

Besides the chondrocutaneous structure, there are intrinsic and extrinsic auricle muscles that stabilize the auricle and allow limited ear movement of no functional significance.

The intrinsic muscles are thus named because their origin and insertions are within the auricle itself. The ones located on the anterior surface of the ear are the tragus, antitragus, and major and minor helix. The intrinsic muscles on the posterior surface of the ear are the intrinsic transverse and oblique muscles.

The two extrinsic muscles have their origins outside the auricle, and they insert on it. These muscles are thin and normally hypo- or atrophic and include the following:

1. The auricular anterosuperior muscle, which is made of two portions: the anterior part, which is triangular-shaped, originates from the galea of the temporal region in front of the auricle and inserts on the helix and the concha; and the superior part, a triangular-shaped muscle with the base facing upward, originating from the galea of the temporal region superior to the auricle and inserting into the cymba and superior margin of the helix.
2. The auricular posterior muscle originates from the mastoid region and inserts into the concha.

Because of their origins from the galea aponeurotica, both the extrinsic auricular muscles are agonistic with the fronto-occipitalis muscle. The minimal auricular movements, when present, are normally associated mainly with the concomitant action of the fronto-occipitalis muscle rather than with a very rare proper function.

Vessels and Nerves

The vascular supply to the auricle comes from branches of the posterior auricular artery and superficial temporal artery. The anterior and posterior branches of the great auricular nerve and the auriculotemporal nerve are responsible for the innervation of the mandibular brachial arch structures (tragus and helical crus) and of the hyoid arch (the rest of the ear), respectively.

The Biomechanics of Ear Cartilage and Its Surgical Implications

The cartilage tissue exists in various forms and performs a range of functions in the human body. Cartilage is composed of the extracellular matrix enriched by two main types of macromolecules, glycosaminoglycans and proteoglycans. These are able to interact with elastic and collagen fibers. Depending on the different compositions of these macromolecules, elastic and collagen fibers, cartilages are classified into three main types as follows:

1. Articular cartilage, also called *hyaline cartilage*. The most common cartilage type in the human body, it is mainly composed of collagen type II fibers. This tissue is present in freely moveable synovial joints (dysarthroses), with its main function being as a binder surface between bones that permits smooth motion between adjoining bony segments.
2. *Fibrocartilage*. This is present in fibrocartilaginous joints with limited movement, such as the intervertebral disc and pubic symphysis, with a main function of bearing between-bone surfaces. The features of this tissue are being between the hyaline cartilage and the dense connective tissue, being mainly composed of collagen type I fibers. This cartilage is always associated with the dense connective tissue, from which it is sometimes histologically indistinguishable.
3. *Elastic cartilage*. This is present in structures such as the ear, Eustachian tube, epiglottis, nasal septum and larynx. Its main function is to maintain a defined shape. Its structure is similar to that of hyaline cartilage, but in addition to the other components, its matrix has elastic fibers and interconnecting sheets of elastic material (Fig. 21.2).

The peculiar structure of the elastic cartilage is responsible for maintaining the shape when a structure undergoes a static and dynamic deformation. When a force is applied on the external ear, it keeps this position as long as the external forces are applied. Once these forces are removed, the elastic properties allow the structure to return to its natural shape. Even though this behavior is characteristic of any elastic structure that ideally follows Hooke's law, in the plastic surgery and otolaryngology literature, this phenomenon is known as the "intrinsic memory of cartilaginous elasticity."

According to Hooke's law, an ideal elastic structure follows the rule

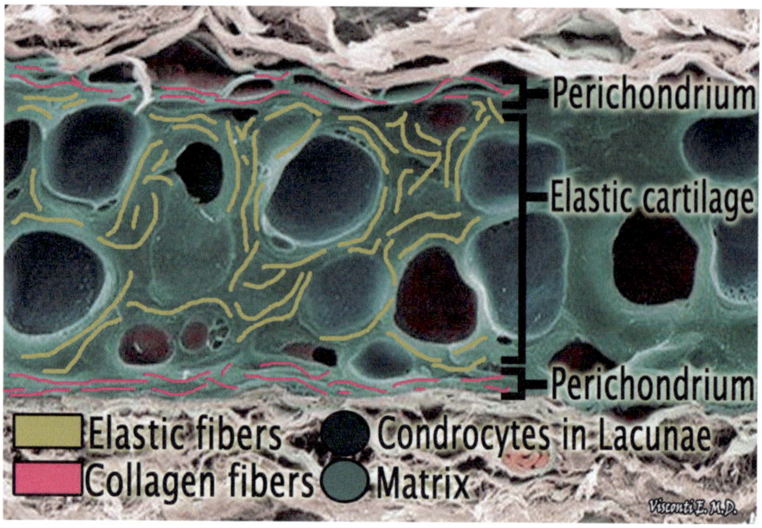

Fig. 21.2 A schematic section of ear cartilage. On the periphery, the grey tissue is the skin and subcutis. The blue tissue is the elastic ear cartilage

$$F = -k\Delta s$$

where the elastic force (F) elicited by an elastic tissue with an elastic constant (k) depends on the amount of tissue deformation (Δs) impressed.

This elastic model is valid when the elastic structure integrity is maintained. Applying any kind of cartilage breaking force capable of disrupting the elastic network integrity, a permanent modification of the elastic properties occurs. The manifestation of this phenomenon will depend on the characteristics of the breaking force applied.

However, the composition of human cartilage makes it a viscoelastic-fibrous rather than an ideal elastic structure. The biomechanical properties of viscoelastic tissue can be surgically analyzed by referring to four main physical parameters: the breaking or bursting strength, suture-type tearing forces, the tissue stress relaxation, and the tissue creep.

Regarding the biomechanics of human ear cartilage in otoplasty, the breaking or bursting strength is of limited value as this is normally not an issue. The suture-type tearing force is similar to the breaking strength but is more clinically relevant as it evaluates the forces that are applied on a specific suture material to pull the suture out of the sample.

The tissue stress relaxation is the tension created with a constant stretch. It is measured by applying a constant force to the tissues for a period of time to obtain a certain amount of tissue distortion (deformation or elongation). During this time, the decrease in tissue tension measured defined the stress relaxation. This method serves to evaluate the elasticity of a tissue. If the tissue is not elastic and completely viscous, it will relax (distort), and the decrease in tissue tension will be high. If the tissue is totally elastic, it will not relax but will be distorted and lower the decrease in tissue tension measured. This occurs until a critical point (the breaking point) is reached where the force becomes a breaking strength.

The tissue creep is defined as the amount of tissue deformation with a constant load over time. The ear cartilage elasticity is age dependent (Figs. 21.3 and 21.4).

In the *newborn*, till the third day after birth, the cartilage shows a unique malleability that is rapidly lost day by day [4, 5]. Biomechanically, the cartilage shows a virtual absence of the intrinsic elastic memory, and it is in these days that a reliable nonsurgical correction of the ear deformities can be obtained by only molding, as demonstrated by Matsuo et al. [4] and other pediatric series. This unique, virtually only viscous and not elastic framework has been related to the high serum estrogen level that rapidly drops in the next days.

In childhood before the age of 6, the cartilage shows an elastic behavior, still being very pliable and malleable. Biomechanically, it is a balanced viscoelastic structure with high tissue stress

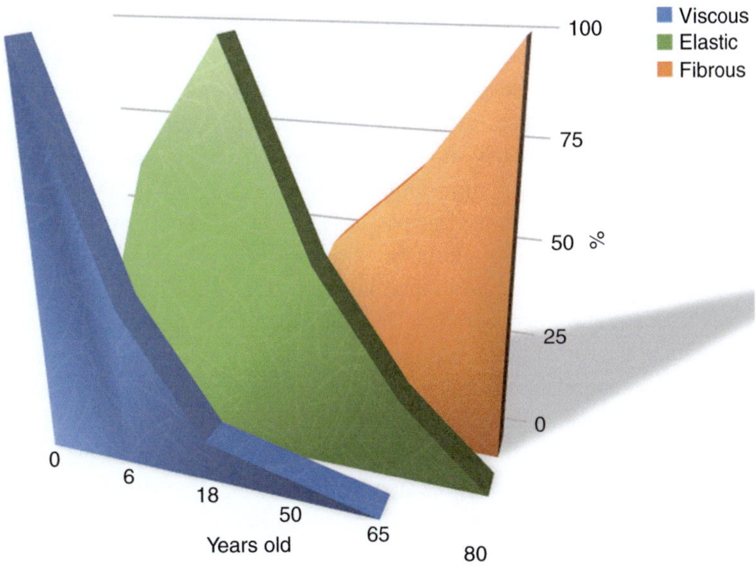

Fig. 21.3 The biomechanical properties of the ear cartilage in relation to age

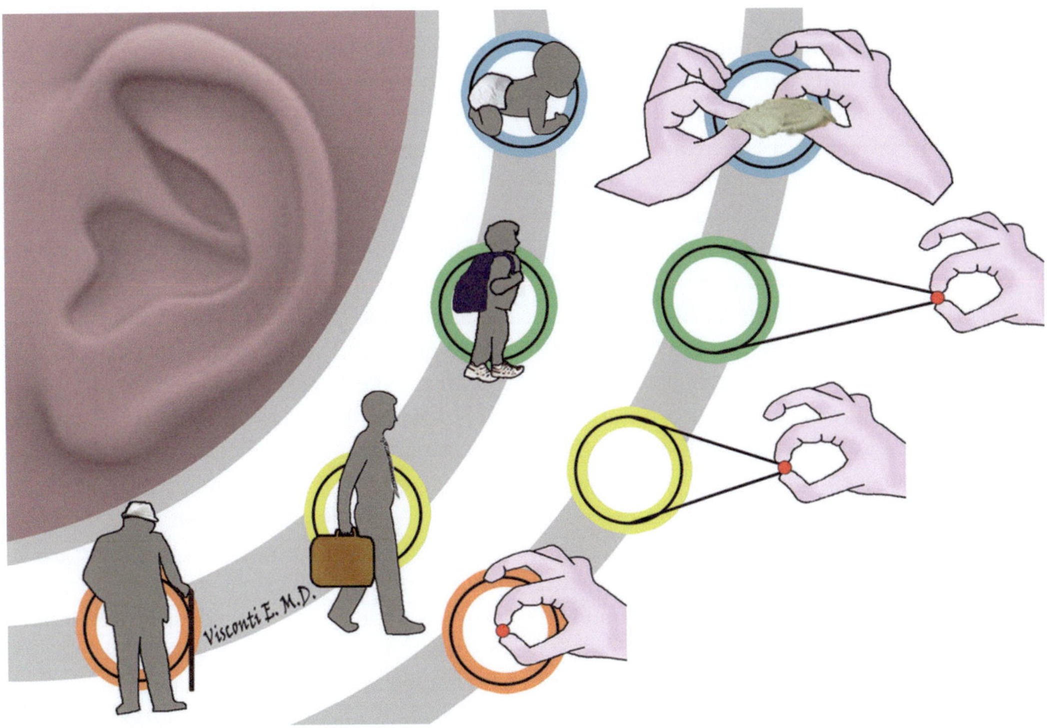

Fig. 21.4 Schematic drawing of cartilage malleability in relation to age. In newborns the cartilage is easily manipulated, like plasticine. From childhood to elderly the elasticity of the cartilage progressively decreases until it is no longer elastic cartilaginous tissue

relaxation and tissue creep and consequent low suture-type tearing forces. This means that it is easier to modify the intrinsic cartilage elastic memory with corresponding good long-term results and a lower rate of deformity relapse, according to evidence in the literature.

In *adolescence and adulthood*, the ear cartilage becomes progressively less pliable and stiffer [6–10]. Its tissue stress relaxation is low, as well as the tissue creep, with a corresponding high suture-type tearing force. This is strictly related to the progressively different composition of the cartilage extracellular matrix, as time passes. The cartilage aging phenomenon starts to settle down. The framework is more elastic than viscous with progressive fibrous degeneration. In this patient population, the ear cartilage is progressively more difficult to manipulate, resulting in less satisfying results and a higher relapse rate.

From *adulthood to the elderly*, the auricular cartilage progressively undergoes significant structural, matrix composition, and mechanical changes with age [6–10]. These phenomena are strictly related to a progressive decline of cell function and of their ability to maintain the tissue, with a consequent imbalance between chondrocyte synthetic and degradative activity. The cartilage matrix consequently undergoes loss and alterations in aggregating proteoglycans, a decrease in water concentration, increased collagen cross-linking, and elastosis. The cartilage becomes stiffer and almost non-pliable. The loss of elastic fibers along with increased fibrosis lead the elastic cartilage to become progressively almost all fibrous-like tissue. It could be not worth to perform otoplasty on these patients, as the otoplasty technique would be hard to apply to this modified tissue. Even if the literature is plenty of examples of different surgical otoplasty techniques, information is lacking on how each technique works biomechanically.

Depending on the type of ear deformity, a cartilage manipulation is usually necessary when performing otoplasty. One of the most common ear deformities is the prominent or bat ear. Its features are the effacement or deficiency of the antihelical fold along with different degrees of overall concha hypertrophy. One of the main goals in the correction of prominent ear is the creation of the missing antihelical fold. In literature, many cartilage manipulation techniques have been reported to address this issue. The techniques can be classified into two groups: the cartilage-sparing and the cartilage-scoring techniques [5–10]. In cartilage-sparing techniques, the cartilage manipulation is performed using only sutures. All these techniques are based on the Mustardé concept of horizontal mattress sutures. Cartilage-scoring techniques, on the other hand, can be divided into two major subgroups. The cartilage-cutting techniques are based on the concept of cartilage "tubing" reported by Becker in 1952 [11]. A pair of parallel incisions on either side of the antihelix are made posteriorly and the edges sutured together to form a smooth, rounded antihelix. The cartilage-abrasion techniques are based on the initial observation by Gibson and Davis [12] that the costal cartilage tends to bend away from the injured surface. Later, Stenstroem [13] and Chongchet [14] applied this concept in otoplasty. Stenstroem [13] reported his experimental observations when rasping the ear cartilage, making the following conclusions:

1. The auricular cartilage, when scratched on one side, bends in the opposite direction.
2. The perichondrium plays no role in this phenomenon.
3. The deeper the scratching is, the higher the bending effect.
4. The tendency to bend, however, becomes smaller in the deeper layers.

The exact physiologic mechanism of the "bending" effect after cartilage abrasion is still not clear. The hypothesis of Gibson and Davis [12] that the bending effect is due to matrix expansion and outer stretched layer contraction has been confuted by Stenstroem [13]. From his clinical observation, he concluded that the bending phenomenon is probably related to the gradually increasing firmness of the rasped cartilage and by a contraction of the opposite, non-injured cartilage. After Weinzweig's [15] histological observation, we now know that a fibrocartilaginous cap develops after cartilage abrasion that favors and stabilizes the bending effect.

One of the major issues in surgical correction of prominent ear is relapse. This complication results in patients with prominent ear after otoplasty, meaning that the surgical technique applied has been not effective in correcting the deformity. The recurrence is mainly due to the intrinsic elastic cartilaginous memory that brings the operated ear back to the original shape. The cartilage manipulation technique aims to hold the ear in its new position until scar formation has stabilized the result. In cartilage-sparing techniques, early disruption of sutures is associated to relapse because of the intrinsic elastic cartilage memory that brings the cartilage back to its initial shape. This is particularly true in less pliable and malleable cartilages. Biomechanically, their elastic constant is higher and tissue stress relaxation is lower. When a load is applied (i.e., sutures), the consequent elastic rebound force generated is high. If the sutures are not able to keep the load till scar formation, the likelihood of relapse is high. After prominent ear correction in patients younger than 6 years old, Mustardé [16] reported a 1.8 % relapse rate with a follow-up period of 10 years. With his technique, however, he experienced a 30 % recurrence rate in patients older than 6 years.

In 2009, Miyamoto et al. [17] investigated the postoperative stresses and shapes of eight prominent ears by using two modified models (scaphal incision and abrasion) along with the no-manipulation model to analyze the antihelical cartilage manipulation biomechanics after the placement of Mustardé sutures. The biomechanics of conchal correction were implemented by using two other modified models (conchal incision and conchal excision) along with the no-manipulation model. They found that the mean maximal stress of the scaphal and abrasion model after Mustardé suture placement was 82 and 95 %, respectively, when compared to the no-manipulation technique. In scaphal incision models, they observed that the position of the helix does not change with load, with a corresponding smaller ear width on lateral view. The cut edges along loads became irregular. So far, while the cartilage-cutting techniques seem more advantageous biomechanically for the lower maximal cartilage stress, they present several limitations in cartilage shaping. The risk of an irregular, non-smooth antihelical fold is high, and there is no surgical control of the helical shape as the continuity between the helix and antihelix is interrupted. This is why a skin excision becomes essential in cartilage-cutting techniques to obtain a helix setback. These issues are generally overcome by the cartilage-abrasion techniques. For these reasons, today cartilage-cutting techniques are only considered because of their historical value and have been generally abandoned.

The mean maximal stresses in the conchal incision and excision model were not different from each other, but significantly different from the no-manipulation model, making both techniques biomechanically valid.

The "Normal" and the "Deformed" Ear

The "Normal" Ear

The correct diagnosis of any type of ear deformity cannot be correctly made without knowledge about the proportions and landmarks of what is defined as the "normal" ear. This information is essential for any surgeon performing aesthetic and reconstructive ear surgery (Table 21.1; Fig. 21.5).

In anthropometric studies [18], the ear is ideally described as a triangular structure called the "auricle triangle;" its base is defined by the anterior part that is directly attached to the most lateral part of the face. This corresponds to the earlobe attachment, such as the tragus and the superior ear attachment. The apex of the triangle is identified in Darwin's tubercle. By connecting the superior and inferior limits of the base with the apex, a triangular structure is obtained.

In anthropometric studies, the auricular index of Topinard is used:

$$\text{AI of Topinard} = (\text{W} \times 100) / \text{L}$$

It is similar to what is called the width (W) to length (L) ratio. The AI is around 60.5 in white males and 59 in white females. In Asians, it is smaller, and it is higher in the black population [18].

The auricular index of Schwalbe

$$\text{AI of Schwalbe} = (\text{base} \times 100) / \text{height}$$

is used to compare the human ear proportions with those of mammals and of anthropoids. When

Table 21.1 Proportions and landmarks of the "normal" ear

1. Superior ear attachment on lateral view is located in the same horizontal plane as the inferior eyebrow border
2. Inferior ear attachment on lateral view corresponds to the earlobe attachment and is located on the same horizontal plane as the columnar base
3. The tragus should be midway between the superior and inferior attachment
4. Ear position is positioned approximately one ear length posterior to the lateral orbit
5. Ear width-to-length ratio: the ear width is approximately between 3.0 and 4.5 cm and the length between 5.5 and 7.0 cm, with a corresponding ear width:length ratio of 0.5:0.6
6. The long axis of the ear is posteriorly inclined approximately 20° from the coronal plane
7. Cephalo-auricle angle designed by helix protrusion from the scalp is approximately 20–30° with a corresponding distance between the lateral helix margin and the head of approximately 1.5–2.0 cm
8. Helix profile on frontal view: the lateral margin of the helix should protrude more laterally than the antihelix for approximately 2–5 mm. The lateral margin of the helix should be smooth and linear and should minimally and gradually angle medially in the cephalocaudal direction
9. Conchal-scaphal angle: the angle defined by two tangential planes passing through the concha and the scapha is approximately 90°
10. Cephalo-conchal angle: the angle defined by the head and the concha is approximately 90°

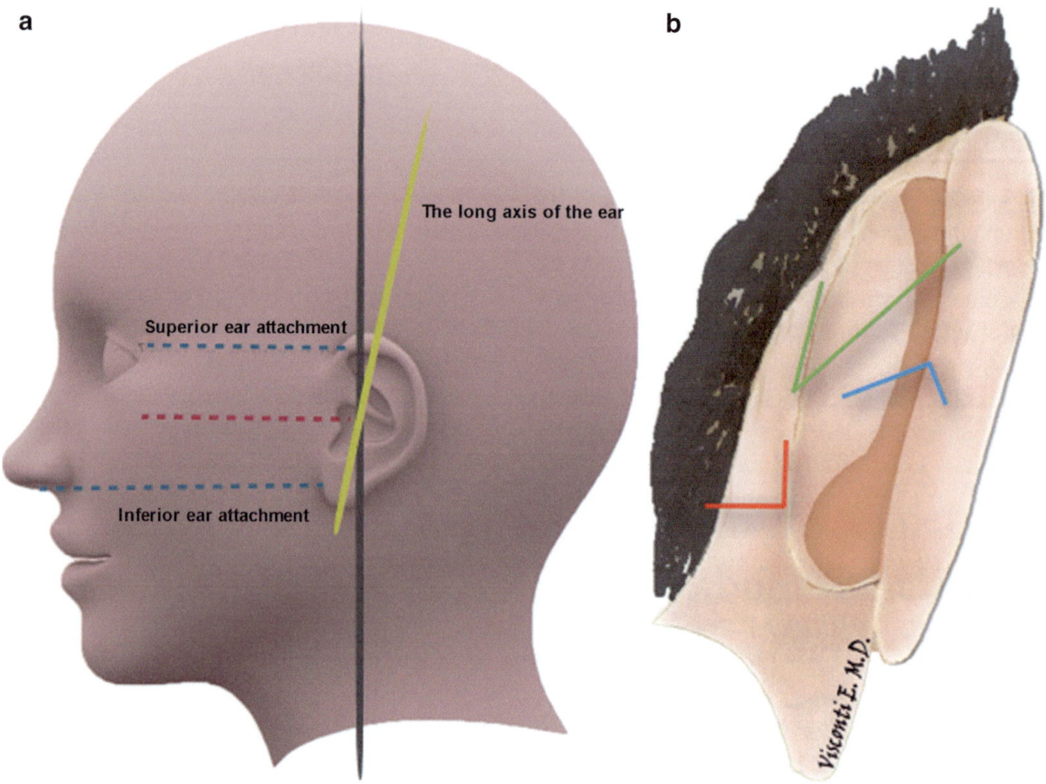

Fig. 21.5 (**a**) The aesthetic landmarks of the "normal" ear. (**b**) Aesthetic proportions of the "normal" ear. The *green* lines identify the cephalo-auricular angle, the *blue* lines the conchal-scaphal angle, and the *red* lines the conchal-mastoid angle

the height is defined by connecting Darwin's tubercle to the anterior auricle incisura, the Schwalbe AI is very low in mammals with long ears. It is higher in anthropoids and even more so in humans with the progressive reduction in ear height (Fig. 21.6) [18].

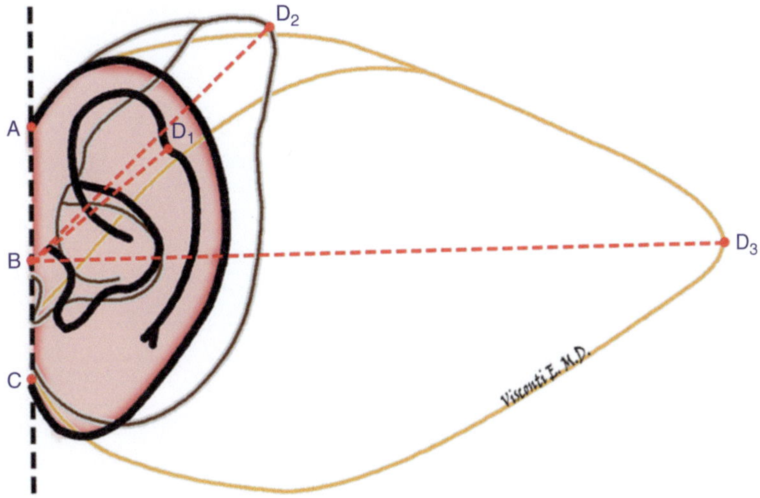

Fig. 21.6 Human external ear (*pink*) compared to the baboon ear (A-D²-C) and the calf ear (A-D³-C). D¹, D², and D³ are Darwin's tubercle of each ear. When each of these points is connected to B (anterior auricle incisura), the auricle height is defined, according to Schwalbe AI. A-B-C is the auricle base

The "Deformed" Ear

Aesthetic otoplasty is mainly restricted to the correction of the external ear deformities. Plastic surgeons treating patients complaining of external ear deformity must keep in mind that the ear is a complex sensory organ made of the external, middle, and inner ear. Thus, a deformed external ear can be associated with middle or inner ear problems that need to be ruled out before performing an aesthetic otoplasty of the external ear. This is particularly true when facing craniofacial syndrome patients.

Ear deformities can be classified into two main categories: congenital and the acquired ear deformities [18, 19].

1. Congenital ear deformities: Congenital ear deformities are conditions existing before and at birth or developing during the first month of life:
   (a) *Malformation* ear deformities: These anomalies develop by the tenth week of gestation and are caused by embryologic maldevelopment. They are also called "true" malformations and consist of deficient supernumerary auricular components, ranging from anotia and microtia to auricular sinuses and tags.
   (b) *Deformation* ear deformities: These anomalies occur on embryologically mature ears and can develop starting from the tenth week of gestation. Their etiology is usually related to abnormal physical forces (from imbalance of auricular muscle action to abnormal positioning) that act on the embryologically mature, malleable framework, altering its shape. They represent the majority of ear deformities, including the prominent or bat ear, which occurs most frequently, the Stahl deformity, cup and lop ear, and others.

The Prominent or Bat Ear

Prominent ear deformity is probably the most frequently encountered congenital malformation (Fig. 21.7). It occurs relatively frequent among Caucasians, with an incidence of approximately 5 %; men and women are equally affected [19, 20]. This condition is genetic, transmitted in an autosomal dominant pattern with varying degrees of penetration [20]. It is universally recognized at a glance and often responsible for psychological problems during childhood. This deformity is usually present at birth. However, Matsuo et al. [4] emphasized that prominent ear can also be an acquired deformity. They observed an increase in the prominent ear deformity rate from 0.4 % at birth to 5.5 % at 1 year of age. They hypothesized that abnormal forces acting on the malleable ear framework, mainly when the baby is in the cradle, can favor its development. In these cases,

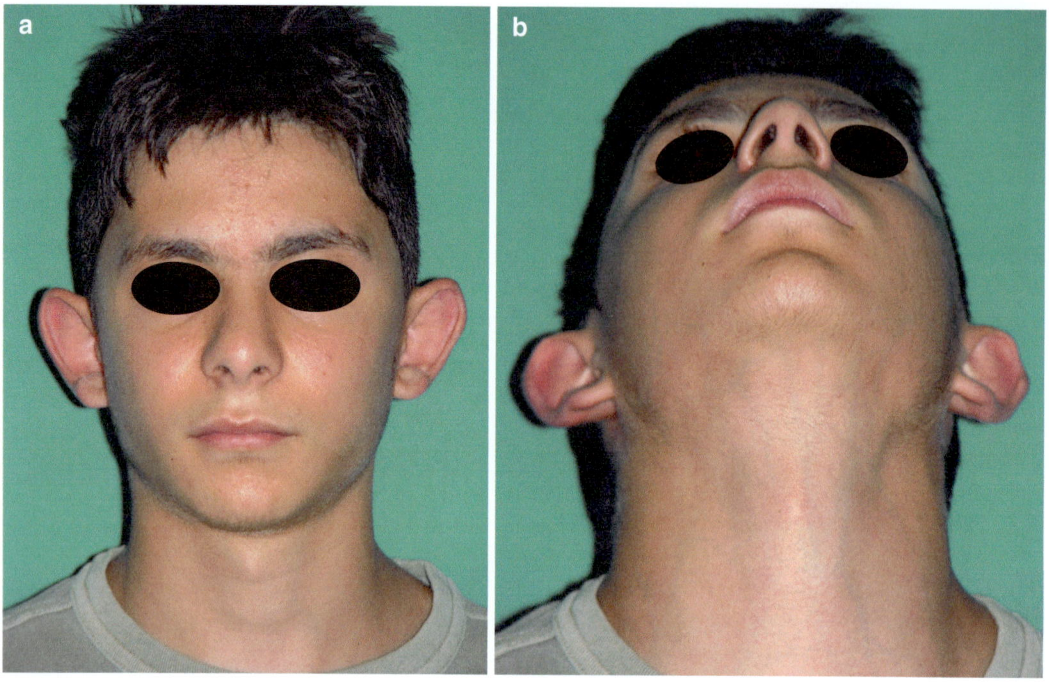

Fig. 21.7 An example of bat ear. The antihelical fold is not present; the helical tail is laterally displaced. The concha is hypertrophied, and the lobules show some grade of protrusion. (**a**) Frontal view; (**b**) inferior view

the prominent ear should be classified as an acquired deformity.

When performing aesthetic otoplasty to treat this condition, the most important step is the correct analysis of each ear and of each different deformity. This condition, in fact, can be monolateral or bilateral. When bilateral, it is not uncommon to be presented with different issues on each side.

One or more of the following features characterize the anatomy of the prominent ear:

1. The anatomical relationship among the superior antihelical crus, scapha, and fossa triangularis is preserved (this differentiates the bat ear from "constricted ears").
2. Effacement or deficient formation of the antihelical fold (the root, superior crus, inferior crus, or complete). Different degrees of inadequate antihelix formation exist, from subtle to complete without definition of the antihelical fold. A confluent concavity from the antihelix to the scapha can be appreciated as well as a lateral and forward displacement of the helix.
3. Various degrees of conchal hypertrophy or shape abnormalities (upper pole, lower pole, or complete). The evaluation of the conchal contribution in the definition of prominent ear is paramount as it represents the base on which the deficient antihelix and the displaced helix are mounted. The correction of the antihelical fold without addressing conchal hypertrophy could lead to unsatisfying and incomplete results. The concha can become completely enlarged. However, conchal hypertrophy can be localized mostly on the upper pole where the conchal cartilage creates a "bar" that pushes away the auricle or on the lower pole at the level of the antitragus where it can ultimately be responsible for earlobe protrusion.
4. Consequent conchal-scaphal angle greater than 90°.
5. Deformity of the skeletal auricular base. The deformities of the underlying skeleton can be responsible for the prominent appearance of the ear even if the two main features of

prominent ear, the inadequate antihelix and conchal hypertrophy, are not present or evident. The skull anomalies can be subtle or minimal in non-syndrome patients or can be the predominant feature in prominent ear like in craniofacial syndromes such as nonsynostotic plagiocephaly and the hemifacial microsomia without microtia.

6. Lobular protrusion. This condition can be isolated even if it is normally related to the lower pole or complete conchal hypertrophy.
7. Lateral displacement of the helical tail.
8. Macrotia. "True" macrotia is a very rare condition characterized by a too large auricle with normal proportions that can be due to an isolated congenital ear overgrowth or to a hemifacial hypertrophy. However, it can be associated with diseases such as neurofibromatosis or vascular anomalies. "Apparent" macrotia is a more common condition in which part of the ear is disproportionately enlarged, with earlobe hypertrophy being the most common.

The Stahl Ear Deformity

In the nineteenth century, Stahl first described a peculiar ear malformation characterized by the presence of an abnormal third antihelical crus extending from the superior helical crus to the edge of the helix, deforming the regular curvature of the upper third of the ear in a triangular structure. This condition, nowadays known as Stahl syndrome or Satiro's ear, is thought to be genetically transmitted as it reaches its highest expression in identical twins. A further etiopathogenesis has been proposed, which hypothesizes that the altered growth or function of the transverse muscle is responsible for the cartilaginous malformation.

It is interesting to analyze Stahl's ear deformity in relation to the evolution of the human species. Satiro's ear can be seen as an anthropogenic ear underdevelopment, as the AI of Schwalbe in Stahl's ear deformity is closer to that of anthropoids than of humans. The ear shape is similar to that of baboons (Fig. 21.6).

Lop and Cup Ear Deformities

Lop and cup ear deformities represent a curious group of auricle anomalies characterized by a "constricted" appearance of the ear. They differ from the prominent ear in that the scapha, fossa triangularis, and superior crus of the antihelix do not have a normal anatomical relationship.

The different terms given to these anomalies have increased the confusion and difficulty in categorizing these malformations. In his 1975 paper, Tanzer [21] coined the generic term "constricted ear" for all ear anomalies that share a degree of overhanging upper third (lop) with a degree of protrusion and the ear tubing in on itself (cup). Then, he classified the constricted ear according to the specific type of deformation and severity:

1. Grade I: the minor form of constricted ear is characterized by an altered helical shape. The helix is flatted or rolled along its superior rim with a corresponding reduction in ear height (lop appearance). It usually lacks cartilage support as the helical cartilage is normally found to be acutely angulated on itself, almost adherent to the scapha.
2. Grade II: the helix and scapha are involved at various degrees. They are divided into two subgroups:
   (a) Grade II A: minor form characterized by a rolled and constricted helix along with conchal enlargement or hypertrophy. Grade II A anomalies are similar to prominent ear deformities as there is also an effacement of the antihelix (Fig. 21.8). They differ from the more severe grade II B deformities as no supplemental skin is needed to cover the expanded cartilage during reconstruction.
   (b) Grade II B: a more severe form of grade II constricted ear with a more pronounced helix rolling along with a sharply reduced ear height. The antihelix and its crura are not folded with a corresponding protruding or constricted ear appearance. It normally needs additional skin to cover the reconstructed cartilaginous framework.

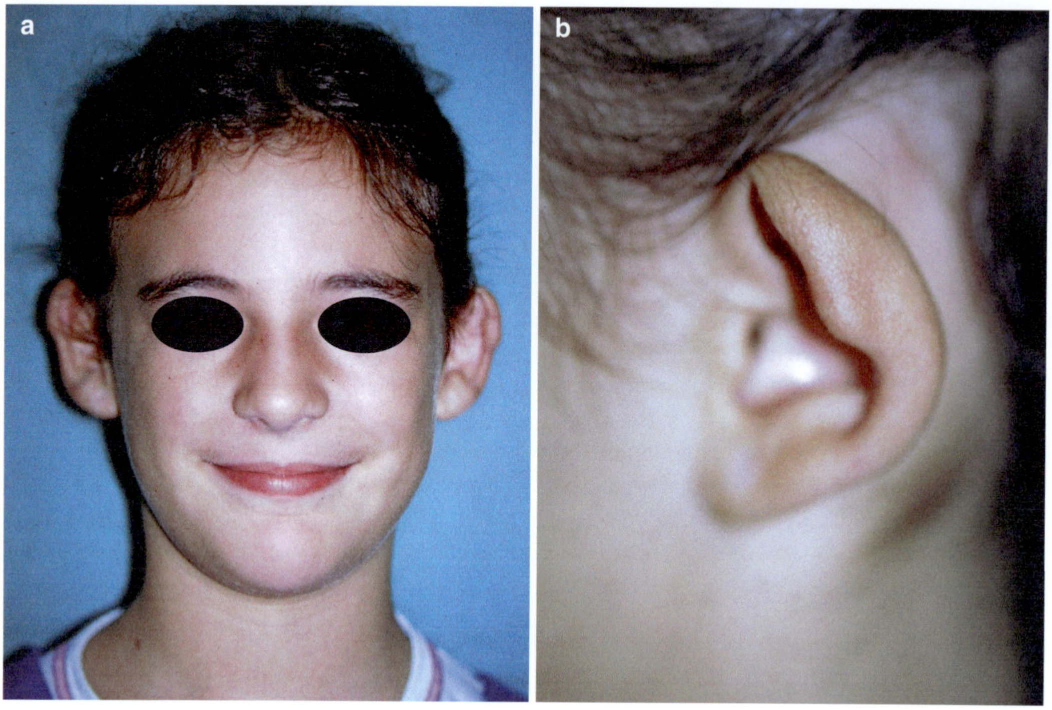

Fig. 21.8 Patient with moderate II A constricted left ear. The minimal helical altered shape and the moderate cupping appearance are accompanied by the anatomical features of the prominent ear. (**a**) Frontal view; (**b**) lateral view

3. Grade III: the most severe form of constricted ear characterized by an extreme cupping appearance. The auricle is rolled like a tube in a pouch-like fashion. The anterior margin of the helix is almost in contact with the earlobe. It is often associated with a mislocated auricle (almost always low set), forward tilt, stenosis of the external auditory canal, and deafness. It is not easy to deal with grade III anomalies. This condition is better handled by plastic surgeons well trained in ear reconstruction in collaboration with an expert otorhinolaryngologist for the exploration and, eventually, reconstruction of the middle third, which can result in distortions. Both external and middle ear alterations contribute to the hearing impairment in these patients.

Patient Evaluation and Surgical Indications

Many of the patients coming to the outpatient clinic for the first time are children accompanied by their parents, who are often highly motivated to have their child operated on to reduce the potential social embarrassment. This is particularly true when the child is around 3–6 years old and is going to start school. However, there are other types of patients, adolescents and adults, who have overcome the psychological impact of the deformity and are seeking surgery for other reasons.

While adolescents and adults are offered otoplasty under local anesthesia plus intravenous sedation, for children operating under general anesthesia is preferred because of minimal patient cooperation.

There are few contraindications to otoplasty. Children usually tolerate the operation well. However, some children are particularly worried about the operation, seeing the doctor, and entering a clinic. In this case, the operation is better delayed until the child's awareness of the deformity arises and the child openly requests the procedure. The adult population requesting otoplasty, however, has greater need of a thorough psychological analysis than the pediatric population. As the social embarrassment is normally of minor concern to these patients, it is important to understand their motivation as well as to make sure that their request for surgery is based on realistic expectations.

Medical contraindications are skin diseases, chondritis, acute otitis media, and chronic ear infections [6–10, 19, 22]. The presence of ear piercing can also be a problem that needs to be addressed. The pierced area represents a full-thickness skin and cartilage defect. If it is located exactly on the area of interest for surgery, this will limit cartilage manipulation in that area, thus influencing the result. Moreover, this area could be a source of bacterial contamination and subclinical infection, increasing the risk of skin infection and chondritis. All of these issues should be taken into account before operating on a patient with ear piercing, and a detailed and thorough informed consent on the limits of surgery and on the increased risk of infection is essential.

Nonsurgical Correction and Timing of Surgery

During the first days of life, the ear cartilage presents unique biomechanical features. It is particularly malleable and more viscous than elastic structures. It seems not to have developed the "intrinsic elastic cartilaginous memory" yet. This concept is the basis of nonsurgical correction of prominent ear. Literature reports from Japan and the UK have demonstrated that it is possible to achieve satisfying long-term correction of prominent ear by simple auricular molding if this is started within the first 3 days of birth and continued till the first 6 months [4, 5]. The high serum maternal estrogen level has been postulated to be responsible for the unique biomechanical ear features in this specific period of life. As the estrogen serum level starts to decrease (from 3 days after birth until reaching normal levels by 6 weeks), the result of nonsurgical correction is poor, as demonstrated by Matsuo [4]. So far, the nonsurgical prominent correction is of limited value if applied later than the first 3 days of life.

The rationale for the correct timing of surgery requires a balance between the ear growth state and patient age. It is preferable to operate before the child reaches school age in order to reduce the psychological embarrassment and teasing by peers. In the literature, no general agreement exists on the exact timing of surgery. Even though there is a general opinion among surgeons worldwide that the best age is around 5–6 years for the reasons explained above, some authors advocate that the operation can be safely performed even at 4 years old without altering the physiological ear growth. Gosain et al. [5] demonstrated that children can safely undergo otoplasty before the age of 4 years and as early as 9 months. Furthermore, they stressed the biomechanical concept that at this age the highly malleable ear is more compliant to correction with a consequently higher rate of successful long-lasting results.

The authors encourage surgery before the child reaches school age, and we reassure the parents, when needed, that there are no risks of interference with the physiological ear growth.

Goals of Correction

The general goal of otoplasty is to restore the anatomy and the shape of the ear to look like a "normal" ear in an aesthetically acceptable and permanent way. McDowell [23] defined the basic goals of otoplasty in his paper (Table 21.2). Besides the McDowell goals of otoplasty, some anatomical goals should be kept in mind when treating protruding ears:

1. The antihelical fold should be shaped in a round and smooth way along with the superior crus.
2. Conchal-scaphal angle of 90°.

Table 21.2 McDowell goals of otoplasty

1. All trace of protrusion in the upper one-third of the ear must be corrected. Some remaining protrusion in the middle or lower third may be acceptable provided that the superior aspect is thoroughly corrected; however, the reverse may not be true
2. From the front view, the helix of both ears should be seen beyond the antihelix (at least down to the mid-ear and preferably all the way)
3. The helix should have a smooth and regular line throughout
4. The postauricular sulcus should not be markedly decreased or distorted
5. Protrusion should measure between 15 and 20 mm from the helix to the head
6. Position of the two ears: the distance from the lateral border to the head should be within 3 mm at any given point

3. Reduction of conchal excess and reduction of the angle between the concha and mastoid.
4. Reduction of the cephalo-auricular distances.
5. Correction of an abnormal position of the lobule (if the lobule projection is beyond the helical rim).

Acquired Ear Deformities

Acquired ear deformities occur during a patient's lifetime, with trauma being the main etiology. The most common source of trauma is earring avulsion, burns, human bites, infection, accidents, shotgun wounds, and cutting weapons. The upper third of the ear is the most frequent site of ear trauma in male patients, whereas the earlobe is the most frequent site of trauma in women (earring avulsion). With the exception of some conditions (i.e., earring avulsion) that are easily addressed, acquired ear deformities usually require complex reconstructive operations.

Combined Technique in Aesthetic Otoplasty

Preoperative evaluation of the ear deformity to be corrected is essential to achieve a tailored result able to address the specific type of deformity. The specific type of deformity along with the cartilage shape and consistency of both ears is evaluated in detail as are comprehensive 3D ear proportions and symmetry.

The external ear is a bilateral structure that usually is not symmetrical. When treating a case of severe deformity on one side with a minimal anomaly on the other side, we prefer to operate on both sides to achieve a more symmetrical result. When a unilateral deformity is present with a "normal" contralateral ear, we still prefer to operate on both ears to achieve symmetry. Rare cases presenting a contralateral "normal" ear with maximum setback are operated only on the affected side.

The operation is usually performed under local anesthesia plus intravenous sedation except in young children, in whom general anesthesia is required because of minimal patient compliance. The local anesthesia solution (xylocaine 2 % and epinephrine 1:100,000) is used on both the posterior surface of the ear and the anterior surface over the antihelix and concha with the aim to achieve both a bloodless surgical field and hydrodissection. Before anesthesia induction, systemic broad-spectrum prophylactic antibiotics are administered.

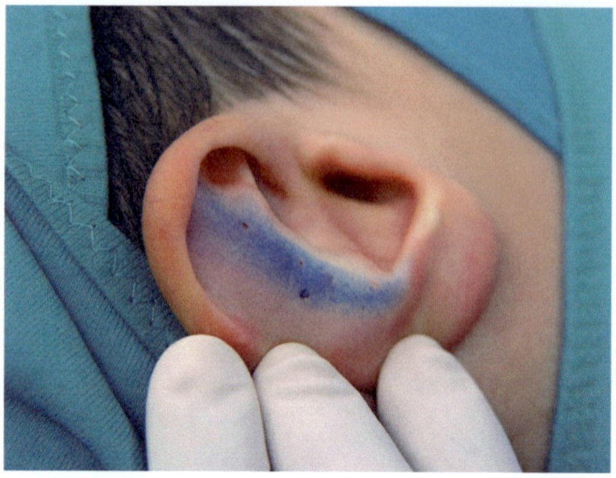

Fig. 21.9 Manual maneuver of folding back the helical rim toward the head to visualize the position of the antihelical fold that is then marked with methylene blue

The helical rim is folded back against the head to visualize the position of the antihelix to reconstruct. This is marked with methylene blue (Fig. 21.9). The posterior projection of the new antihelix is marked on the posterior surface of the ear. This defines the linear surgical incision that is normally located 1–1.5 cm above the retroauricular fold. The length of the skin incision extends from a few millimeters above the tail of the antihelix inferiorly to a few millimeters above the bifurcation of the lateral and medial antihelical crus superiorly. No skin is excised. By using our technique, this maneuver is not needed to address the ear deformity (Fig. 21.10).

A straight, full-thickness, skin-subcutis linear incision is performed following the marked line on the posterior ear surface. Then the posterior ear skin is undermined up to the tail of the antihelix inferiorly, laterally toward the helix margin, and toward the postauricular sulcus medially. Thus, the posterior cartilage surface is widely exposed (Fig. 21.11). This allows an easier positioning of the Mustardé sutures in order to bend

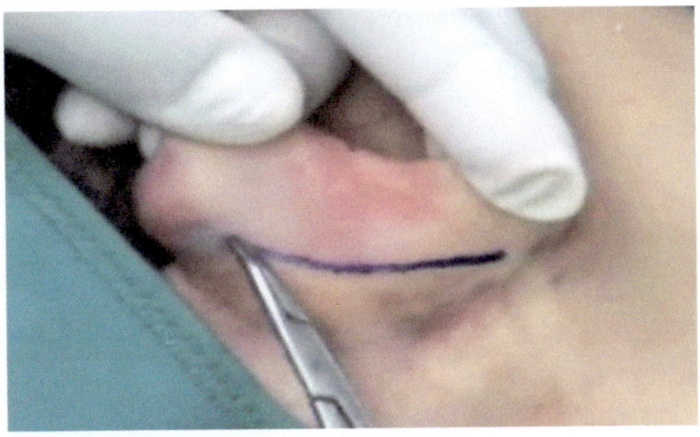

Fig. 21.10 The skin incision being marked

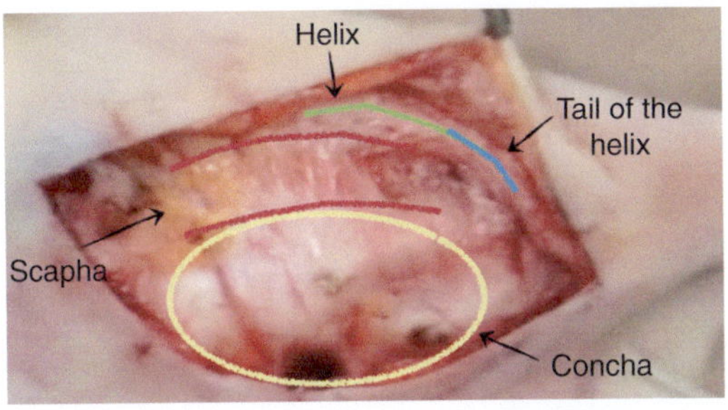

Fig. 21.11 The posterior ear cartilage exposed after blunt soft tissue undermining. The ear structures come into view

the cartilage of the antihelix. Accurate hemostasis is achieved.

At this point, the anterior cartilage is approached by creating a blunt tunnel with a mosquito through the antitragus-helical fissure. A Stenstroem otoabrader is inserted in this tunnel and is directed toward the anterior surface of ear following the marked new antihelix position (Fig. 21.12). The otoabrader needs to be gently advanced in order to first bluntly divide the skin from the cartilage.

Then, the perichondrium and the antihelical and scapha cartilage are carefully abraded in order to weaken the anterior surface elastic fiber cartilage network and obtain the "bending-away" effect. Precise cartilage scoring is also performed at the tail of the antihelix and medially toward the concha. At this level, the cartilage is thicker than in the upper third of the ear. The resulting "bending-away" effect at this level allows a posterior rotation of the tail of the antihelix with a resulting desirable retroposition of the earlobe.

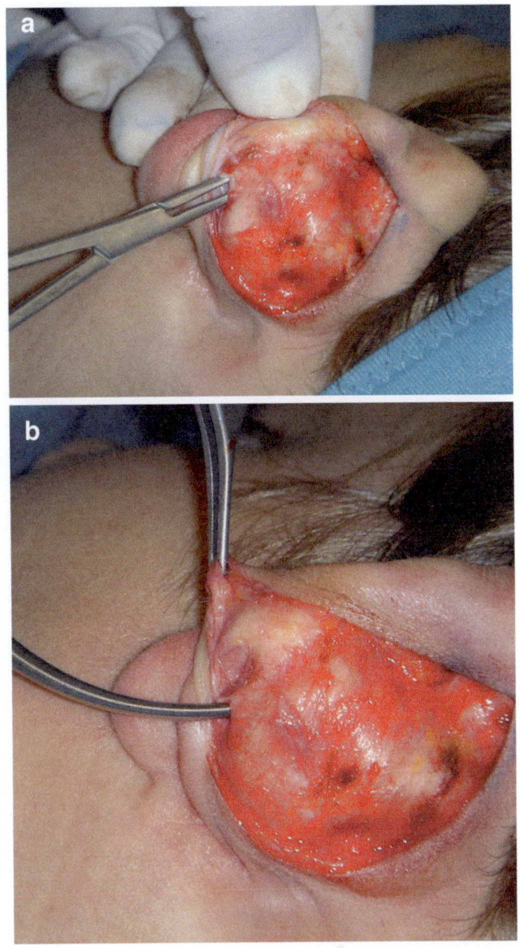

Fig. 21.12 (**a**) The mosquito used to approach the anterior cartilage surface through the antitragus-helical fissure. (**b**) The Stenstroem otoabrader is inserted

The helix is manually pressed toward the mastoid to create the correct fold of the antihelix.

Straight needles dipped in methylene blue are passed through repeatedly to mark the cartilage posteriorly with three pairs of points:

1. The first straight needle is passed inferiorly through the tail of the antihelix on the scaphal and the conchal side.
2. The second straight needle is passed midway at the antihelix bifurcation on the scaphal and the conchal side.
3. The third straight needle is passed superiorly between the triangularis fossa and the scapha to delineate the superior crus of the antihelix (Fig. 21.13).

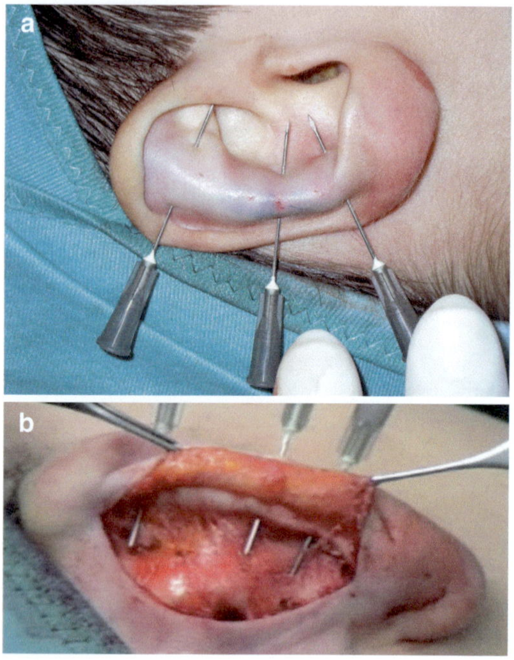

Fig. 21.13 (**a**, **b**) Three straight needles have been used to position the antihelix

On the posterior cartilage surface, the three pairs of points identify the exact position of the three horizontal mattress Mustardé sutures to define the new antihelical fold.

Three 3-0 Vicryl sutures are now passed through the posterior cartilage surface with a partial-thickness bite placed exactly on the blue points. Starting inferiorly and progressing superiorly, each suture is tied, determining the bending of the antihelix (Fig. 21.14).

The correct position of these mattress sutures is a key point of the operation. With the inferior suture, we both rotate the helical tail medially toward the concha, decreasing the conchal-scaphal and the cephalo-auricular angle, and, at the same time, an earlobe setback is achieved. In fact, the earlobe fibrofatty tissue is a natural downward continuation of the helical tail, and, being a completely viscous structure, it follows the movement of the helical tail. The midway and the superior sutures serve to shape the antihelical fold in two critical points: before the bifurcation in the superior and inferior crus and to correctly shape the superior crus at the triangular fossa.

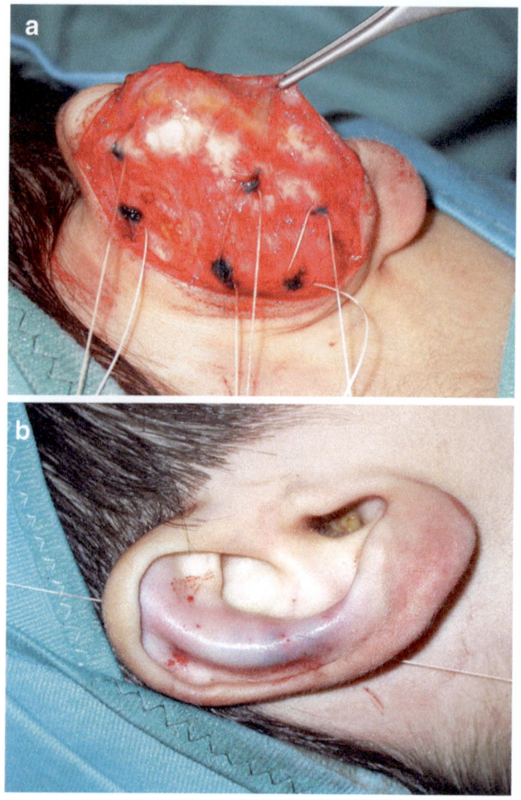

Fig. 21.14 (**a**, **b**) Three 3-0 Vicryl sutures have been placed with partial-thickness bites

When facing with a very deep and hypertrophied concha, the authors prefer to add a small crescent full-thickness cartilage excision (width ranging from 2 to 6 mm) at the junction of the floor and posterior wall of the concha. The edge of this crescent is widely undermined from the skin to favor the natural alignment without placing sutures.

The posterior linear skin incision is now closed with a few interrupted 4-0 Vicryl rapid sutures to allow eventual blood drainage in case of minimal bleeding (Fig. 21.15). Three 5-0 transfixing Prolene sutures over tulle gras are placed on the anterior surface of the ear to stabilize the result and to further reduce tension on the Mustardé sutures (Fig. 21.16). These sutures are removed after 10 days (Figs. 21.17 and 21.18).

The patient is instructed to wear a light bandage for 10 days for stabilization and to protect

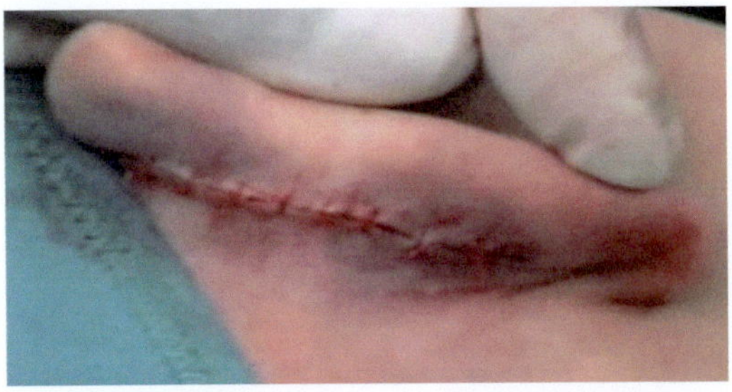

Fig. 21.15 A few interrupted 4-0 Vicryl rapid sutures close the skin in a tension-free fashion. No excess skin is present

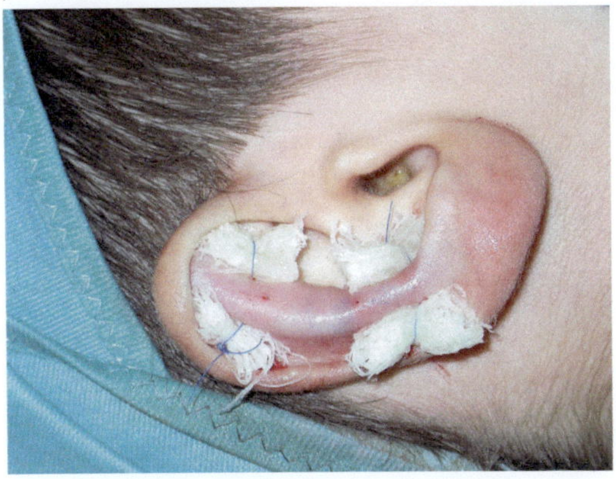

Fig. 21.16 Ear appearance at the end of surgery before wound dressing

the ear from unintentional movements and position (such as during sleeping) that could jeopardize the surgical result. After 10 days, the patient is instructed to wear an elastic band for 15 days. Arnica-based medications along with instructions to sleep between two pillows are prescribed to reduce postoperative edema. Broad-spectrum oral antibiotics and painkillers are prescribed as well.

Complications

In otoplasty we should distinguish early complications that can occur within the first 14 days postoperatively and late sequelae that can occur from the 15th day postoperatively onward. Overall, the complication rates in otoplasty are low, and when complications occur, they are often minor complications [6–10, 20].

Early Complications

1. Hematoma: Limandjaja et al. [20] found this complication to range from 0 to 7.5 % in the literature. Insufficient hemostasis is the main cause of hematoma development. Rarely, it can be due to a rebound vasodilatation effect from local anesthesia, hypertension, postoperative trauma, and coagulopathy. It can be recognized as the patient usually reports excessive, disproportionate, persistent unilateral pain a few hours postoperatively. Continuous bleeding from the surgical wound can be associated as well. Hematoma is fraught with the risk of cartilage and skin necrosis due to excessive pressure. It requires prompt and immediate intervention. If encountered, the first thing to do is remove the sutures and drain the hematoma. In case of ongoing bleeding, the patient has to be taken back to the operating room or the hemostasis controlled.
2. Infection: This complication is rarely reported in otoplasty as the extensive auricular blood supply represents a sufficient protective system. However, insufficient sterility as well as hematoma and wound dehiscence can favor infection. It can be clinically recognized by a deep, continuous pain along with skin erythema, swelling, and pus formation. This condition needs to be readily recognized to establish an appropriate systemic antibiotic therapy to control it in order to avoid its eventual progression to perichondritis and chondritis, which can lead to cartilage necrosis and acquired malformation.
3. Bleeding. Bleeding from the surgical wound can be a minor complication managed by bandage changes. However, it has to be viewed as a warning signal for a possible hematoma requiring immediate surgical intervention.
4. Skin necrosis. This rare complication can occur when there is a subdermal plexus venous discharge impairment normally related to undue pressure applied on the auricle (i.e., thigh dressings, hematoma). It can also be experienced as the final stage of an infection.
5. Wound dehiscence.

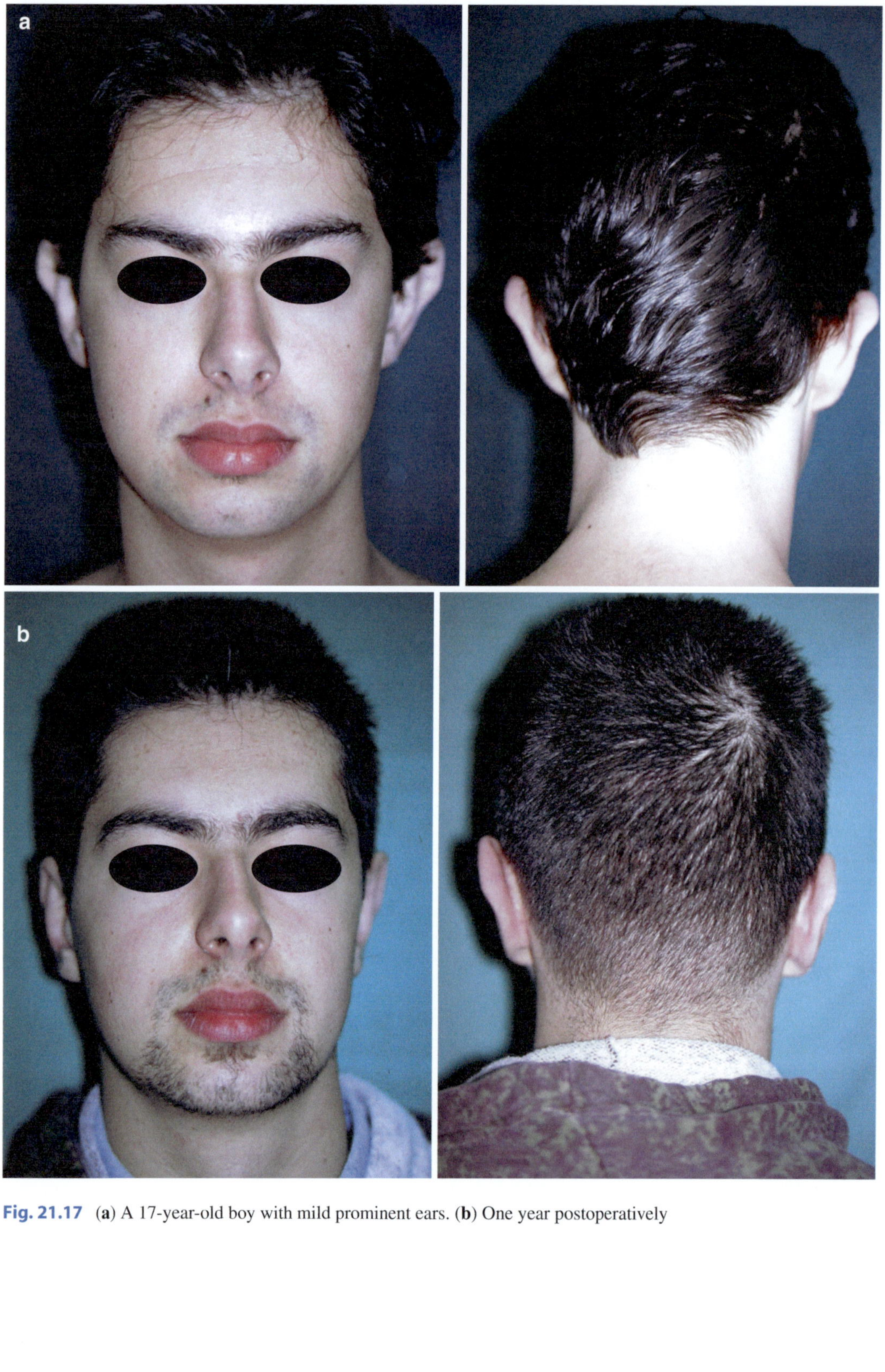

Fig. 21.17 (**a**) A 17-year-old boy with mild prominent ears. (**b**) One year postoperatively

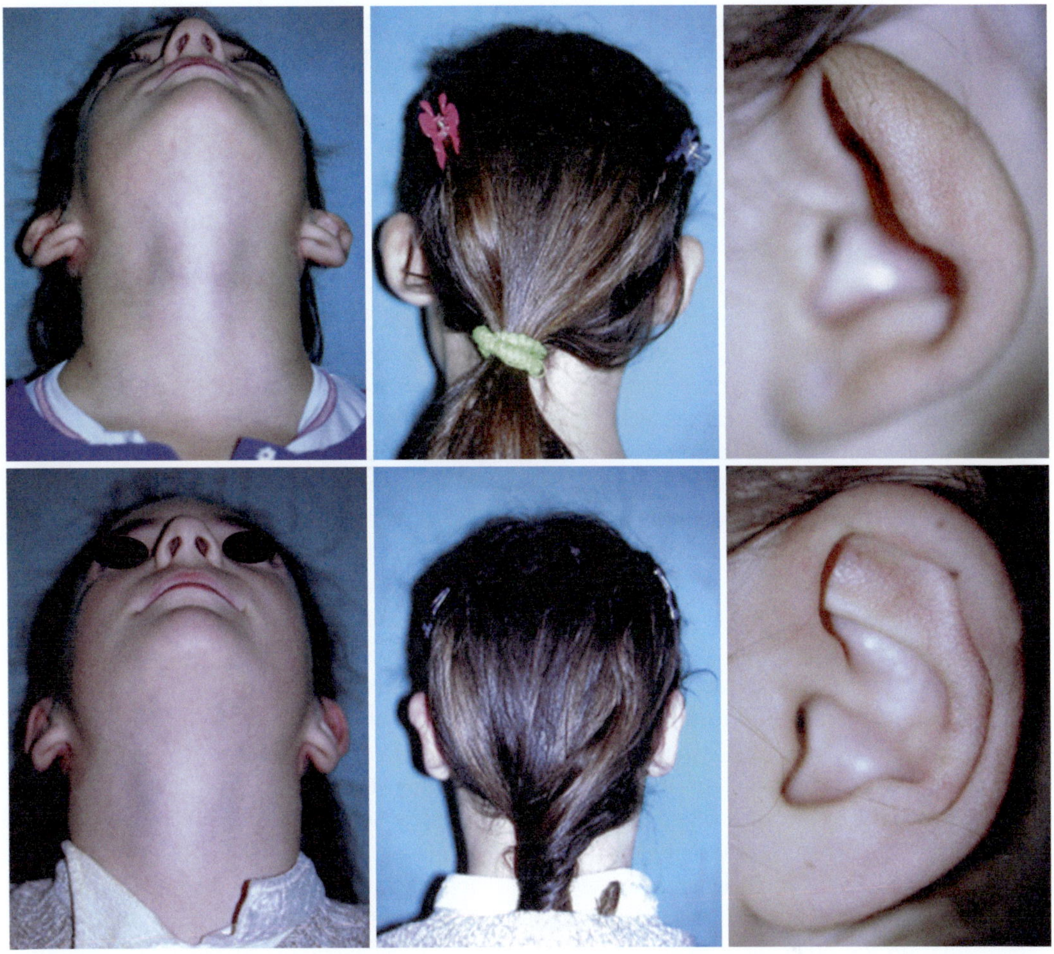

Fig. 21.18 (*Above*) A 9-year-old girl with right prominent ear and left cup ear of mild degree, preoperatively. (*Below*) Result 6 months postoperatively. The constricted *left* ear has been corrected

Late Complications

1. Unsatisfactory cosmetic outcomes. Under this category, many different conditions can be experienced:
   (a) Relapse: The recurrence of ear deformity after surgery is normally directly related to the age of the patient and the technique used. It is more frequent after non-combined techniques as the cartilage recoil will defeat the forces applied by the surgery and return to the original condition. In combined techniques, insufficient cartilage weakening and suture failure are the main causes of relapse. The relapse rate increases with the age (less frequent in children under 6 years old and more frequent in adolescents and adults) and is far higher for techniques relying solely on skin excision than on cartilage manipulation.
   (b) Undercorrection: Undercorrection is recognized as a failure in some steps of the surgical technique with a corresponding insufficient correction of the deformity. The ear will appear less prominent, for example, but it is still possible to recognize the features of bat ear.
   (c) Overcorrection: Contrarily, overcorrection is also a failure of some steps of the surgical technique with corresponding

results going beyond the goals of the otoplasty. The classic example of overcorrection is a "pinned-back" appearance with the auricle flattened against the head, with a corresponding cephalo-auricular angle of less than 20° and the helix no longer visible in the frontal view.

(d) Cartilage irregularities (Fig. 21.19): Acute crests and irregular contours along the fold of the antihelix with a tendency to overcorrection are typical deformities seen with the cartilage-cutting techniques, which require a full-thickness cartilage incision. These residual deformities require secondary correction surgery. Frequently seen in the past, these complications are rarely found now as cartilage-cutting techniques have generally been abandoned.

(e) Telephone ear (Fig. 21.20): This peculiar deformity is the result of both undercorrection of the upper and lower third of the ear and overcorrection of the mid-ear. This complication is usually experienced with the skin excision technique when a classic lozenge excision pattern is used.

(f) Reverse telephone ear: This complication, on the other hand, is the result of both overcorrection of the upper and lower ear third and undercorrection of the mid-ear. This is frequently the result of an undercorrection of a very deep and hypertrophied concha. Like the telephone ear deformity, it is more frequently experienced with the skin excision technique with a modified pattern, such as the dumbbell pattern. A millimeter underestimation in skin excision will lead to this deformity.

(g) Asymmetry: This condition is physiologically present in people with both normal and deformed ears. The goal of otoplasty is the achievement of a pleasant and symmetrical result. Asymmetry can be considered acceptable when minimal (hardly appreciable by the patient) and when already evident preoperatively.

2. Suture extrusion. This complication can be experienced when sutures are placed in too close proximity to the skin, when using permanent sutures, when there is too much tension on the sutures, and in case of infection. According to Limandjaja et al. [20], the suture extrusion rate is from 0 (absorbable sutures) to 22.2 %. Interestingly, according to their review, suture extrusion has been experienced mainly by surgeons using permanent nylon sutures. Since the first description by Horlock et al. in 2001 [24], the use of the postauricular fascial flap has been popular in otoplasty. This flap serves as an intervening tissue layer between the cartilage and the skin with the aim to reduce the suture extrusion complication rate. However, some series have demonstrated that this complication is still possible when using this technique. The real issues in suture extrusion seems to be the type of material used (permanent vs. absorbable sutures) and the tension applied.
3. Scarring. Dystrophic scars, such as hypertrophic scar and keloids (Fig. 21.21), can occur in otoplasty, especially when using a posterior approach, as this part of the body is normally prone to abnormal scarring. In black people, the rate of this complication is higher. Abnormal scarring can be prevented by using a tension-free closure. This is also the reason why we prefer the postauricular skin incision over other skin excision patterns.
4. Hypersensitivity. Some patients describe a sense of postauricular tenderness. This condition is related to axon regeneration and tends to disappear within months.

The Evolution of the Combined Technique

Postauricular Skin Incision or Excision?

The postauricular approach is largely favored when performing an aesthetic otoplasty because it allows good exposure of the auricular cartilage, direct and indirect access to anterior and posterior

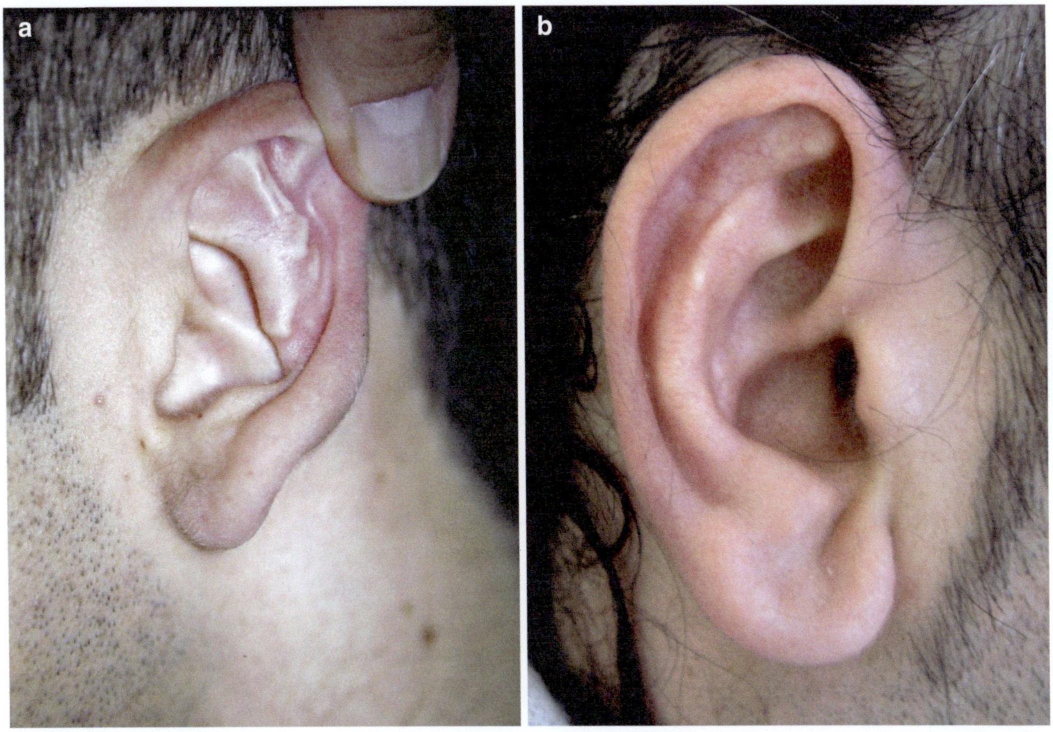

Fig. 21.19 (**a**, **b**) Two examples of sharp cartilage edges with acute crests and irregular contour, signs of the cartilage full-thickness cutting technique

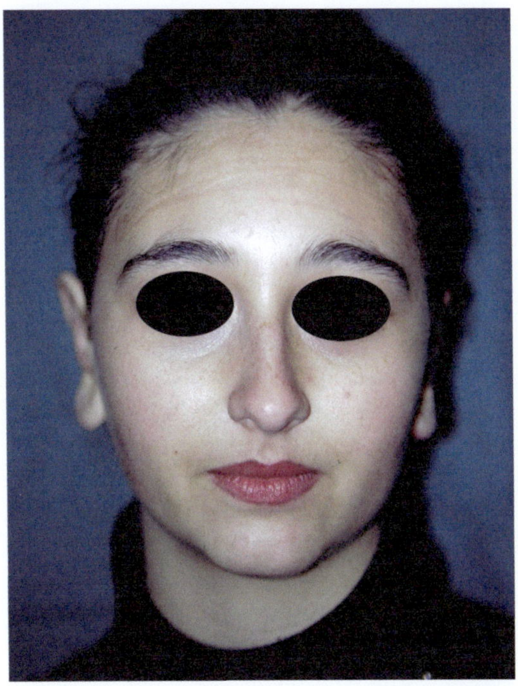

Fig. 21.20 An example of telephone ear. Note the upper and severe lower ear third protrusion and the mid-ear retroposition

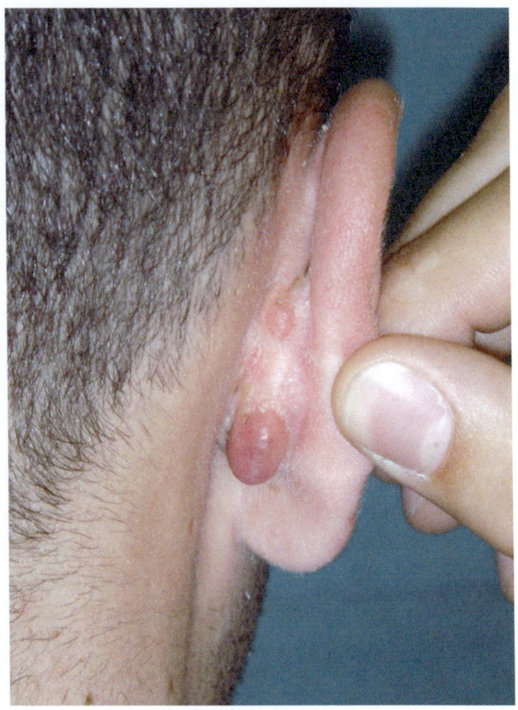

Fig. 21.21 A keloid at the retroauricular scar

cartilage surfaces, and the final scar is not visible as it is hidden postauricularly.

Both postauricular skin incision and skin excision allow the same advantages. Much has been written regarding variously shaped postauricular skin excision patterns to facilitate wound closure and to improve the surgical correction of a prominent ear [6–10]. By using a skin excision pattern, it is believed that the final skin closure will also contribute to the auricle and earlobe setback. However, the retroauricular skin excision is frequently responsible for poor cosmetic outcomes, leading to dystrophic scars and iatrogenic complications, such as the telephone ear.

In our opinion, the postauricular skin excision should generally be avoided as it does not add any benefit to prominent ear correction. Considering the anatomy of bat ear, skin excess is not an issue. We firmly believe that the skin should be preserved in order to compensate for excessive skin retraction, which can lead to posterior sulcus obliteration and to unexpected and uncontrollable mid-ear setback with a consequent telephone ear deformity. However, when the skin excision pattern is reduced in the mid-third to avoid telephone ear, the excessive undercorrection can lead to a reverse telephone ear deformity. Moreover, the likelihood of dystrophic scars and keloid formation is higher as the skin is not closed in a tension-free fashion.

By using a linear postauricular skin incision, normally located 1–1.5 cm over the retroauricular fold, we have been able to offer satisfactory otoplasty to all our patients without experiencing the common drawbacks of a skin excision. Moreover, by preserving all the postauricular soft tissues, good soft tissue coverage is provided over the Mustardé sutures, thus minimizing bow stringing and suture extrusion.

A skin excision pattern should be performed only in very rare cases, in which skin excess is a real issue, such as in adulthood and in the elderly. In this limited subset of patients, the skin has lost its elasticity and can be redundant. However, it is always better to start with a skin incision and to customize the skin excision when performing the final skin closure.

Surgery of the Antihelix

When treating prominent ears, some subtypes of constricted ear and Stahl ear deformities, the effacement or misdevelopment of the antihelical fold is normally an issue. A practical and effective way to evaluate the amount of antihelical shaping is to manually bend the auricle against the head and then mark how the new antihelix should look like.

Surgery of the antihelix can be divided into two major schools of thought: the cartilage-sparing and the cartilage-scoring techniques.

The cartilage-sparing techniques rely on the Mustardé concept of posteriorly located full-thickness horizontal mattress sutures to create the antihelical fold [26]. These sutures are tightened accordingly to the extent required to obtain a pleasant antihelical fold shape. The main issues with the Mustardé technique are the relatively high rate of relapse, especially in patients over 6 years old, and the possible stitch extrusion.

Relative to the relapse rate, Mustardé [16] retrospectively reviewed his otoplasty patients, reporting a relapse rate of 1.8 % in patients younger than 6 years old and a very high recurrence rate of 30 % in patients older than 6 years old. His findings are in line with the biomechanical properties of the auricle. The hypothesized mechanisms are that, the insufficient suture load for holding the cartilage in its new position together with the consequent cartilagineous recoil, increase the suture load and breaks the sutures. A further explanation could be the suture tearing forces, also known as the "cheese wire" effect. It is possible that an incorrectly placed suture (not full-thickness) and/or a high suture tearing force in a cartilage with low stress relaxation causes the suture to have a cutting effect on the cartilage with the consequent loss of suture load on the cartilage itself.

Relative to the suture extrusion rate, two main factors can contribute to this complication: the type of suture material used and the tension on the Mustardé sutures. Concerning the type of suture material, the extrusion rate is definitely higher for permanent sutures. In our otoplasty series, we never experienced suture extrusion, confirming that our choice of using absorbable sutures is advantageous.

Concerning the tension applied and the soft tissue covers, some authors sustain that the skin excision technique favors suture extrusion because of a tenting effect and the minimal soft tissue coverage over the Mustardé sutures. To overcome the issue of insufficient tissue coverage, the postauricular fascia flap has been advocated by many authors since its first description by Horlock et al. in 2001 [24, 25]. In our opinion, these drawbacks can be avoided by combining a skin incision pattern with the use of absorbable sutures.

The cartilage-scoring techniques can be further divided into two main subgroups: the cartilage-cutting and the cartilage-abrasion techniques.

1. The cartilage-cutting techniques are based on the initial report by Luckett [6] that creates the new antihelical fold by excising a crescent segment of cartilage posteriorly and approximating the remaining edges to each other. Following this report, the concept of cutting the cartilage in a full-thickness fashion to create the antihelical fold was popularized in the 1960s, after Becker introduced the tube-like shaping of the antihelix. He incised the cartilage by using two parallel incisions on either side of the antihelix and sutured these edges in order to make a tube of the intervening cartilage to form the antihelical fold. Other popular techniques are those of Converse et al., Farrior, and Pitanguy. Nowadays, the cartilage-cutting techniques have been abandoned because they produce sharp, visible, not natural-looking ridges on the antihelical fold that are very difficult to correct. Furthermore, by cutting the cartilage, there is no surgical control of the helical protrusion as the cartilage continuity has been interrupted. All these drawbacks favor the use of the cartilage-abrasion techniques.

The cartilage-abrasion techniques rely on the first observation of the bending effect experienced in injured costal cartilage by Gibson and Davis [12]. Later on, Stenstroem [13] and Chongchet [14] applied this concept to aesthetic otoplasty. Many instruments have been used to abrade the cartilage, such as rasps, abraders, Adson-Brown forceps, and hypodermic needles. As with Mustardé sutures, the cartilage-abrasion techniques are effective by themselves when treating prominent ears of children younger than 6 years old. When treating older patients with thicker and more elastic cartilage, the cartilage-abrasion techniques have been reported to have a virtual relapse rate of 100 % [6–10].

Cartilage-abrasion technique are largely preferred to the cartilage-cutting techniques as they avoid the deleterious creation of sharp edges and allow obtaining smooth and round contours [6–10].

Considering the advantages and limitations of both the cartilage-sparing and cartilage-cutting techniques, nowadays many surgeons have refined their otoplasty techniques, which are normally a combination of both cartilage-sparing and cutting methods.

Our technique is a combination of the Stenstroem cartilage-abrasion and Mustardé cartilage-sparing technique. The cartilage is scored with Stenstroem otoabraders in order to define the new shape by the bending effect and to weaken it in order to reduce the tension on the sutures. During the maneuver of cartilage abrasion, the surgeon must assess the cartilage thickness at each level in order to perform an appropriate and non-aggressive abrasion. Furthermore, the abrasion should be performed along the antihelical fold in a rectangular-shaped area and along the superior crus in a fan-shaped area in order to weaken the cartilaginous area to be shaped.

The 3-0 Vicryl Mustardè sutures give the final and permanent shape to the antihelix once it has been correctly weakened. By combining the two techniques with the use of absorbable sutures, we experienced satisfying long-term results with a 0 % rate of suture extrusion. Our findings are in line with the actual biomechanical principles of the ear cartilage.

Surgery of the Concha (Mid-Third of the Ear)

Besides effacement of the antihelical fold, conchal hypertrophy represents another major issue in prominent ears. However, it is rare to find a patient with an isolated conchal hypertrophy and normal antihelix development. A review of current otoplasty techniques by Nuara and Mobley [9] found that the residual conchal prominence is generally addressed after correction of the antihelical fold. Conchal hypertrophy can be managed by using several techniques:

1. Conchal suture setback: Conchal-mastoid sutures were originally described by Owens and Delgado to correct conchal hypertrophy or prominence. However, the modified Furnas technique [27] is the most reported. Furnas used nonabsorbable, full-thickness (till the anterior perichondrium) mattress sutures placed between the conchal cartilage and the mastoid fascia. Three to four sutures are placed in a strict anteroposterior direction in order to gently set back the concha, avoiding its forward rotation and external auditory canal narrowing. As reported by Elliot [28], the concha setback can be more effective if the postauricular muscle and fibrofatty tissue over the mastoid are excised in order to create a hosting pocket. As reported by Furnas, the concha suture setback is effective for mild to moderate cases with a conchal height less than 2.5 cm. In our hands, mild to moderate cases of conchal enlargement are managed by the placement of inferior Mustardè sutures.
2. Excision techniques: The use of these techniques has been advocated when treating concha hypertrophy of higher grades. The cartilage can be incised using either an anterior or posterior approach based on the surgeon's preference. Once the base of the concha cartilage has been dissected from the anterior and posterior skin, the ear is manually retroposed, producing conchal cartilage overlapping. The excess cartilage is marked and excised without skin. The free edges can or cannot be repositioned by sutures [6–10].
3. Scoring techniques: Using the same concept of scoring techniques in defining the antihelix, the conchal anterior abrasion can be used alone or in combination with sutures to allow a conchal setback with lower tension. In fact, the same issues experienced with Mustardé sutures for the antihelical fold, such as relapse and suture extrusion, can be equally experienced with Furnas sutures. Thus, the same concepts applied for Mustardé sutures are valid for the Furnas sutures as well [6–10].

The authors correct mild to moderate concha hypertrophy with inferior mattress sutures. When a very enlarged concha is present after the antihelical shaping has been finished, adding a small crescent, full-thickness cartilage excision (width ranging from 2 to 6 mm) at the junction of the floor and posterior wall of the concha is preferred. The edge of this crescent is widely undermined from the skin to favor the natural alignment, without placing sutures.

The Concept of Helical Tail Setback and Management of Earlobe Protrusion (Lower Third of the Ear)

Earlobe protrusion can be an important issue in prominent ear. The lobule is the natural downward continuation of the upper cartilaginous ear framework. It represents the lower third of the ear and differs from the upper two-thirds because it is a noncartilaginous structure, being made of fibrofatty tissue with different biomechanics, which makes it similar to normal skin (more viscous than elastic structures). Earlobe protrusion is usually a feature of the prominent ear.

The helical tail setback represents an important step in otoplasty to restore a gentle, balanced sweep to the helical rim as well as to correct the earlobe protrusion [8].

Many different techniques are reported for the helical tail setback, most of them relying on pexy sutures between the helical tail and the concha, besides Mustardé sutures.

In our technique, the helical tail setback is an important maneuver. It is achieved by correctly moving the skin toward the helix margin and the helical tail, by abrading the helical tail itself and by precisely placing the lowest Mustardè suture without adding other sutures. The authors do not normally perform any direct earlobe procedure to correct a prominent earlobe as a precisely performed helical tail setback is effective in correcting the earlobe protrusion.

Other authors prefer to approach the earlobe protrusion directly by using different patterns of postauricular skin excision to posteriorly displace the earlobe. This maneuver is effective because of the viscoelastic properties of the earlobe, with a low-elastic spring, allowing obtaining long-lasting results as the new position is typically maintained.

Conclusions

Over 200 otoplasty techniques have been described, each of them with its own advantages, disadvantages, and limits. The authors present a technique that combines the principle of the cartilage-sparing techniques with those of the cartilage-abrasion techniques. This technique adapts well to different types of prominent ears as well as to some subtypes of constricted ear (type I and some IIA) and lobule protrusion, allowing pleasant and satisfying results for both the patients and surgeon with low complication rates.

Acknowledgment Thanks to Emiliano Visconti, MD, (www.emilianovisconti.it) resient in training, Department of Bioimages and Radiological Sciences, Catholic University of "Sacro Cuore," University Hospital "A. Gemelli," for his contribution to the digital artwork.

References

1. Dieffenbach JE. Die operative Chirurgie. Leipzig: FA Brockhause; 1845.
2. Ely ET. An operation for prominence of the auricles. Arch Ophtalmol Otolaryngol. 1881;10:97.
3. Salgarello M, Gasperoni C, Montagnese A, Farallo E. Otoplasty for prominent ears: a versatile combined technique to master the shape of the ear. Otolaryngol Head Neck Surg. 2007;137(2):224–7.
4. Matsuo K, Hayashi R, Kiyono M, Hirose T, Netsu Y. Nonsurgical correction of congenital auricular deformities. Clin Plast Surg. 1990;17(2):383–95.
5. Gosain AK, Kumar A, Huang G. Prominent ears in children younger than 4 years of age: what is the appropriate timing for otoplasty? Plast Reconstr Surg. 2004;114(5):1042–54.
6. Janis JE, Rohrich RJ, Gutowski KA. Otoplasty. Plast Reconstr Surg. 2005;115(4):60e–72.
7. Adamson PA, Litner JA. Otoplasty technique. Otolaryngol Clin North Am. 2007;40(2):305–18.
8. Kelley P, Hollier L, Stal S. Otoplasty: evaluation, technique, and review. J Craniofac Surg. 2003;14(5):643–53.
9. Nuara MJ, Mobley SR. Nuances of otoplasty: a comprehensive review of the past 20 years. Facial Plast Surg Clin North Am. 2006;14(2):89–102.
10. Petersson RS, Friedman O. Current trends in otoplasty. Curr Opin Otolaryngol Head Neck Surg. 2008;16(4):352–8.
11. Becker OJ. Correction of protruding deformed ear. Br J Plast Surg. 1952;5:187.
12. Gibson T, Davies W. The distortion of autogenous cartilage graft: its cause and prevention. Br J Plast Surg. 1958;10:257–74.
13. Stenstroem SJ. A "natural" technique for correction of congenitally prominent ears. Plast Reconstr Surg. 1963;32:509–18.
14. Chongchet V. A method of antihelix reconstruction. Br J Plast Surg. 1963;16:268–72.
15. Weinzweig N, Chen L, Sullivan WG. Histomorphology of neochondrogenesis after antihelical fold creation: a comparison of three otoplasty techniques in the rabbit. Ann Plast Surg. 1994;33(4):371–6.
16. Mustardé JC. The treatment of prominent ears by buried mattress sutures: a ten-year survey. Plast Reconstr Surg. 1967;39(4):382–6.
17. Miyamoto J, Nagasao T, Tamaki T, Nakajima T. Biomechanical evaluation of surgical correction of prominent ear. Plast Reconstr Surg. 2009;123(3):889–96.
18. Lambertini G. Manuale di Anatomia dell'Uomo. Padova: Piccin-Nuova; 1972.
19. Pitanguy I. Congenital and acquired deformities of the ear. In: Pitanguy I, editor. Aesthetic plastic surgery of the head and body. Heidelberg: Springer; 1981.
20. Limandjaja GC, Breugem CC, van der Mink Molen AB, Kon M. Complications of otoplasty: a literature review. J Plast Reconstr Aesthet Surg. 2009;62(1):19–27.
21. Tanzer RC. The constricted (cup and lop) ear. Plast Reconstr Surg. 1975;55(4):406–15.
22. Richards SD, Jebreel A, Capper R. Otoplasty: a review of the surgical techniques. Clin Otolaryngol. 2005;30(1):2–8.
23. McDowell AJ. Goals in otoplasty for protruding ears. Plast Reconstr Surg. 1968;41(1):17–27.
24. Horlock N, Misra A, Gault DT. The postauricular fascial flap as an adjunct to Mustardé and Furnas type otoplasty. Plast Reconstr Surg. 2001;108(6):1487–90.
25. Sinha M, Richard B. Postauricular fascial flap and suture otoplasty: a prospective outcome study of 227 patients. J Plast Reconstr Aesthet Surg. 2012;656(3):367–71.
26. Mustarde JC. Correction of prominent ears using buried mattress sutures. Clin Plast Surg. 1978;5(3):459–64.
27. Furnas DW. Correction of prominent ears by conchamastoid sutures. Plast Reconstr Surg. 1968;42(3):189–93.
28. Elliott Jr RA. Otoplasty: a combined approach. Clin Plast Surg. 1990;17(2):373–81.

Incisionless Otoplasty

22

Yaşar Çokkeser

Introduction

Prominent ear may cause major psychological problems for school-age children. A study performed by Bradbury et al. [1] in 1992 showed that 10 % of patients requiring prominent ear surgery needed psychiatric therapy.

Prominent ear deformation is a condition with an autosomal dominant trait and a prevalence of 5 % in the white race. It emerges for two anatomical reasons: underdevelopment of the antihelical fold and lateral overdevelopment of the conchal bowl (Fig. 22.1) [2].

Multiple anatomical problems may coexist together in prominent ear deformation. Various surgical methods have been developed to address these problems. Since otoplasty was first defined by Ely in 1881 [3], more than 200 surgical techniques have been defined. These techniques can be classified as those forming an antihelix and those addressing the conchal bowl and lobule [4, 5].

A traditional open otoplasty can give rise to surgical difficulties and complications in the postoperative period, especially in the area of incision, with the potential for hematomas, abscess formation, and perichondritis.

The incisionless otoplasty technique presents an easy and direct approach to bending the nondeveloped antihelix. It is convenient to use in flexible, thin, malleable ears, but can also be applied in to ears with strong cartilage with scoring. If lateral overdevelopment of the conchal bowl exists, excess cartilage removal should be addressed first. Management of a hypertrophic conchal bowl was presented in another study including cartilage excision of a semilunar shape together with similar suture fixation as described in this technique [6]. According to our technique, a new antihelical fold is acquired with hidden subdermal pulling sutures, providing backward bending of the helix and forming a new antihelical fold, in full view, with a direct anterior approach used for non- or underdeveloped antihelical fold problems (Fig. 22.2).

There are several advantages of the incisionless hidden suture technique. These are:

1. Easy and rapid correction of an underdeveloped antihelical fold with an incisionless technique using hidden sutures
2. Easy adjustment of posterior bending of the antihelical fold by tightening of the hidden sutures
3. Local or general anesthesia can be used
4. Direct control of ear contours
5. Providing suturing compatible with the antihelical fold

Surgical Technique

Before surgery, photographs are obtained.

The surgical technique can be applied under general or local anesthesia. Permanent folding

Y. Çokkeser, M.D.
ENT Department, Mustafa Kemal University,
Tayfur Sökmen Ata Medical School,
Tayfur Sökmen Ata Campus,
Serinyol Antakya, Hatay, Turkey, 31000
e-mail: ycokkeser@yahoo.com

M.A. Shiffman (ed.), *Advanced Cosmetic Otoplasty*,
DOI 10.1007/978-3-642-35431-1_22, © Springer-Verlag Berlin Heidelberg 2013

Fig. 22.1 Auricular anatomy

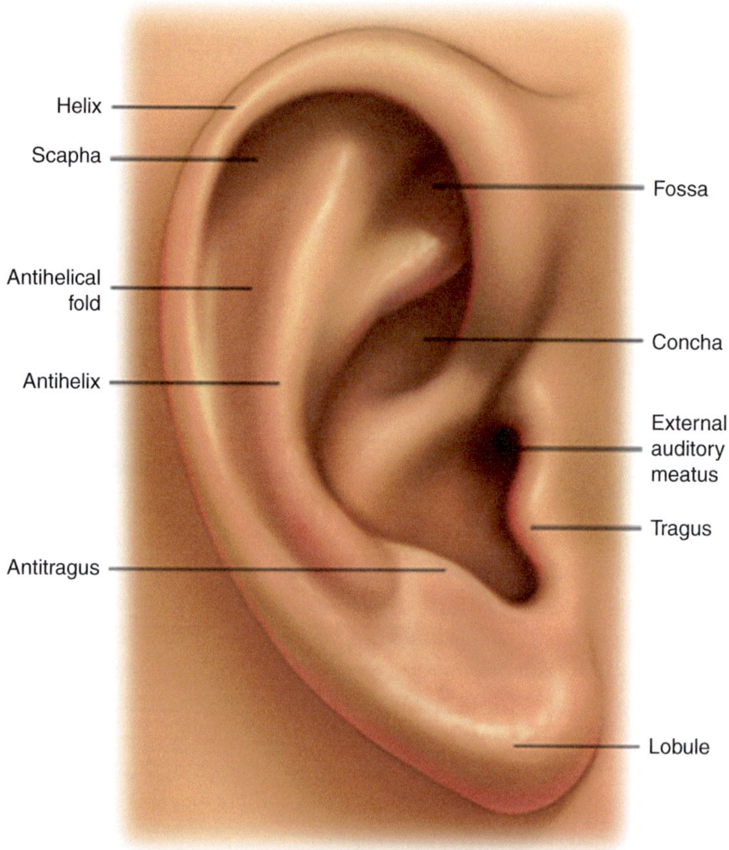

can be achieved with 3/0–4/0 Prolene 26-mm cutting sutures (Ethicon, Turkey) for antihelix formation using hidden sutures for young patients with soft, foldable cartilage having no lateral hypertrophy of the conchal bowl cartilage and needing no cartilage excision. This technique involves Mustardé asymmetric quadrangular suturing (Fig. 22.3), which is wider at the periphery and narrower on the medial side in proportion to the antihelical fold to the medial conchal level.

By manually bending the pinna, the surgeon defines where the planned antihelix will be. If the cartilage spring resists bending, then scoring should be done (Fig. 22.4). A 20-gauge phlebotomy needle, bent at the tip and serving as a microknife, is used to produce scoring along the anterior surface of the cartilage. The needle enters through the skin in only two places horizontally; then, it is turned perpendicularly to scratch the cartilage (Fig. 22.5). Cartilage scoring with the bent-tip needle passes between the cartilage and the skin anteriorly over the planned antihelical fold. Weakening of the newly formed antihelix (Fig. 22.5) allows a good rim of antihelix (Fig. 22.5) if the cartilage is strong enough to resist suture bending.

The suturing procedure (Fig. 22.6) starts by passing the needle through the conchal bowl anteriorly through the skin, perichondrium, and cartilage to the posterior face of the auricular cartilage under the posterior perichondrium, then passing it through between the cartilage and the perichondrium in the posterior face, and then turning it back again through the cartilage, perichondrium, and skin, exiting between the helix and the newly formed antihelix anteriorly. In the next phase, the needle is inserted in the same hole as it exited perpendicular to the previous needle axis, moving superiorly and passing in the same manner as previously done, then passing between

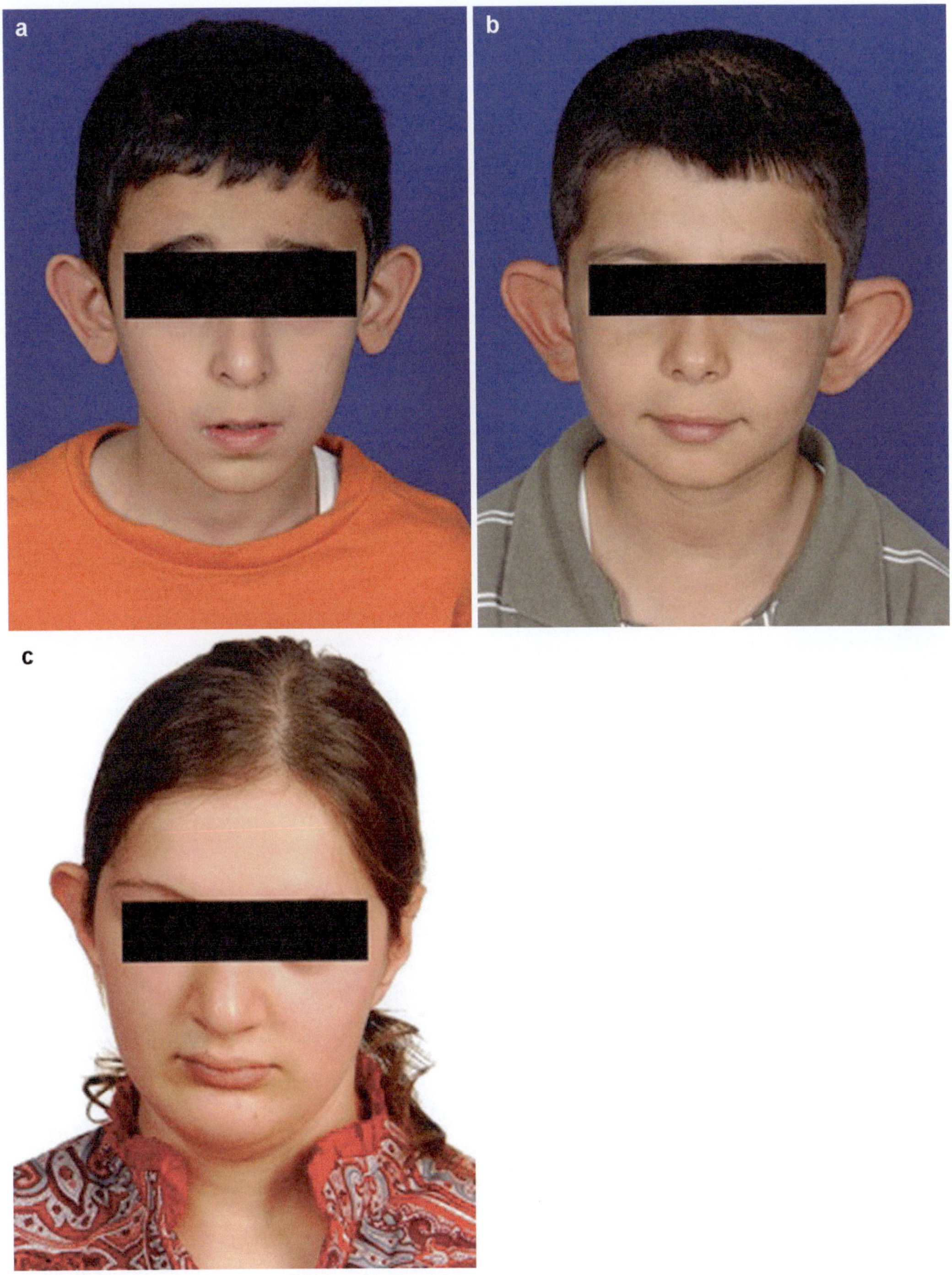

Fig. 22.2 Presurgical diagnosis and assessment of the pathological anatomic structure is vital. (**a**) Overdeveloped conchal bowl. (**b**) Overdeveloped conchal bowl together with dimensional problem. (**c**) Lack of antihelical fold in the right ear

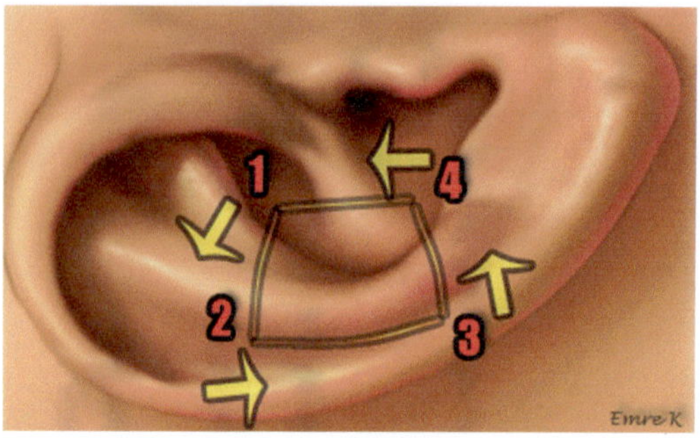

Fig. 22.3 Asymmetrical, quadrangular suture needle entry points. *1* the first needle entry point, consequtively other needle entry points

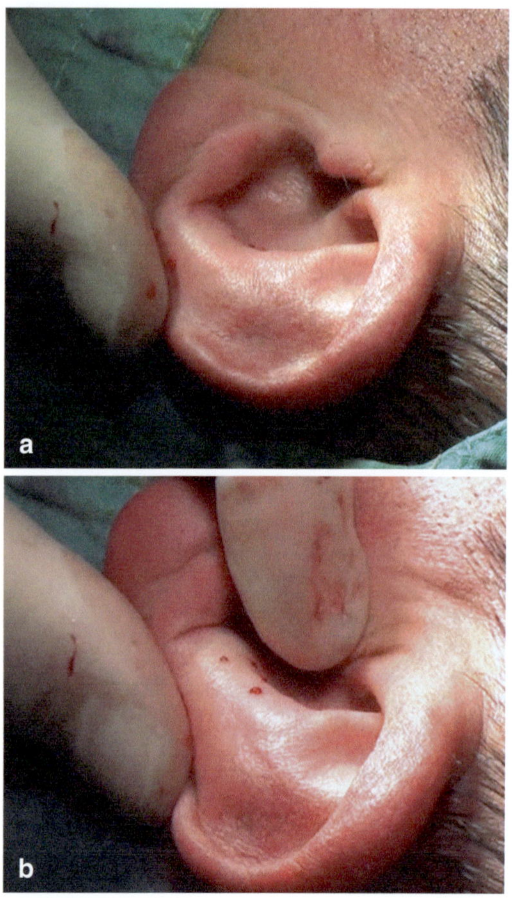

Fig. 22.4 (**a**) Strong ear cartilage. (**b**) Resistance to bending by this strong ear cartilage

the cartilage of the posterior face and the posterior side of the perichondrium. This needle exits 1 cm superiorly between the antihelix and helix. The needle again is inserted in the same hole as

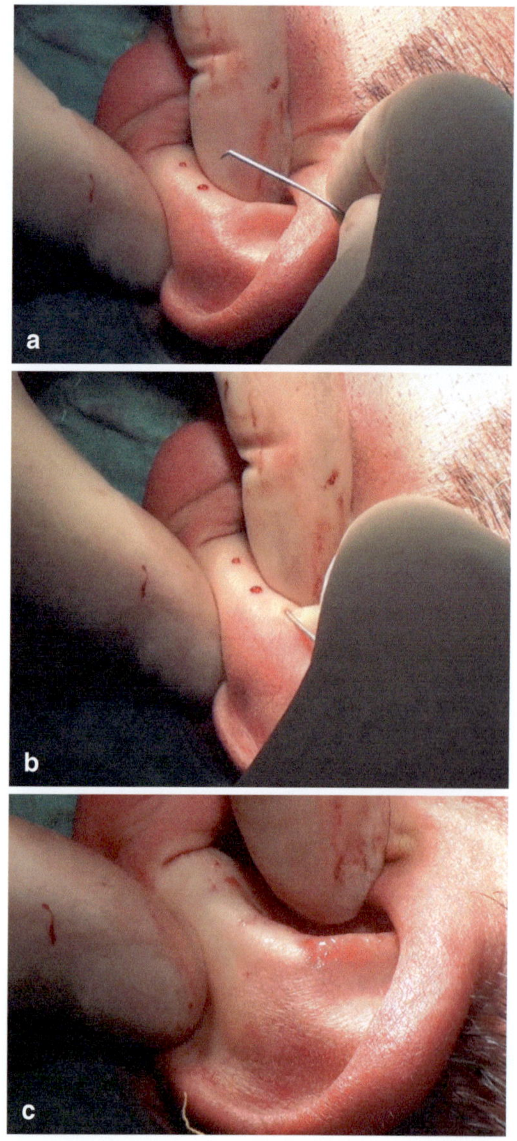

Fig. 22.5 (**a**) Scoring on the anticipated antihelical ridge for easy bending by the suture. (**b**) Scoring by 20-gauge needle bent at the tip. (**c**) Pliable ear cartilage after scoring bends easily

it exited, this time moving medially. The process is repeated without exiting from the skin in the posterior face from superior to inferior. The same point is reached and exited where it started. Then, the knot is tied as tightly as necessary. In the third phase, the ear cartilage is bent, and a nicely formed antihelical fold is seen (Fig. 22.7). The final ear position should be slightly overcorrected to "aesthetic normal" to ensure patient satisfaction (Fig. 22.8). The suturing can be repeated if necessary. Generally, only one suture is sufficient; if necessary, two or more quadrangular sutures can be applied.

The operation is completed using bending sutures with 3/0–4/0 polypropylene and no bandages or dressing is necessary.

All cases achieved satisfactory results, without no incisions or cartilage removal. Two cases

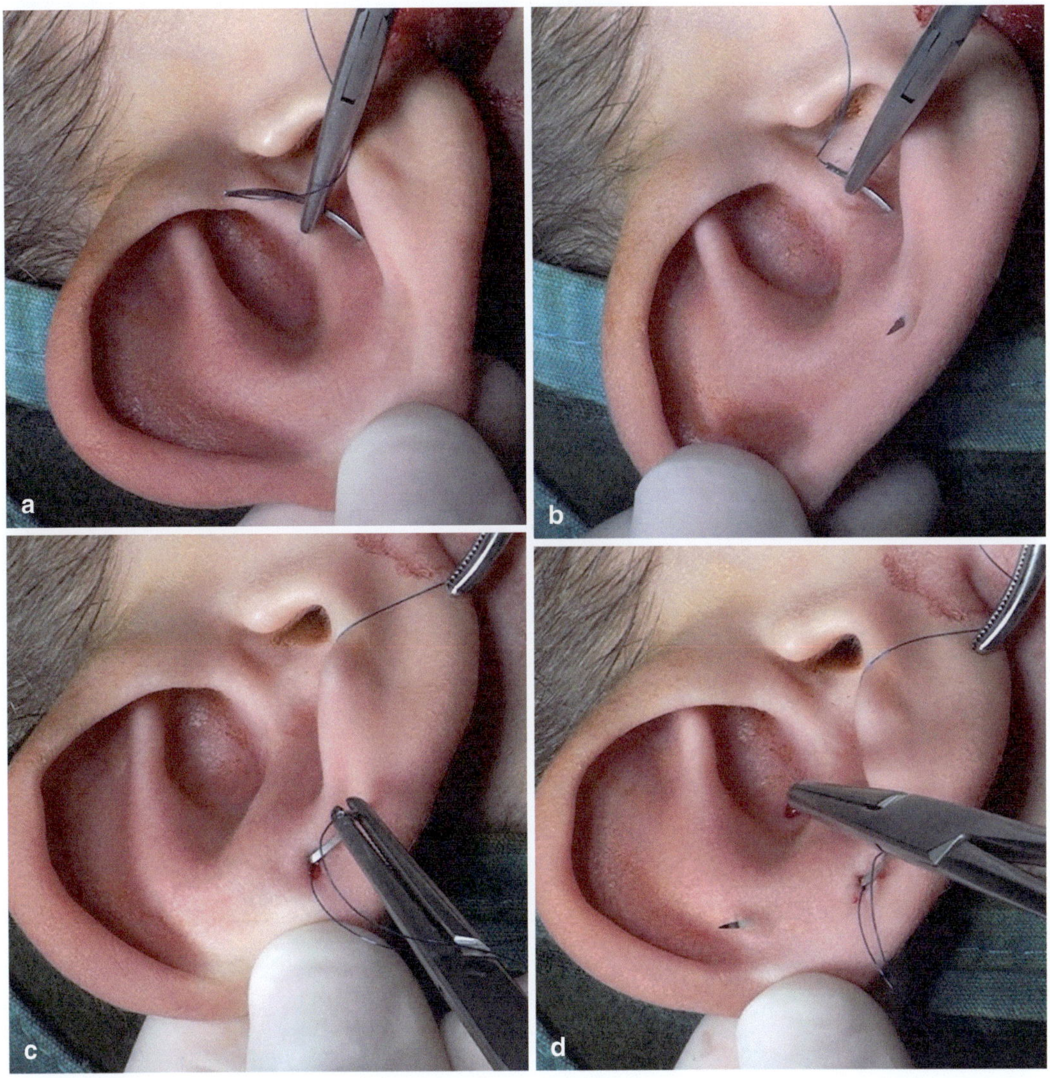

Fig. 22.6 Surgical technique: (**a**) The needle passes through the conchal bowl anteriorly through the skin, perichondrium, and cartilage to the posterior face of the auricular cartilage under the posterior perichondrium then is passed through between the cartilage and the perichondrium in the posterior face; it then is turned back again through the cartilage, perichondrium, and skin, exiting between the helix and the newly formed antihelix anteriorly. (**b–d**) The needle is inserted in the same hole as it exited perpendicular to the previous needle axis, moving superiorly and passing in the same manner as previously, then passing between the cartilage of the posterior face and the posterior side of the perichondrium. This needle exits 1 cm superiorly between the antihelix and helix. (**e**, **f**) The needle again is inserted in the same hole as it exited, moving medially this time. (**g**) The process is repeated without exiting from the skin in the posterior face from superior to inferior. The same point is where the sutures were started is reached and exited. (**h**) Then, the knot is tied as tightly as required

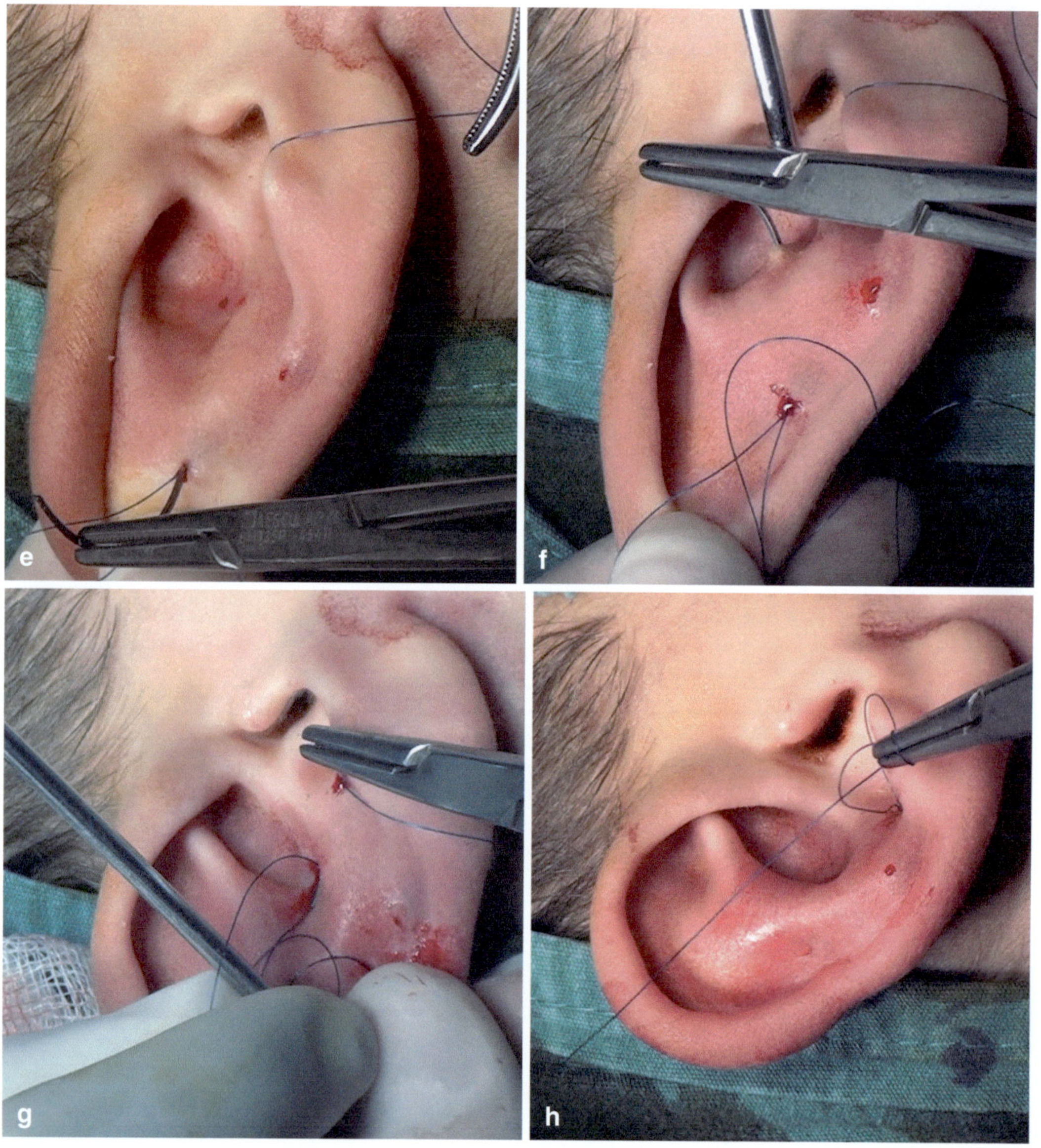

Fig. 22.6 (continued)

required resuturing because of suture disruption, 1 h and 1 week later. Intraoperative suture disruption is immediately resolved with resuturing. None of the needle entry or exit points are visible, and they healed well, without noticeable scarring.

Discussion

Prominent ear deformation is a significant cosmetic problem. For this important reason, many surgical techniques have been developed. One of the widely used techniques is the conchal mastoid suture technique, which is known as the "classic conchal setback technique" defined by Furnas in 1968 [7]. In this technique, permanent sutures are applied between the periosteum and conchal cartilage by applying a wide retroauricular incision. In this technique, a wide incision is needed for the posterior part, and the nonnatural auricle fixation is carried out with permanent sutures.

For the correction of the lack of antihelical folding, Stenströem [8] defined the antihelix formation technique with a loop through the non-scored face

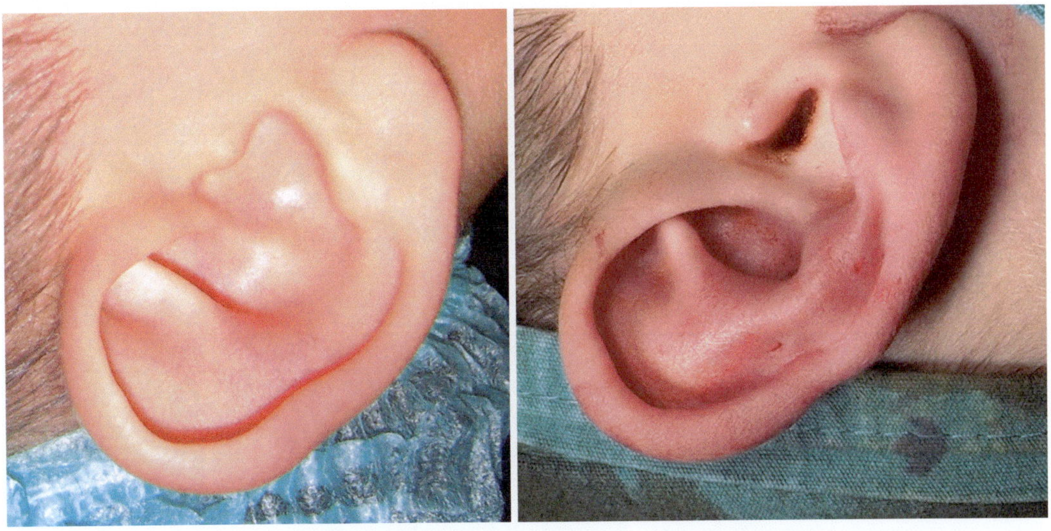

Fig. 22.7 (*Left*) Preoperative. (*Right*) Postoperative. Note the nicely formed antihelical fold

Fig. 22.8 The final ear position should be slightly overcorrected from "aesthetic normal" to ensure patient satisfaction

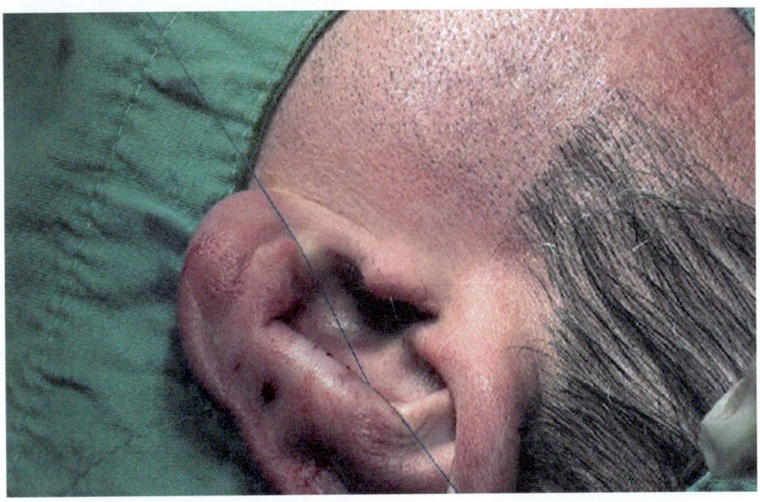

using the anterior scoring method. This technique fails, giving no reliable results, and also cartilage necrosis can be encountered in patients with thin cartilage. Two procedures come from Mustardé for correction of the missing antihelical fold.

In the method defined by Gibson and Davis [9], folding is provided by scoring of the counter side of the cartilage. In our technique, permanent monofilament polypropylene sutures are used for antihelix bending and fixation. If strong cartilage resists bending, scoring of the anterior face of the cartilage is applied, and the cartilage is folded to the side where the perichondrium is intact.

In incisionless suture placement, it is very important for the needle to reenter the skin through exactly the same puncture site from which it exited in order to ensure that no squamous epithelium is buried subcutaneously and to prevent dimpling of the skin.

In the author's technique, a natural helix and antihelical fold are obtained without an incision or dissection.

Limitations of this technique are that strong, thick ear cartilage in adult patients can resist bending with asymmetric quadrangular mattress sutures; this problem is solved by scoring. Also, without correction of the lateral hypertrophy of the conchal cartilage, this technique may result in an unnaturally evident antihelix. So if there is lateral hypertrophy of the conchal

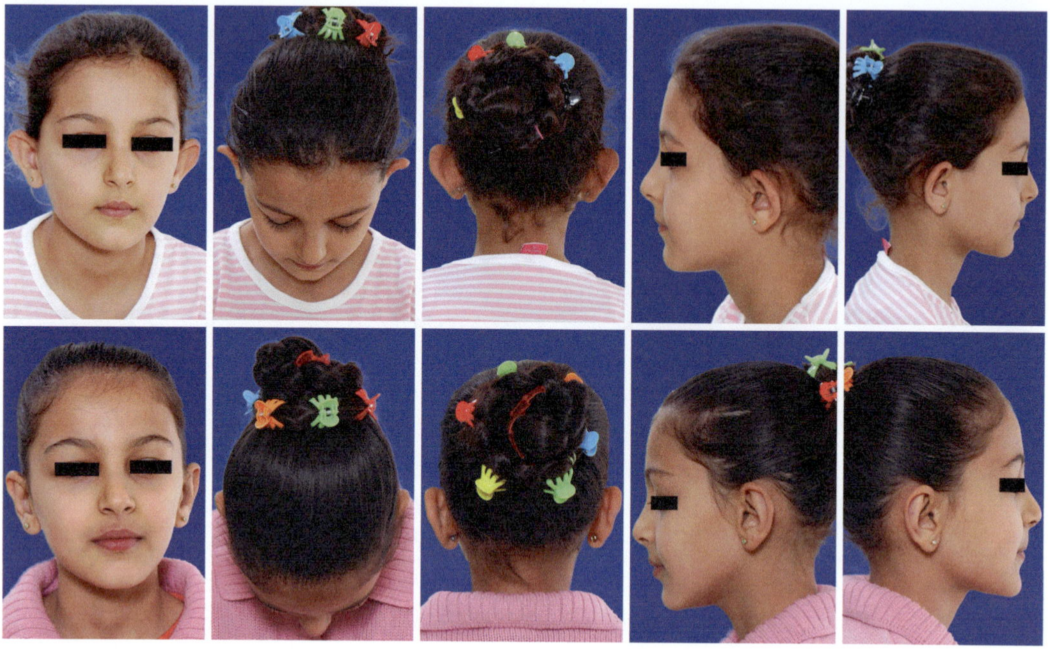

Fig. 22.9 (*Top*) Preoperative. (*Bottom*) Postoperative

cartilage, it is recommended to perform conchal surgery first and afterwards to correct the antihelical pathology [10]. Semilunar cartilage incision and excision in the lateral conchal bowl are required to provide good antihelical folding by reducing resistance and obtaining a more malleable, pliable, nonresistant formation with sutures and a natural-looking new lateral conchal level [6]. In the anterior approach technique, both pathologies can be solved in the same operation [6].

Widely observed early complications after otoplasty are hematoma and infection. Late complications are suture rupture and patient dissatisfaction. Since there is no wide dissection to adjacent regions by operating from the subperichondrial area, there is almost no risk of hematoma compared to other surgical techniques. Again, for the same reasons, the frequency of infection will be less. Therefore, no significant complications, including hematoma, were observed in any of our cases. Only in two cases did the sutures open; resuturing was carried out without a problem.

The incisionless otoplasty technique results in excellent cosmetic effects with a minimal manipulation and few complications. It does not require postoperative bandaging, and no maintenance efforts are required of the patient or suture care of the physician.

The defined technique for prominent ear surgery is shown to be satisfying for both the surgeon and patient (Figs. 22.9, 22.10, 22.11, 22.12 and 22.13).

Conclusions

The incisionless otoplasty operation corrects underdeveloped antihelical fold deformities. In addition, conchal bowl problems can be addressed in conjunction with the same suture placement. Incisionless otoplasty is an outpatient procedure of minimum morbidity, needing minimal postoperative care, and it is well tolerated by patients. Over 15 years of experience with this operation has proven its long-term reliability, low complication rate, cost-effectiveness, and great appreciation by patients.

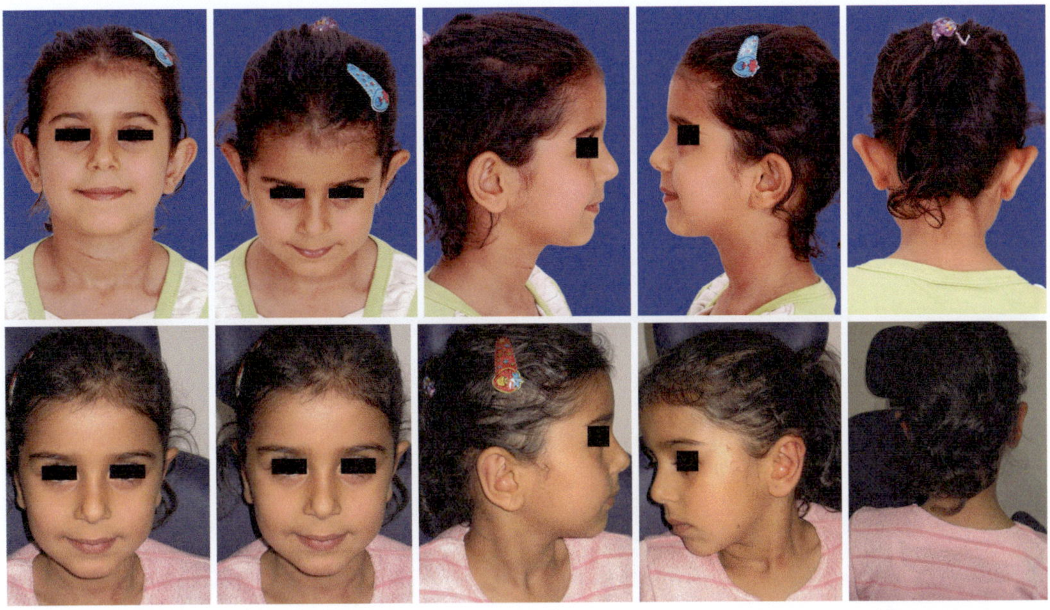

Fig. 22.10 (*Top*) Preoperative. (*Bottom*) Postoperative

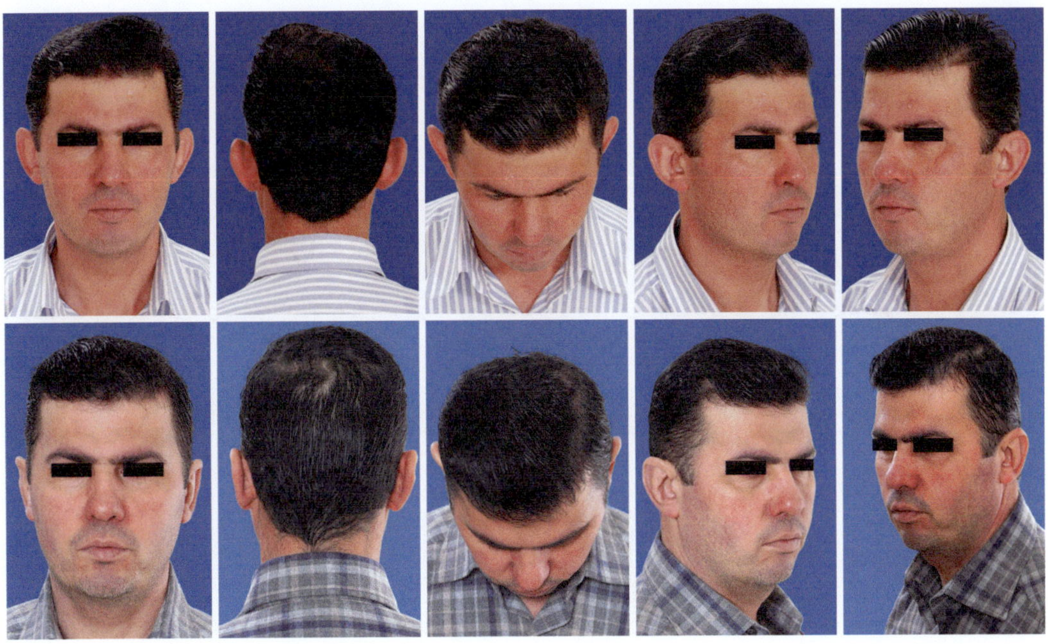

Fig. 22.11 (*Top*) Preoperative. (*Bottom*) Postoperative

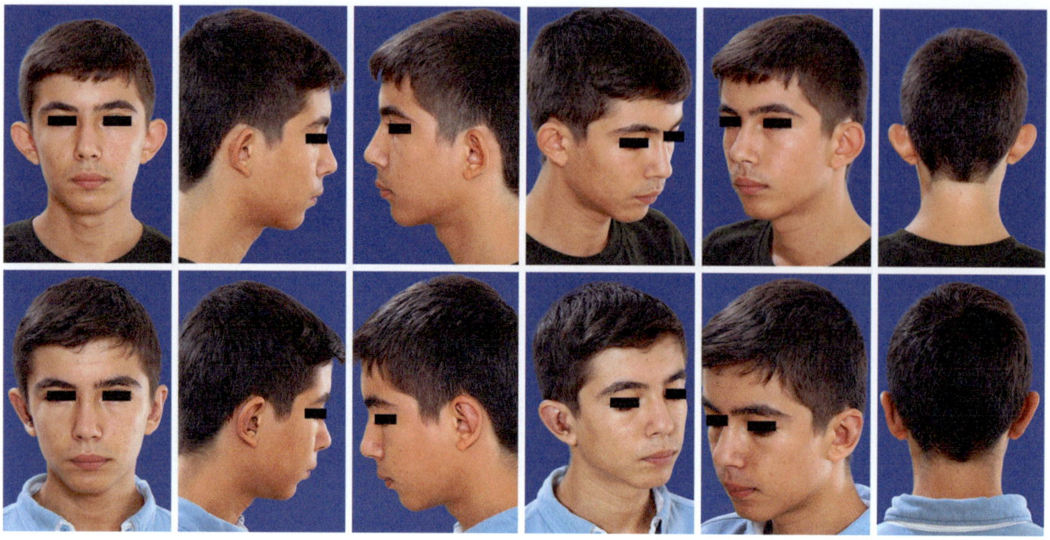

Fig. 22.12 (*Top*) Preoperative. (*Bottom*) Postoperative

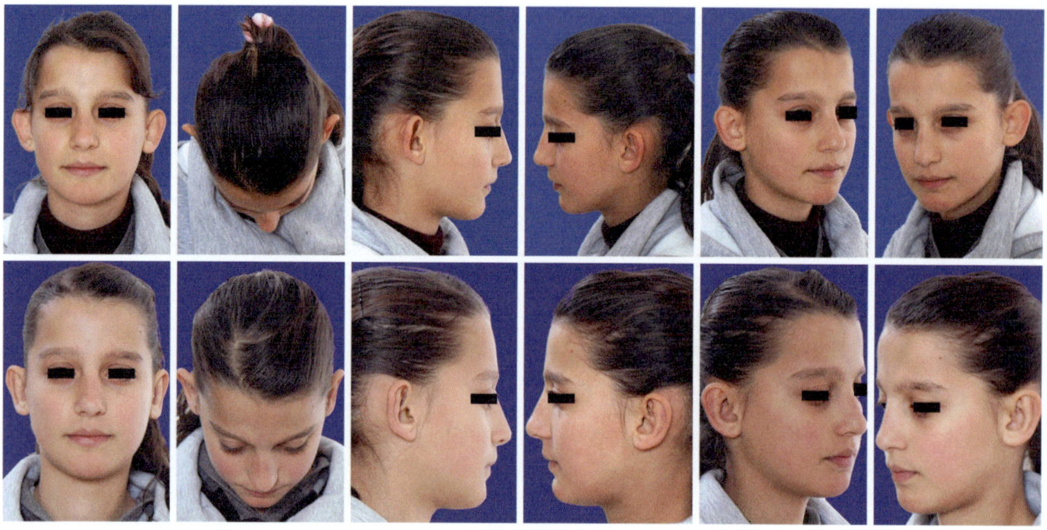

Fig. 22.13 (*Top*) Preoperative. (*Bottom*) Postoperative

References

1. Bradbury ET, Hewison J, Timmons MJ. Psychological and social outcome of prominent ear correction in children. Br J Plast Surg. 1992;45:97–100.
2. Adamson PA, Strecker HD. Otoplasty techniques. Facial Plast Surg. 1995;11:284–300.
3. Ely ET. An operation for prominence of the auricles. Arch Otolaryngol. 1881;10:97–9.
4. Campbell AC. Otoplasty. Facial Plast Surg. 2005;21(4):310–6.
5. Janis JE, Rohrich RJ, Gutowski KA. Otoplasty. Plast Reconstr Surg. 2005;115(4):60–72.
6. Cokkeser Y, Karaoglu E. Anterior approach technique in otoplasty (how I do it). Kulak Burun Bogaz Ihtis Derg. 2011;21:349–55.
7. Furnas DW. Correction of prominent ears by concha-mastoid sutures. Plast Reconstr Surg. 1968;42: 189–93.
8. Stenstroem SJ. A "natural" technique for correction of congenitally prominent ears. Plast Reconstr Surg. 1963;32:509–18.
9. Gibson T, Davis WB. The distortion of autogenous cartilage grafts: its cause and prevention. Br J Plast Surg. 1958;10:257–74.
10. Burres S. The anterior-posterior otoplasty. Arch Otolaryngol Head Neck Surg. 1998;124:181–5.

Incisionless Otoplasty

23

Michael H. Fritsch

Introduction

The aim of incisionless otoplasty technique is to create a cosmetically pleasing pinna. There are two steps necessary to create a pleasing pinna. First, percutaneous needle modeling of the cartilage breaks the cartilage memory spring and establishes a specifically weakened tract in the cartilage which will bend in a certain way so as to create a new pinna form. Secondly, permanent sutures are percutaneously placed in order to hold the cartilage during the scar healing process. Separate incisionless techniques deal with the antihelical fold, lobule, and conchal bowl. Each of these techniques can be used alone or in combination for any specific patient's ear deformity. Individualization of treatment, effectiveness and reproducibility, and atraumatic techniques leading to a low complication rate make incisionless otoplasty an excellent choice for correction of the lop ear deformity. Using these tried methods, a reliable otoplasty procedure with pleasing results can be accomplished.

M.H. Fritsch, M.D., FACS
St Vincent Medical Center,
9002 N. Meridian st., suite 204,
Indianapolis, IN 46260, USA
e-mail: mfritschmd@gmail.com

Technique (Figs. 23.1, 23.2, 23.3, 23.4, 23.5, 23.6, 23.7, 23.8, 23.9, and 23.10)

There is a sequence of surgical events that is best suited for successful incisionless otoplasty. Initially, all of the percutaneous needle cartilage modeling work for all of the to-be-corrected areas is performed. The cartilage weakening and breaking is completed before any sutures are placed. The entire cartilage modeling work is completed first in order not to cut any already placed retention sutures. Thereafter, the retention sutures for the conchal bowl, lobule, and then the antihelical fold are placed. The order of conchal bowl, lobule, and antihelical fold suture placement progresses from the conchal foundation to the lowered antihelical shape.

Conchal Bowl Correction

In almost all cases of otoplasty, there is a significant abnormality of the conchal bowl. The conchal bowl is the foundation for the otoplasty repair. If the antihelix is corrected without attention to the conchal bowl, then there is often an unnatural appearance to the correction. The main reason for this is that the antihelix will need to be overcorrected to compensate for the conchal bowl problem. The unnatural appearance is best characterized as an "angularity" to the finished otoplasty. Therefore, an overall reduction in conchal bowl prominence translates to a more natural-appearing antihelical correction.

M.A. Shiffman (ed.), *Advanced Cosmetic Otoplasty*,
DOI 10.1007/978-3-642-35431-1_23, © Springer-Verlag Berlin Heidelberg 2013

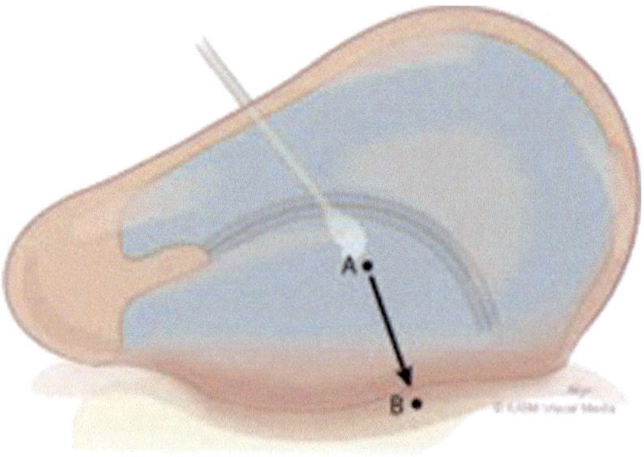

Fig. 23.1 To begin an incisionless technique, conchal recession procedure of the left ear, suture anchor points of maximal effectiveness are chosen by using a cotton swab to simulate the correction

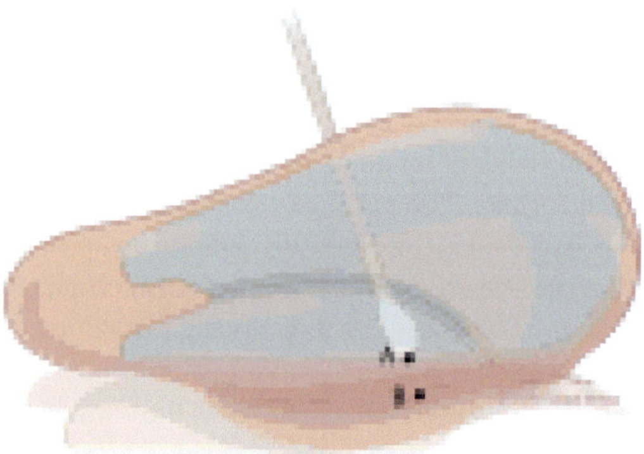

Fig. 23.2 Once the points have been found, an ink dot is placed to accurately guide the surgeon's needle placement

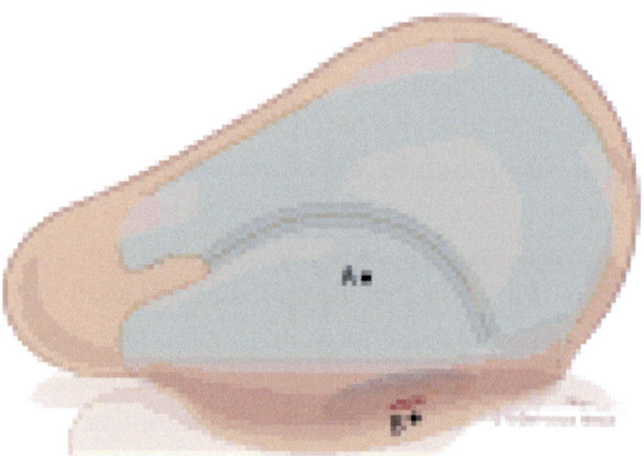

Fig. 23.3 A 3-mm stab opening is created. It almost always is in the area of the postauricular muscle

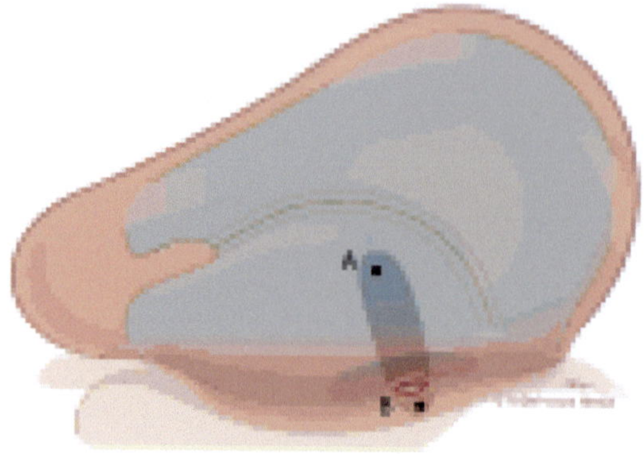

Fig. 23.4 Tissue between the conchal cartilage and mastoid is removed through the 3-mm opening using needle-tip monopolar cautery and iris scissors. This broadly undermined area will create a scar tissue anchor plane

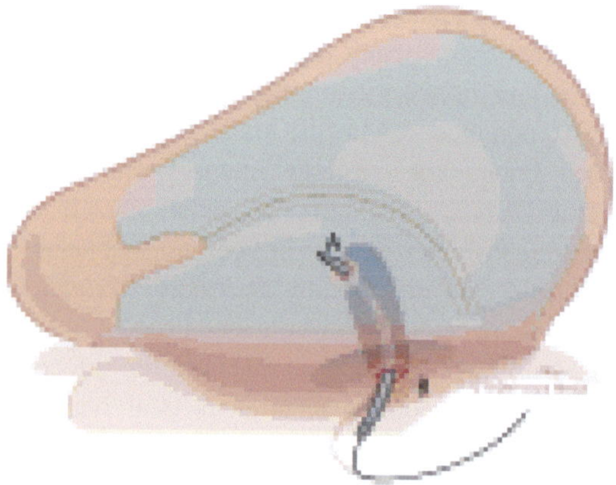

Fig. 23.5 Undermining of the skin above the perichondrium creates a scar tissue tunnel that, in addition to the sutures, will help firmly and permanently secure the correction

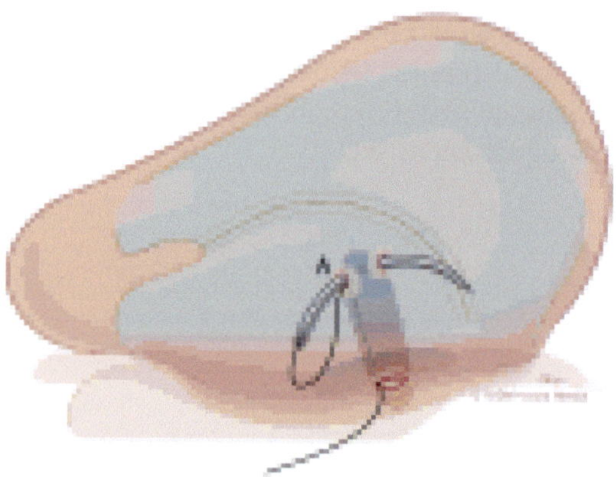

Fig. 23.6 The first limb of the four-sided incisionless retention suture loop begins. The needle exits through the posterior skin surface

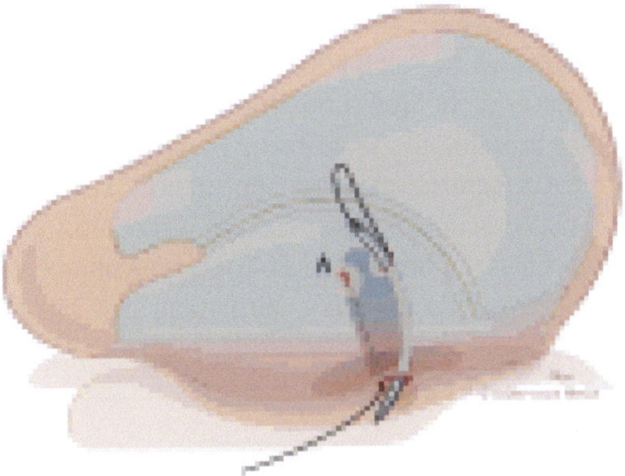

Fig. 23.7 Since the needle exits and enters the same needle tract at a 90° angle to the skin surface, there is no dimpling or skin inclusion cyst formation. On exiting the skin, as the skin surface is approached by the curved needle, the 90° exit from the skin is achieved by "back-scratching" the undersurface of the skin

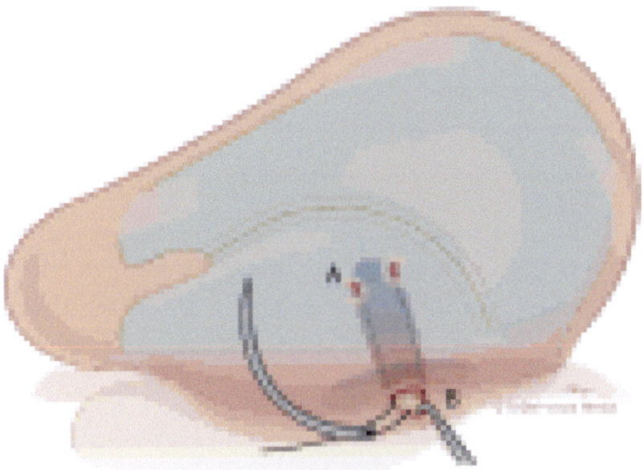

Fig. 23.8 Reentry through the same needle hole and tract is performed before the needle is guided through the tunnel and out of the stab opening

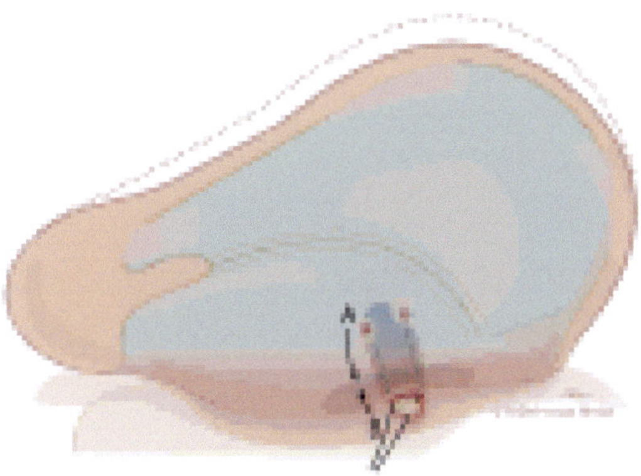

Fig. 23.9 A very firm anchor into the mastoid periosteum of 5–6 mm width and depth is made in order to retain the conchal cartilage as the scar tissue planes mature

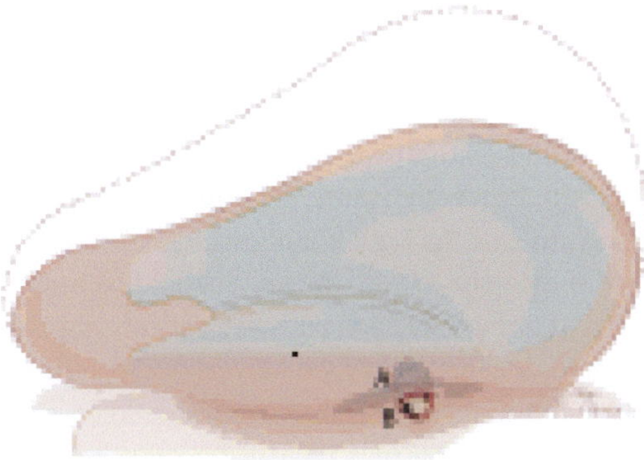

Fig. 23.10 After placement of the conchal bowl, lobule, and antihelical sutures, the conchal bowl suture is tightened. Points *A* and *B* are near each other as predicted by the initial cotton swab simulation

The conchal bowl correction proceeds through several steps: Initially, the suture anchor points for maximal correction are found; then, excess soft tissue is removed from between the conchal bowl and mastoid bone; next, a plane for scar tissue development is created; and lastly, the retention suture is placed and very firmly anchored to the mastoid.

Antihelical Correction

After the conchal bowl and lobule have received retention sutures, the antihelical sutures are placed. All of the percutaneous retention sutures are placed before any sutures are tightened.

As with all incisionless corrections, of prime technical importance are that the retention sutures enter and exit from the same needle holes at a 90° angle to the skin surface and also that they follow the same needle tract on entering and exiting. These two aspects are important in order to prevent skin inclusion cysts and skin dimpling by allowing all sutures to slip below the skin surface and down to the perichondrium.

There are several other technical issues to remember. On the posterior pinna surface, the best entry point to start the four-cornered retention suture loop is the medial superior corner; this allows the suture knot to be buried deeply under thicker skin. The needle is guided as deeply under the skin throughout the entire course of the suture loop as possible; the perichondrium is even picked up along the needle course in order to better anchor the suture to the cartilage – this prevents suture bridging under the skin. Since the suture is permanent, only the unraveling of the knot could endanger the integrity of the suture loop; the knot should be redundantly knotted. As each patient's ears are slightly symmetrical between themselves, the final tightening of the suture retention loop should be done by a combination of a measuring ruler and surgeon's perspective as this gives rise to the greatest accuracy and symmetry in aesthetic form. Lastly, the antihelical work is always overcorrected as there is a tissue relaxation that takes place and will loosen the correction over the 6-month postoperative time. By overcorrecting, the end result will meet the patient's expectations and please the patient.

Conclusions

Through a systematic use of incisionless otoplasty techniques, the protuberant lop ear can be brought into an aesthetic position and shape for a natural, pleasing appearance. The incisionless process is relatively atraumatic and avoids the many possible complications of open otoplasty. Thus, the patient and physician are both well served by use of the incisionless otoplasty.

General References

1. Fritsch MH. Incisionless otoplasty: early techniques without address of the cartilage spring. Laryngoscope. 1995;105(5 Pt 3 Suppl 70):1–11.
2. Fritsch MH. Incisionless otoplasty. Otolaryngol Clin North Am. 2009;42(6):1199–208.

Carbon Dioxide Laser-Assisted Cartilage Reshaping Otoplasty for Prominent Ears

24

Ahmed Ragab

Laser and the Auricular Cartilage

Throughout thinking in correction of outstanding ears, working as sculpture artists can push us forward towards the aim of putty auricle and face. The auricle has a perfect suite which is the skin and skeleton, i.e., the cartilage. What is underneath the skin surface constitutes the puzzling of otoplasty sculpture. Cartilage is an avascular tissue that consists of chondrocytes and an extensive extracellular matrix produced and maintained by chondrocytes. Extracellular matrix accounts for 90 % of the composition. Cartilage matrix is composed predominantly of aggrecan and type II collagen. It is believed that type II collagen is primarily responsible for tensile strength, while aggrecan molecules, entrapped within the type II collagen lattice, provide compressive strength. The highly sulfated glycosaminoglycan side chains of chondroitin sulfate and keratan sulfate enable the matrix to structure large amounts of water and thereby create a large osmotic pressure [1]. Long chains of hyaluronan are present throughout the matrix and serve to specifically bind aggrecan and to link protein to retain the aggrecan molecules within the cartilage extracellular matrix [1].

Reshaping the skeleton (the cartilage) in permanent forms with the least trauma and complications remains the gold standard of care in reshaping otoplasty [2]. Multiple surgical operations were used in correction of deformed outstanding auricles (Table 24.1). Otoplasty techniques are either cartilage-sculpting (cutting) [3], cartilage-sparing (suturing) [4, 5], or composite techniques (combining sutures and sculpting) [6, 7]. Different complications can take place according to the used technique (Fig. 24.1). Recurring problems, suture extrusion, and some loss of correction over time were associated with techniques relying only on cartilage suturing procedures [8, 9]. Thick cartilage and its tricky reshaping is another difficult task in suture techniques. Alternatively, cutting techniques can permanently distort the shape of the ear [10] with the possibility of sharp edgings [11, 12], cartilage irregularities [12, 13], and difficulty in revision surgery [2].

Using other methods in cartilage reshaping, e.g., electrothermal or laser, became an area of research during the last years aiming to achieve otoplastic surgeons' aims adequately. Application of laser to cartilage results in changes of its ultrastructure (chondrocytes, febrile components of type 2 collagen, and intercellular matrix material of proteoglycans and hyaluronic acid) and subsequently in change of its biophysical belongings [14, 15].

Laser-mediated cartilage reshaping (thermochondroplasty) is a non-ablative low-intensity

A. Ragab, M.D., Ph.D. (Brussels)
Department of ORL Head and Neck Surgery, Menoufia University Hospital, Shibin El Kom, Egypt
e-mail: ahmedragab2000@hotmail.com

M.A. Shiffman (ed.), *Advanced Cosmetic Otoplasty*,
DOI 10.1007/978-3-642-35431-1_24, © Springer-Verlag Berlin Heidelberg 2013

interaction in which heat accelerates stress relaxation in mechanically deformed cartilage specimens, resulting in shape change. Cartilage can be reshaped when heated to approximately 60–75 °C [3]. Sobol et al. [14] pioneered the development of this procedure and suggested that stress relaxation is owing to a phase transformation of water molecules from a bound state (binding to proteoglycans or collagen) to a free or mobile state. Microscopic findings showed distortion of the proteoglycans and alterations in the collagen skeleton. It was then suggested that laser energy would destroy the water-binding ability of proteoglycans and lead to uneven reduction in the tensile stresses within the cartilage. The collagen network resists tensile and shear stresses and strains, while the fluid component resists the high hydrostatic compressive stresses that are generated. The cartilage cells are directly attached to the extracellular matrix and are part of the fluid continuum of the tissue. The cells do not provide any special structural resistance, but their cellular shapes, pressures, and chemical environments

Table 24.1 Surgical procedures used in correction of prominent ear deformity

Recreation of underdeveloped antihelix
Suture techniques: conchascaphal sutures
Cartilage sculpting techniques: incising, wedge excisions, scoring, abrading, filing
Composite technique: combining sutures and sculpting
Correcting conchal protrusion
Suture techniques: Furnas' conchamastoid sutures
Cartilage sculpting techniques: excision
Composite technique (combining sutures and sculpting)

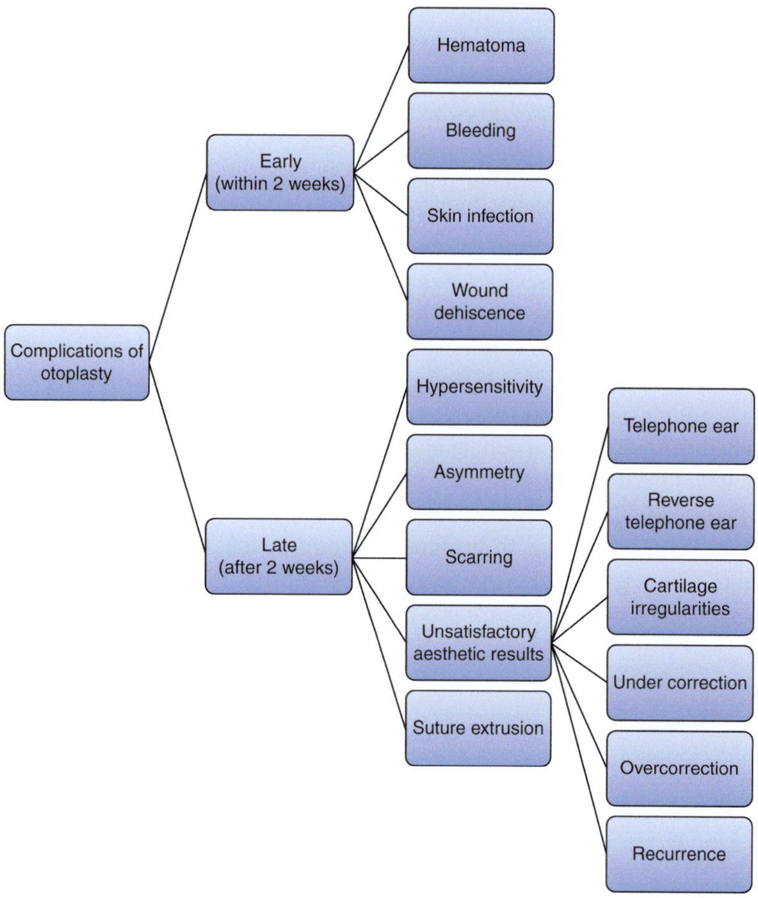

Fig. 24.1 Complications of different types of otoplasty operations

are directly altered by deformations created in the extracellular matrix and by local fluid pressure and flow [13].

The contribution of collagen to cartilage internal stresses is more important than is generally believed. In addition, collagen plays a key role in the cartilage laser-reshaping effect, and it may be the primary cartilage constituent responsible for cartilage transformation. More specifically, (1) in the plane of histological section, many collagen fibers seemed shorter than normal, (2) the number of ring-shaped collagen components was significantly increased, and (3) the collagen fibers, which normally have a symmetric orientation, especially around the borders of the chondrocyte nests and in the vicinity of the perichondrium, lost their spatial orientation in the irradiated areas [15].

Another effect of laser is decreasing the mass of chondroitin sulfate and diffusion of macromolecules into the medium. Also it induces detaching of proteoglycan units from hyaluronic acid backbones [15].

Also affection of the cartilage cells is another effect of laser. Partially laser-ablated auricle regenerated by newly formed cartilaginous tissue originated mainly from chondrocytes present in preserved parts of the vaporized cartilage and, to a lesser extent, from perichondrial fibroblasts. The exact mechanism of the chondrocyte stimulation is not fully understood as yet. One plausible explanation is the activation of cell surface receptors, especially β1 integrin. This factor, supposed to transmit mechanical signals from the extracellular matrix to the cytoskeleton and type II collagen, may then alter gene expression as well as upregulate proteoglycan and collagen synthesis [16].

Alternatively, laser irradiation could stimulate the chondrocyte metabolism by affecting pore structure and water permeability of the matrix strong proliferation of perichondrium with numerous fibroblasts and their transition into chondrocytes on the side opposed to the laser application.

Ayhan et al. [17] studied histomorphological changes in the rabbit auricle cartilage, modeled either with erbium:yttrium–aluminum–garnet (Er:YAG) laser or classical scalpel incisions. They stated that partial laser ablation caused a thermal effect in non-vaporized deeper layers of the cartilage, resulting in its necrosis and degeneration. These alterations healed by formation of fibrosis-free young cartilage of permanent shape. Regeneration of the laser wound differed from that induced by classical scalpel in that the latter consisted mainly of fibrosis of the underlying connective tissue. The explanation of that difference was that the mechanical cartilage incisions did not cause changes in deeper layers of the cartilage.

Jones et al. [18] used a Ho:YAG laser to form the porcine auricle cartilage into a U shape. Histological analysis performed 3, 8, and 16 weeks later revealed that, depending on the energy delivered, slight, moderate, or heavy alterations of the chondrocytes and matrix were present. In all specimens, any inflammatory reaction was lacking, and there was marked proliferation of perichondrial cells away from the side to which the laser had been applied.

All these effects depends on the laser wavelength, pulse duration, irradiance, and tissue thermal and optical properties. The Nd:YAG laser light penetrates the tissue deeply and is evenly scattered and absorbed. Power densities between 10 and 30 W/cm^2 and energies of 100 J, resulting in an enhanced matrix, do not meet the formal criteria of low-level laser therapy anymore because the tissue has been heated up. A cellular tolerance by pulsed heating using a CO_2 laser system has been described. It was manifested that, if there was a specific parameter constellation (2 W, 16 W/cm^2, 60 s, 120 J), an enhanced matrix synthesis can be observed [19]. In an experiment on ten rabbits, 8-W carbon dioxide (CO_2) laser evaporation of the perichondrium, together with part of cartilage thickness of the auricle cartilage, was performed by Janík et al. [16]. The regeneration process, originating from chondroblasts as well as from perichondrium cells, was strongly stimulated by the laser energy delivered [16].

Sequencing of Laser-Assisted Cartilage Reshaping Otoplasty (Table 24.2)

Assessment and Surgical Planning

Evaluation of normal measurements and protrusion of the auricle: The ear occupies a zone from the brow superiorly to the base of the columella inferiorly. The base of the tragus begins approximately a single ear length lateral to the lateral orbital rim (6.5–7.5 cm in adults). The average length of the adult ear varies from 5.5 to 6.5 cm. The width of the ear is approximately 50–60 % of the length. The vertical axis is inclined 15–30° posterior [20].

Protrusion from the skull must be analyzed carefully. Protrusion can be described in terms of measurements from points along the lateral-most projection of the helical margin to points directly perpendicular on the skull. On average, the upper third of the helical rim measures 1–1.2 cm from the scalp, the middle third measures 1.6–1.8 cm at the midpoint of the helix, and the lobule is located 2.0–2.2 cm from the mastoid region. According to anthropometric evaluation, the normal angle between the helical rim and the scalp covering the mastoid is 25–35° and that between concha and scaphoid fossa is 80–90° [20].

The normal concha can be described as a hemispherical bowl with a sharply defined rim. Normal conchal depth is less than 1.5 cm [5]. The angle between concha and scalp over the mastoid ranges from 45 to 90°. The scapha–helix complex emanates from the margin of the concha, creating the antihelix [6, 7]. The antihelical fold forms an acute angle between the concha and scapha, measuring less than 90° in the normal ear [5]. The antihelix starts at the antitragus and continues in an uninterrupted, smooth fashion superiorly to eventually form superior and inferior crura. Ideally, the helical rim and antihelical contours are parallel so that the helix is visible beyond the antihelix from the front. Approximately 50 % of persons demonstrate up to 3-mm variation in the horizontal and vertical positioning of the ear.

Table 24.2 Sequences of carbon dioxide laser-assisted cartilage reshaping otoplasty

Assessment and surgical planning
a. Evaluation of normal measurements and protrusion of the auricle
b. Evaluation of the type of deformity
c. Evaluation of the cartilage characters and thickness
Laser assisted cartilage reshaping otoplasty
a. Time of Surgery
b. Goal of Surgery
c. Anesthesia and draping
d. Marking, injection and skin incisions
e. Skin excision and elevation of the post-auricular surface
f. Preparation of the postauricular surface and identification of the tail of the helix
g. Laser reshaping of the scapha
h. Internal splint and securing of the new antihelix
i. Laser reshaping and repositioning of the concha
j. Management of the helical tail and control of the lobule
k. Skin closure and postoperative dressings

Table 24.3 Characteristics of prominent ear deformity

Characteristics of protruding ears
Underdeveloped or absent antihelical fold
Increased distance between the helical rim and scalp
Increased angle between the mastoid and helical rim
Overdeveloped concha with deep conchal wall
Protruding lobule

Evaluation of the Type of Deformity

The outstanding ears result from two basic causes: underdevelopment of the antihelix and/or a large conchal bowl (Table 24.3). Obtuse angles represent poor development of the antihelix, promoting lateralization of the helix. Prominence of the ear is also promoted by the presence of a deep conchal bowl (>1.5 cm) or anterior rotation of the conchal bowl. Various degrees of both can coexist. Secondary anomalies can also exist with the above deformities, including (1) excessively prominent helical root, (2) over-projected lobule (lobule, cavum concha, cauda helix), (3) excessive antitragal protrusion, (4) insufficient curling of the helix (shell ear), (5) cup ear deformity, (6) Darwin tubercle, (7) telephone ear deformity, (8) Stahl ear, and (9) macrotia. Other causes can include cranial abnormalities (that influence the base on which the ear rests) must be evaluated

[21]. Clearly, projection beyond the average values can be considered prominent to some, but much of the final opinion is derived from objective and subjective evaluation by the physician, patient, and the family in relation to facial morphology.

In the day of surgery, preoperative photographs are usually taken in front, posterior, and each ear lateral and oblique views.

Evaluation of the Cartilage Characters and Thickness

Expectation of the internal cartilage characters according to the age of the patient is vital in choice of otoplasty technique. Auricular elastic fibers in the young group were relatively homogeneous in diameter thickness with little branching and fragments, whereas in the aged group, highly branched elastic fibers were observed frequently and deviation in thickness, such as the occurrence of small fragments and large masses, was conspicuous. In the aged group, fine fibrous structure was frequently found in elastic fibers and the territorial matrix. The number of chondrocytes per unit area in the aged group was significantly less than in the young group. Moreover, collagenous fibers increased in number around the boundary of the territorial matrix where multivesicular bodies were also increased. All this factors must be in mind when dealing with cartilages in different age groups. So difficulties in bending and recurrence are anticipated with upgrading years of life. So using laser techniques reaching to the deeper layers of cartilages with nonabsorbable internal splinting is preferred.

Also evaluation of the cartilage thickness at the helix and antihelix is crucial. In very thin cartilages, curling of the cartilages is difficult and bending at one site may create deformity at another area. In such circumstances, cartilage-cutting techniques are preferred. While in normal cartilages, laser cartilage reshaping can afford the needed curvature with absorbable internal splints. Application of laser in thick can be highly advantageous when reaching to more depths with increasing thickness and support with nonabsorbable internal splints.

The biological principles when applying cartilage forces, e.g., scoring on one side, lead to: (1) auricular cartilage bends away from the scored surface, (2) bending properties are intrinsic to the cartilage and are independent of the perichondrium, and (3) deeper furrowing results in more profound bending. Weinzweig et al. [22] discovered from histologic studies in rabbits that a fibrocartilaginous cap develops after cartilage scoring that promotes and stabilizes cartilage bending.

Technique of Laser-Assisted Cartilage Reshaping Otoplasty

(a) Time of Surgery

The rapid development of the ear to approximately 90 % of adult dimensions by age 3 years allows for early surgical intervention for auricular anomalies. Also operating at younger ages does not retard the growth of the ear [23, 24]. So the author recommends like many surgeons operating on prominent ears when children are aged 3–6 years, before the start of school. The goal is to minimize the malformation before the period of socialization to avoid ridicule by other children. The psychosocial distress created by prominent ear has been previously documented in the literature [24]. The child perception of the anomaly is preferred as they are likely to be more agreeable and compliant in their treatment. Often surgery can be delayed safely for a child who does not perceive the deformity until adequate maturity is obtained.

(b) Goal of Surgery

McDowell in 1968 [25] and Wright 1970 [26] identified that regardless of the used technique, the following requirements should be fulfilled:

- The operative technique should be applicable to all age groups.
- The results must have postoperative symmetry of both ears.
- Good auricular proportions should be achieved.
- The helix-to-mastoid distance should be 10–12 mm at the superior helix, 16–18 mm at the midpoint, and 20–22 mm at the lobule.

- The elimination of protrusion in the upper third of the ear.
- The helix earlobe curve should run parallel to the mastoid surface.
- The posterior sulcus should be well formed.
- No sharp ridges should be visible.
- The earlobe should be set back to the same extent as the rest of the auricle.

(c) Anesthesia and Draping

General anesthesia is preferred for any child aged less than 10 years. Mature children and adults can receive sedation and regional anesthesia (1 % lidocaine with 1:100,000 epinephrine) with little discomfort. Contrary to intuition, the procedure is typically not associated with a great deal of pain, and use of Marcaine has not proven fruitful.

A cerebellar headrest is used for positioning and exposure; the face, ears, and hair are scrubbed with chlorhexidine gluconate solution. Hair is positioned out of the operative field using sterile surgical gel, and the drapes are applied. A central drape is also applied to cover the nose, mouth, and the tube. Draping in this manner provides simultaneous exposure of the ears and midface required for intraoperative comparison. Intraoperative assessment of the deformity is an important step (Fig. 24.2) with trial of bending to evaluate the forthcoming procedure (Fig. 24.3).

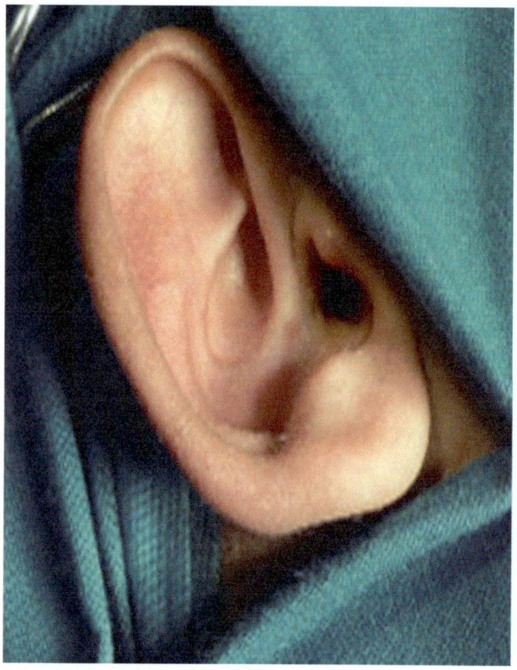

Fig. 24.2 Evaluation of intraoperative prominent ear deformity characteristics

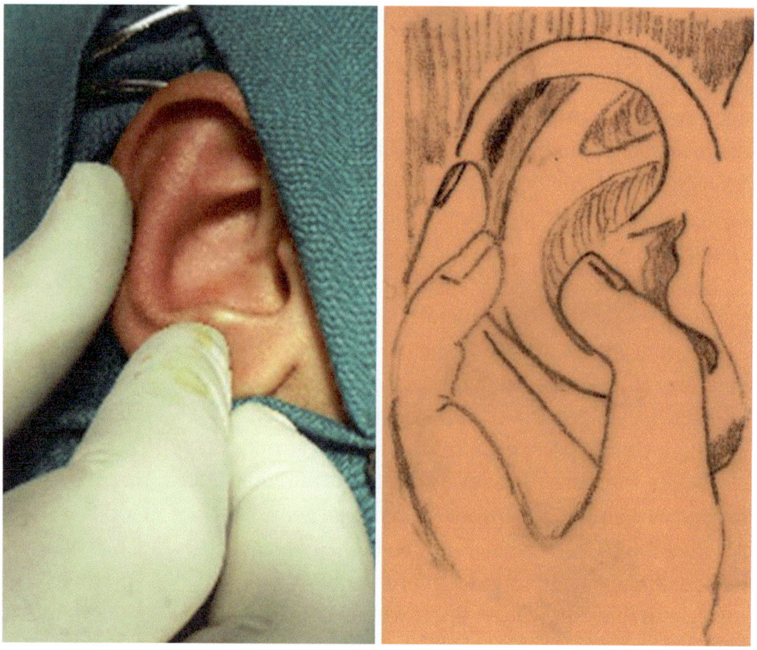

Fig. 24.3 Intraoperative folding of the proposed new antihelix

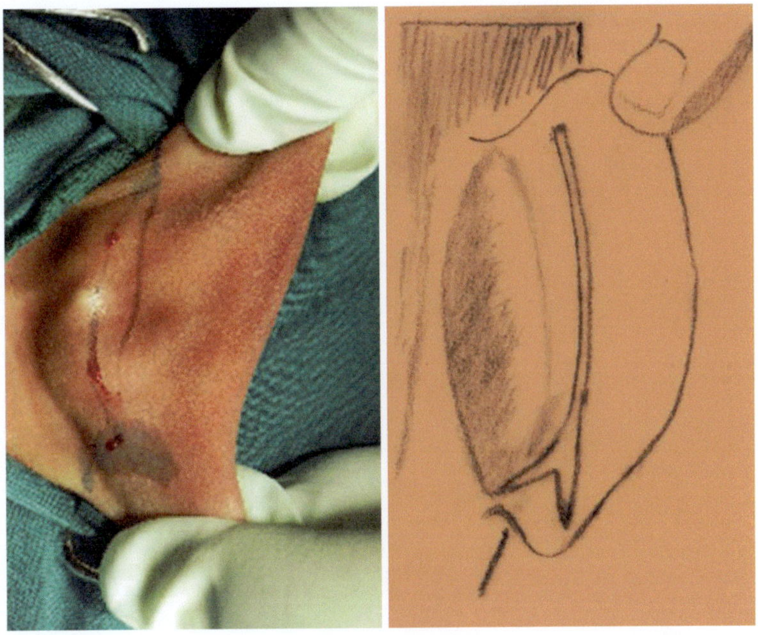

Fig. 24.4 Marking of fish-shaped medial surface skin incision

(d) Marking and Skin Incisions
Retroauricular fish-shaped incision was demarcated at the proposed incision site at the dorsal aspect at the concha (Fig. 24.4). Its transverse dimensions are decided by dorsal measurements of the needle length between the medial and lateral border of the proposed antihelixes. The tail thickness was determined according to the lobule protrusion. Four small, sharp cutting needles tattooed with methylene blue were pinned through the skin and the cartilage from the lateral surface at the posterior border of the proposed new antihelix (scaphal line) and passed to superior crus (fossa line) and the anterior border of the proposed antihelix (conchal line) (Fig. 24.5). Local anesthesia (lignocaine with 1 in 200,000 adrenaline) was infiltrated into the medial surfaces of the auricle. Local anesthesia enhances hemostasis and demarcates the plain of dissection.

(e) Skin Excision and Elevation of the Postauricular Surface
Retroauricular fish-shaped excision (Figs. 24.6 and 24.7) was carried out. Fashioning of such shape allowed decreasing the dead space and subsequent hematoma formation. Also it allows dressing the resized cartilage in adequate fashion without redundancy of skin. Repositioning a protruding lobule utilizing an eccentric excision of posterior, lobule skin, and fibrofatty tissue is another advantage of such incision and excision. It gives your blessing to extensive setback in adults when the skin lacks elastic recoil. This is followed by standard wide postauricular supraperichondrial undermining for exposing all the medial surface of the auricular cartilage reaching to the helix border and its perichondrium. In the present technique, the retroauricular open approach allocated precise laser application and control of the auricular reshaping process and at the same time passed up skin laser interactions.

(f) Preparation of the Postauricular Surface and Identification of the Tail of the Helix
Hemostasis can be done after elevation of the skin. Elevation can be accomplished when reaching to the anterior antihelix border and reaching to the postauricular area (Fig. 24.8). Dissection and identification of the tail of the helix can allow better use of laser and fixation in a proper position and positioning of the lobule.

(g) Laser Reshaping of the Scapha
The laser beam was delivered by means of a TEKA SL 250S (Italy) CO2 laser at a wavelength of 15,600 nm to the medial surface of the auricular cartilage. The laser beam was con-

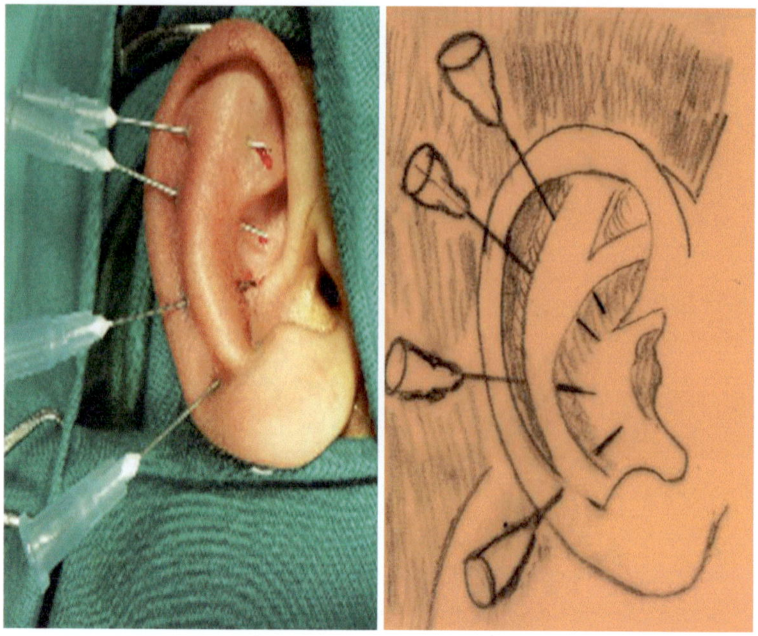

Fig. 24.5 Marking of the antihelix with needles tattooed with methylene *blue* pinned from scaphal to conchal lines and fossa line

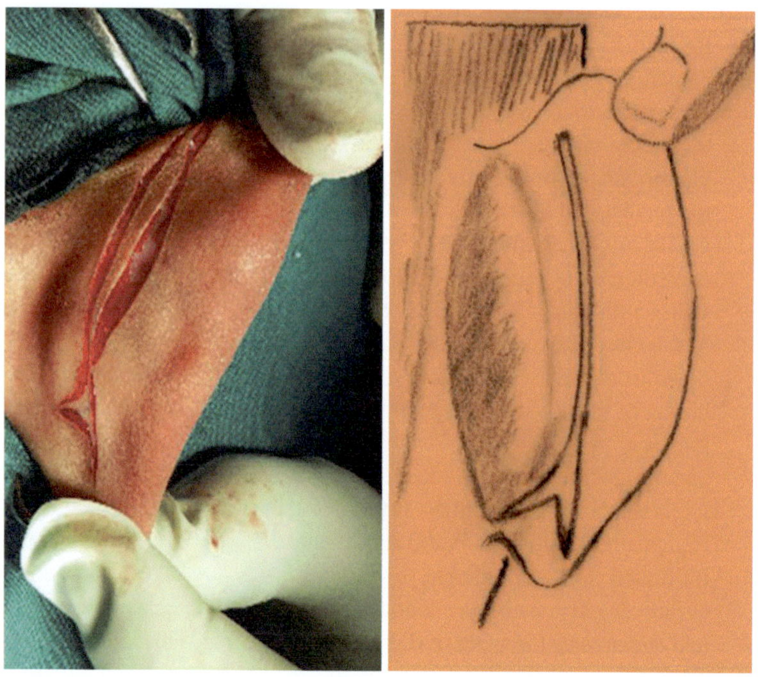

Fig. 24.6 Fish-shaped medial surface skin incision

trolled with the micromanipulator with a focal length of 200 mm, mounted on a surgical microscope (Karl Zies, Germany). Carbon dioxide (CO2) laser evaporation (Figs. 24.9 and 24.10) of the posterior perichondrium, together with partial thickness of the auricular cartilage, was carried out on the medial surface of the proposed new auricular antihelix and the superior crus and guarded by the scaphal line posteriorly and conchal line anteriorly (Figs. 24.9 and 24.10) [27]. The laser beams of evaporation were applied parallel to Frankfort line, e.g., perpendicular to

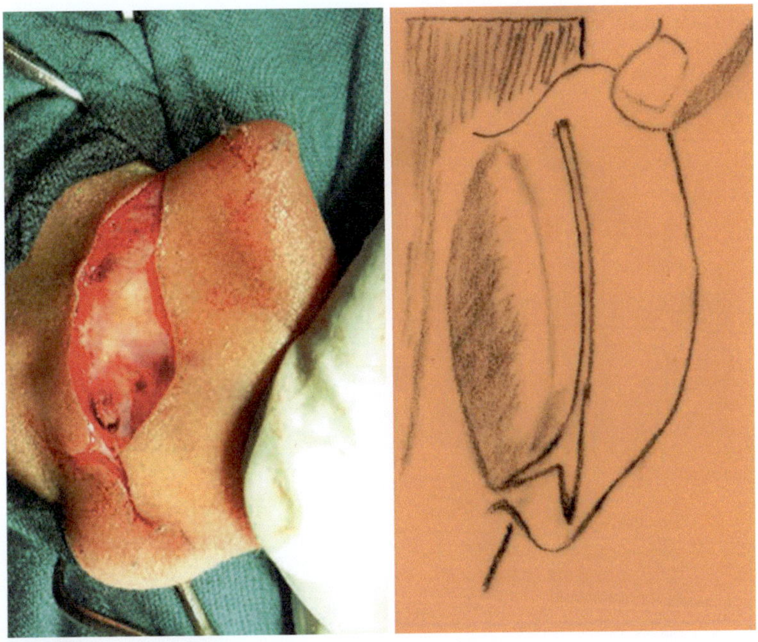

Fig. 24.7 Excision of skin

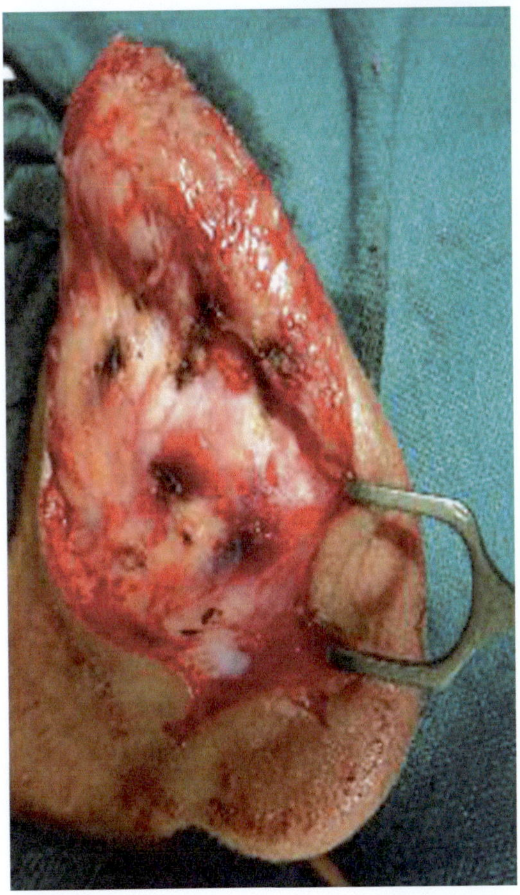

Fig. 24.8 Exposure of the medial surface of the auricle

the axis of the proposed antihelix (Figs. 24.9 and 24.10). With such application, curling and folding of the antihelix can be observed. The depth of penetration was determined according to age and cartilage thickness. In normal cartilages and age less than 6 years, the depth of laser is only one third the thicknesses. While in thick cartilages and children over 6 years, the thickness reaches from one half to two thirds thickness. A pair of parallel laser incisions with a focused laser beam (Figs. 24.9 and 24.10) was performed (reaching to a deeper thickness of the auricular cartilages and leaving the ventral perichondrium intact) on either side of the antihelixes and superior crus (at scaphal line, fossa line, and conchal line) (Figs. 24.9 and 24.10) [27]. To permit better optimal angle of curling with smooth curvature of the cartilages, laser cartilage incisions were carried out with preservation of the lateral perichondrium. Laser incisions can be healed by formation of fibrosis-free young cartilage of permanent shape in comparison to classical scalpel incisions that consisted mainly of fibrosis. The assistant always looks to the lateral surface of the auricle with each laser application. Pressure and cooling with wet gauzes that were applied against the scapha allowed curling of the superior crus and the antihelix all through the procedure.

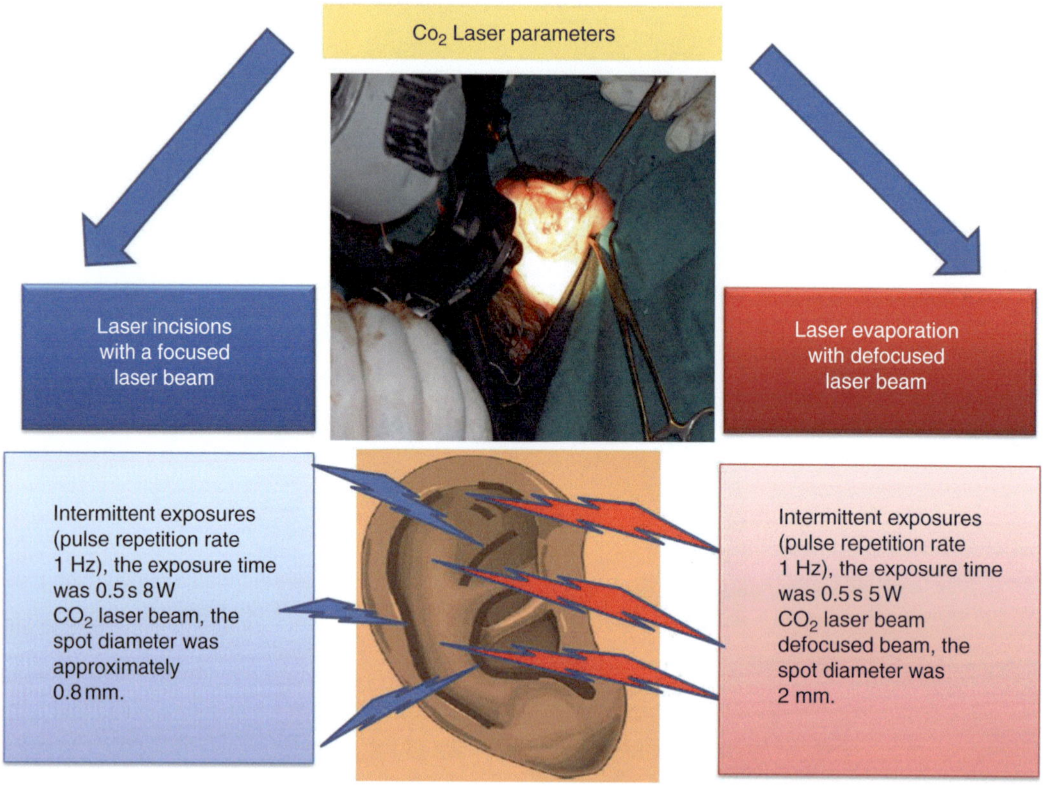

Fig. 24.9 Carbon dioxide laser parameters used in carbon dioxide laser-assisted cartilage reshaping otoplasty

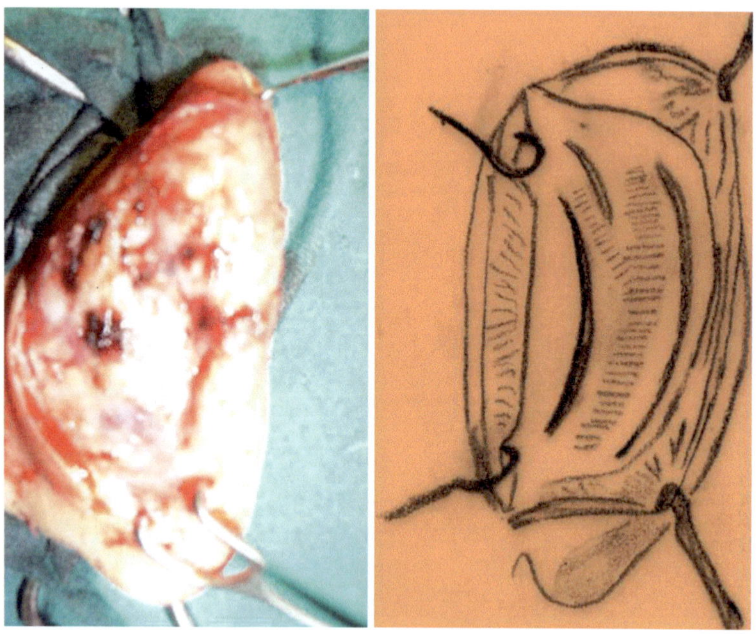

Fig. 24.10 Sites of laser vaporization of the antihelix and laser incisions in scaphal and conchal lines with intraoperative shape of the cartilage after laser-assisted cartilage reshaping otoplasty

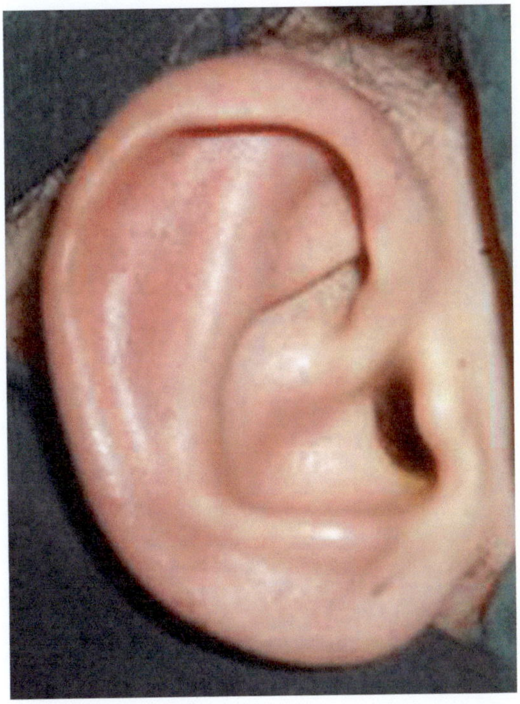

Fig. 24.11 Intraoperative shape of the auricle after application of laser

Assessment of the results is essential after laser application (Fig. 24.11).

(h) Suture Internal Splints and Securing of the New Antihelix

The cartilage is fixed by absorbable 4-0 Prolene sutures (Fig. 24.12) which act as an internal mold that allow smooth tense curve of the antihelix without postoperative prolonged solid mold wearing. An inter-suture distance of 4–6 mm usually produces a soft, natural fold. These sutures function as markers obviating needle and ink tattooing and as traction levers for positioning. Three to four mattress sutures were applied: one was above the junction of the crura, the second was just below the junction of the crura to fold the superior antihelix, and the third and forth (when needed) were to fix the inferior part of the antihelix as distant as needed.

(i) Laser Reshaping and Repositioning of the Concha

A poorly defined, "unfolded" antihelix in conjunction with an abnormally deep concha, possessing a prominent posterior wall, characterizes the majority of ears. When this combination of anomalies is encountered, surgical correction of the concha is performed first by concha–mastoid suturing, as described by Furnas [5]. The postauricular muscle and ligament are divided. The dissection is continued downward until the cartilaginous insertion (ponticulus) of the postauricular muscle is identified. After exposing the ponticulus, the skin and subcutaneous tissues are elevated off the mastoid fascia for approximately 2 cm. With deep concha more than 2.5 cm, excision of postauricular muscles reaching to the periosteum or laser ablation of the postauricular tissue is advised. The concha is mobilized down to its junction with the mastoid bone. A laser incision with a focused laser beam was performed (reaching to a deeper thickness of the auricular cartilages and leaving the ventral perichondrium intact) on the lateral border of the concha [27].

When the combination of "unfolded" antihelix in conjunction with an abnormally deep concha anomaly is encountered, surgical correction of the concha is performed first by concha–mastoid suturing, as described by Furnas [5]. The concha is rotated to the mastoid bone and fixed on the periosteum of the mastoid bone by two to three 4-0 on a half-round, atraumatic Prolene needle. The concha–mastoid sutures are oriented in the strict anteroposterior direction. This alignment draws the concha gently back and reduces forward rotation and external auditory canal narrowing produced by more radial-oriented sutures. The sutures are synched down with half-hitch knots to gauge the effect with the middle suture addressed last.

(j) Management of the Helical Tail and Control of the Lobule

Excessive anterolateral projection of the earlobe is a frequent contributor to prominent ear. The magnitude of this deformity is often exacerbated by the production of the new antihelical fold. The lower pole of the ear possesses moderate elastic recoil and typically maintains the position produced by fishtail excision of skin and fibrofatty tissue from the lobule (Figs. 24.13 and 24.14). The forgiving nature of the lower third of the ear is the basis of several posterior skin excision techniques. Using

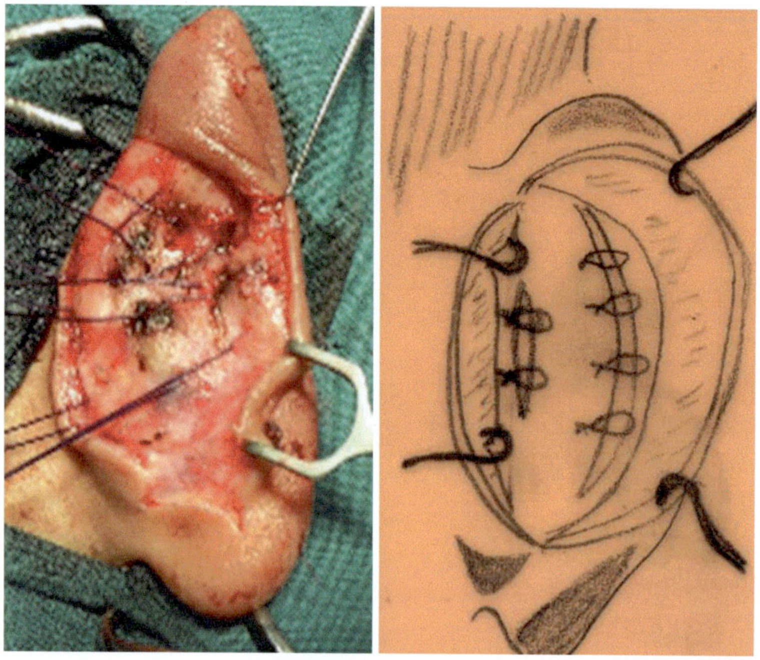

Fig. 24.12 Internal molding of the antihelical fold and concha using mattress nonabsorbable 4-0 sutures

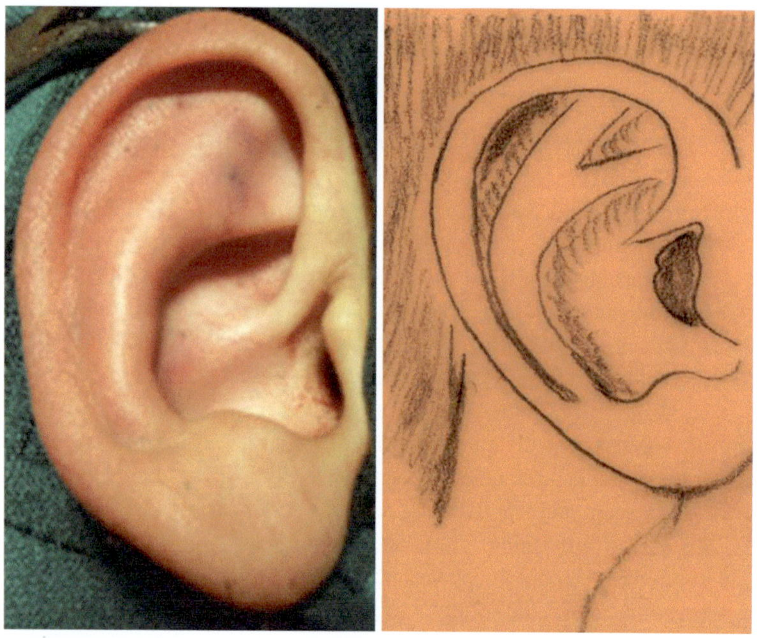

Fig. 24.13 Intraoperative shape of the auricle after application of laser and internal fixation with sutures

a "training suture" can protect the lobe position following skin excision setback. We use single lobe–muscle suture extending from the fibrofatty tissue of the lobe to the postauricular muscles.

(k) Skin Closure and Dressing

Postauricular skin closure is the surgeon's signature. This anatomic area is cosmetically "silent" but should be closed with the same attention to detail that is given to any other

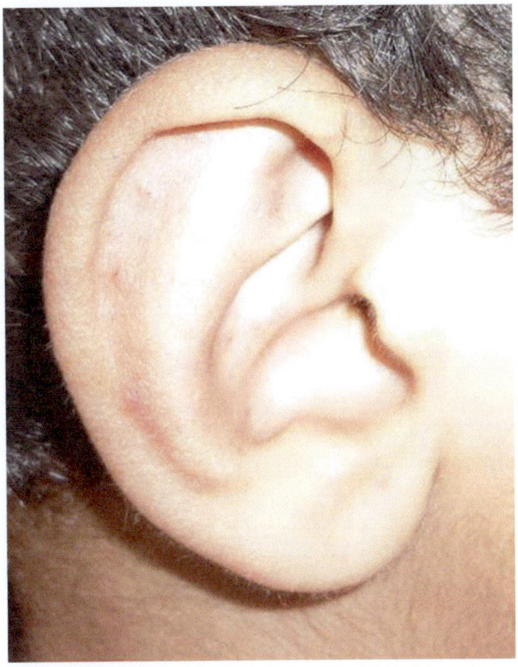

Fig. 24.14 Postoperative auricle after laser-assisted cartilage reshaping otoplasty

wound. Skin closure is performed with subcuticular absorbable 4-0 Vicryl sutures. That is bathed starting on the seventh postoperative day and dissolves very shortly thereafter. It obviates the discomfort of suture removal, especially in children. Drains should not be needed if adequate hemostasis has been achieved. Then a fluffed, dry, all-cotton gauze dressing is wetted and carefully placed into the new antihelical folds and the concha and soaked with an antibiotic-containing preparation and fixed by a head bandage. Control of the new ear contours in the early postoperative period is very important. The effects of shear, especially in the younger patient, can be disastrous. The gauzes are held in place with cling wrap. At the first postoperative visit, the entire dressing is removed. The new dressing remains in place for 7 days. The patient is then instructed to wear an ear protector (either a swimming ear protector or a tennis sweatband) each night

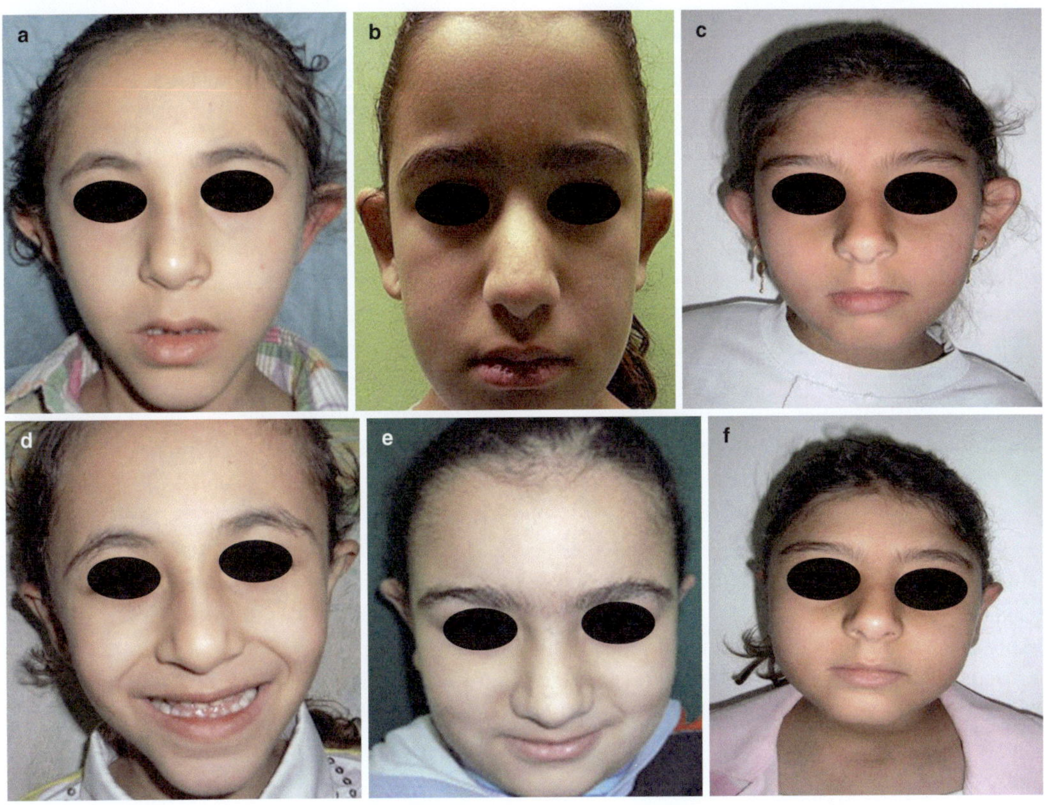

Fig. 24.15 (*Upper*) Preoperative prominent ear deformity children. (*Lower*) Postoperatively after laser-assisted cartilage reshaping otoplasty

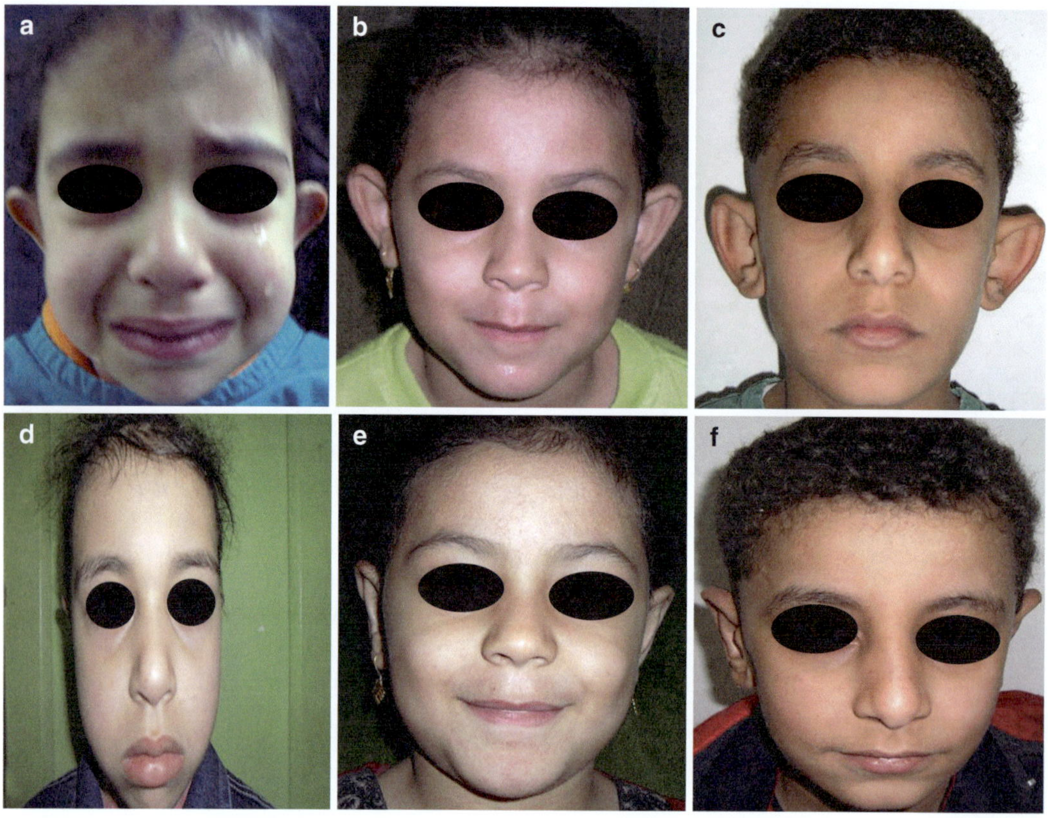

Fig. 24.16 (*Upper*) Preoperative prominent ear deformity children. (*Lower*) Postoperative after laser-assisted cartilage reshaping otoplasty

for a month to prevent accidental stresses on the ear during sleep (Fig. 24.7). Vigorous activities such as sports and dancing are permitted 1 month from the day of surgery. After the dressing is removed, showers and shampooing are allowed. Gentle scrubbing of the postauricular suture line is necessary to encourage suture dissolution. Postoperative photographs are taken at the 2-month visit.

Results and Complications

After early and late follow-up, no complications or sequel, e.g., hyperpigmentation or thermal injuries, was observed (Figs. 24.15, 24.16, 24.17, 24.18, and 24.19).

According to patient satisfaction with the results in terms of shape and symmetry 13 (81.3 %) and 14 (87.5), patients were pleased in early and late assessment, respectively (Figs. 24.7, [27]). Using doctor satisfaction outcome 12 (75 %) and 13 (81.3 %), patients were good in early and late assessment, respectively. With objective McDowell's basic goals in early and late assessment, the score was 4–6 and the mean was 5 from 6 (Figs. 24.15, 24.16, 24.17, 24.18, and 24.19) [27].

The mean immediate postoperative change of protrusion was 13.42 mm and the mean change of protrusion found at last follow-up was 15.45 mm. In last postoperative follow-up, the number of ears where there was an increase of protrusion from the early postoperative follow-up was 5 (15.6 %) [27].

Fig. 24.18 (*Upper*) Preoperative children with prominent ear. (*Lower*) Postoperatively after laser-assisted cartilage reshaping otoplasty

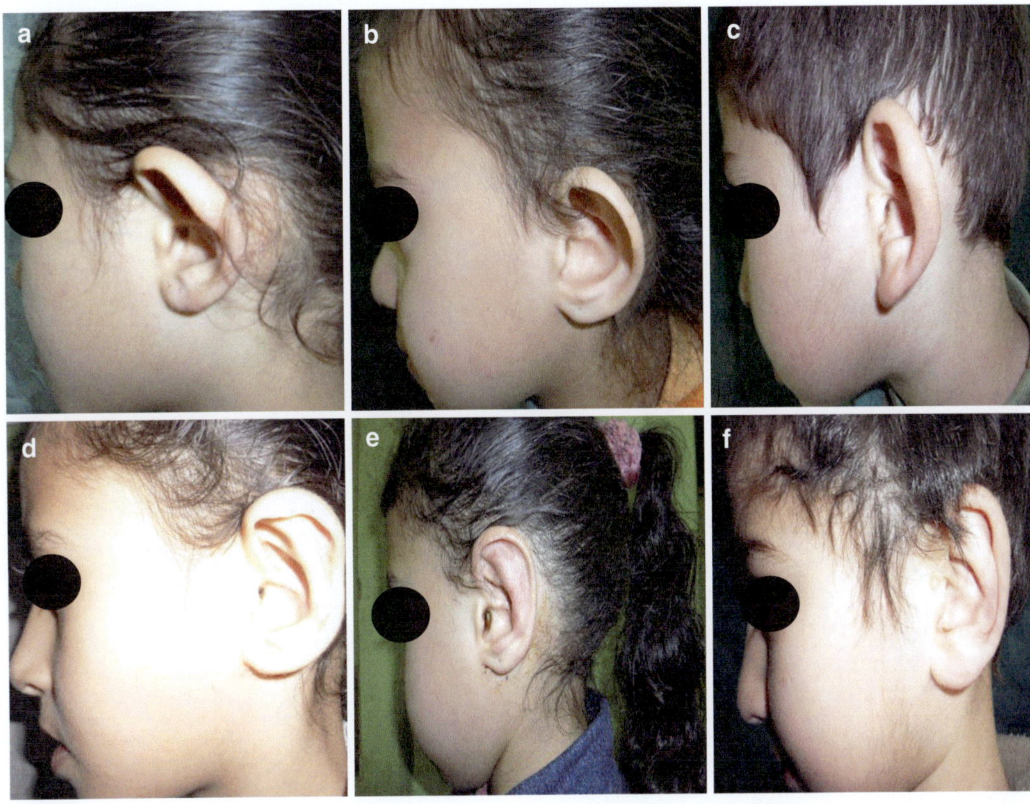

Fig. 24.17 (*Upper*) Preoperative prominent ear in children. (*Lower*) Postoperatively after laser-assisted cartilage reshaping otoplasty

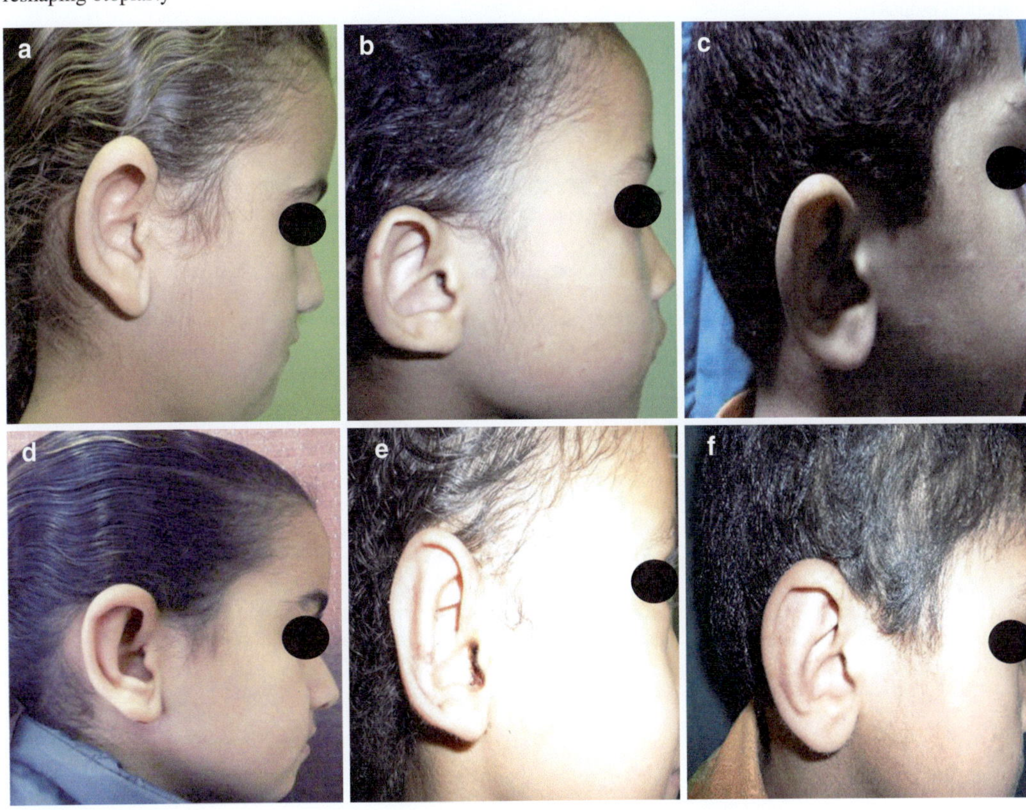

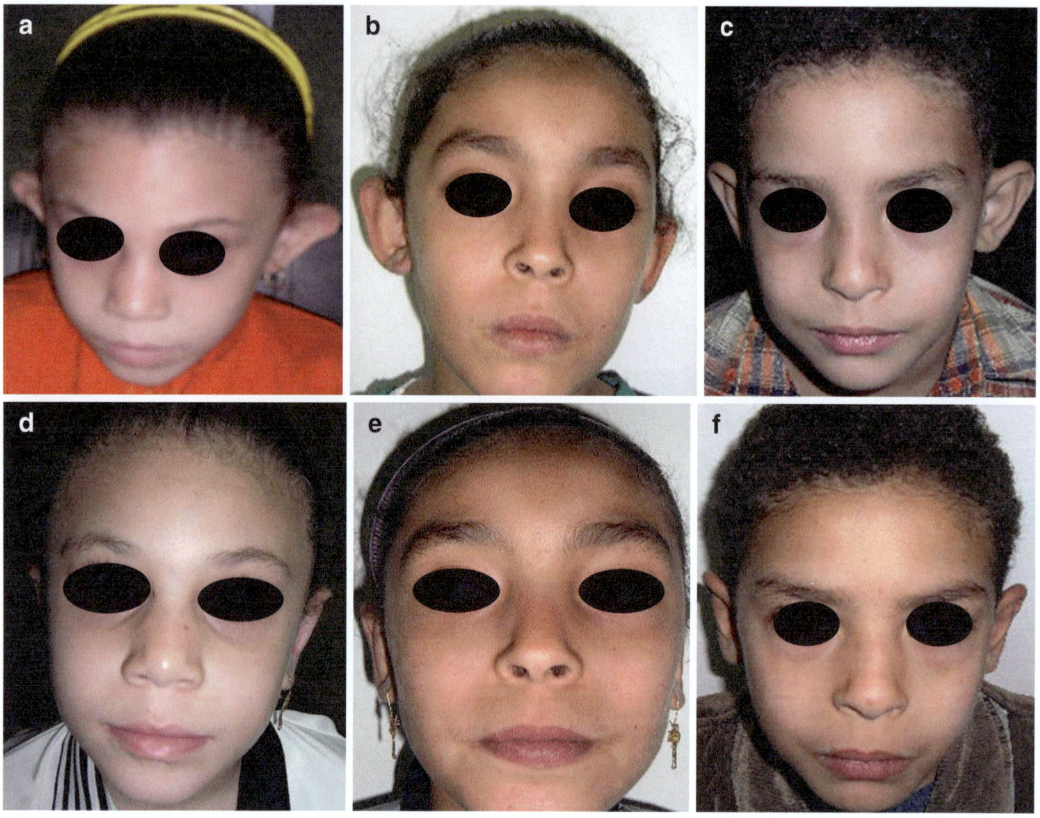

Fig. 24.19 (*Upper*) Preoperative children with prominent ear. (*Lower*) Postoperatively after laser-assisted cartilage reshaping otoplasty

References

1. Bichara DA, O'Sullivan NA, Pomerantseva I, Zhao X, Sundback CA, Vacanti JP, et al. The tissue-engineered auricle: past, present, and future. Tissue Eng Part B Rev. 2012;18(1):51–61.
2. Widgerow AD. Revision otoplasty: the contracted antihelical fold. Plast Reconstr Surg. 2002;110(3):827–30.
3. Stenstrom SJ. A "natural" technique for correction of congenitally prominent ears. Plast Reconstr Surg. 1963;32:509–18.
4. Mustardé JC. The treatment of prominent ears by buried mattress sutures: a ten-year survey. Plast Reconstr Surg. 1967;39(4):382–6.
5. Furnas DW. Correction of prominent ears by conchamastoid sutures. Plast Reconstr Surg. 1968;42(3): 189–93.
6. Walter C. Plastic surgery of protruding ears. HNO. 1998;46(3):193–4.
7. Converse JM, Wood-Smith D. Technical details in the surgical correction of the lop ear deformity. Plast Reconstr Surg. 1963;31:118–28.
8. Owsley TG, Biggerstaff TG. Otoplasty complications. Oral Maxillofac Surg Clin North Am. 2009;21(1):105–18.
9. Tan KH. Long-term survey of prominent ear surgery: a comparison of two methods. Br J Plast Surg. 1986; 39(2):270–3.
10. Nachlas NE. Otoplasty. In: Papel ID, Larrabee W, Holt GR, et al., editors. Facial plastic and reconstructive surgery. 2nd ed. New York: Thieme; 2002. 309–31.
11. Vuyk HD. Cartilage-sparing otoplasty: a review with long-term results. J Laryngol Otol. 1997;111(5): 424–30.
12. Olivier B, Mohammad H, Christian A, Akram R. Retrospective study of the long-term results of otoplasty using a modified Mustardé (cartilage-sparing) technique. J Otolaryngol Head Neck Surg. 2009;38(3): 340–7.
13. da Silva Freitas R, Shin JH, Persing JA, Alonso N, Busato L. Solving the sharpness borders in otoplasty. Plast Reconstr Surg. 2009;123(6):197e–9.
14. Sobol E, Omel'chenko A, Mertig M, Pompe W. Scanning force microscopy of the fine structure of cartilage irradiated with a CO2 laser. Lasers Med Sci. 2000;15:15–23.

15. Holden PK, Chlebicki C, Wong BJ. Minimally invasive ear reshaping with a 1450-nm diode laser using cryogen spray cooling in New Zealand white rabbits. Arch Facial Plast Surg. 2009;11(6):399–404.
16. Janík I, Stárek I, Hlozek Z, Hubácek J, Novotný R, Dvorácková J. Histomorphological transformation of the auricular cartilage after carbon dioxide laser-assisted Mustardé otoplasty. An experimental study. Lasers Med Sci. 2009;24(3):433–7.
17. Ayhan M, Deren O, Görgü M, Erdogan B, Dursun A. Cartilage shaping with the Er:YAG laser: an in vivo experimental study. Ann Plast Surg. 2002;49(5):527–31.
18. Jones N, Sviridov A, Sobol E, Omelchenko A, Lowe J. A prospective randomised study of laser reshaping of cartilage in vivo. Lasers Med Sci. 2001;16(4):284–90.
19. Baumann M, Jörgensen B, Rohde E, Bindig U, Müller G, Scheller EE. Influence of wavelength, power density and exposure time of laser radiation on chondrocyte cultures – an in-vitro investigation. Med Laser Appl. 2006;21:191–8.
20. Farkas LG. Anthropometry of the head and face. 2nd ed. New York: Raven; 1994.
21. Kelley P, Hollier L, Stal S. Otoplasty: evaluation, technique, and review. J Craniofac Surg. 2003;14(5):643–53.
22. Weinzweig N, Chen L, Walter GS. Histomorphology of neochodrogenesis after antithelical fold creation: a comparison of three otoplasty techniques in the rabbit. Ann Plast Surg. 1994;33(4):371–6.
23. MacGregor FC. Ear deformities: social and psychological implications. Clin Plast Surg. 1978;5(3):347–50.
24. Balogh B, Millesi H. Are growth alterations a consequence of surgery for prominent ears? Plast Reconstr Surg. 1992;90(2):192–9.
25. McDowell A. Goals in otoplasty for protruding ears. Plast Reconstr Surg. 1968;41(1):17–27.
26. Wright WK. Otoplasty goals and principles. Arch Otolaryngol. 1970;92(6):568–72.
27. Ragab A. Carbon dioxide laser-assisted cartilage reshaping otoplasty: a new technique for prominent ears. Laryngoscope. 2010;120(7):1312–8.

Sutureless Otoplasty: Anterior Scoring of the Antihelical Fold

25

Asif Zubair Bhatti and Muhammad Ijaz

Introduction

The first time this concept was introduced was by Gibson and Davis in 1958 [1] based on the principle that the injured cartilage tends to fold away from the injured site. This was used successfully by Stenstrom [2] and Chongchet [3]. Chongchet's technique used sharp scoring of the lateral scaphal cartilage (with a scalpel) to form an antihelix. Stenstrom, in contrast, used a rasp to score the antihelix blindly.

In 1967, Kaye [4] combined Stenstrom's anterior scoring technique with Mustarde's [5] posterior suture placement technique. This technique, which later became very popular, involved using the vertical curvilinear striations of the anterior perichondrium to weaken the cartilaginous "spring," followed by the creation and securing of the new antihelical fold by placement of posterior mattress sutures. Kaye also advocated the use of nonabsorbable sutures to avoid recurrence after failure of a knot. The knot was often prominent beneath the thin antihelical skin, which was a problem, so few other surgeons adopted anterior placement.

Minimal access anterior scoring has been described using dedicated cartilage scoring instruments, toothed forceps, endoscopic carpal tunnel release instruments, and a bent hypodermic needle. The latter technique described by Mahler used a needle with a bend in one axis for scoring.

The authors use scoring as a way to shape the antihelix. Scoring the anterior surface of the cartilage facilitates the formation of the antihelical fold. A noc. 15 surgical blade is used at an angle of 45 along a predetermined line on our future antihelix. The depth of the incision was two-thirds the depth of the cartilage until it twisted through 180°.

Indication

Patient age range from 8 to 20 years, where the predominant anatomic defect is underdevelopment of antihelical fold.

Operative Technique (Figs. 25.1, 25.2, and 25.3)

Under local or general anesthesia, the patient is prepared and draped.

Local anesthetic with adrenaline is infiltrated along the line of the desired position of the refashioned antihelix between the cartilage and the subcutaneous tissues both anteriorly and posteriorly. A 21G needle dipped in methylene blue solution is used to mark the skin over the cartilage in the line of the new antihelical fold.

A.Z. Bhatti, M.D., MBBS, BSc (✉) • M. Ijaz, M.D.
Plastic, Reconstructive, Hand and Cosmetic Surgery, Saad Specialist Hospital, Prince Faisal Bin Fahd Road, 30353, 31952 Alkhobar, Eastren Province, Kingdom of Saudi Arabia
e-mail: asif1025@yahoo.com; drbhatty@doctors.org.uk; muhammadijazdr@gmail.com

M.A. Shiffman (ed.), *Advanced Cosmetic Otoplasty*,
DOI 10.1007/978-3-642-35431-1_25, © Springer-Verlag Berlin Heidelberg 2013

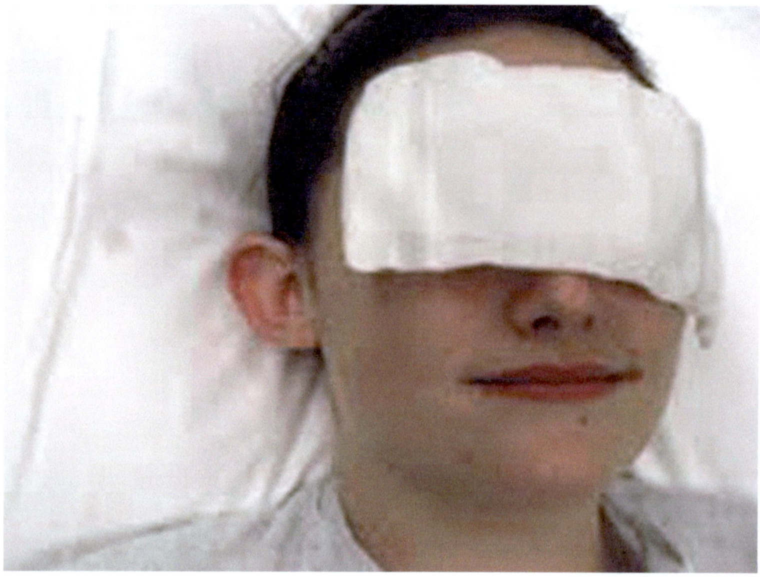

Fig 25.1 Preoperative prominent ear and absent antihelix

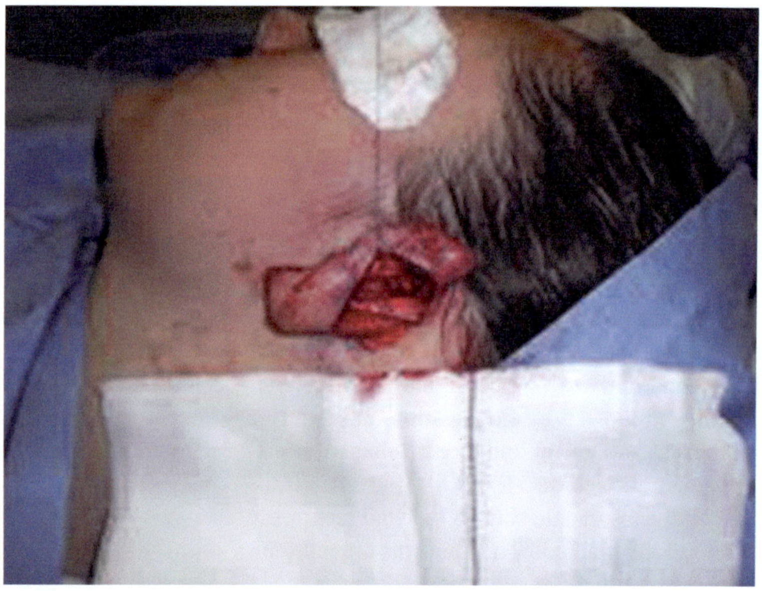

Fig. 25.2 Perioperative curved cartilage

A conservative dumbbell-shaped skin excision is made posteriorly, and the tissue is dissected to expose the points on the cartilage that mark the new antihelical fold. The cut is made starting about 2 mm from the marked areas. A no. 15 surgical blade is held in a curved angle of 45 and is used to cut the two-thirds depth of cartilage until it curves completely 180°. Fine diathermy is then used at the edges of the fold so that the antihelix keeps its shape and contour. No suture is used at any stage. After the cartilage has been curved to the desired position, hemostasis is secured.

Special care must be taken not to score over the same point twice as one may cut through the cartilage. If that happens, the cartilage must be repaired to avoid an unsightly ridge under the skin. Repeated milking of the anterior surface of the antihelical fold removes any collection throughout the procedure.

The skin is closed using 5/0 absorbable (Monocryl) poliglecaprone vertical mattress sutures.

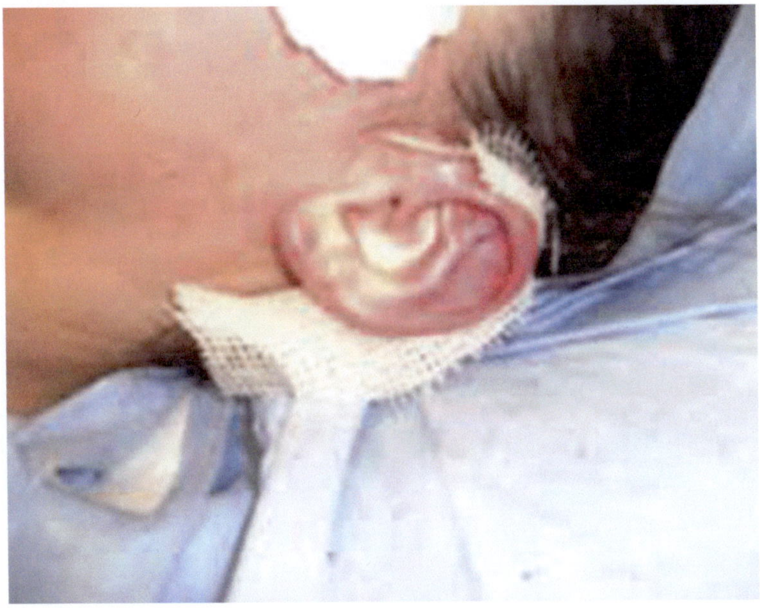

Fig. 25.3 Postoperative after closure

The cavum concha, cymba concha, scapha, triangular fossa, and the retroauricular sulcus are packed with cotton wool soaked in paraffin. A tailored piece of tulle gras is placed over the ears and the skin around the auricle. Turban dressing is applied with two rolls of crepe with a scalpel. Bandage is applied, kept slightly loose at the lower edge so that the ears may be examined postoperatively.

Postoperative Care

There are a number of advantages to this form of dressing (turban dressing): it is easy to put on, tends not to fall off, is cool in hot weather, and has no risk of pressure ulceration. This is left in place for a week. The use of a headband during the night is advised for 6 weeks after the operation.

Complications

Infection 1(1.45 %)
Hemorrhage 2(2.9 %)
Hypertrophic scarring 0
Residual deformity 1(1.45 %)
Palpable sutures 0
Skin problems 1(1.45 %)

Discussion

The correction of prominent ears has been shown by Bradbury et al. [6] to improve happiness and confidence and is therefore a worthwhile operation. Many techniques have been published in an attempt to improve the cosmetic outcome of correction and reduce the postoperative morbidity. The one described here combines a number of well-established methods of correction, most importantly anterior scoring with some of our own refinements.

Stenstrom [2] showed the advantage of scoring of the anterior cartilage in both cadavers and patients. This was taken further by Chongchet [3]. If diathermy cuts are placed in the desired position, they allow for precise tightening and accurate control of the degree of folding of the antihelix. This requires minimal dissection or degloving of the cartilage of the ear. Mahler [7] described how the hypodermic needle was simply hooked to the desired curvature, but in our technique, a precise cut can be made using the blade. This enables the authors to produce cuts of varying depths depending on the thickness of the cartilage to break its spring adequately but not completely transect it. The entry point for scoring enables the milking of any collection that may have formed anterior to the cartilage. The postoperative morbidity compares well with other published series.

The technique did not allow any potential dead space, so there is less chance of any collection or any swelling. As no suture is used, chances of foreign body reaction, protrusion, and wound breakdown become minimal.

References

1. Gibson T, Davis WB. The distortion of autogenous cartilage grafts: its cause and prevention. Br J Plast Surg. 1958;10:257–74.
2. Stenstrom S. A natural technique for correction of congenitally prominent ears. Plast Reconstr Surg. 1963;32:509–18.
3. Chongchet V. A method of antihelix reconstruction. Br J Plast Surg. 1963;16:268–72.
4. Kaye BL. A simplified method for correcting the prominent ear. Plast Reconstr Surg. 1973;52(21):184.
5. Mustarde JC. The treatment of prominent ears by buried mattress sutures: a ten-year survey. Plast Reconstr Surg. 1967;39(4):382–6.
6. Bradbury ET, Hewison J, Timmons MJ. Psycho logical and social outcome of prominent ear correction in children. Br J Plast Surg. 1992;45(2):97–100.
7. Mahler D. The correction of the prominent ear. Aesthetic Plast Surg. 1986;10(1):29–33.

Anterior Scoring of the Upper Helical Cartilage as a Refinement of the Chong-Chet Technique in Otoplasty

26

Corrado Rubino, Franceso Farace, and Mario Faenza

Anatomical Considerations

The ear is composed mainly by cartilage and skin; its shape is oval and flat, with the upper extremity larger than the lower one and positioned on the lateral surface of the cranium with an angle between 20° and 25°. The length of the ear is between 5.5 and 6.5 cm, whereas its width is between 3.0 and 3.5 cm. The auricular pavilion presents an anterior and a posterior aspect. The anterior aspect is represented by helix, fossa of the helix, triangular notch, antihelix, concha, antitragus, tragus, intertragic notch, and lobule.

1. Helix is the most prominent and peripheral aspect of the ear; it originates from the concha (crus of the helix) then courses upward to the ascending helix until its insertion on the skull. The point where the ascending helix separates from the skull is called superior otobasion. The inferior portion of the helix is melted with the cranial aspect of the lobule.
2. Antihelix is a curve prominence that originates inferiorly from the antitragus and then courses upward parallel to the helix until it divides into superior and inferior crus.
3. Triangular notch is a space between the superior and the inferior crus of the antihelix.
4. Fossa of the helix is a space between the helix posteriorly and the antihelix anteriorly.
5. Concha is the widest and deepest central depression; anteriorly it surrounds the external auditory meatus whereas posteriorly is delimited by the antihelix. The concha is divided into a narrow upper part (cymba) and a wide lower part (cavum) that continues directly into the external auditory meatus.
6. Tragus is a small prominence with a triangular shape sited in front of the concha and, together with it, completes the external auditory meatus.
7. Antitragus is the downward and forward extension of the antihelix, from which it is separated by a depression. It shows an ovoid shape and is located behind the tragus.
8. Intertragic notch is a depression that separates the tragus from the antitragus.
9. Lobule is the inferior one third of the auricular pavilion, is composed by skin and fat tissue (without cartilage), superiorly originates from the tail of the helix, and then courses downward and forward forming a free semicircular edge. The point in which the lobule is inserted on the skull is called inferior otobasion.

The posterior aspect is represented by two prominences corresponding to the depressions of the anterior aspect, called eminence of the concha and triangular eminence.

C. Rubino, M.D. (✉)
Plastic Surgery Unit, Department of Medicine and Surgery, University of Salerno, Via S Allende 1-84081, Baronissi (Salerno), Italy
e-mail: corubino@uniss.it, crubino@unisa.it

F. Farace, M.D. • M. Faenza, M.D.
Plastic Surgery Unit, Department of Surgical, Microsurgical and Medical Sciences, University of Sassari, V.le San Pietro 43B, Sassari 07100, Italy
e-mail: farace@uniss.it; mfaenza@alice.it

M.A. Shiffman (ed.), *Advanced Cosmetic Otoplasty*,
DOI 10.1007/978-3-642-35431-1_26, © Springer-Verlag Berlin Heidelberg 2013

The auricular pavilion is composed of:

1. Cartilage.
2. Ligaments are divided into intrinsic and extrinsic:
   Intrinsic ligaments are fibrous expansions that join various subunits together.
   Extrinsic ligaments fix the auricular pavilion to the temporal bone.
3. The anterior ligament goes from the spine of the helix and the tragus to the apophysis of the zygomatic bone.
4. The posterior ligament connects the medial aspect of the concha to the mastoid bone.
5. Muscles lie on the ligaments and, as the ligaments, are divided into intrinsic and extrinsic: Intrinsic muscles are bent across the subunits of the auricular pavilion, and their surgical role is secondary.
   Extrinsic muscles are very thin and connect the auricular pavilion to the skull and to the scalp orienting the ear (anterior auricular m., posterior auricular m., superior auricular m.).
6. Adipose tissue is poorly represented on the anterior aspect and well represented on the posterior aspect.
7. Skin.

Vascular Supply

Arterial Blood Supply

1. Superficial temporal artery (STA) is the terminal branch of the external carotid artery; it courses upward in front of the pavilion and gives three branches for the lobule, the ascending helix, and the tragus, respectively. These collateral branches move to the external aspects of the mentioned structures and then give anastomosis with perforator branches of the posterior auricular artery.
2. Posterior auricular artery (PAA) is a collateral of the external carotid artery that courses upward between the parotid gland and the stylomastoid process and then continues between the auricular cartilage and the mastoid process giving an inferior branch for the posterior aspect of the lobule. At this point the PAA courses upward under the posterior aspect of the concha, and the posterior auricular muscle, at this level, gives two branches (intermediate and superior) for the posterior aspect of the auricular pinna and the peripheral margin of the helix and then gives anastomosis with terminal branches of STA.

Venous Blood Supply

1. Anteriorly the superficial veins drain into the venous plexus of the cheek, whereas the deep veins drain into the temporal vein superiorly and into the deep veins of the parotid gland inferiorly.
2. Posteriorly superficial veins drain into superficial occipital veins, the posterosuperior veins drain into the deep temporal vein, and the middle and the inferior veins join together in a posterior arch that drains into the deep parotid veins.

Nerve Supply

The motor innervation of the auricular pavilion is provided by the facial nerve; its temporal branch innervates anterior auricular muscle, superior auricular muscle, and intrinsic muscles of the anterior aspect. The posterior auricular branch innervates the posterior auricular muscle and the intrinsic muscles of the posterior aspect. Sensitivity innervation is provided by:

1. Great auricular nerve originates from cervical plexus (C2–C3) and gives two branches for the inferior half of the auricular pavilion.
2. Minor occipital nerve originates from cervical plexus and innervates the superior one third of the pavilion.
3. Arnold's nerve originates from vagus nerve and innervates the concha and the external auditory meatus (Ramsay-Hunt area).
4. Auriculotemporal nerve originates from the mandibular nerve (branch of the trigeminal nerve) and innervates the ascending portion of the antihelix and tragus.

Anatomical Considerations in Auricular Deformities

Angles between the auricular pavilion and the skull are expressed by codified values, whose knowledge may suggest which surgical treatment is most indicated.

There are three angles that we consider during the clinical evaluation of an auricular pavilion:

1. Cephaloconchal angle is delimited between two lines, one which passes through the mastoid bone and the other one runs tangential to the concha. Normal values are included between 80° and 90°. Malformations occur when this value is increased for more than 10°.
2. Scaphoconchal angle is delimited by the intersection of the conchal and the scaphal planes, which rules the angulation of the helix on the antihelix. Normal values are included between 85° and 90°. In "loop deformities" this angle may be more than 150°.
3. Cephaloauricular angle is described as the space between the mastoid bone and the posterior aspect of the auricular pavilion. Normal values are included between 20° and 30°. An increase in this angle of more than 10° causes an aesthetic deformity.

Anesthesia

A peripheral nerve block of the auricular pavilion is performed together with a direct intraconchal infiltration (Ramsay-Hunt area) with 0.5 % bupivacaine with 1:200,000 epinephrine. No sedation is required for the adult patients, whereas it is necessary for pediatric patients. The patient should be positioned in a comfortable supine position in order to facilitate the procedure.

The procedure consists of three different steps:

1. After an accurate disinfection of the area, the needle is inserted at the level of the superior otobasion and then is pushed toward the tragus. After a progressive infiltration of the local anesthetic, the needle is retracted, but not disinserted from the skin, and is pushed backward along the superior portion of the cephaloauricular sulcus, and another infiltration is performed.
2. Once the superior aspect of the pavilion is blocked, the needle is inserted at the level of the inferior otobasion and then is pushed upward along the caudal aspect of the cephaloauricular sulcus. After a progressive infiltration of the local anesthetic, the needle is retracted, but not disinserted from the skin, and is pushed forward to the tragus, and another infiltration is performed.
3. The needle is inserted directly in the Ramsay-Hunt area, and the local anesthetic is infiltrated.

The peripheral block of the auricular pavilion is easy to perform. The only trap could be represented by the accidental cannulation of the superficial temporal artery. If this happens, a fast disinsertion of the needle and a mechanical compression for at least 30 min should be performed. The infiltration must not be performed without previous aspiration, in order to check directly if the needle is positioned inside a vessel.

Surgical Technique [1]

The concept of otoplasty concerns hundreds of different techniques. This means that there is not a single standard surgical procedure. Anyway, inside this wide technical reservoir, three different groups could be defined: the "cartilage-incision" procedures, the "suture-placement" procedures, and the "combined" procedures.

Scoring of the anterior surface of the auricular cartilage represents one of the most common techniques in otoplasty. The authors have reported a further refinement to the Chong-Chet anterior scoring technique [2], which involves anterior scoring of the upper helical cartilage to correct helical radix upper prominence and prevent postoperative residual deformity. The principle is the same: the restoration of the antihelix fold by incising the cartilage trough by anterior scoring technique.

The patient is positioned in a supine fashion with the head lying on a silicone ring in order to prevent the deformation of the auricular pavilion by the weight of the skull. With pressure applied medially to the prominent helix by fingers, the ideal missing antihelical fold is created on the anterior aspect of the auricular pavilion, and then three dots are drawn on a line on the posterior auricular cartilage and skin by passing three 21 G needles dipped in methylene blue through the cartilage on an imaginary line between the helix and the future antihelix (Fig. 26.1). This line indicates the point in which the cartilage will be incised.

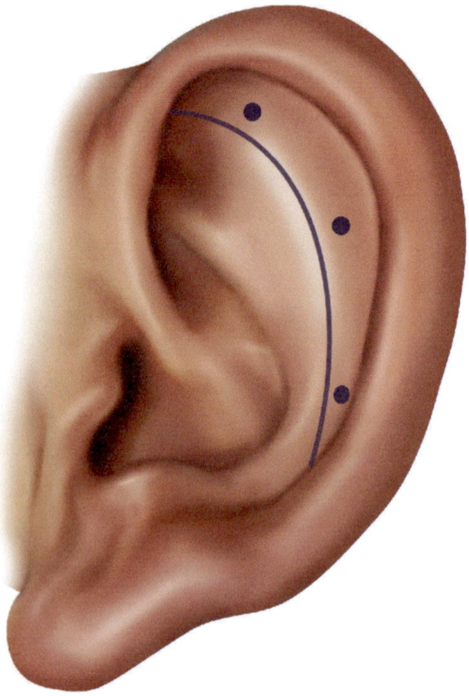

Fig. 26.1 With pressure applied medially to the prominent helix by fingers, the ideal missing antihelical fold is created on the anterior aspect of the auricular pavilion, and then three dots are drawn on a line on the posterior auricular cartilage and skin by passing three 21 G needles dipped in methylene blue through the cartilage on an imaginary line between the helix and the future antihelix

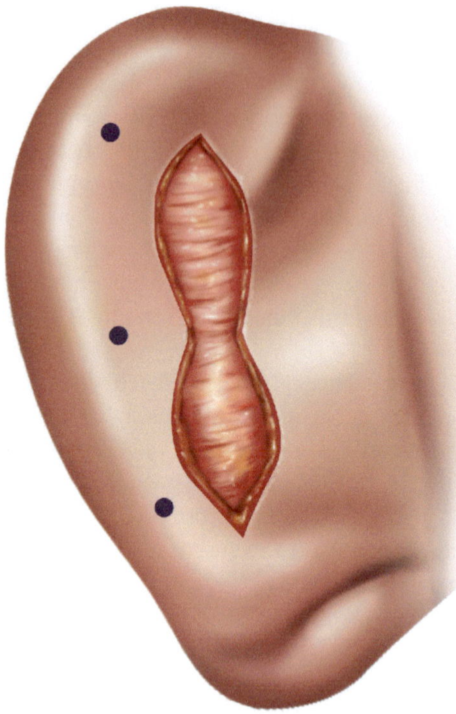

Fig. 26.2 A 3 cm clepsydra-shaped strip of skin is excised from the posterior aspect of the auricular pavilion between the free edge of the pinna and the cephaloauricular angle

A 3 cm clepsydra-shaped strip of skin is excised from the posterior aspect of the auricular pavilion between the free edge of the pinna and the cephaloauricular angle (Fig. 26.2). Soft tissues are removed also, and the underlying cartilage is exposed. Posterior undermining of the remaining soft tissues is performed in order to expose the blue dots on the cartilage (Fig. 26.3). Cartilage then is incised from the superior antihelical crus to the tail of the future antihelix. Skin and soft tissues from the anterior aspect of the pavilion are now detached from the cartilage which is rotated back after the creation of a cartilaginous flap by prolonging the incision in a conchal direction (Fig. 26.4).

The back-rotated anterior surface of the cartilage is weakened by scoring it with parallel and cross-hatched cuts; in this way the cartilage folds spontaneously (Fig. 26.5). The newly restored antihelix is then fixed by two 4/0 white Vicryl rolling sutures in its upper and lower parts (an extra suture could be placed in the middle part if necessary).

A small portion of soft tissues on the upper anterolateral aspect of the radix of the helix prominent area is undermined without cartilage exposure on a line which is a direct continuation of the neo-antihelix on the upper helix cartilage to weaken also a part of the helix curve. This area is weakened by anterior scoring in the antihelical area (Fig. 26.6). The skin closure is performed by four nonabsorbable 4/0 horizontal mattress stitches, whereas the inferior part of the skin is left not sutured for 0.5 cm of length (Fig. 26.7).

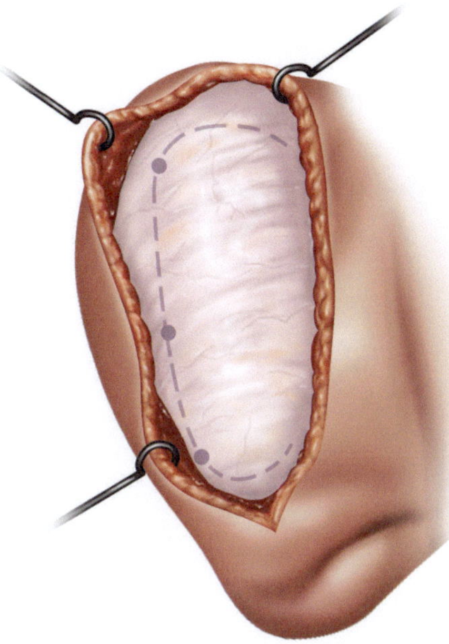

Fig. 26.3 With the soft tissues removed and the underlying cartilage exposed, posterior undermining of the remaining soft tissues is performed in order to expose the blue dots on the cartilage

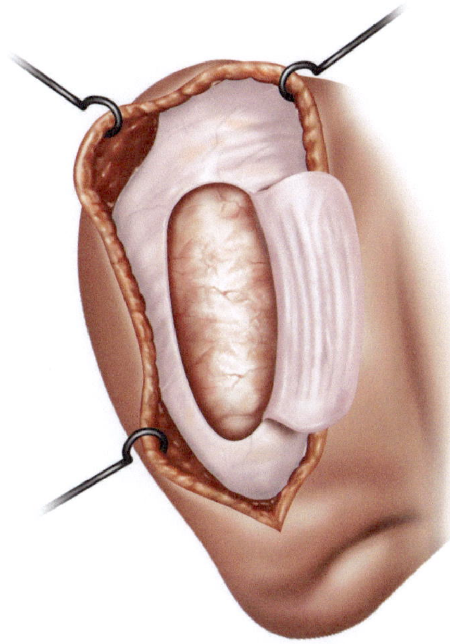

Fig. 26.4 Skin and soft tissues from the anterior aspect of the pavilion are detached from the cartilage that is rotated back after the creation of a cartilaginous flap by prolonging the incision in a conchal direction

The procedure could be bilateral or monolateral depending on the clinical case.

The ears are dressed by stuffing of the triangular fossa, concha, and scapha with nonadherent gauze, which is placed also on the suture line on the posterior aspect of the pavilion. A cotton wool piece covers both the ears, and dry gauze covers the cotton. An elastic bandage holds the dressing in place for 7 days. Early postoperative check should be performed after 3 days.

Discussion

The authors have treated 36 patients affected by prominent ears with bilateral otoplasty using anterior scoring of the upper helical cartilage. These patients were followed with regard to the final outcome (residual upper third prominence or recurrence) and occurrence of complications. An antimicrobial prophylaxis with amoxicillin and clavulanic acid was administered orally to all the patients. Follow-up was at 3, 7, and 15 days and then 3, 6, and 12 months after surgery. No postoperative complications occurred, except for physiological mild ecchymosis due to the procedure. None of the patients developed postoperative hematoma, infection, or hypertrophic scars. No residual or recurrent prominence of the ear/of the upper third or cartilage irregularities at the last follow-up control.

Elasticity and memory are most representative features of the auricular cartilage. The anterior scoring technique described by Chong-Chet in 1963 [2] alters these two characteristics and controls the degree and the final position of the antihelical fold. An 8 % of residual cartilage deformity treated with this procedure has been described in literature [3]. Intraoperative undercorrection is responsible for this kind of complication [4].

The cartilage of the upper third of pinna is likely to have more memory than the middle

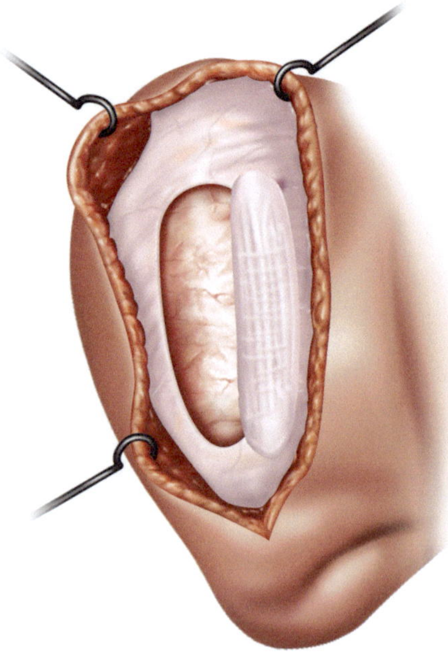

Fig. 26.5 The back-rotated anterior surface of the cartilage is weakened by scoring it with parallel and cross-hatched cuts; in this way the cartilage folds spontaneously

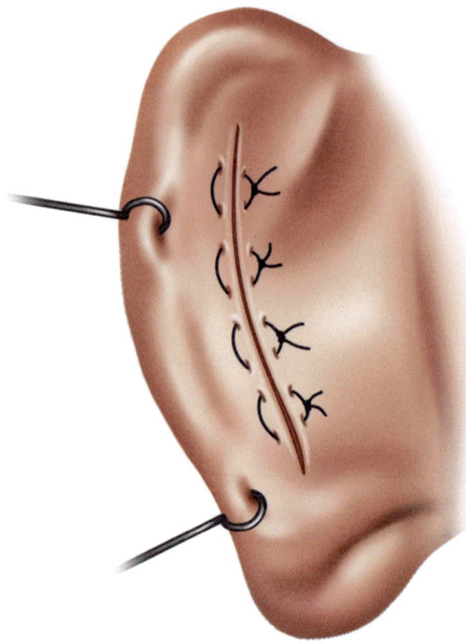

Fig. 26.7 The skin closure is performed by four nonabsorbable 4/0 horizontal mattress stitches, whereas the inferior part of the skin is left not sutured for 0.5 cm of length

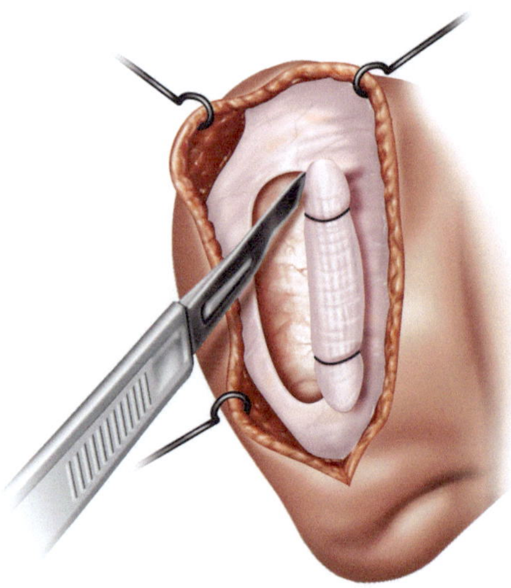

Fig. 26.6 A small portion of soft tissues on the upper anterolateral aspect of the radix of the helix prominent area is undermined without cartilage exposure on a line which is a direct continuation of the neo-antihelix on the upper helix cartilage to weaken also a part of the helix curve. This area is weakened by anterior scoring in the antihelical area

third; in fact, residual deformities are more common in the pinna than in other components of the pavilion. To prevent this late complication, the authors use the Chong-Chet modified technique [5] associated with anterior scoring of the upper helical cartilage. This means that it is necessary to cut the cartilage up to a few millimeters from the helical rim (without interrupting it) in order to harvest a cartilage flap that simulates the antihelix. This flap also reduces the height of the concha. The correction of the upper helical prominence with one or two sutures between the helix and the antihelix, as described by Mustarde [6], does not really weaken the cartilage, but it just bends the apical part of the pinna leading to a higher risk of undercorrection or recurrence of the deformity. Our refinement is based on the principles described by Gibson and Davis [7].

The authors perform anterior scoring of the radix of the helix, weakening a part of the cartilage usually left untouched by other techniques.

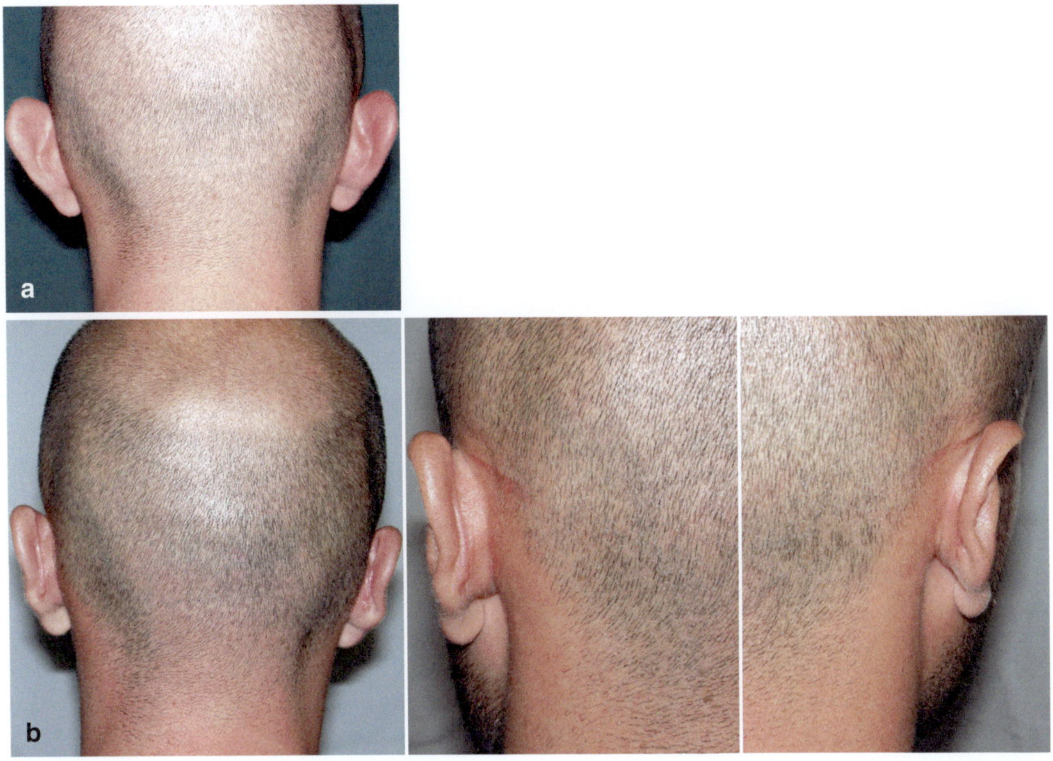

Fig. 26.8 (**a**) Preoperative. (**b**) Postoperative

This procedure leads to a complete correction of prominent ears, avoiding the suturing of the cartilage. This refinement could be used in the management of the recurrent deformities after primary correction or even in the management of deformities due to an incomplete development of the antihelix (Fig. 26.8).

Conclusions

The authors' refinement in combination with classic otoplasty techniques may prevent upper third prominence and may be useful in secondary procedures. The technique is safe, fast, and easy to perform, adding more or less 5 min to the standard procedure. It gives good and reproducible aesthetic results with no complications.

References

1. Rubino C, Farace F, Figus A, Masia DR. Anterior scoring of the upper helical cartilage as a refinement in aesthetic otoplasty. Aesthetic Plast Surg. 2005;29(2):88–93.
2. Chongchet V. A method of antihelix reconstruction. Br J Plast Surg. 1963;16:268–72.
3. Calder JC, Naasan A. Morbidity of otoplasty: a review of 562 cases. Br J Plast Surg. 1994;47(3):170–4.
4. Jeffrey SL. Complications following correction of prominent ears: an audit review of 122 cases. Br J Plast Surg. 1999;52(7):588–90.
5. Pancrazi E, Campus GV, Rubino C. Correzione delle orecchie ad ansa con la tecnica di Chongchet modificata. Riv Ital Chir Plast. 1999;31:35–9.
6. Mustarde JC. The correction of prominent ears using simple mattress sutures. Br J Plast Surg. 1963;16:170–8.
7. Gibson T, Davis WB. The distortion of autogenous cartilage graft: its cause and prevention. Br J Plast Surg. 1958;10:257–74.

Anterior Scoring Technique in Otoplasty

27

Louise Caouette-Laberge and Patricia Bortoluzzi

Introduction

Corrective otoplasty is a commonly performed procedure aiming at changing the shape of the auricular cartilage to decrease the lateral projection of the auricle (Fig. 27.1). Many techniques use anterior scoring of the cartilage to take advantage of the natural tendency of the cartilage to curl in a direction opposite to the side weakened [1–4]. The depth of the scoring varies with the thickness of the cartilage, and it has proven particularly helpful in cases where the cartilage is thick and difficult to handle with suture techniques. There are many published methods to access and score the anterior surface of the ear cartilage through an anterior or a posterior approach, ranging from a limited exposure combined with suture techniques (cartilage sparing) to a wide exposure of the anterior surface of the cartilage and scarification under direct vision. Scoring of the cartilage can be achieved with partial-thickness incisions done with a blade, a needle, toothed forceps, or even abrasion with a rasp or a burr/obrader.

L. Caouette-Laberge, M.D. (✉) • P. Bortoluzzi, M.D.
Division of Plastic Surgery, CHU Sainte-Justine,
3175, Cote Sainte-Catherine, Room 7907,
Montréal (Québec) H3T 1C5, Canada

University of Montreal,
Montréal (Québec), Canada
e-mail: caouette-laberge@umontreal.ca,
louise_laberge@ssss.gouv.qc.ca;
patricia_bortoluzzi@ssss.gouv.qc.ca

Review of Surgical Techniques

1. Combined Techniques with "Minimal Access" Anterior Cartilage Scoring. Anterior scoring or weakening of the auricular cartilage can be achieved with a limited anterior skin incision (Fig. 27.2): small incisions either in the scapha or along the edge of the helix are done where the superior crus of the antihelix is anticipated [5–8]. With these techniques, a periosteal elevator or curved scissors are inserted to create a small tunnel to allow the insertion of a rasp, an abrader, a toothed forceps, or a needle that will be used to make the scarifications to weaken the cartilage of the antihelix without direct vision. The thickness of the scarifications may be difficult to assess. Other authors [2, 5, 9–13] use a posterior skin incision and access the anterior aspect of the cartilage via an incision at the lower aspect of the ear in the antitragohelicine fissure. An elevator or scissors are then used to create the tunnel on the anterior surface of the cartilage for the scarifications (Fig. 27.3). The majority of these authors use permanent sutures with the scoring/weakening of the cartilage to maintain the desired fold of the antihelix.
2. Anterior Scoring with Wide Exposure of the Anterior Surface of the Cartilage. Erol [14] uses an anterior skin incision in the concha (Fig. 27.2). This incision serves two purposes: it allows a resection of cartilage with or without anterior skin to lower the concha, and it provides access to elevate the anterior skin/perichondrium flap on the antihelix area to facilitate the scarifications/

M.A. Shiffman (ed.), *Advanced Cosmetic Otoplasty*,
DOI 10.1007/978-3-642-35431-1_27, © Springer-Verlag Berlin Heidelberg 2013

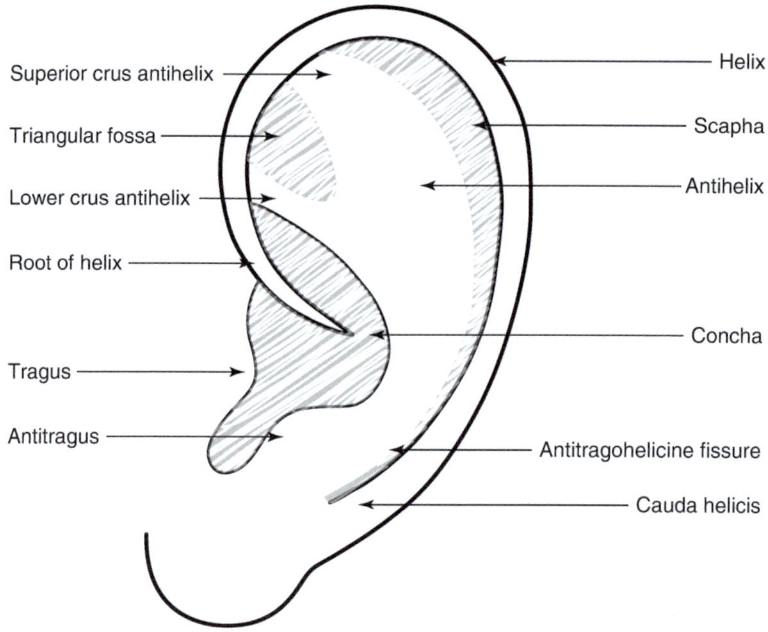

Fig. 27.1 Nomenclature of the ear components

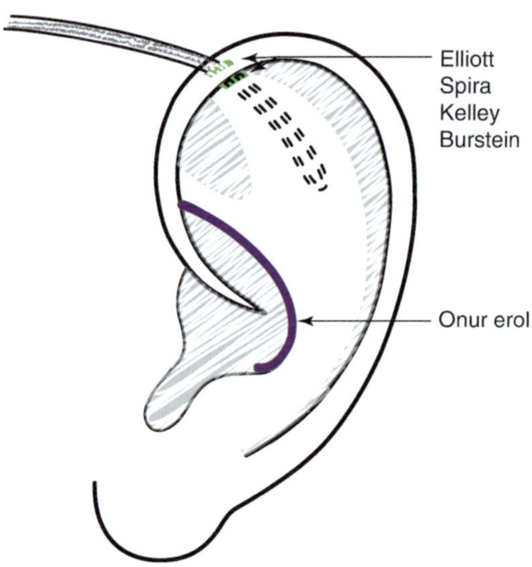

Fig. 27.2 Anterior skin incisions to access the anterior surface of the cartilage

abrasions under direct vision. More authors make a posterior skin incision combined with a transcartilaginous incision (Fig. 27.4) to gain access to the anterior surface of the ear cartilage [15–22]. The lower limit of this incision is often the antitragohelicine fissure, and it continues superiorly in the scapha, to different extents depending on the technique. Some continue this transcartilaginous incision to the superior crus of the antihelix [16, 17, 21] or to the fossa triangularis [19, 20]. Others continue to section the helix either at the level of the superior crus of the antihelix 18 or beyond at the origin of the helix [15, 22]. With these techniques, the skin with or without the perichondrium is lifted from the cartilage widely to expose the antihelix and the superior portion of the concha. The cartilage incision does not lie on the antihelical fold but rather at the periphery of the antihelix in the scapha. Partial-thickness cartilage incisions (scarifications, scoring) or abrasions (obrader, rasp) are done in a vertical or curved direction to obtain folding of the superior crus of the antihelix either unidirectionally (vertical scoring) or bidirectionally (curved scoring). Some authors add sutures to maintain the antihelix in this corrected position [20].

Author's Preferred Method

Preoperative Evaluation

Preoperatively the ear is examined from the frontal view. It is important to recognize that the distance between the auricle rim and the

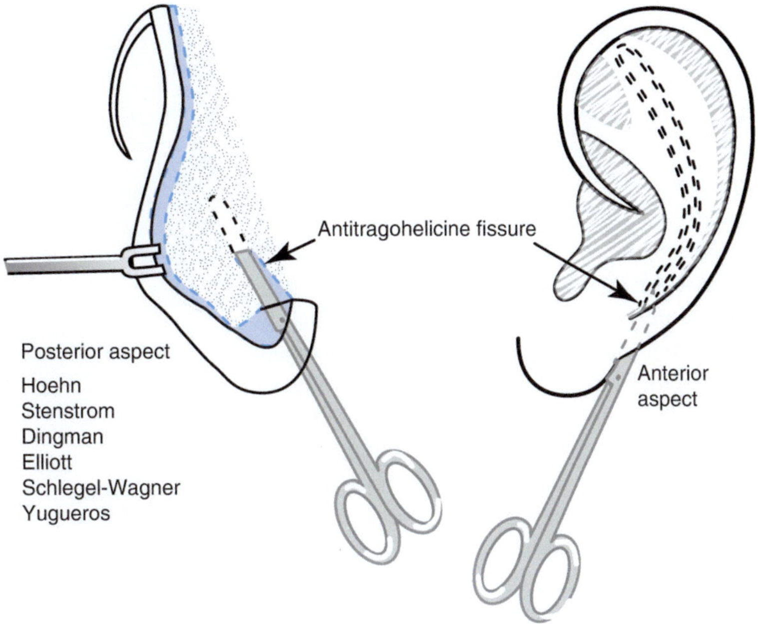

Fig. 27.3 Posterior access through the antitragohelicine fissure to the anterior surface of the cartilage

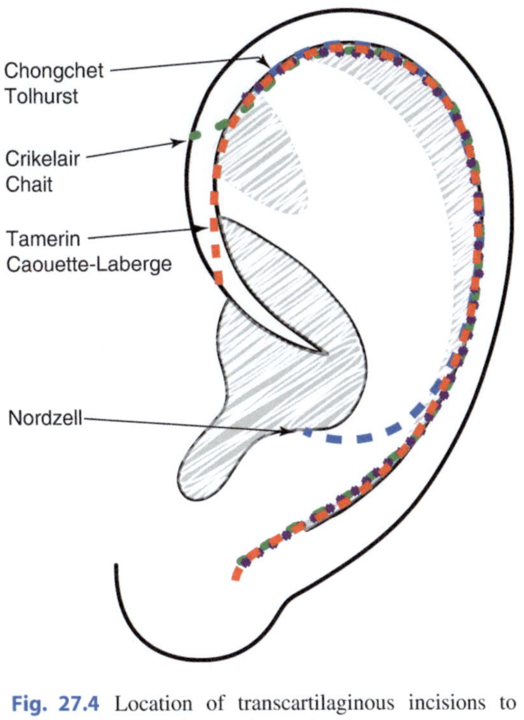

Fig. 27.4 Location of transcartilaginous incisions to expose anterior surface of the cartilage

cranium and mastoid area varies with the age of the patients. It is not uncommon to see an adult with normal projection of the auricle from the frontal view and very little retroauricular space due to a large mastoid. Another important fact is that the proportion of the ear to the face is different in 7-year-old children since the ear reaches near-normal adult size in children well before the age of 7, while the lower face matures at the end of puberty. Therefore, the ear is more noticeable in a young child, particularly if the ears are large and the face is narrow. If the shape of the ear and the frontal projection are normal, the parents should be reassured that the ear will progressively "fit" the child's face, and aggressive reduction of the lateral projection of the ear will make the child look strange as he grows older. An excellent description of the "normal ear" projection and measurements was published by Kelly et al. [7].

During the preoperative evaluation, the child is asked to stand in front of a mirror while the parents stand behind to observe the change in the shape of the ear that is proposed with the surgery. It is important that everyone understands the necessity to preserve lateral projection of the auricle, with the newly formed antihelix, the helix, and lobule on a straight line, and the middle third of the auricle as the most projecting part of the ear. Families are asked to notice the retroauricular space that is necessary to obtain normal frontal projection in a young child.

It is also a good time to point out any asymmetry in size or shape of the ears and explain what features of the ear will be corrected with the procedure and what will not (e.g., asymmetry in size). It is however more difficult to detect asymmetry after the surgery because of a lesser degree of lateral projection; both ears are not so easily visible and comparable from the frontal view. Irregularities of the helix and the presence of a Darwin's tubercle are also discussed so that the parents have realistic expectations and understand better the limitations of the procedure. Minor helical irregularities are often best left alone since they become less noticeable postoperatively when the helix is not facing anteriorly. If Darwin's tubercle is to be removed, a separate skin and cartilage resection on the helical rim is necessary. The scar is usually very discrete.

The presence of an accessory fold of the antihelix (Stahl's ear) (Fig. 27.5) produces an irregularity of the helix (unfolding) that should also be discussed as it often persists even after correction of the antihelix. It may be improved with a wedge resection of the helix at the cost of an additional scar. Constricted ears (cup ear deformities) may have a deficient or absent lower crus of the antihelix and absent fossa triangularis. Again, pointing this to the parents before the surgery will help them understand the shape of the newly formed antihelix with the deficient fossa triangularis postoperatively. It is important to recognize the presence of a preauricular sinus because the surgical technique used requires a sharp section of the root of the helix. Given the dissection in this area, the presence of a preauricular sinus and underlying cyst increases the risk of infection, and the sinus should be removed completely before undertaking the otoplasty. The authors often combine the two surgeries in the same setting but suggest that antibiotics be used in these selected cases.

The concha may also be prominent and produce a marked elevation of the middle third of the auricle. It is often due to the fact that the concha is missing the normal fold that is present where the concha meets the scapha in the middle third of the ear [6]. Finally the shape and position of the lobule is assessed. When a large bulky lobule is present, one should be particularly hesitant to lower the middle one-third of the ear because it does easily produce a more conspicuous lobule. It is also particularly important in these cases to keep the lobule at the same level than the rest of the ear, so it is not visible from the frontal view.

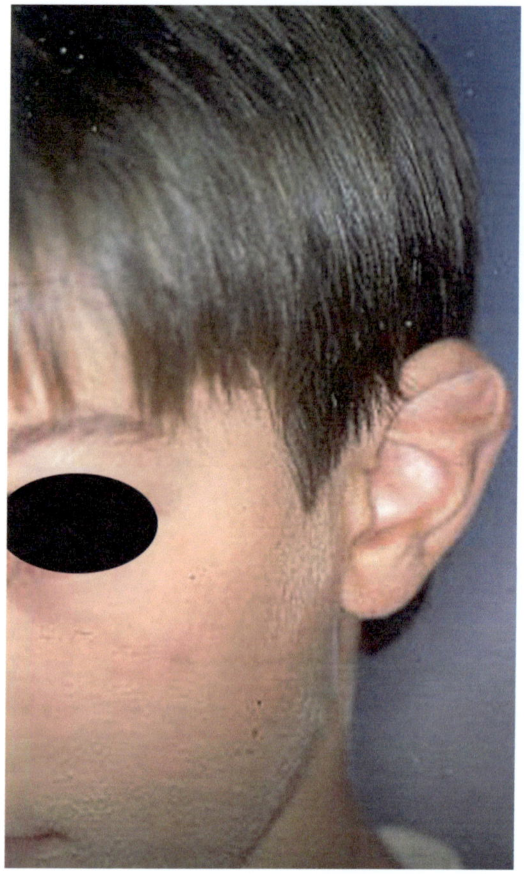

Fig. 27.5 Accessory fold of the antihelix (Stahl's ear) produces an irregularity of the helix (unfolding)

This privileged time in front of the mirror with the child and family gives the surgeon a good idea of the child's motivation and cooperation for the surgery. The procedure can be performed under local anesthesia without any sedation in a 5- or 6-year-old child who is motivated since the total duration of the procedure including anesthesia is generally under 1 h.

Surgical Technique

The parents are requested to wash the patient's hair and auricle with particular care the day before surgery. No antiseptic soap is used. The surgery is done in day surgery under local or general anesthesia as requested by the parents and depending on the cooperation of the child. Antibiotics are not given routinely. In the operating room, the face is prepped with chlorhexidine-aqueous solution, and the auricular area and scalp are prepped with Betadine except for the children done under local anesthesia where chlorhexidine-aqueous solution alone is used for all areas prepped. A head drape is placed, leaving both ears and face exposed. It is particularly important not to cover the patient's face when working under local anesthesia to keep a good contact with the patient and alleviate any potential anxiety with having the face covered. The ears are then infiltrated with Xylocaine 1 % with epinephrine 1/100,000. A total of less than 10 cc is used for both ears. The same infiltration is done whether the surgery is under local or general anesthesia. This hydrodissection (Fig. 27.6) facilitates the procedure and lessens the bleeding. A 30-gauge needle and a very slow infiltration of anesthetic are particularly helpful in children who often do not feel the needle prick but rather the tissue distension from the infiltration. A 3.5 cm posterior auricular incision is located 1 cm from the helical rim (Fig. 27.6) so that it lies in the concavity created by the antihelical fold and therefore is hidden.

No skin excision is done. It is not necessary to excise skin to control the cartilaginous correction of the auricle. Very little skin undermining is done on the posterior aspect of the ear since the skin incision lies close to the proposed transcartilaginous incision (Fig. 27.7). This lessens the risk of postoperative hematoma. The cauda helicis and the antitragohelicine fissure are located, and a transcartilaginous incision is made in the scapha, parallel to the border of the helical rim superiorly into the upper one-third of the auricle (Fig. 27.6). It can be useful to mark the location of the scapha from the anterior surface of the ear with tattoo marks that will allow easy location of the transcartilaginous incision on the posterior surface of the cartilage. Access to the anterior surface of the concha and antihelix is then provided (Fig. 27.6) by elevation of the anterior skin and perichondrium using a periosteal elevator and continued with scissors in the upper portion of the antihelix (Fig. 27.6). It is important to make this dissection deep to the perichondrium where there is a relatively avascular plane, ensuring minimal bleeding and preserving the blood supply to the skin. The use of the cautery is seldom needed. Very little dissection is required in the concha since only modest reduction of the conchal height is necessary (often no reduction is done). The incision between the helical rim cartilage and the antihelix cartilage is continued subcutaneously with scissors up to the origin of the helix maintaining a constant helical width (Fig. 27.6). The section of the origin of the helix is mandatory (Fig. 27.7) if the helical rim is to follow the posterior rotation of the antihelical fold which will be created. The helical cartilage becomes like a "handle" that can freely follow the new position of the antihelix and, because it is completely sectioned, it does not tend to "spring back" anteriorly and cause protrusion of the upper one third of the auricle.

After the section of the origin of the helical cartilage, the skin and perichondral elevation on the anterior surface of the antihelix and triangular fossa is completed the antihelical cartilage is completely exposed up to its origin (Fig. 27.6) and scarifications consisting of partial-thickness cartilage incisions (scoring) are then done with a number 15 blades (Figs. 27.7 and 27.8). The directions of these incisions are important in order to have a normal appearing "fan-shaped" antihelix that will curve both superiorly and posteriorly (Fig. 27.6). These partial-thickness incisions are bidirectional, the first following the curvature of the newly formed antihelical fold allows for the posterior curvature of the cartilage where the concha reaches the scapha and the second fan-shaped perpendicular ones that meet at the middle third of the ear, allowing for anteroposterior roundness, particularly superiorly. At the very caudal part of the newly formed antihelix, the incision is full thickness so that the cartilage can be folded sharply upon itself at the appropriately chosen conchal height (Figs. 27.6 and 27.8). This can effectively correct any conchal excess. Care should be taken to avoid lowering excessively the height of the concha at

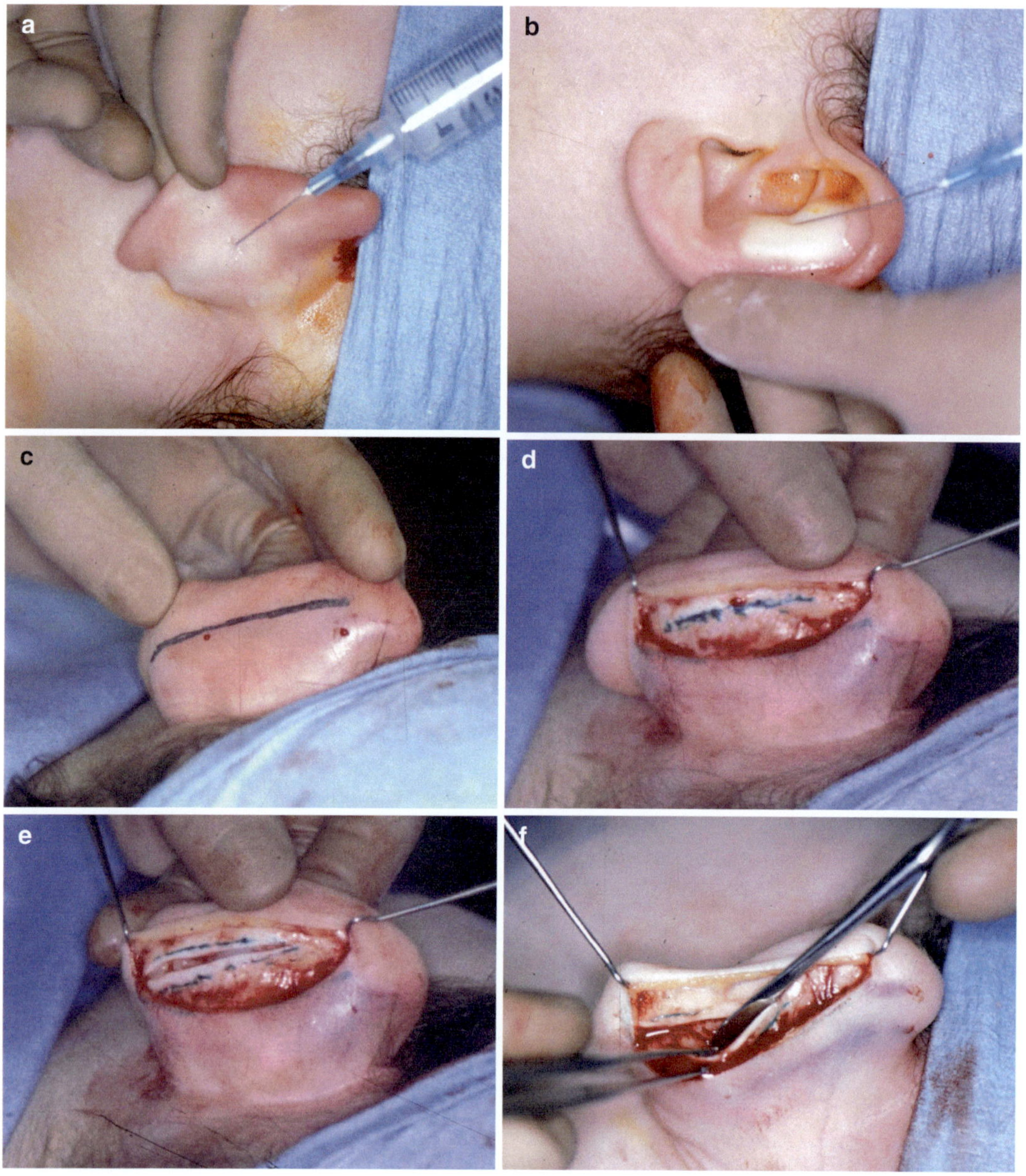

Fig. 27.6 Operative procedure: (**a**, **b**) Hydrodissection. (**c**) 3.5 cm posterior auricular incision. (**d**, **e**) The cauda helicis and the antitragohelicine fissure are located, and a transcartilaginous incision is made in the scapha, parallel to the border of the helical rim superiorly into the upper one-third of the auricle. (**f**) Access to the anterior surface of the concha and antihelix is then provided. (**g**, **h**, **i**) Access to the anterior surface of the concha and antihelix is then provided. (**j**, **k**, **l**) The incision between the helical rim cartilage and the antihelix cartilage is continued subcutaneously with scissors up to the origin of the helix maintaining a constant helical width. (**m**) The antihelical cartilage is completely exposed up to its origin. (**n**) The directions of the incisions are important in order to have a normal appearing "fan-shaped" antihelix that will curve both superiorly and posteriorly. (**o**) At the very caudal part of the newly formed antihelix, the incision is full thickness so that the cartilage can be folded sharply upon itself at the appropriately chosen conchal height. (**p**, **q**) Two sutures of 5-0 plain catgut are used to keep the sharp fold of the caudal end of the new antihelix and to insure a smooth cartilage shape in this area where the overlying skin is particularly thin and any cartilage irregularity will be noticeable. (**r**) The lobule's position is controlled by fixing the cartilage of the cauda helicis posteriorly behind the conchal cartilage. (**s**) The skin is then closed with a running horizontal mattress 5-0 plain catgut. (**t**) The skin is carefully molded on the cartilage framework, and a 5-0 plain gut suture is inserted percutaneously from the fossa triangularis to the scapha to prevent any anterior displacement of the helical rim. (**u**) Dressing is then applied, starting with one thin gauze covered with Xeroform dressing in the posterior auricular sulcus. (**v**) A moistened elongated gauze is placed to conform the concha, fossa triangularis, and scapha. (**w**) Fluffed and Kling gauze complete the dressing. (**x**) Fluffed and Kling gauze is usually left in place for 7–10 days

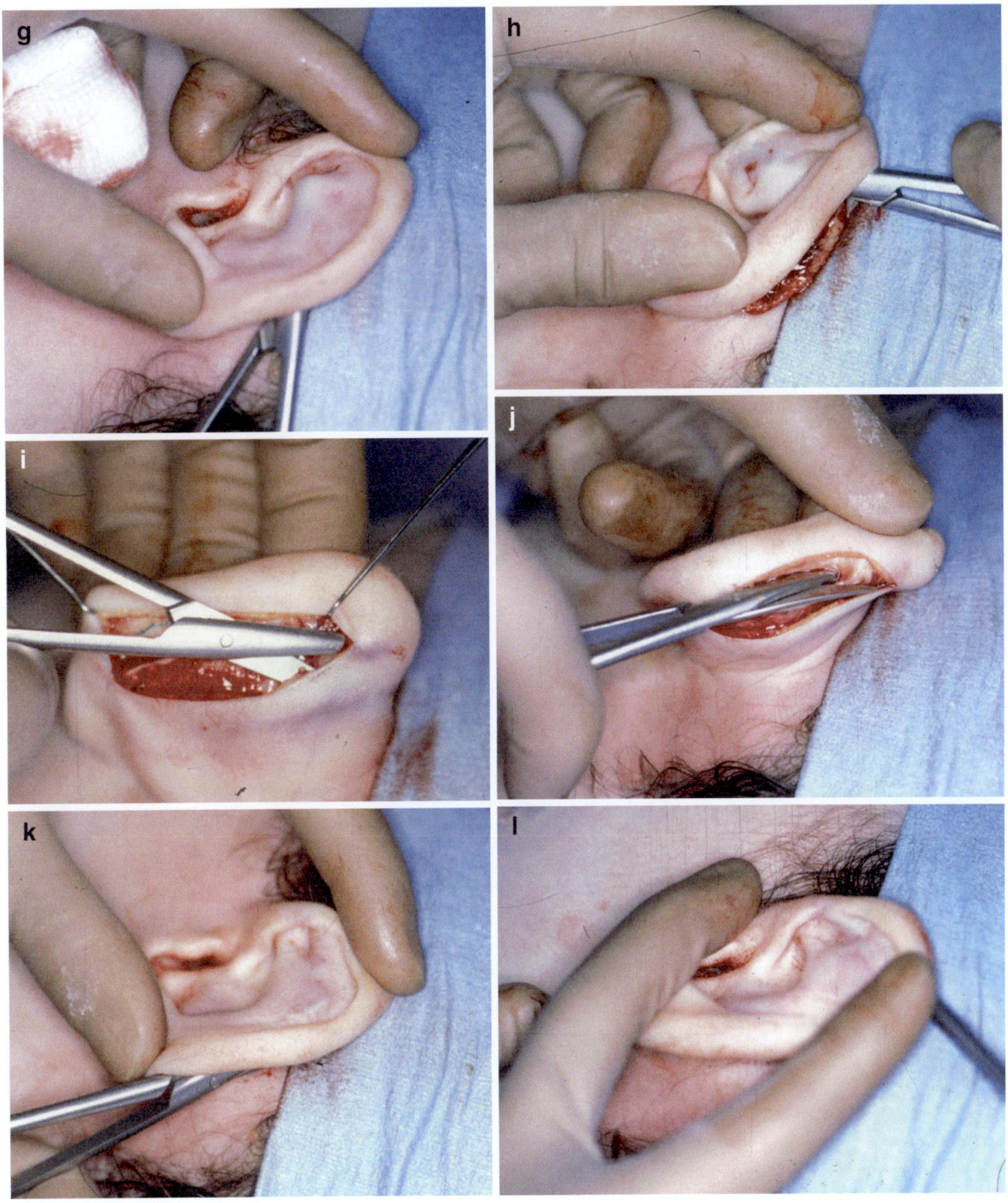

Fig. 27.6 (continued)

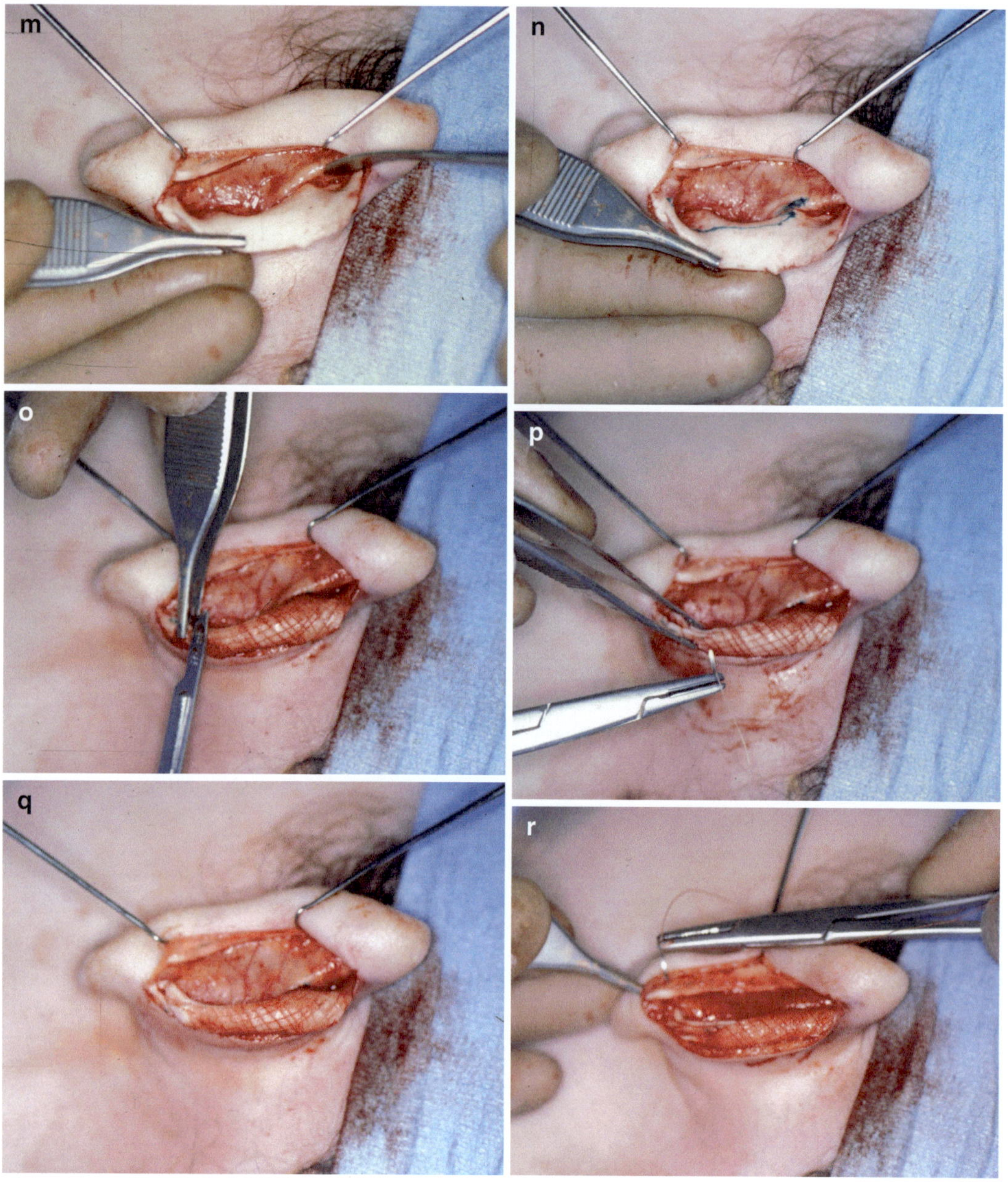

Fig. 27.6 (continued)

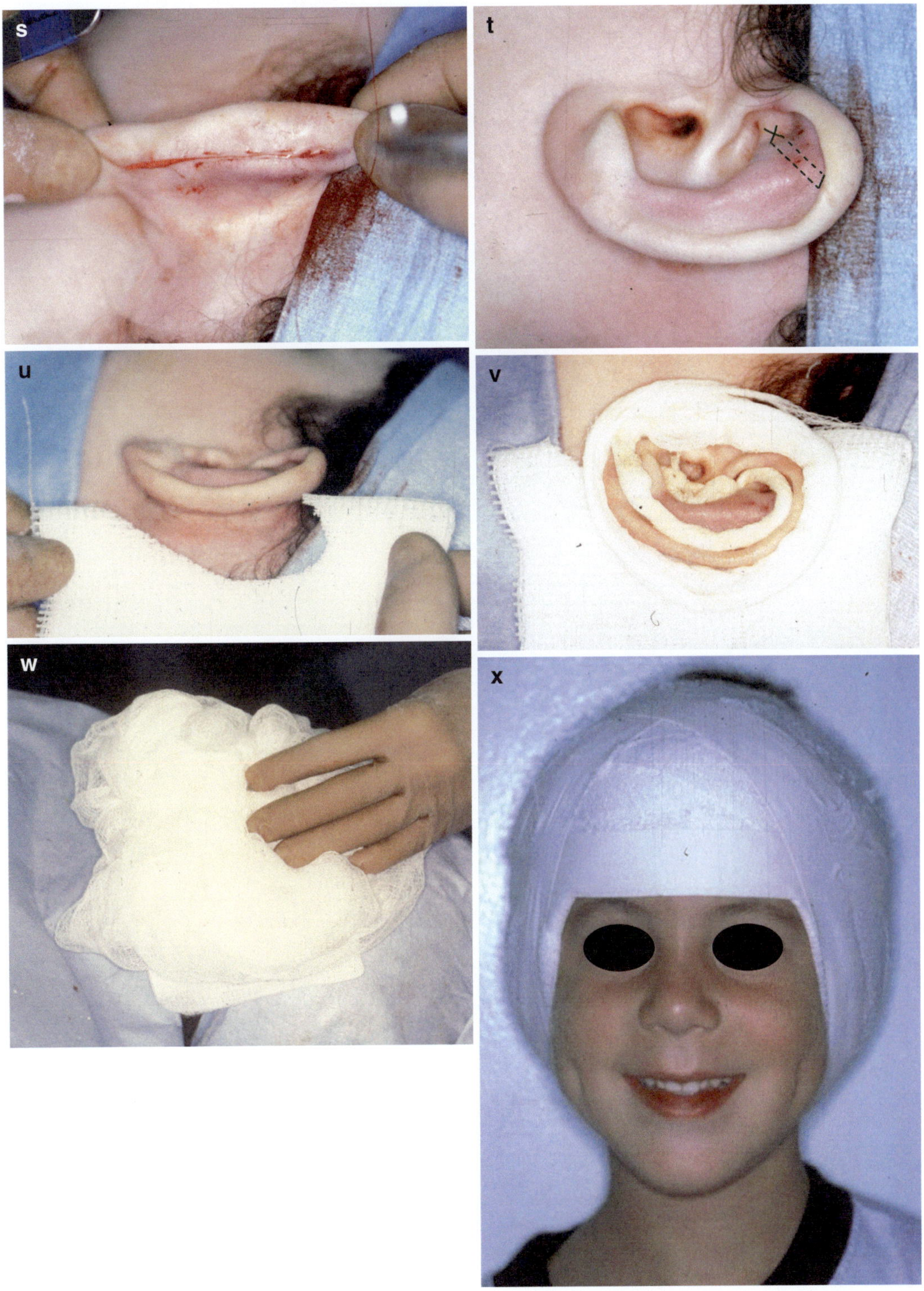

Fig. 27.6 (continued)

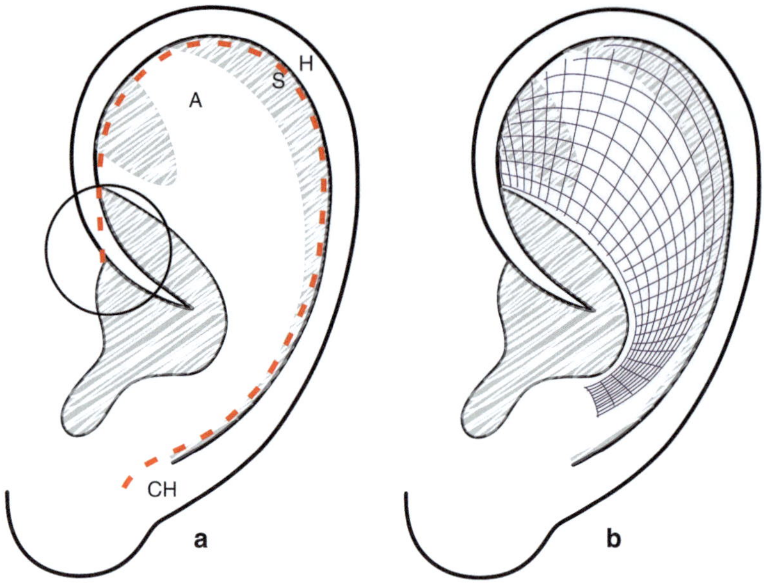

Fig. 27.7 (**a**) Location of transcartilaginous incision (*red dotted line*) *H* helix, *S* scapha, *A* antihelix, *CH* cauda helicis (encircled section of the root of helix). (**b**) Orientation of the partial-thickness scoring incisions on the anterior aspect of the auricular cartilage

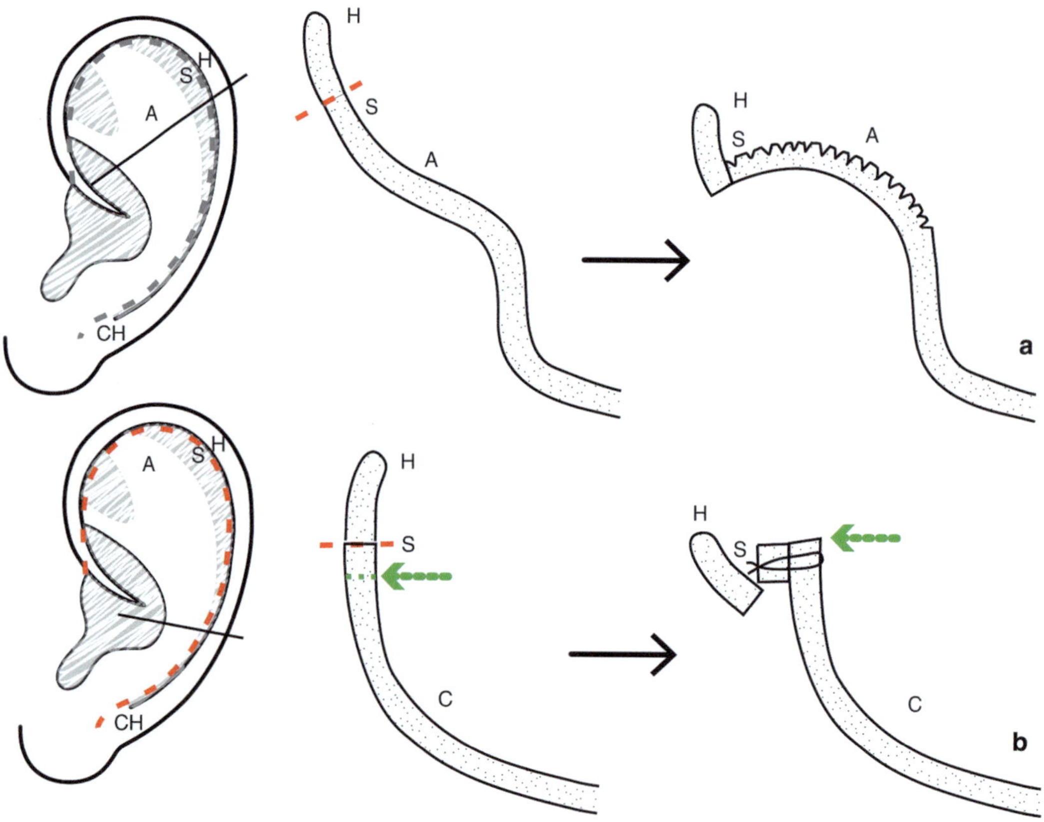

Fig. 27.8 (**a**) Upper third: partial-thickness cartilage scoring creating a regular antihelical fold. (**b**) Sharp fold of cartilage (*green arrow*) at the junction of antihelix and scapha. *A* antihelix, *CH* cauda helicis, *H* helix, *S* scapha with cartilage section

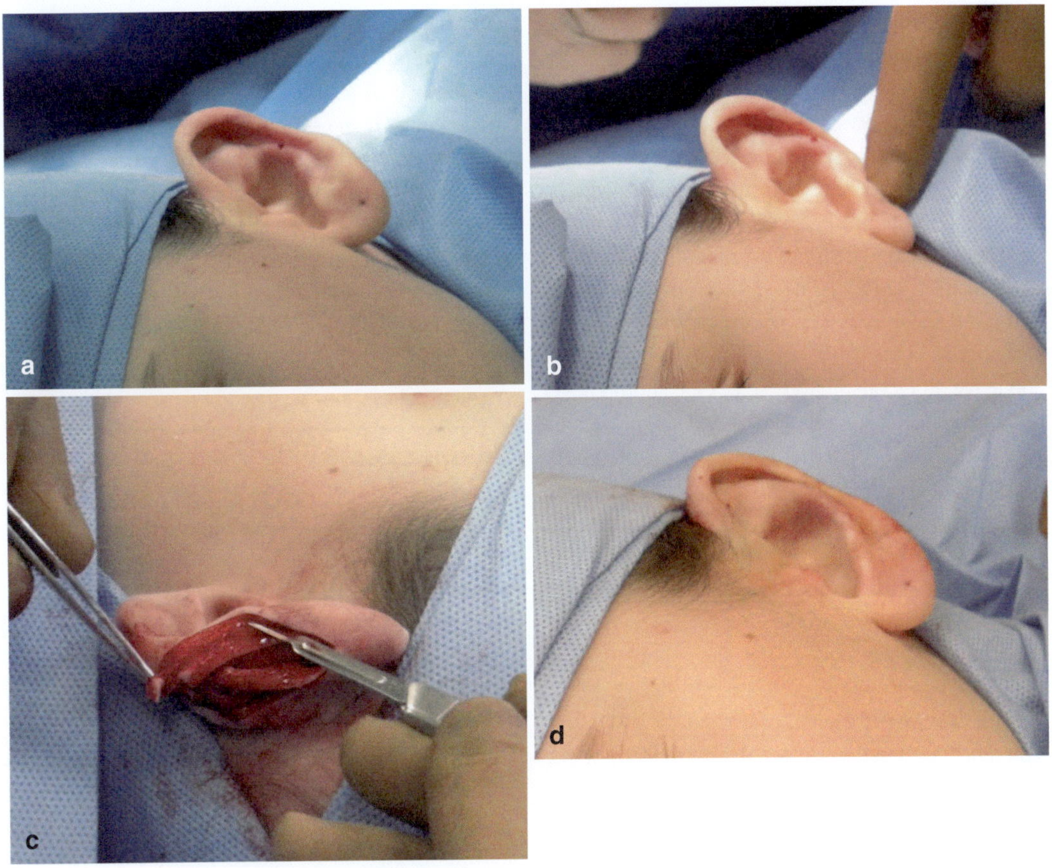

Fig. 27.9 (**a**) C-shaped helix with upper and lower third prominence. (**b**) Lowered cauda helicis behind the concha (upper third prominence). (**c**) A 3 mm closing wedge of cartilage is resected immediately above cauda helicis. (**d**) Resulting straight helix

this point. Once these cartilaginous incisions are done, the cartilage should stay in the desired position without the help of any suture material since its natural elasticity and intrinsic memory have been overcome. Two sutures of 5-0 plain catgut (Fig. 27.6) are used to keep the sharp fold of the caudal end of the new antihelix and to insure a smooth cartilage shape in this area where the overlying skin is particularly thin and any cartilage irregularity will be noticeable. When necessary, the antitragus can easily be exposed and lowered. The helical rim and anterior skin flap are then returned to their original position, and the projection of the lobule is examined. The lobule is prominent in most cases. Its position is controlled by fixing the cartilage of the cauda helicis (Fig. 27.6) posteriorly behind the conchal cartilage. A limited undermining of the skin is done on the anterior aspect of the cauda helicis to preserve the contact between the cauda helicis and the anterior lobule skin. The posterior aspect of the concha is exposed, and a 5-0 plain catgut suture is used to secure the cauda helicis to the conchal cartilage producing a posterior and superior transposition of the cauda helicis. It is not necessary to place a nonresorbable suture. Occasionally, in constricted ears with a small helical circumference, it is necessary to use a suture that will be retained longer, such as a 5-0 Maxon (Davis & Geck). One notices at this point that the more prominent lobule being set back tends to produce an elevation of the upper one-third of the helical cartilage (i.e., with one structure in continuity, lowering one end will elevate the other) (Fig. 27.9). When this is the case, it is necessary to interrupt the continuity of the helical cartilage. This is done by removing a 2–3 mm closing wedge of cartilage immediately above the cauda helicis (Fig. 27.9) where the anterior skin is thickened with subcutaneous tissue. This discontinuity in the inferior helix allows posterior and superior positioning of the lobule without elevation of the rest of the helix giving a harmonious redraping of the helix around the antihelix (Fig. 27.9). The skin is then closed with a running horizontal mattress 5-0 plain catgut (Fig. 27.6). No skin is excised. Although there may be an apparent skin excess particularly in the lower third, it will rapidly flatten and leave an inconspicuous scar. One should never rely on skin to correct the ear shape. Skin excision in an attempt to correct inadequate cartilaginous remodeling will only lead to recurrent deformity. At the completion of the procedure, the skin is carefully molded on the cartilage framework, and a 5-0 plain gut suture is inserted percutaneously from the fossa triangularis to the scapha to prevent any anterior displacement of the helical rim (Fig. 27.6).

The dressing is then applied, starting with one thin gauze covered with Xeroform dressing in the posterior auricular sulcus (Fig. 27.6) and one moistened elongated gauze to conform the concha, fossa triangularis, and scapha (Fig. 27.6). Care is taken to ensure that this conforming gauze does not cross any auricular prominences but remains in the depths of the new concha and scapha so as not to cause any pressure wounds on the vulnerable undermined skin. Fluffed and Kling gauze complete the dressing (Fig. 27.6), which is usually left in place for 7–10 days (Fig. 27.6). Routine analgesics (acetaminophen and codeine) are used only during the first 12–24 h. The parents are advised to return for evaluation should the pain require any medication after this time. Complications such as hematoma, infection, or necrosis can be diagnosed early when unusual pain is present, and the dressing is then removed for early ear inspection. The parents are also advised to return should the dressing be displaced.

The dressing is removed 7–10 days after the surgery, and parents are requested to wash the hair and auricle. Antibiotic ointment is placed on the remaining resorbable 5-0 plain gut sutures daily for 1 week, and the parents are instructed to rub off the sutures to help dissolution. No dressing or headband is used after dressing removal, but the use of a nightcap, often the Lycra swimming caps, is recommended for a week. Some ecchymosis and edema may be present for the following week, and definitive result is usually obtained after 3 months (Fig. 27.10). Sports including swimming are permitted after dressing removal with the exception of contact sports. Helmet protection is then suggested.

Complications

Five hundred cases were operated on with this technique [22] and evaluated to assess the complication rates. When compared with other series, the complication rates were similar or lower in our study. The early complications were bleeding (2.6 %) and hematoma (0.4 %). There were no infections or ear necrosis. A 2–3 mm cutaneous wound was present on the anterior skin in three patients (0.6 %), and there was one wound dehiscence (0.2 %). Late complications were keloids in two cases and inclusion cysts in three cases. Residual deformity was noted in 22 cases (4 %) and asymmetry in 28 cases (5.6 %). Secondary surgery was performed in six cases. A long-term follow-up was obtained through a questionnaire answered by 77.4 % of the patients 2–5 years after the surgery. The satisfaction rate was 94.8 % even if 18.4 % of the patients were able to see some degree of residual asymmetry. Some patients (7.5 %) found the ear more sensitive to touch or cold, while 3.9 % found their ear less sensitive to touch. No permanent sutures are used with this technique since the natural elasticity of the cartilage has been overcome. This inherently eliminates any risks of chronic sinuses or loss of correction as previously reported with permanent suture techniques [23–30]. There is no need for overcorrection since there is no relapse as may happen after a suture correction technique [24]. This technique also has the advantage of giving access to all areas of the ear and therefore can be used for many different forms of ear anomalies.

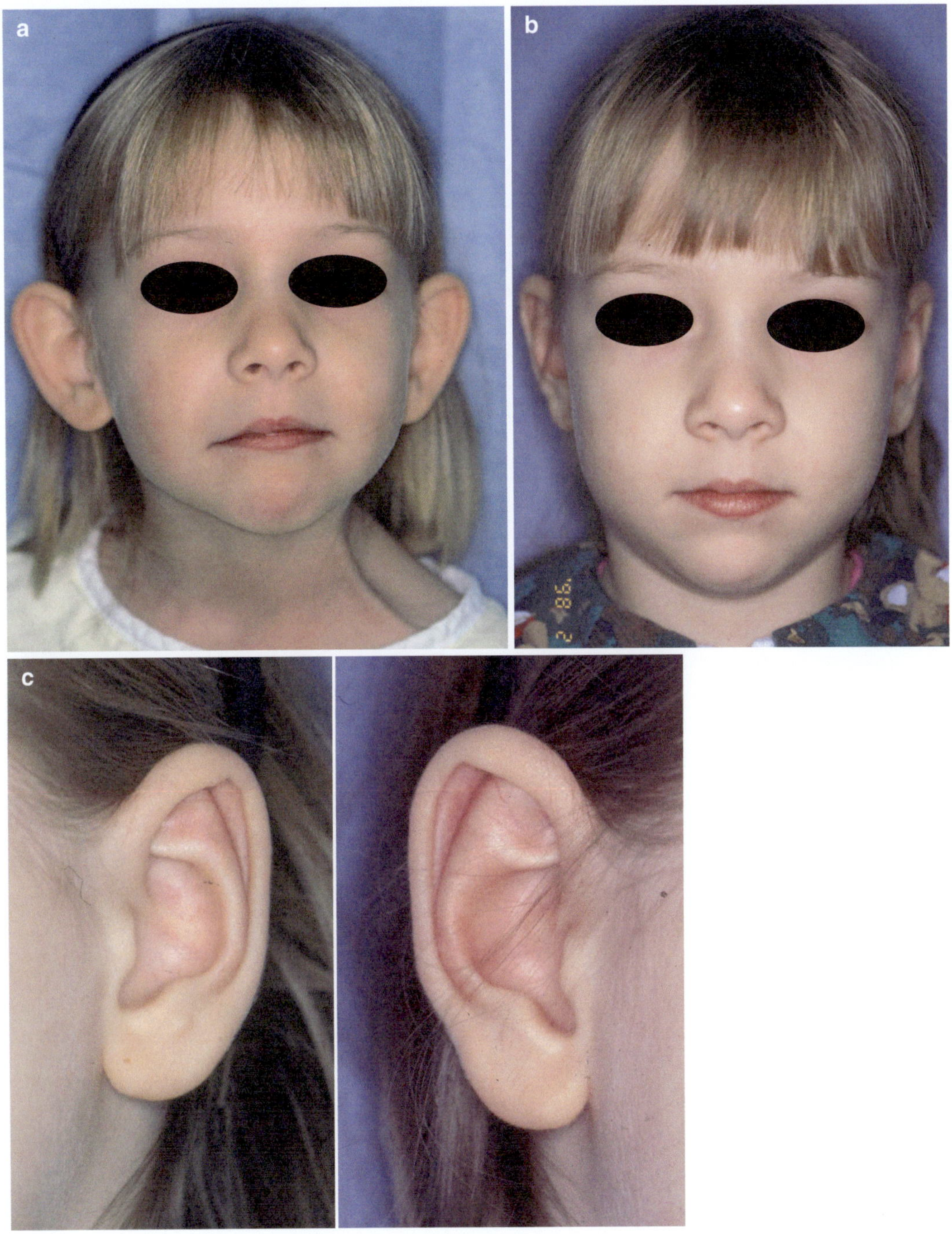

Fig. 27.10 (**a**) Preoperative. (**b**, **c**) Postoperative

Avoidable Technical Pitfalls in Otoplasty

Prominent Upper Third (Helix)

This deformity can occur if the section of the root of the helix (Fig. 27.7) is not complete so that helix can freely follow the antihelical fold. Rubino [31] does not section the root of the helix as we propose but rather makes scarifications on the helical cartilage at this level. Calder [17] cautions against a section of the helix because of the risk of producing a pointed squared ear; this can be seen if the helix is sectioned at the level of the superior crus of the antihelix, but not when the section is done at the level of the root of the helix as in our technique. Some authors correct the prominent upper third by adding a suture from the root of the helix to the temporalis fascia (Hatch suture) [7, 32] through the posterior incision or another incision at the root of helix.

Another reason to have a prominent upper third is a misplaced transcartilaginous incision that leaves a wide rim of cartilage on the helix and too little cartilage to create the normal antihelix [17]. In so doing, the superior crus of the newly created antihelix is too small to make a complete fold, and the wide cartilage of the antihelix cannot hold posteriorly since the antihelical fold is deficient (Fig. 27.11). To correct this deformity, a strip of cartilage has to be removed from the helix and sutured to the antihelix to restore the normal anatomy.

It is also possible to see a protruding upper third due to an anterior dislocation of the helical cartilage (Fig. 27.11). To prevent this deformity we now

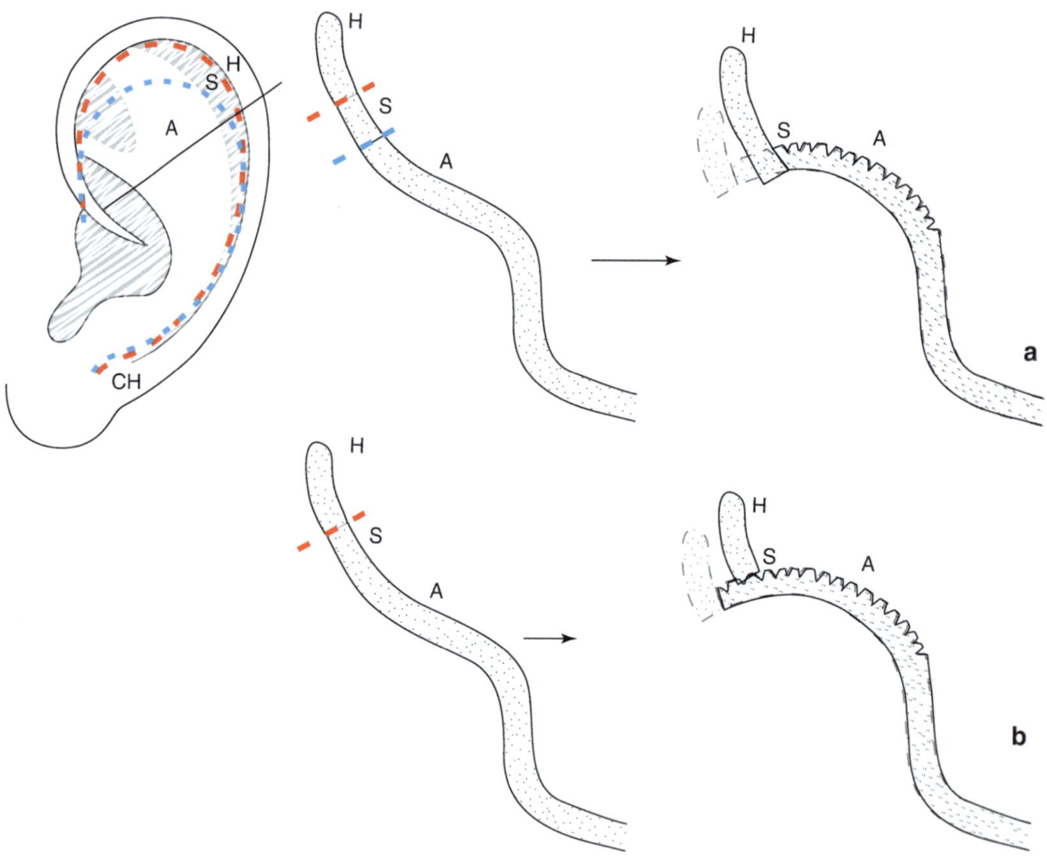

Fig. 27.11 Prominent upper third. (**a**) Transcartilaginous incision located too low (*blue dotted line*) below the scapha, remaining antihelix too narrow for complete curve and helix too wide and prominent. (**b**) Helix anterior dislocation: faulty repositioning of helix (*orange dotted lines*) at the completion of the procedure. *A* antihelix, *H* helix, *S* scapha

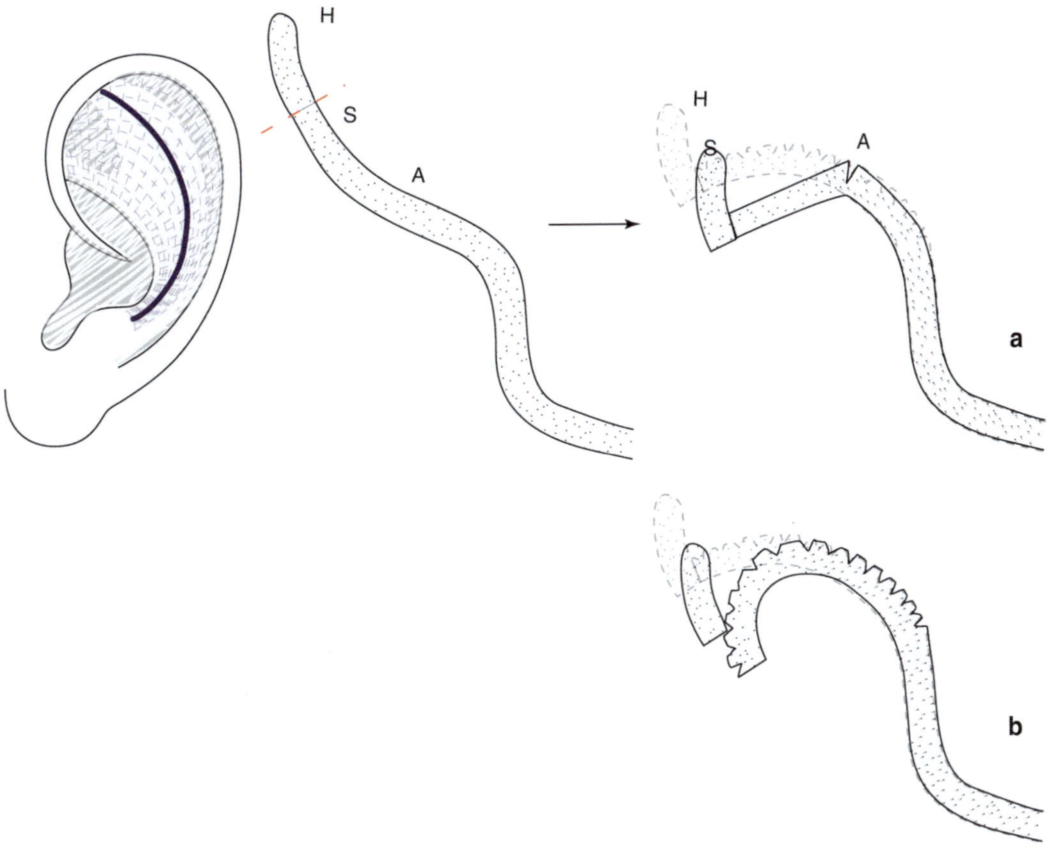

Fig. 27.12 Narrow ear. (**a**) Sharp fold of antihelix. (**b**) Excessive folding of antihelix reducing the transverse diameter of the ear

routinely use a percutaneous 5-0 plain gut suture from the triangular fossa to the scapha (Fig. 27.6). If present, the deformity can be corrected by repositioning the helix and fixing it behind the antihelix as suggested by Nordzell [21].

Narrow Ear

Reduction of the width of the auricle can be seen when the scarifications or abrasions of the newly constructed antihelix are too deep and create a sharp fold rather than the normal fan-shaped appearance of the antihelix (Fig. 27.12). It can also be seen if the curl of the antihelical cartilage is exaggerated (Fig. 27.12). The same problem may occur if too much skin has been excised from the posterior incision or when the sutures used to obtain the antihelical fold are too tight. This deformity is not easily corrected since expanding a constricted fold is difficult. Some authors suggest the addition of a mastoid fascia flap or cartilage graft [33] interposed on the posterior surface of the antihelix to widen the constricted antihelical fold. If there is also a shortage of retroauricular skin, a full thickness skin graft or mastoid skin advancement flap can be done.

Vertical Antihelical Fold

The superior crus of the antihelix should curve anteriorly to obtain a normal folding of the auricle in two planes bringing the superior third closer to the temporal area and the middle third closer to the mastoid area. When only the vertical portion of the antihelical fold is done, with sutures or with scoring, it creates an unnatural appearance

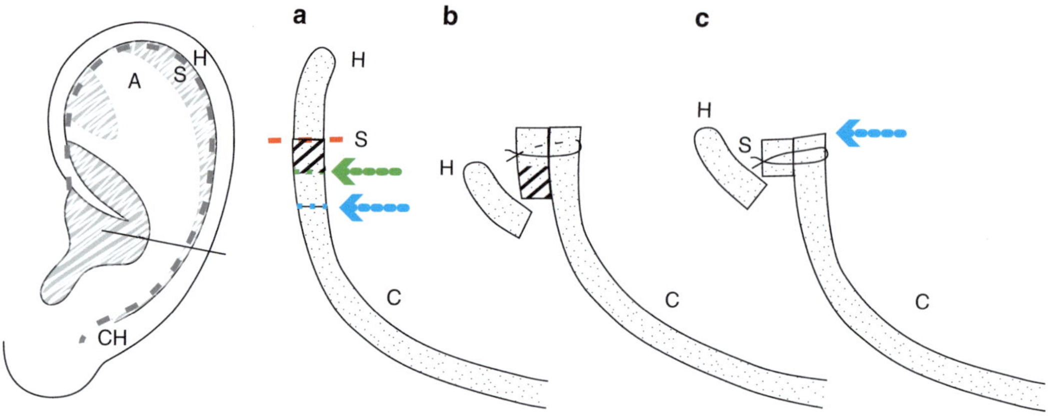

Fig. 27.13 Disappearing helix. (**a**) Location of the sharp fold of cartilage to lower concha (*blue dotted arrow*). (**b**) Wide strip of cartilage folded behind the concha causing a low position of the helix (disappearing helix). Cartilage to be resected (*green arrow and striations*). (**c**) Position of helical rim after cartilage resection

of the ear from the frontal view with protruding upper third away from the temporal area exposing this anomalous "vertical post" shape and evident triangular fossa.

Disappearing Helix

Although some authors state that the helical rim should always be visible from the frontal view, it is normal to find that the helix slowly disappears from the frontal view in the middle third of the ear. However, the position of the helix should not be too far behind the antihelix creating a deep scapha in the middle third. To avoid this deformity, the cartilage folded on itself to set the height of the concha can be trimmed to reduce the height of the scapha and the location of the helical rim (Fig. 27.13). Aggressive retroauricular skin excision can also produce a posterior displacement of the helix. The authors prefer not to remove any skin during the otoplasty; it is not necessary when the shape of the cartilage has been corrected.

Irregular Helix

The "buckled" helix is a well-documented complication of suture technique corrections [5]. It can also happen in techniques where the helix is completely freed from the antihelix since there is a risk of weakening of the helical cartilage and creation of irregularities (or waves, sharp angles) of the helical cartilage. It is particularly true in young children with thin pliable cartilage, and caution should be taken to preserve enough width of helical cartilage, particularly in the presence of a narrow area seen preoperatively. One should also resist the temptation to reduce the size of a large ear by excising a strip of cartilage at the periphery of the antihelix. When the antihelix is significantly reduced in diameter, the helical rim becomes too wide to fit the reduced antihelix. It loses its normal support and can easily become irregular. To correct this problem, an excision of a wedge of the helical rim (skin and cartilage) can be done.

Prominent Lobule/C-Shaped Helix

The authors agree with many authors [5, 24, 34–36] that the key to the position of the lobule is the cartilage of the cauda helicis as long as the attachment to the anterior skin flap is maintained. The tail of the cauda helicis is transposed posteriorly and superiorly and fixed behind the concha cartilage. This creates a posterior rotation of the lobule to place it in a straight line with the rest of the auricle. It is important to observe the shape of the helix preoperatively to predict the location of the lobule after correction of the antihelix. When the helix has a C-shape facing anteriorly, it is natural that after the antihelical fold is created and the ear faces laterally, the C-shaped helix will face laterally with protrusion of the upper third and the lobule. As the correction of the protrusion of the upper third is obtained (see above), the protrusion of the lower third (the lobule) will only be more prominent since it is one structure in continuity. To be able to correct this C-shaped helix, we recommend excising a small wedge of helix, immediately above the cauda helicis fixed behind the concha. This closing wedge will allow maintenance of the lowering of both the upper and lower portions of the ear simultaneously (Fig. 27.9).

Conclusions

Anterior scoring of the auricular cartilage in otoplasty has been used for many decades to create the antihelical fold. The technique the authors use provides a wide exposure of the anterior surface of the auricular cartilage to weaken and remodel the cartilage so as to produce a smooth regular antihelical fold without the addition of any permanent sutures. It also provides a simultaneous correction of the height of the concha. The position of the helix is corrected by a subcutaneous section of the root of the helix to control the prominence of the upper third, and the cauda helicis is fixed behind the concha to correct the position of the lobule. It is a versatile technique that can be used to correct many ear deformities since every part of the auricle is accessible. Long-term follow-up shows that the correction obtained is stable. The duration of the procedure is generally less than 1 h, and it can be performed under local anesthesia in children as young as 5 years of age.

References

1. Gibson T, Davis WB. The distortion of autogenous cartilage graft: its cause and prevention. Br J Plast Surg. 1958;10:257–74.
2. Stenströem SJ. A "natural" technique for correction of congenitally prominent ears. Plast Reconstr Surg. 1963;32:509–18.
3. Hagerty TA, Barone EJ, Cohen IK. Endoscopic otoplasty in the rabbit model: effect of mechanical abrasion on ear cartilage deformation. Plast Reconstr Surg. 1998;101(2):487–93.
4. Weinzweig N, Chen L, Walter GS. Histomorphology of neochodrogenesis after antihelical fold creation: a comparison of three otoplasty techniques in the rabbit. Ann Plast Surg. 1994;33(4):371–6.
5. Elliott Jr RA. Complications in the treatment of prominent ears. Clin Plast Surg. 1978;5(3):479–90.
6. Burstein FD. Cartilage-sparing complete otoplasty technique: a 10-year experience in 100 patients. J Craniofac Surg. 2003;14(4):521–5.
7. Kelley P, Hollier L, Stal S. Otoplasty: evaluation, technique and review. J Craniofac Surg. 2003;14(5):643–53.
8. Spira M. Otoplasty: what I do now- a 30-year perspective. Plast Reconstr Surg. 1999;104(3):834–40.
9. Wright WK. Otoplasty goals and principles. Arch Otolaryngol Head Neck Surg. 1970;92(6):568–72.
10. Dingman RO, Peled I. Corrective cosmetic otoplasty: a simple and accurate technique. Ann Plast Surg. 1979;3(3):250–2.
11. Hoehn JG, Ashruf S. Otoplasty: sequencing the operation for improved results. Plast Reconstr Surg. 2005; 115(1):5e–16.
12. Schlegel-Wagner C, Pabst G, Müller W, Linder T. Otoplasty using a modified anterior scoring technique :standardized measurements of long-term results. Arch Facial Plast Surg. 2010;12(3):143–8.
13. Yugueros P, Friedland JA. Otoplasty: the experience of 100 consecutive patients. Plast Reconstr Surg. 2001;108(4):1045–51.
14. Erol OO. New modification in otoplasty: anterior approach. Plast Reconstr Surg. 2001;107(1):193–202.
15. Tamerin JA, Mirehouse O. Reconstruction of the antihelix and scapha in selected cases of protruding ears. Arch Otolaryngol Head Neck Surg. 1959;70:597–606.
16. Chongchet V. A method of antihelix reconstruction. Br J Plast Surg. 1963;16:268–72.
17. Calder JC, Naasan A. Morbidity of otoplasty: a review of 562 consecutive cases. Br J Plast Surg. 1994;47(3): 170–4.
18. Tolhurst DE. The correction of prominent ears. Br J Plast Surg. 1972;25(3):261–5.
19. Crikelair GF, Cosman B. Another solution for the problem of the prominent ear. Ann Surg. 1964;160: 314–24.
20. Chait L, Nicholson R. One size fits all: a surgical technique for the correction of all types of prominent ears. Plast Reconstr Surg. 1999;104(1):190–5.
21. Nordzell B. Open otoplasty. Plast Reconstr Surg. 2000;106(7):1466–72.
22. Caouette-Laberge L, Guay N, Bortoluzzi P, Belleville C. Otoplasty: anterior scoring technique and results in 500 cases. Plast Reconstr Surg. 2000;105(2):504–15.
23. Adamson PA. Complications of otoplasty. Ear Nose Throat J. 1985;64(12):568–74.
24. Adamson PA, McGraw BL, Tropper GJ. Otoplasty: critical review of clinical results. Laryngoscope. 1991;101(8):883–8.

25. Adamson PA, Strecker HD. Otoplasty techniques. Facial Plast Surg. 1995;11(4):284–300.
26. Feuerstein SS. Revision techniques in otoplasty. Evaluation and management. Otolaryngol Clin North Am. 1974;7(1):133–44.
27. Mustarde JC. The correction of prominent ears using simple mattress sutures. Br J Plast Surg. 1963;16:170–8.
28. Furnas DW. Complications of surgery of the external ear. Clin Plast Surg. 1990;17(2):305–18.
29. Goode RL, Proffitt SD, Rafaty FM. Complications of otoplasty. Arch Otolaryngol Head Neck Surg. 1970;91(4): 352–5.
30. Weerda H, Siegert R. Complications in otoplastic surgery and their treatment. Facial Plast Surg. 1994; 10(3):287–97.
31. Rubino C, Farace F, Figus A, Masia DR. Anterior scoring of the upper helical cartilage as a refinement in aesthetic otoplasty. Aesthetic Plast Surg. 2005;29(2): 88–93.
32. Sénéchal B, Chauffeté JP, Sénéchal G. Complications et échecs des otoplasties. Ann Otol Rhinol Laryngol. 1983;100(7):493–8.
33. Widgerow AD. Revision otoplasty: the contracted antihelical fold. Plast Reconstr Surg. 2002;110(3):827–30.
34. Webster GV. The tail of the helix as a key to otoplasty. Plast Reconstr Surg. 1969;44(5):455–61.
35. Goulian Jr D, Conway H. Prevention of persistent deformity of the tragus and lobule by modification of the Luckett technique of otoplasty. Plast Reconstr Surg. 1960;26:399–404.
36. Gomulinski L, Maudy M, Saterre J. Our experience of otoplasty based on the study of the cartilaginous frame, especially the tail of the helix. Ann Chir Plast Esthet. 2005;50(3):206–15.

Prevention of Intra-Auricular Deformity in Prominent Ear Correction

28

Tomohisa Nagasao

Introduction

In surgical correction of prominent ears, the Mustarde technique – a technique to fold the antihelix – is frequently performed. The Mustarde technique effectively reduces the prominence of the ear and produces an antihelix. On the other hand, the Mustarde technique has two disadvantages. First, the contour of the helix develops irregularity after its application. Second, antihelixes produced with the Mustarde technique tend to present excessively linear shapes compared with ordinary antihelixes. The first problem can be solved by softening the scapha by scoring or thinning it. To enhance the usefulness of the Mustarde technique, this chapter introduces some troubleshooting methods addressing these disadvantages. In particular, theoretical rationales of the troubleshooting technique for the first problem – reduction of the contour irregularity of the helix – are minutely explained.

Morphological Pathology of Prominent Ear

Prominent ear is the condition where the auricle forms an excessive angle with the temporal region. Among congenital auricular deformities, prominent ear has the greatest incidence, with 5 % occurrence per population [1]. Prominent ears usually occur on both sides. High incidence in certain lineages implies genetic influences in the occurrence of the condition [2].

Cultural differences exist in esthetic views of prominent ears. In Asian countries, big ears are associated with wealth, and consequently, excessive prominence of the ear isn't viewed as unfavorable, as in Western countries. Hence, persons with prominent ears do not necessarily seek treatment. On the other hand, prominent ears are disliked in Western countries, since the features may be associated with demons. Consequently, the frequency of patients seeking treatment is greater for Western countries than in Oriental countries.

The prominence of the ear can be quantitatively evaluated by referring to two morphological parameters. The first parameter is the cephalo-auricular angle – the angle between the auricle and temporal region; the second parameter is the scapho-conchal angle – the angle between the concha and scapha. In auricles of prominent ear patients, both of these parameters are greater than normal [2]. Freitas [3], in his measurement study of these parameters in adolescents and adults, reports that the cephalo-auricular angles and scapho-conchal angles for normal persons are $31° \pm 6°$ and $106° \pm 19°$, respectively; with prominent ear patients, these values are $47° \pm 10°$ and $132° \pm 18°$, respectively. The difference between normal auricles and auricles of prominent ear patients is demonstrated in Fig. 28.1. Because of these morphological

T. Nagasao, M.D.
Department of Plastic and Reconstructive Surgery, School of Medicine, Keio University Hospital, Shinjuku-Ward Shinanomachi 35, Tokyo, Japan
e-mail: nagasao@sc.itc.keio.ac.jp

M.A. Shiffman (ed.), *Advanced Cosmetic Otoplasty*,
DOI 10.1007/978-3-642-35431-1_28, © Springer-Verlag Berlin Heidelberg 2013

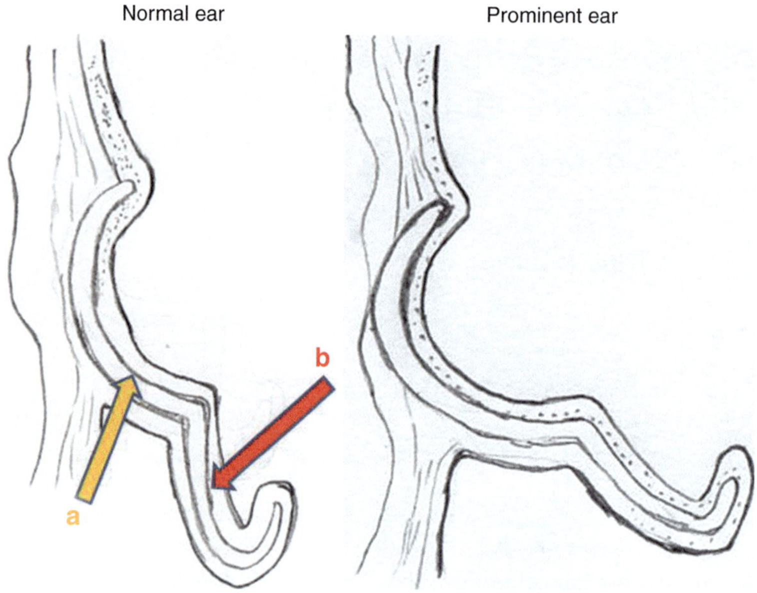

Fig. 28.1 Prominence of the ear is defined by two factors: the cephalo-auricular angle (*a*) and the scapho-conchal angle (*b*). These angles are greater than normal in prominent ear patients

abnormalities, the auricles of prominent ear patients protrude outward, presenting an odd impression. Furthermore, although inner structures of the auricle, such as the antihelix and concha, are invisible to the frontal view with normal persons, they are visible with prominent ear patients, which adds to a curious impression.

Besides the positional abnormality, auricles of prominent ear patients present two abnormal features in terms of intra-auricular geometry (Fig. 28.2). First, the antihelix is hypoplastic and inconspicuous. Because of the hypoplasia, the upper part of the auricle presents flat features. Second, the horizontal length of the auricle is longer than normal. In performing correction for prominent ears, not only the prominence of the ear but also these intra-auricular abnormal features need to be appropriately corrected.

Mustarde Technique

In surgical correction for prominent ears, two purposes need to be achieved. First, the auricle should be moved closer to the temporal region, so that these two structures form a smaller angle. Second, the antihelix needs to be reshaped to present a more natural form.

The first purpose of reduction of the auricular prominence can be achieved to some extent by working on the concha. The distance between the lateral part of the auricle and the temporal region is reduced by removing part of the concha and suturing the defect (Fig. 28.3). For cases with severe protrusion, a sizable piece of cartilage needs to be removed from the concha. In suturing the margins of thus-made defects, the edges of the defect often develop unsightly contours at their junction. Furthermore, natural-looking antihelixes cannot be produced by merely depending on this maneuver.

To solve the problems with the above-stated maneuver on the concha, Mustarde [4] invented a technique for surgical correction of prominent ears. The Mustarde technique, also called the "in-suture technique," was reported in 1962 (Fig. 28.4). Although a long time has passed since the technique was initially reported, it still remains important for the correction of prominent ears. Actual application of Mustarde technique consists of two or three pairs of points that are marked on the parts of the concha where the internal edge of the

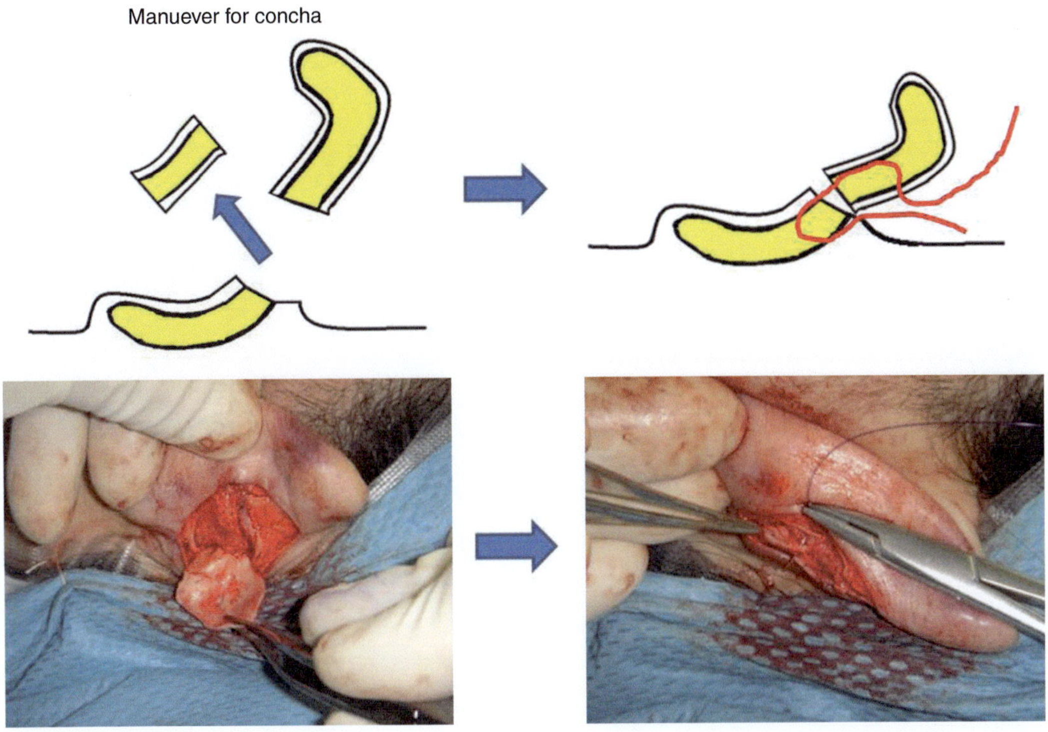

Fig. 28.2 Characteristic features of the prominent ear

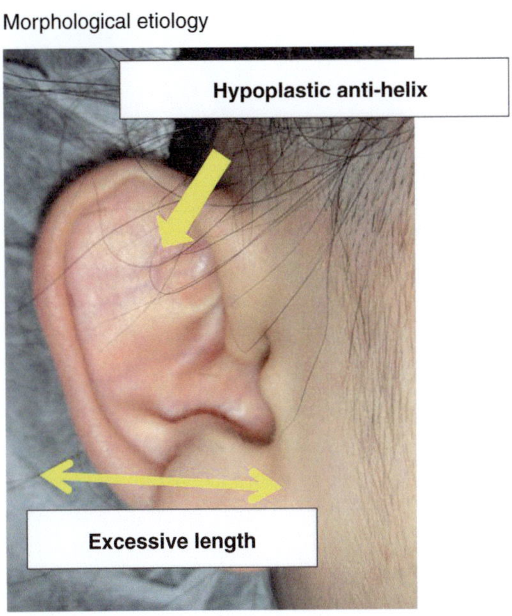

Fig. 28.3 Ear prominence is reduced to some extent by removing part of the concha

inferior crus and exterior edge of the superior crus are to be produced (Fig. 28.5). After the skin is dissected from the auricular cartilage, threads are introduced into the space connecting the paired points. Threads made of nonabsorbable materials – such as nylon – should be used for this maneuver, to avoid postoperative recurrence of ear prominence. As these stitches are tied, the paired points approach one another, forming the antihelix. After the antihelix is produced, rolled bandages are applied to secure its shape. These are removed about a week postoperatively.

Problems with Mustarde Technique

Although the Mustarde technique is an effective and frequently used surgical method for the correction of prominent ears, it also has its share of disadvantages. There are two main disadvantages with the Mustarde technique. First, the contour of the helix often develops irregularity after the Mustarde technique is applied. A typical example

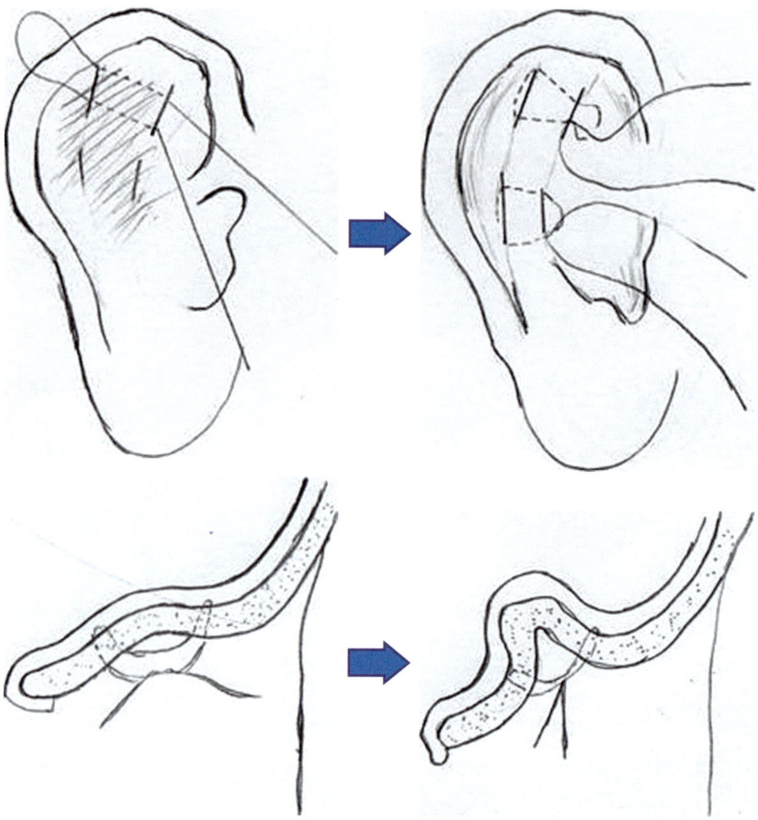

Fig. 28.4 The Mustarde technique. (*Left*) Sutures are applied to the antihelix region. (*Right*) As the threads are tied, the auricle is folded, enhancing the antihelix

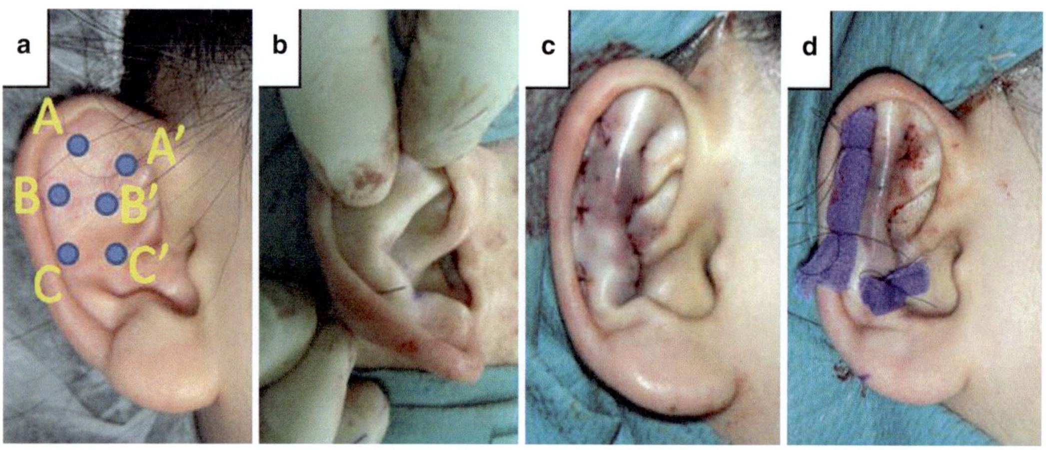

Fig. 28.5 Actual application of the Mustarde technique. (**a**) Paired points are marked. (**b**) Threads are introduced to connect the paired points. (**c**) The threads are tied. (**d**) Rolled gauzes are applied to maintain the shape of the antihelix

of the irregularity is demonstrated in the left picture of Fig. 28.6. Because the helix is pulled inward by the threads of the Mustarde suture, the part of the helix indicated with the arrow presents a concavity. As the second disadvantage, naturally looking antihelixes are difficult to achieve

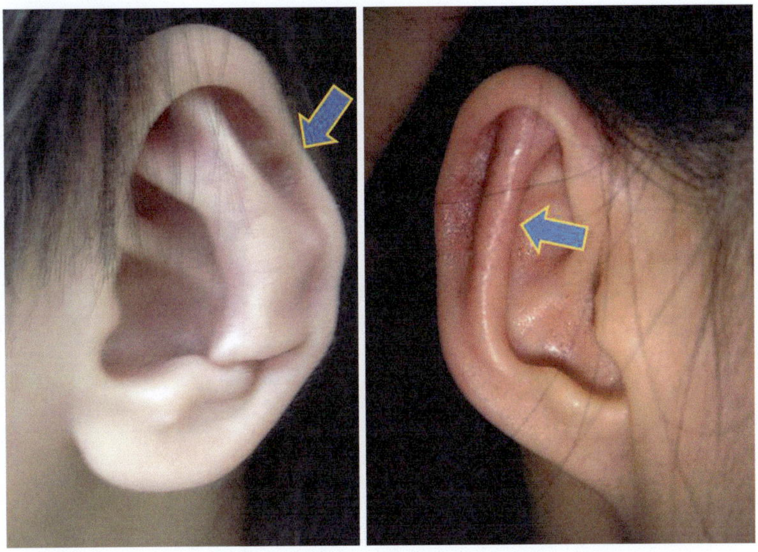

Fig. 28.6 Problems with the Mustarde technique are indicated with *arrows*. (*Left*) Irregularity of the helix contour. (*Right*) Unnaturally linear antihelix

with the Mustarde technique. Although the antihelix presents a smooth curvature in ordinary ears, antihelixes produced with the Mustarde technique often have unnaturally straight features (Fig. 28.6).

Irregularity of the Helix

Biomechanical Etiology

How can the first problem of irregularity of the helix be avoided? Herein, causative mechanisms for the irregularity are first clarified to provide solutions to this problem. The cross-section of the transformation pattern the auricle presents on application of the Mustarde technique is demonstrated in the Fig. 28.7. As the sutures connecting the paired points are tied, a fold appears on the auricle. Subsequently, the sutured part of the helix is pulled inward by the distance *a* in the picture. As a result of this, the edge of the helix near the sutures collapses. Since the antihelix, scapha, and helix form a united entity, they are modeled as three connected plates. A, S, and H in the diagrams indicate the antihelix, scapha, and helix, respectively. As the antihelix is folded by the application of the Mustarde technique, the length of the antihelix is reduced. According to this change, the helix is pulled inward and develops the irregularity (Fig. 28.6).

Prevention of Irregularity

Transmission of the dynamic effect generated in the antihelix is the causative factor for the irregularity of the helix. Hence, the irregularity is avoided by blocking transmission of the dynamic force from the antihelix to the helix. This can be achieved by working on the scapha, because it functions as the dynamic interface between the antihelix and helix. The basic principle for this idea is explained by referring to Fig. 28.8. When the Mustarde technique is applied in an ordinary fashion, the edge of the helix is pulled inward (Fig. 28.8).

However, when the scapha is softened, its flexibility increases. Accordingly, even when the antihelix is folded by the application of the Mustarde technique, the transformation is absorbed in the scapha and is smoothly transmitted to the helix (Fig. 28.8). The difference in the movement presented by the helix in response to the Mustarde technique is demonstrated in the

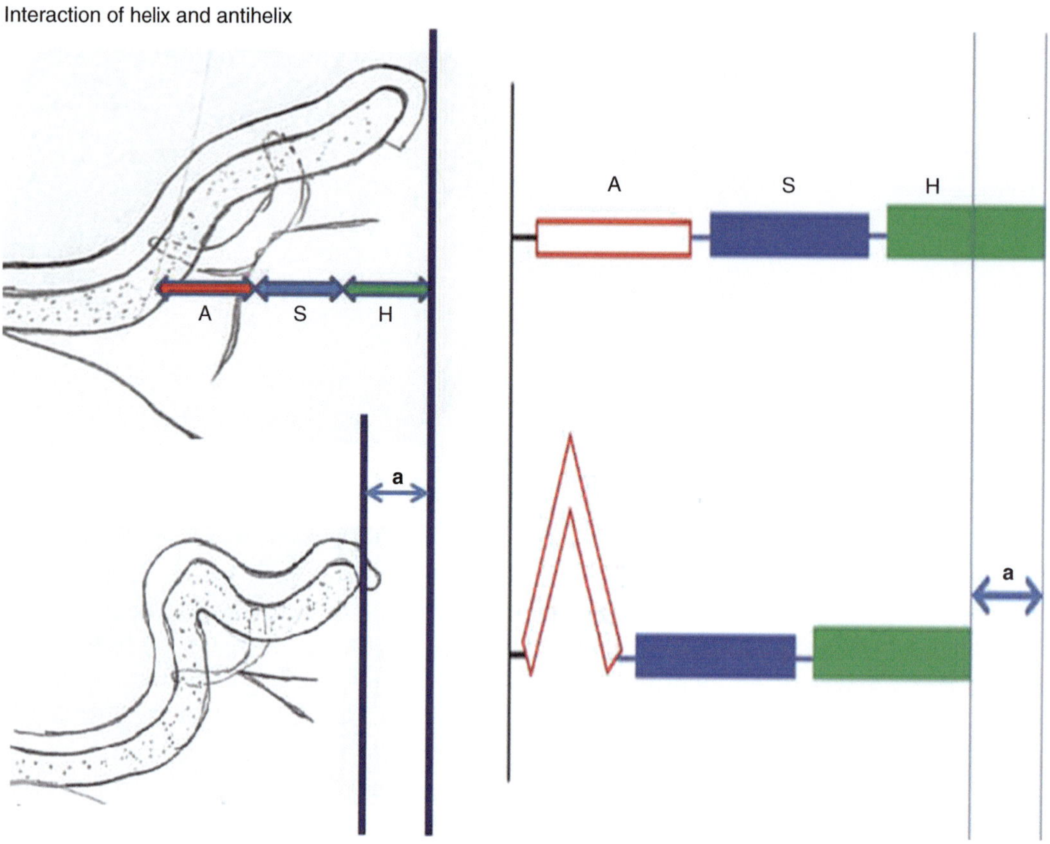

Fig. 28.7 Diagram of the transformation in response to the Mustarde technique. As the antihelix region is folded, the helix is pulled inward by the distance *a*

lower row pictures of Fig. 28.8, where *a*′ is smaller than *a*.

Softening of the scapha is achieved by scoring it or by abrading it. Scoring is the maneuver of making slits on the surface of the cartilage, which can be performed with a scalpel [5, 6]; abrasion is the maneuver of thinning the cartilage using operative devices such as diamond bars [2, 7, 8]. These techniques, originally developed for the purpose of preventing postoperative recurrence of ear prominence (Fig. 28.9), are usually performed after the surface of the auricular cartilage is exposed by separating it from the overlying skin. However, if needles are used instead of scalpels, scoring can be achieved without exposing the cartilage [9]. Similarly, abrasion can be performed under endoscopic observation without exposing the auricle [10].

Experimental Evaluation of the Method's Effectiveness

The effectiveness of scapha softening in reducing the helix irregularity in response to the Mustarde technique is theoretically proven by means of computer simulation in the author's previous study [11]. Herein, the essence of the study is introduced.

First, the basic principles for the study's method are explained, referring to an example problem of dynamic transformation of boards in response to application of forces (Fig. 28.10). When material properties such as thickness and hardness of this board are available, the transformation pattern this board presents in response to a certain force can be predicted by performing a relatively simple dynamic calculation.

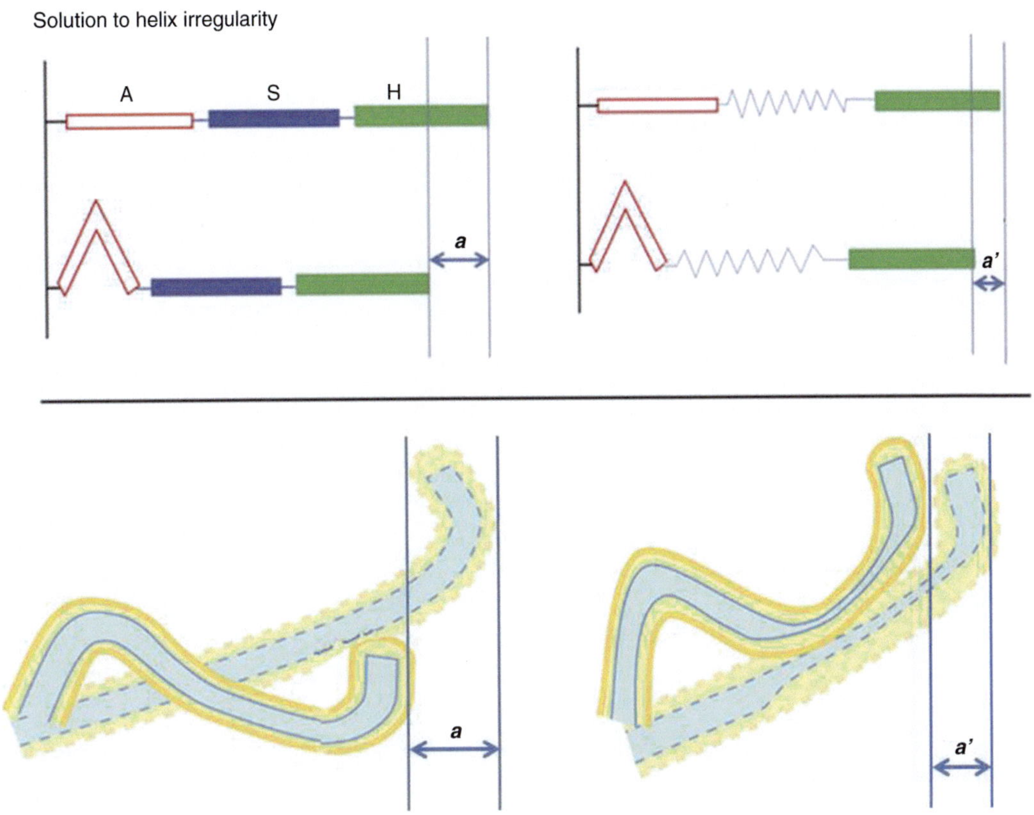

Fig. 28.8 (*Left*) As the antihelix is folded, the helix moves by *a*. (*Right*) When the scapha is softened, the effect of the folding is buffered by the scapha. Accordingly, the helix moves by *a*′, a smaller value than *a*

Next, another board consisting of the same material, but presenting a larger size and curved shape, is assumed (Fig. 28.10). Although the shape of the latter board is complicated compared with the former board, the transformation pattern the latter presents in response to forces can also be predicted by dividing it into small pieces, performing dynamic calculation with each piece as was done with the former, and accumulating the calculated results.

This technique, where an object with a complicated shape is viewed as a unity of multiple small pieces with simple geometries and calculation results from each piece are accumulated, is called finite element analysis. Finite element analysis is an established technique in biomechanical studies and is used for dynamic analyses of various organs – such as facial bones [12], thoraces [13], and skulls [14].

In the author's previous study, finite element analysis is used to prove the effectiveness of the scapha-softening technique. Although the auricle is geometrically a piece of plate, the degree of concavity varies according to location. Therefore, the auricle is divided into numerous small elements to make analysis applicable (Fig. 28.11). Furthermore, to take the difference in local thicknesses into consideration, thicknesses of actual auricles of cadavers were measured. Thereby, a "thickness map" – a map indicating local thicknesses for auricles – was produced (Fig. 28.12). According to the thickness map, appropriate thicknesses are allocated to each element. Through these considerations, three-dimensional models are produced that can accurately reflect dynamic behaviors of the original auricles.

Application of the Mustarde technique is simulated with these three-dimensional models.

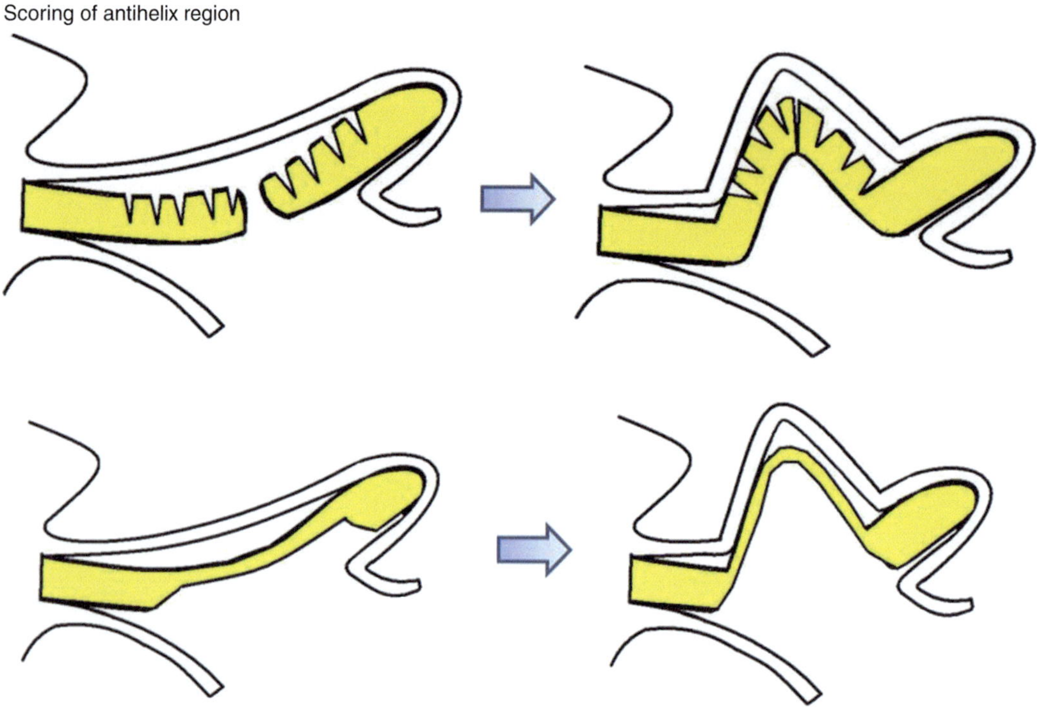

Fig. 28.9 (*Above*) With scoring technique, slits are made on the surface of the cartilage. (*Below*) With abrasion technique, the cartilage is thinned

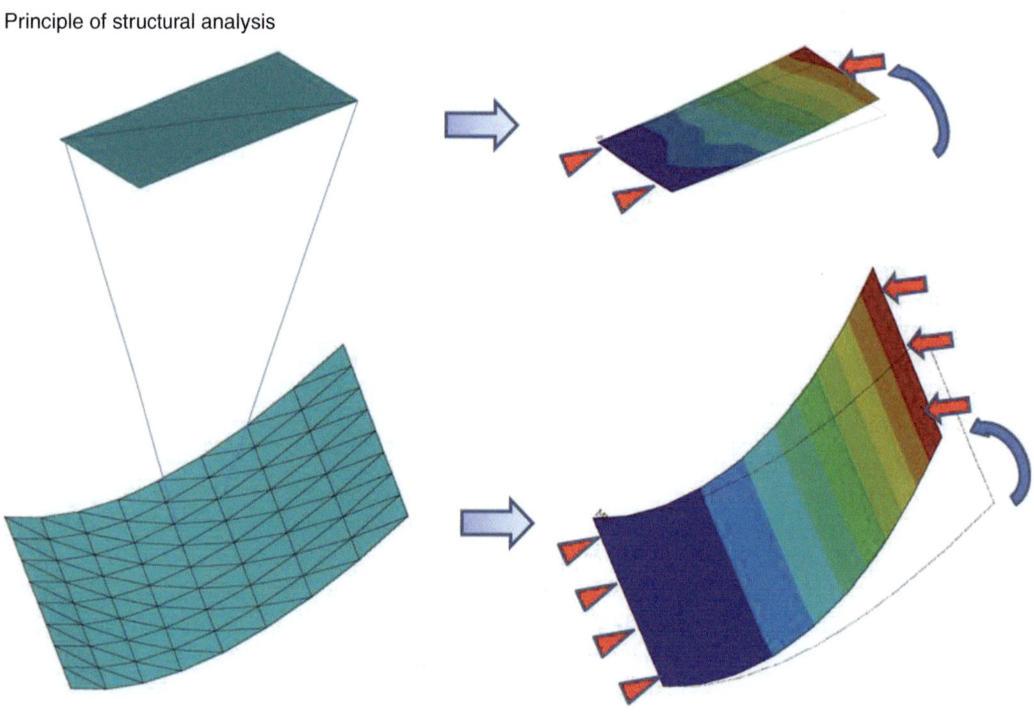

Fig. 28.10 Basic principle of finite element analysis. (*Left*) Calculation results with small components are accumulated to (*Right*) predict dynamic behavior of the whole entity

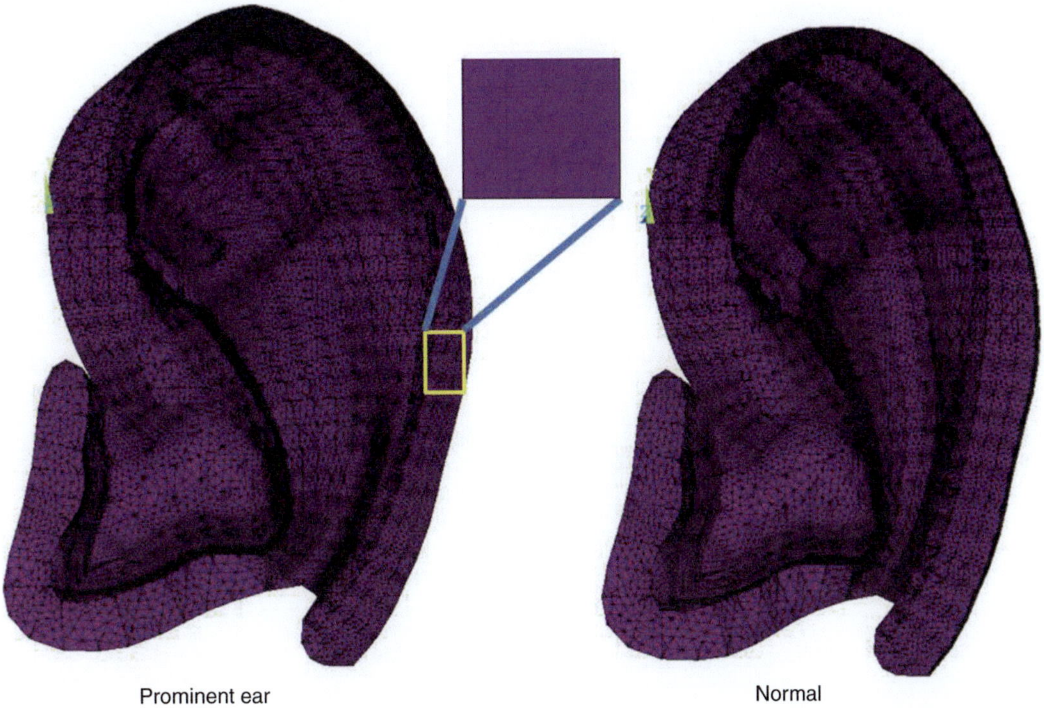

Fig. 28.11 (*Left*) Three-dimensional dynamic models representing a prominent ear and (*Right*) normal ear. The models consist of numerous small elements as shown in the magnified box

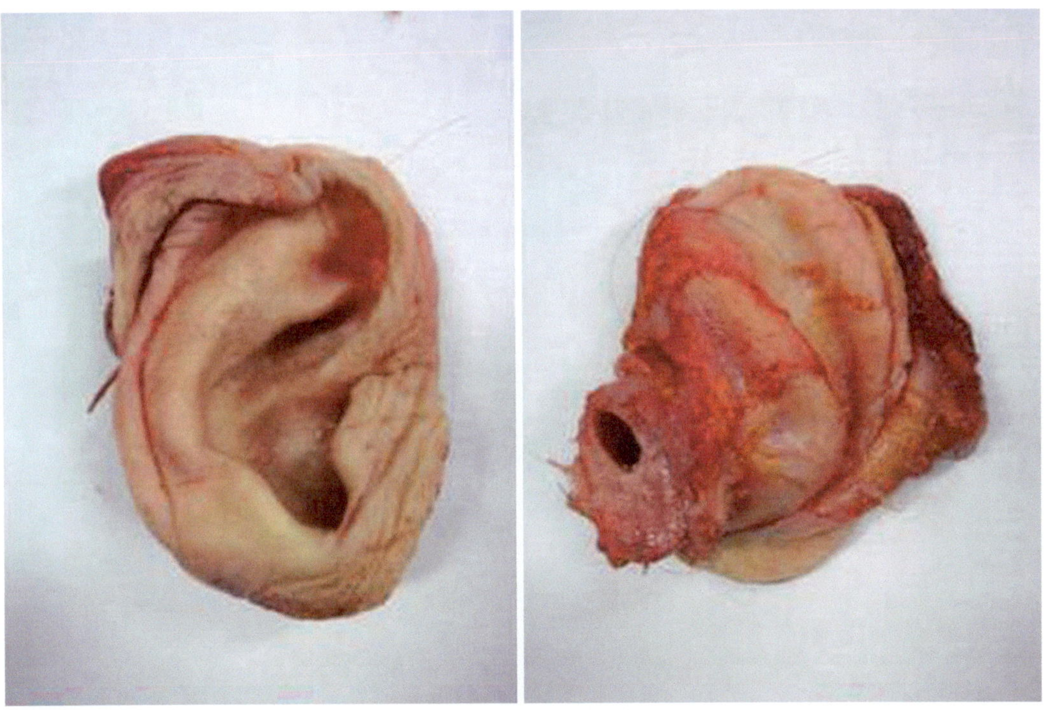

Fig. 28.12 To evaluate differences in local thicknesses, auricles were taken from cadavers and measured. Thereby, thickness maps were produced

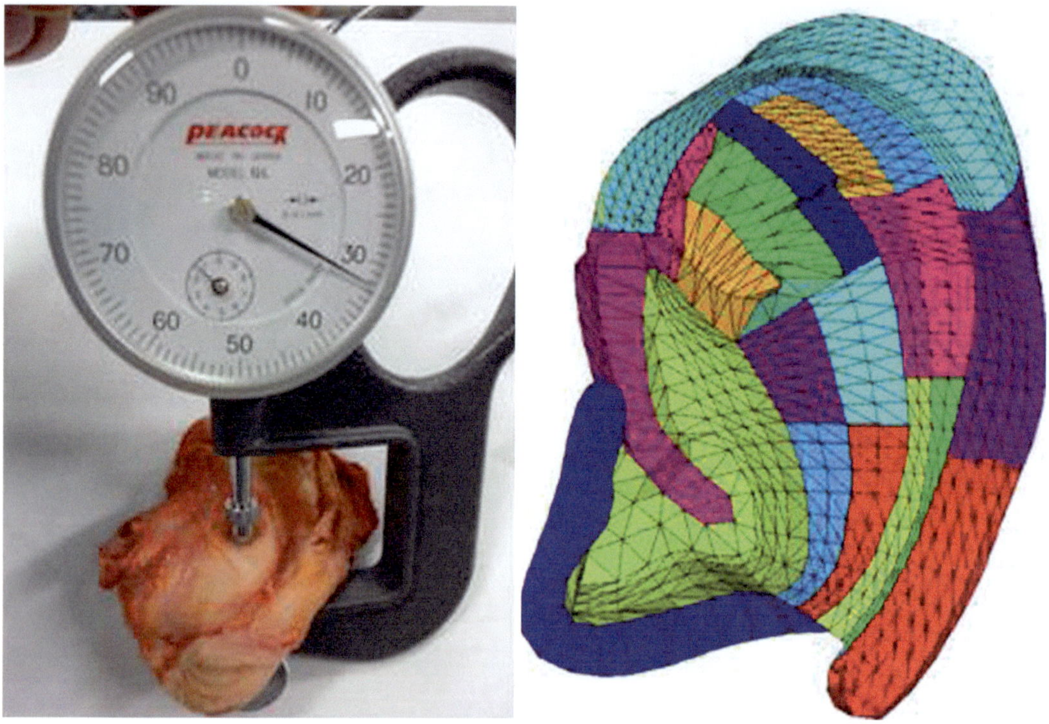

Fig 28.12 (continued)

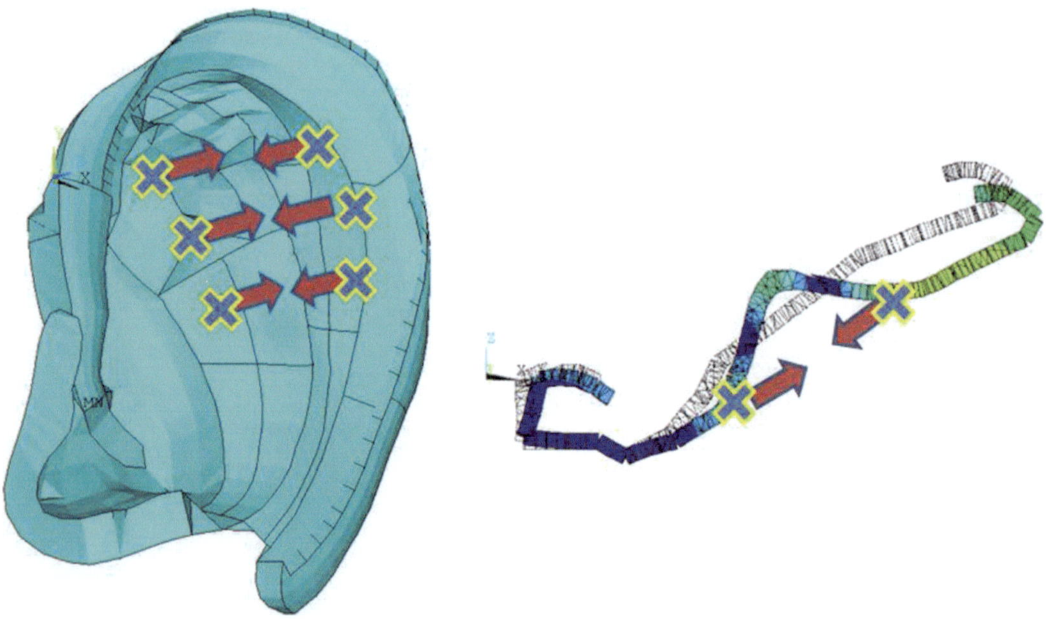

Fig. 28.13 Simulation of auricle transformation in response to the Mustarde technique

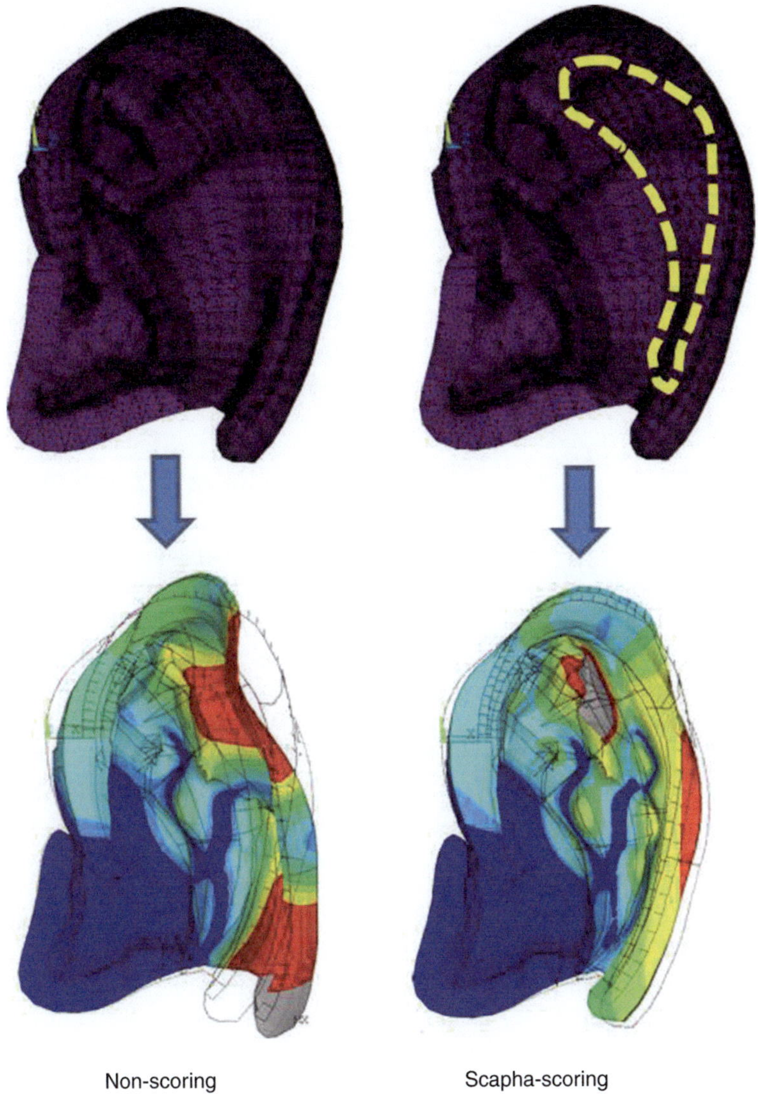

Fig. 28.14 (*Left*) Responding to the Mustarde technique, the contour of the helix develops irregularity. (*Right*) Auricles in which the scapha is softened present little irregularity of the helix

Two or three pairs of points are marked on the antihelix region of the models. Then, forces are applied on these models so that the points of each pair approach each other (Fig. 28.13). In response to the applied forces, the auricle transforms. The transformed shape is the auricular shape after the application of the Mustarde technique.

Using this theoretical method, the effect of the scapha-softening technique is examined. Two models are produced. The first model represents a prominent ear without any surgical treatments (Fig. 28.14). With the second model, the thickness of the scapha is reduced by half, simulating a prominent ear with the scapha softened by scoring or abrasion (Fig. 28.14). Application of the

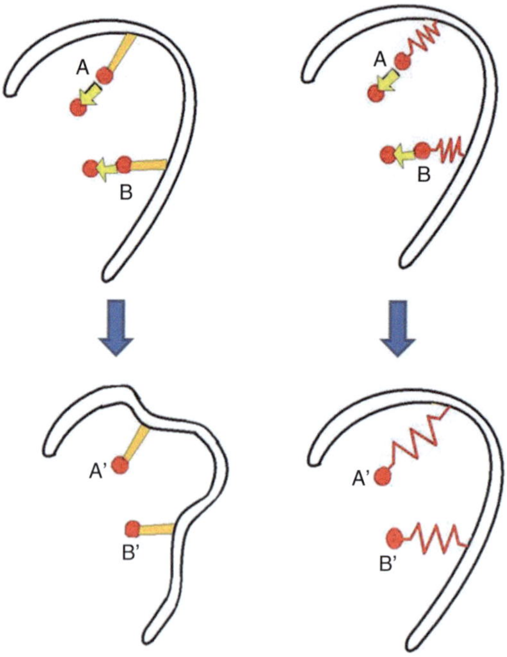

Fig. 28.15 Schematic explanation of the scapha-softening effect. (*Left*) As the antihelix part is folded with the Mustarde technique, the curve of the helix is distorted. (*Right*) When the flexibility of the scapha is increased, dynamic effects generated in the antihelix region are absorbed by the scapha region

Mustarde technique is simulated for each of these models to examine the transformation of the helix. With the former model, the contour of the helix presents obvious deformity. By comparison, the helix contour doesn't present great deformity with the latter model.

Theoretical Consideration

The results indicate that softening of the scapha prevents helix irregularity in response to the Mustarde technique. Herein, mechanisms for this prevention effect are reviewed.

When the Mustarde technique is performed, the part of the helix near the applied sutures is pulled inward and bends. Namely, in Fig. 28.15, as the points A and B move to points A′ and B′, respectively, this dynamic event is transmitted through the scapha (indicated with orange-colored bars) to the helix, and the affected parts of the helix move inward, accordingly (Fig. 28.15). However, with auricles where the scapha was softened by abrasion or scoring, the inward movement is buffered by the scapha. Hence, the helix receives less dynamic effect from the antihelix, presenting less irregularity than the helixes of ears that didn't undergo scapha softening.

Arrangement of Antihelix Shape

Besides the helix irregularity, another problem with the Mustarde technique is the unnatural appearance of the antihelix. Antihelixes produced with the Mustarde technique tend to present linear shapes, which give odd impressions (Fig. 28.6). To make the antihelix look natural, alterations can be made to the antihelix so that it presents a smooth curvature. This is achieved by performing tissue grafting. After some fat tissues or fascias are taken from the temporal region, they are placed beneath the folded cartilage (Fig. 28.16). This maneuver prevents the antihelix from presenting linear and narrow shapes when the Mustarde suture is applied, and helps the antihelix to form a smooth curvature (Fig. 28.17).

Conclusions

Although the main concern in the treatment of prominent ear is the correction of the prominence, care should also be taken to produce beautiful features of the ear. In particular, irregularity of the helix and unnaturally linear features of the antihelix should be avoided. The author hopes surgeons find the techniques introduced in this chapter useful in achieving these purposes.

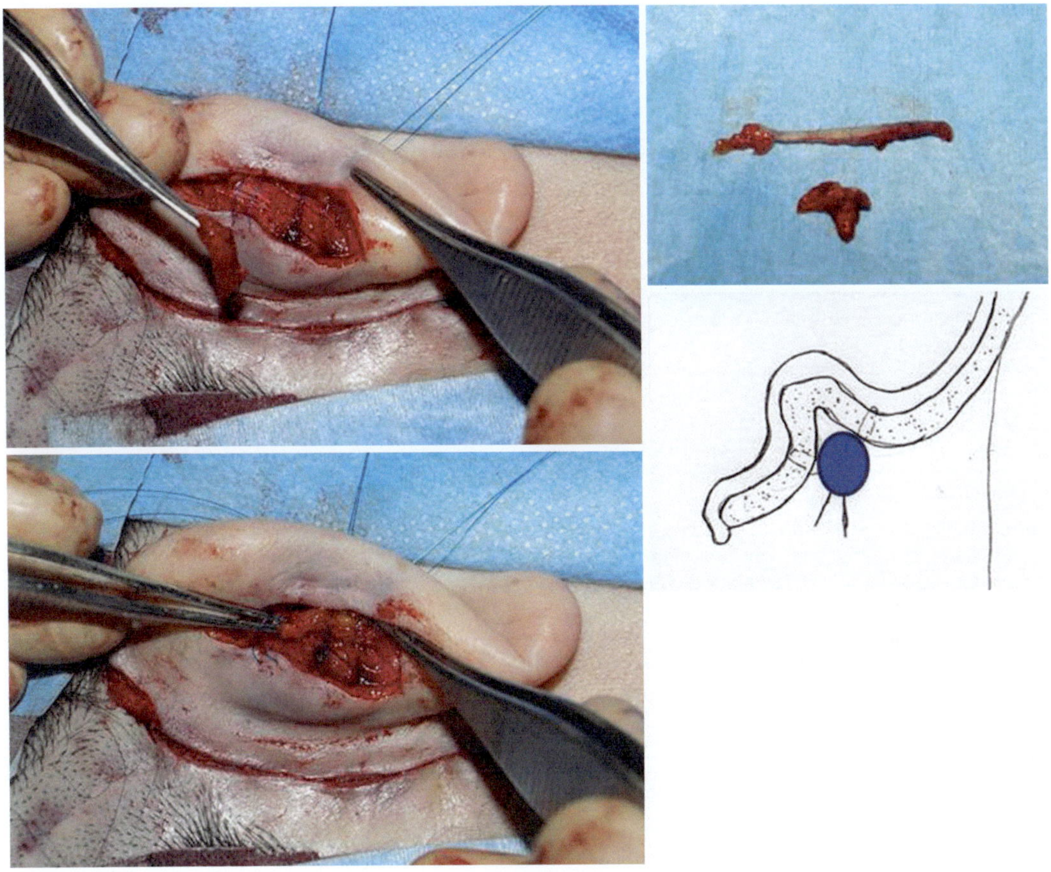

Fig. 28.16 Tissue grafting in the space beneath the antihelix

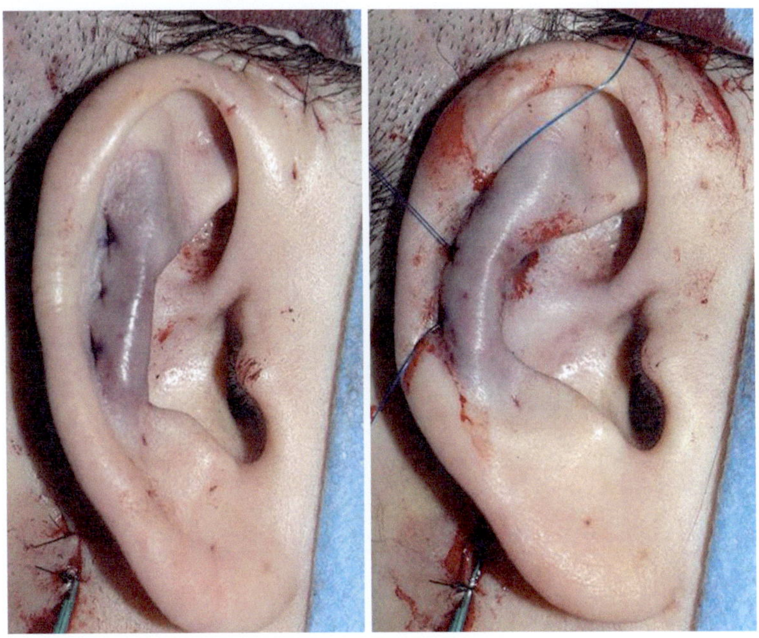

Fig. 28.17 Postoperative appearances of the antihelixes with (*Left*) and without (*Right*) tissue grafting

References

1. Hassanpour SE, Moosavizadeh SM. Posterior scoring of the scapha as a refinement in aesthetic otoplasty. J Plast Reconstr Aesthet Surg. 2010;63(1):78–86.
2. Brent B. Reconstruction of the auricle. In: McCarthy JG, editor. Plastic surgery. Philadelphia: Saunders; 1990. p. 2094–152.
3. da Silva Freitas R, Sanchez ME, Manzotti MS, Baras F, Ono MC, de Oliveira e Cruz GA. Comparing cephaloauricular and scaphaconchal angles in prominent ear patients and control subjects. Aesthetic Plast Surg. 2008;32(4):620–3.
4. Mustarde JC. The correction of prominent ears using simple mattress sutures. Br J Plast Surg. 1963;16: 170–8.
5. Erol OO. New modification in otoplasty: anterior approach. Plast Reconstr Surg. 2001;107(1): 193–202.
6. Lazaridis N, Tilaveridis I, Dimitrakopoulos I, Karakasis D. Correction of the protruding ear with a modified anterior scoring technique. J Oral Maxillofac Surg. 1998;56(3):307–13.
7. Dicio D, Castagnetti F, Baldassarre S. Otoplasty: anterior abrasion of ear cartilage with dermabrader. Aesthetic Plast Surg. 2003;27(6):466–71.
8. Oneal RM. Correction of the prominent ear with cartilage abrasion and concha-mastoid sutures. Aesthet Surg J. 1997;17(5):338.
9. Bulstrode NW, Huang S, Martin DL. Otoplasty by percutaneous anterior scoring. Another twist to the story: a long-term study of 114 patients. Br J Plast Surg. 2003;56(2):145–9.
10. Graham KE, Gault DT. Endoscopic assisted otoplasty: a preliminary report. Br J Plast Surg. 1997;50(1):47–57.
11. Nagasao T, Miyamoto J, Shimizu Y, Kasai S, Kishi K, Kaneko T. Effective scoring of scapha prevents helix irregularity in prominent ear correction—a biomechanical study. J Craniomaxillofac Surg. (in press).
12. Nagasao T, Miyamoto J, Nagasao M, Ogata H, Kaneko T, Tamaki T, et al. The effect of striking angle on the buckling mechanism in blowout fracture. Plast Reconstr Surg. 2006;117(7):2373–81.
13. Nagasao T, Miyamoto J, Kokaji K, Yozu R, Jiang H, Jin H, et al. Double-bar application decreases postoperative pain after Nuss procedure. J Thorac Cardiovasc Surg. 2010;140(1):39–44.
14. Nagasao T, Miyamoto J, Uchikawa Y, Tamaki T, Yamada A, Kaneko T, et al. A biomechanical study on the effect of premature fusion of the frontosphenoidal suture on orbit asymmetry in unilateral coronal synostosis. Cleft Palate Craniofac J. 2010;47(1):82–91.

29 Can Diathermy Enhance Scoring in Otoplasty?

Terry Gourlay and Ekpemi Irune

Introduction

Several otoplastic techniques, over 200, have been described by numerous surgeons as a remedy for auricular abnormalities. This very fact alludes to the lack of a single procedure being seen as absolute in tackling this problem. The use of permanent retention sutures [1], excision and incisions [2–4] of auricular cartilage, and combination techniques [1, 5] have all been described. More recently, the use of scoring of cartilage with the use of the surgical scalpel [6, 7].

Previous studies [8] have demonstrated the use of diathermy – monopolar and bipolar – in scoring the auricular cartilage, to produce comparable effects in deflecting segments of auricular cartilage, as with scalpel scoring. One recent study goes further to carry out the comparisons in whole porcine auricular cartilage. In addition, whilst previous exercises only provided information on 2-dimensional effects on cartilage scoring, the authors discuss the novelty of examining the 3-dimensional changes that occur with diathermy scoring compared with scalpel scoring in intact pig ears.

The Clinical Problem: Auricular Anomalies

Abnormalities of the auricle, whilst less of a physiological problem, often create a huge psychosocial dilemma for its sufferers. The auricles are symmetrical appendages that contribute profoundly to the aesthetic aspects of an individuals' facial structure. Often, subtle symmetrical variations in size or shape go unnoticed, but certain anomalies, especially when unilateral, are manifest. The social consequences often culminate in an emotionally distressed individual, as a result of ridicule from members of society. Thus, in order to avoid such psychological pressures, which can lead to the development of personality disorder, surgical correction of prominent ears should preferably be performed at or before the start of schooling [9].

The only difference between the neonatal ear and the adult ear is that, in the neonate, the cartilage is more malleable and soft. Otherwise, the anatomy is the same [10]. The ear attains approximately 85 % of its adult size by age 3 years [11] with attendant calcification of the cartilage with increasing age. This influences the kind of correction (operative or otherwise) that can be offered if at all and also highlights the importance of early intervention in the management of auricular anomalies.

T. Gourlay, Ph.D., BSc (Hons), FIBiol (✉)
Bioengineering Unit,
University of Strathclyde,
Wolfson Building, Glasgow G4 oNW,
Scotland, UK
e-mail: terry.gourlay@strath.ac.uk

E. Irune, MBChB, MRCS, MSc
Department of Otolaryngology,
Head & Neck Surgery,
Royal Hallamshire Hospital,
Sheffield, UK
e-mail: e_irune@hotmail.com

M.A. Shiffman (ed.), *Advanced Cosmetic Otoplasty*,
DOI 10.1007/978-3-642-35431-1_29, © Springer-Verlag Berlin Heidelberg 2013

Classification of Auricular Anomalies

Auricular abnormalities, as with most other structural anomalies of the body, can be broadly described as congenital and acquired, with these anomalies occurring as part of syndromes or independently. The incidence of congenital anomalies is unknown, although it varies between racial groups [12]. Based on the current knowledge of embryology, congenital anomalies are further divided into malformation or deformation types [13].

Malformations are structural abnormalities that result from abnormal embryologic development [12]. They are defects that occur as a result of a deficiency, absence, or excess of components of auricular structure.

Deformation, which may occur in utero or postnatally, is not caused by embryologic maldevelopment but results from abnormal physical forces applied to a normal structure. Similarly, a deforming force may be applied to a malformed ear [12]. In essence, deformational abnormalities may be corrected by manipulation of the tissues as complete and mature components of the cutaneous and cartilaginous tissues are present. Examples include prominent ear (also known as bat's ear), cryptotia (upper auricular sulcus hidden in scalp), lop ear (folded superior portion of helical rim) and Stahl's ear (aka Stahl's bar – a third crux between superior and inferior crura of the antihelix).

Deformational Abnormalities: The Prominent Ear

The most common of the deformational abnormalities is the prominent ear. Prominent ears are relatively common, with an incidence in Caucasians of about 5 %. It is inherited as an autosomal dominant trait and is commonly caused by a combination of two defects: (1) underdevelopment of antihelical folding and (2) overdevelopment of the conchal wall [14].

In 2007, Furnas and Lin [15] wrote "An ear appears prominent or protruding if it projects more than 15–20 mm or more than 21°–30° from the temporomastoid plane of the skull. The mean length of the ear (sa-sba, i.e., superaural to subaural) in boys is 55 mm when aged 6 years, 60 mm when aged 12 years, and 62 mm when aged 18 years. In girls, the values are 54, 58, and 58 mm at ages 6, 12, and 18 years, respectively. The mean width of the ear (pra-pa, i.e., preaural to postaural) is 34, 35 and 36 mm in boys and 33, 34 and 34 mm in girls at ages 6, 12, and 18 years, respectively. One standard deviation in width is 2.0–2.5 mm and in length is 3.0–3.5 mm. An ear that is two or more standard deviations from the mean is viewed as abnormally large (macrotia). Excessive projection is a far more frequent problem than excessive size."

The authors [15] also mentioned other contributory factors in the development of the prominent ear, for example, abnormal underlying skeletal structure in the form of a prominent mastoid process. In addition, the presence of prominent ear as part of other anomalies, such as Stahl's ear or macrotia, should be borne in mind.

Management of the Prominent Ear

Prominent ears may be managed conservatively, without any intervention to the use of splints to correct the deformation in the very early stages of life. In addition, surgery may also be employed. Below, the use of surgical means is discussed in more detail.

Cartilage Weakening: Scalpel Versus Diathermy Cartilage Scoring

The foundations of otoplasty were essentially laid before the nineteenth century. Thus, today, most surgeons use a combination of techniques borrowed from the pioneers of otoplasty. Ballenger and Snow [16] are keen to state that "Mastery of the precise anatomy of the auricle (anterior and posterior), combined with a knowledge of Becker's dissection technique and Mustarde's mattress suture technique, modified by Tardy and Trenta, allows the surgeon a wide latitude in achieving natural correction of the many varieties of outstanding ear. No single technique suffices" [16].

Thus, in recent times, studies have been carried out to examine the technique of cartilage weakening, paying particular attention to cartilage scoring. It attempts to assess the 3-dimensional effect of diathermy (monopolar) scoring on ear cartilage obtained from the landrace pig. A comparison is made with scalpel scoring.

Quereshi et al. [8] compared the use of bipolar diathermy against scalpel scoring of porcine ear cartilage (it has a similar thickness to human cartilage). The outcome measurements were bend force and deflection angle using the two instruments. They concluded that there was no statistically significant difference between the two mediums – scalpel and diathermy (varied settings) – when used independently. However, when used together on either side of the porcine cartilage (i.e., scalpel scoring on one side and diathermy on the reverse side), the result was a statistically significant increase in the outcome measurements of bend force and angle of deflection [8]. This is explained as a synergistic effect as scalpel scoring will enable deflection away from the surface scored and diathermy, towards the surface scored.

The team postulated that though the diathermy caused necrosis of the cartilage at the direct point of contact, there was a secondary conduction of heat generated that resulted in the contraction of the intact cartilage beyond the area of the burn, the consequence being an increased bend force and angle of deflection.

Prior to this study, investigated the effects of dehydration on strips of cartilage. They carried out similar experiments as in Quereshi et al. [8], utilizing bend angle and bend force as outcome measures in estimating the effects of cartilage scoring with scalpel and diathermy (monopolar and bipolar). In addition, they investigated the effects of skin present on the anterior cartilage surface and cartilage orientation, on these outcome measures. They concluded that dehydration produces a significant deflection of cartilage towards the posterior surface. They found bend angle and force were superior in strips of cartilage scored without skin, that with anterior skin present. In addition, scalpel scoring produced increasingly bigger bends for increasing amounts of scoring on a cartilage surface in all groups. Bipolar and monopolar diathermy did not follow this pattern. Finally, they deduced that scalpel scoring, bipolar scoring, and monopolar scoring are not equally effective in deflecting strips of porcine ear cartilage: Variations are dependent on orientation of the cartilage strip and the surface scored.

More recently, Irune and Gourlay compared the 3-dimensional effects of scalpel and monopolar diathermy scoring on porcine auricular cartilage. They utilized whole landrace pig ears which were acquired immediately after death (Figs. 29.1 and 29.2). A 3-dimensional model of each was digitally reproduced using a 3-dimensional laser scanner: the PICZA® 3D Laser Scanner LPX-250 (Roland DGA, California, USA). During the experiment, identical set of maneuvres were carried out on each intact porcine ear, using a scalpel in one group and monopolar diathermy in the other. The study attempted to mimic true otoplastic techniques, and thus trauma to the cartilage was carried out on the posterior surface of the auricular cartilage following elevation of the posterior skin flap only (Fig. 29.3). Surrounding temperature was controlled to prevent warping of the cartilage from dehydration – a fact already established by Millington and Gourlay. Thus, the porcine ears were stored appropriately in moisture preserving conditions and at temperatures of –4 °C. This was essential during transport from the abattoir and in-between carrying out experiments on each ear. In addition, all measurements were taken immediately following scoring by scalpel or monopolar diathermy technique. The latter was done using the same power settings as in previous studies by Qureshi et al. [8].

These ears were then re-scanned after scoring of the auricular cartilage with a scalpel and monopolar diathermy in Groups A and B, respectively. No scoring was done in the control Group C.

Three-dimensional scanners serve to create 3-dimensional likeness or models of an actual object or environment. Thus, a laser-generated likeness of the porcine ear and a second image of the same ear following either scalpel (Figs. 29.4, 29.5, 29.6, and 29.7) or diathermy (Figs. 29.8, 29.9, 29.10, and 29.11) scoring were created. Digital images as well as outcome

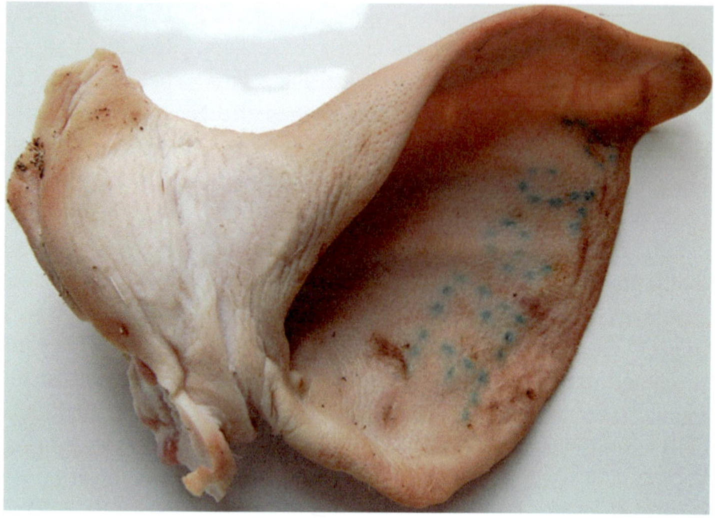

Fig. 29.1 Whole landrace pig ear – anterior

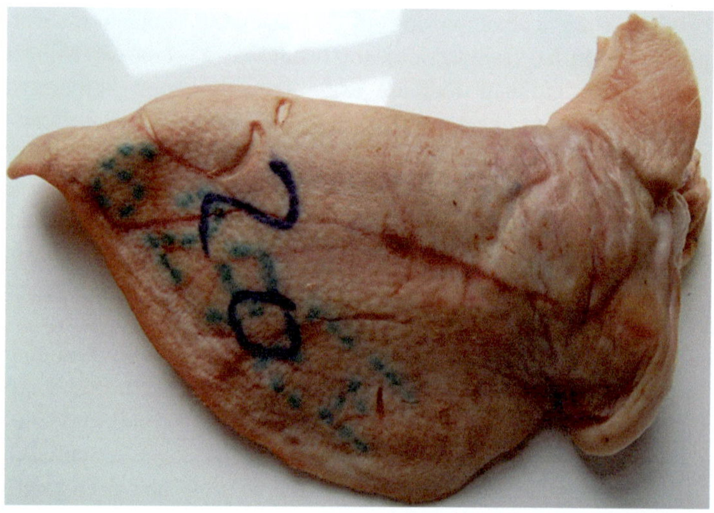

Fig. 29.2 Whole landrace pig ear – posterior

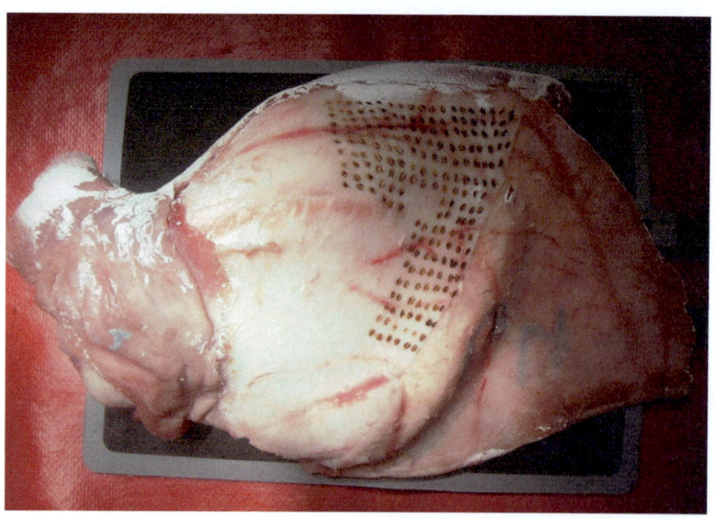

Fig. 29.3 Posterior of whole ear with reflected posterior flap demonstrating underlying porcine cartilage with completed diathermy score pattern

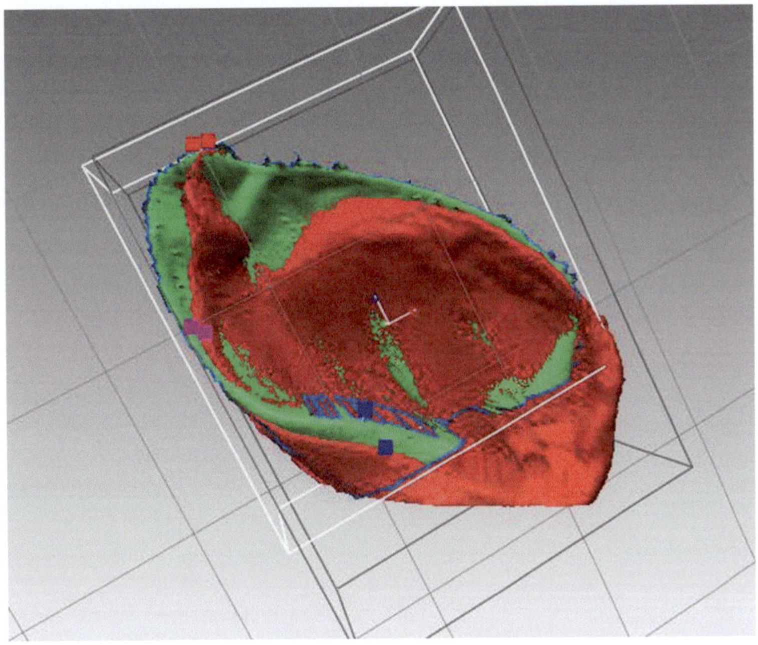

Fig. 29.4 3D Topographical changes: The Scalpel Group. Three-dimensional image of the pre-scalpel and post-scalpel models following overlapping

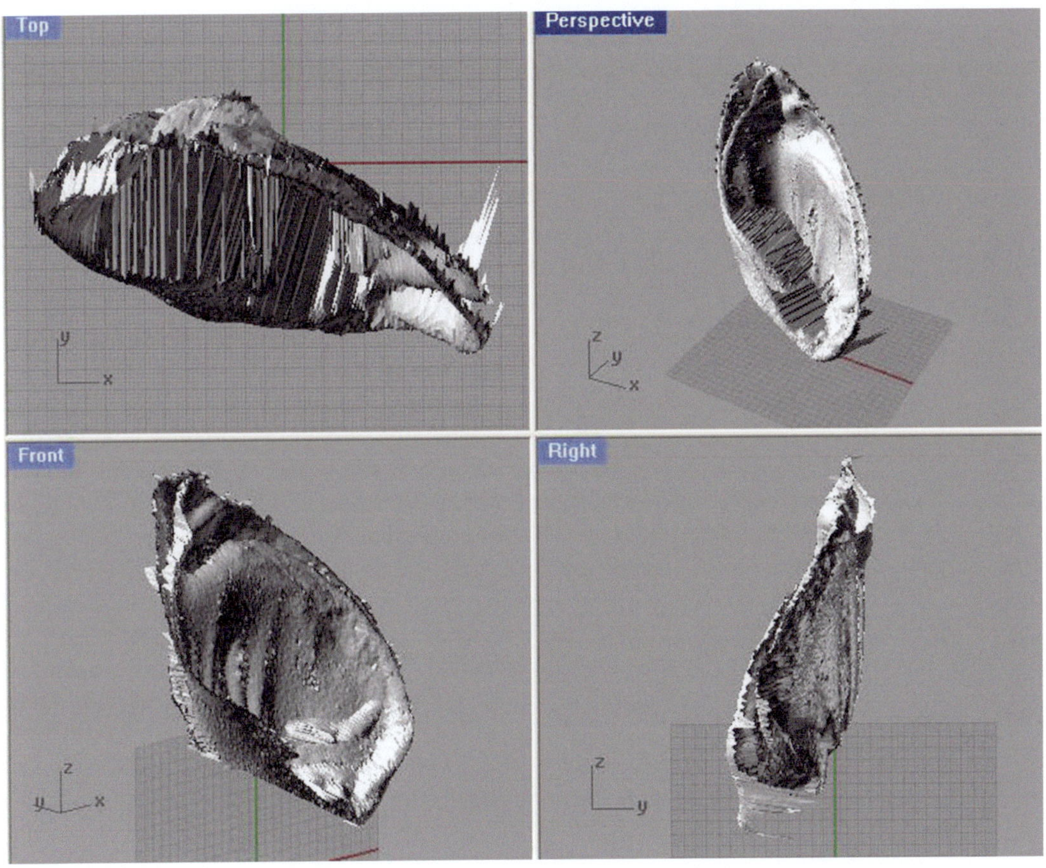

Fig. 29.5 Multi-view point rendered images of the two overlapped models above

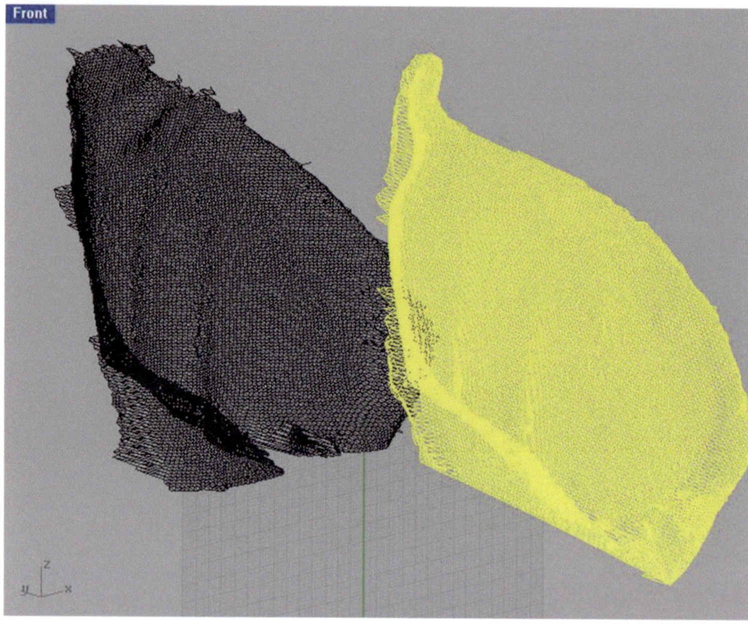

Fig. 29.6 Three-dimensional image of the anterior of the pre-scalpel (*black*) and post-scalpel (*yellow*), images separated

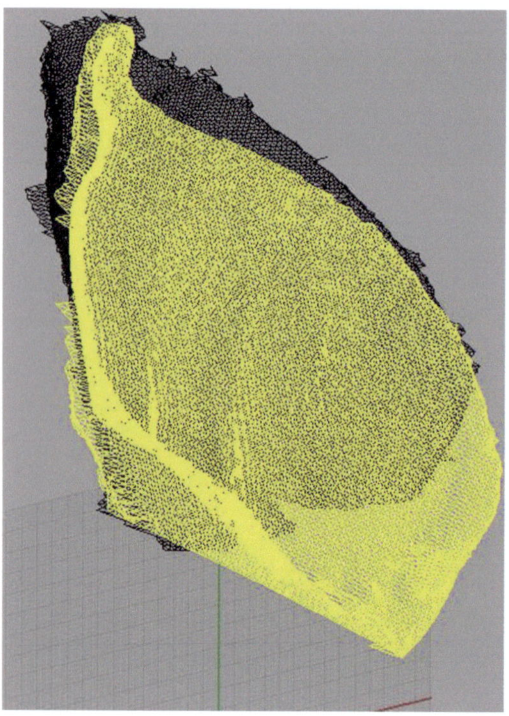

measurements were carried out with the use of the softwares PIXFORM® (Roland DGA, California, USA) and Rhinoceros 4.0® (McNeel, Washington, USA), respectively, outcome measurements being the difference in deflection angle of the cartilage (at two anatomical positions) after scoring by both media and also the gross topographical change of the whole porcine ear upon scoring, as depicted by the overlapping of 3D models of the whole ears, pre- and post-scoring.

Using Rhinoceros 4.0® (McNeel, Washington. USA), a computer-aided design software, a reference line is projected. It is one which lies adjacent and parallel to the largest anatomical area in question (either posterolat-

Fig. 29.7 Three-dimensional image of the anterior of the pre-scalpel (*black*) and post-scalpel (*yellow*), images overlapped

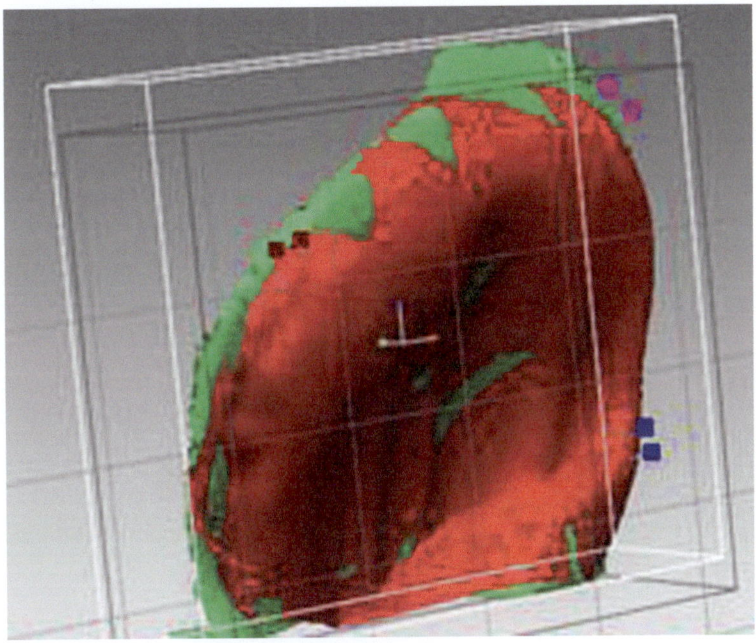

Fig. 29.8 Laser generated likeness of porcine ear

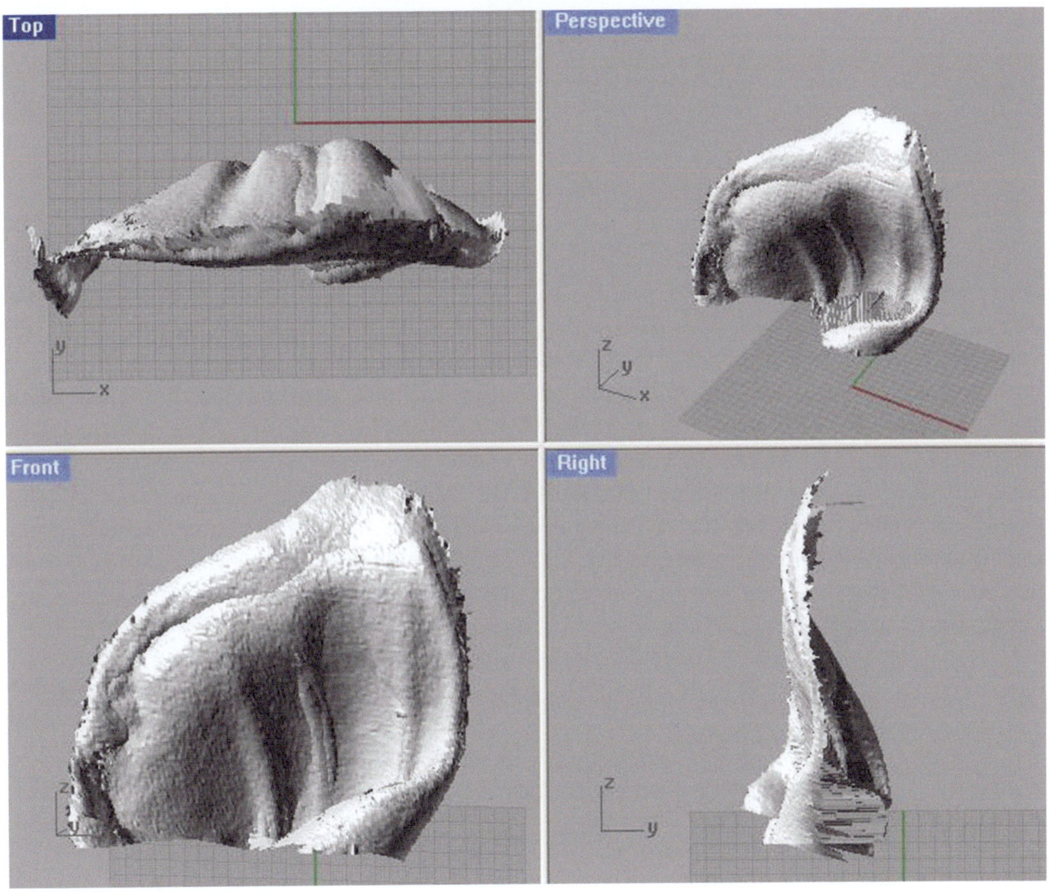

Fig. 29.9 Likeness of ear after scoring

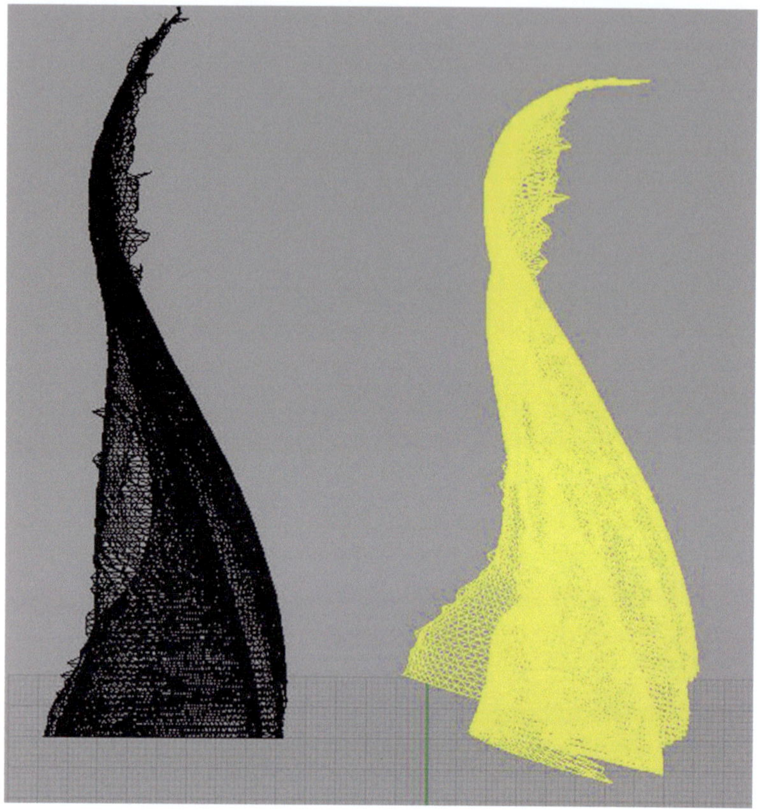

Fig. 29.10 Laser-generated likeness of porcine ear (*Left*). Likeness of porcine ear after scoring with diathermy (*Right*)

eral or superolateral surface) of the whole ear. The angles of deflection was described as that made by a straight line drawn as a tangent to the reference line and was brought about by the curvature of the cartilage following physical scoring by scalpel and diathermy (Figs. 29.12, 29.13, and 29.14). The units were in degrees, and it was also important to note the direction of deflection, in reference to the anatomy of the whole ear, that is, anterior versus posterior.

It was realized that scalpel scoring causes an increase in cartilage curvature away from the scored surface. The scalpel scoring causes a significant difference in deflection angle of whole porcine cartilage $P=0.03$ (SD=6.30). Diathermy causes an increase in cartilage curvature towards the scored surface. In addition, the diathermy insult causes a difference in deflection angle in whole porcine cartilage $P=0.05$ (SD=13.9). Diathermy causes better curvature of the cartilage (Fig. 29.15). However, this isn't statistically significant $P=0.21$ (SD=10.8).

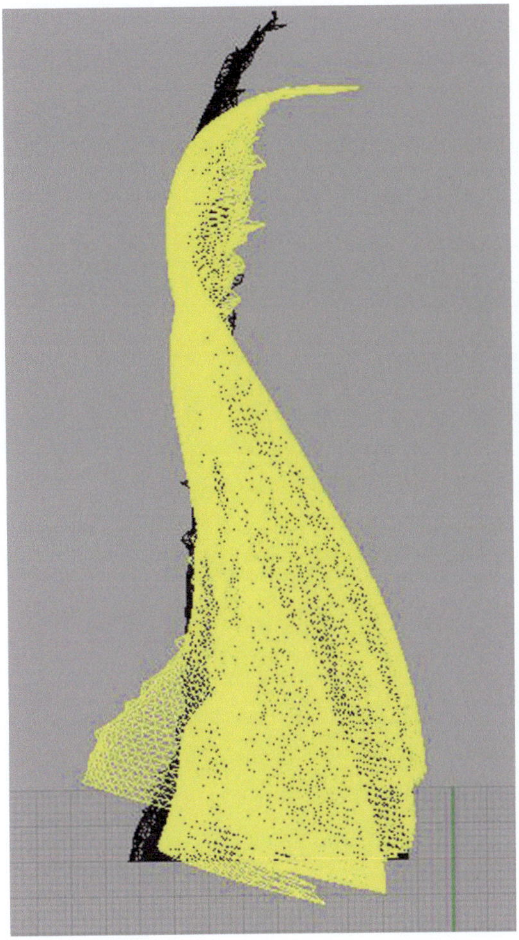

Fig. 29.11 Porcine ear before scoring in *black* and after scoring in *yellow*

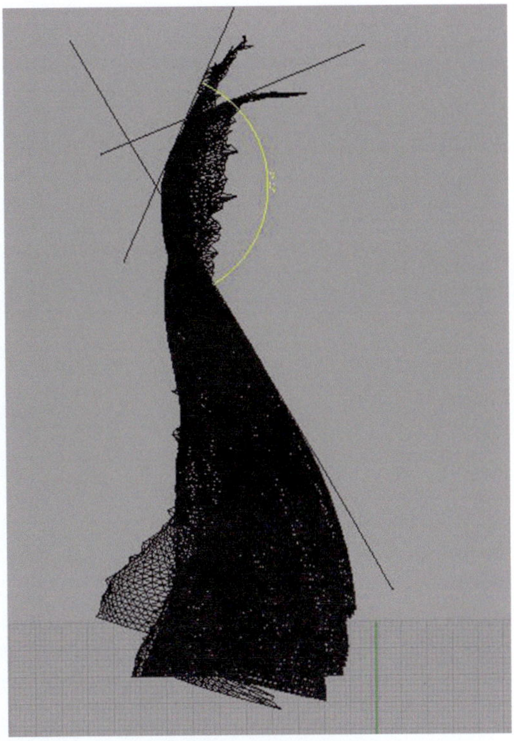

Fig. 29.12 *Yellow line* is angle of deflection

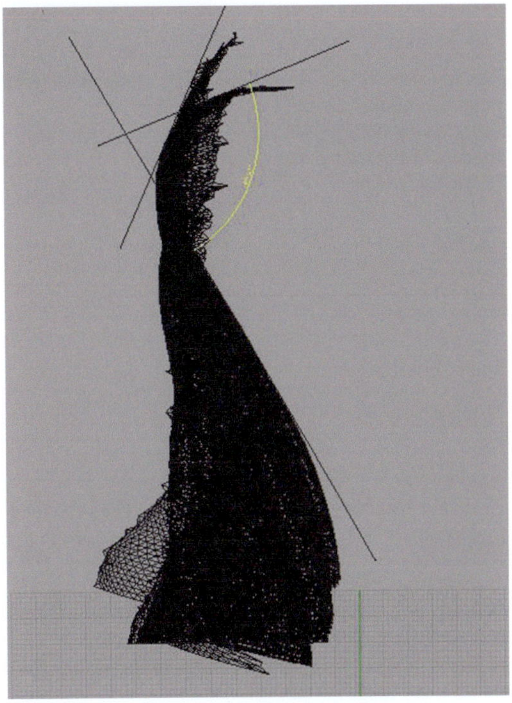

Fig. 29.13 *Yellow line* is angle of deflection

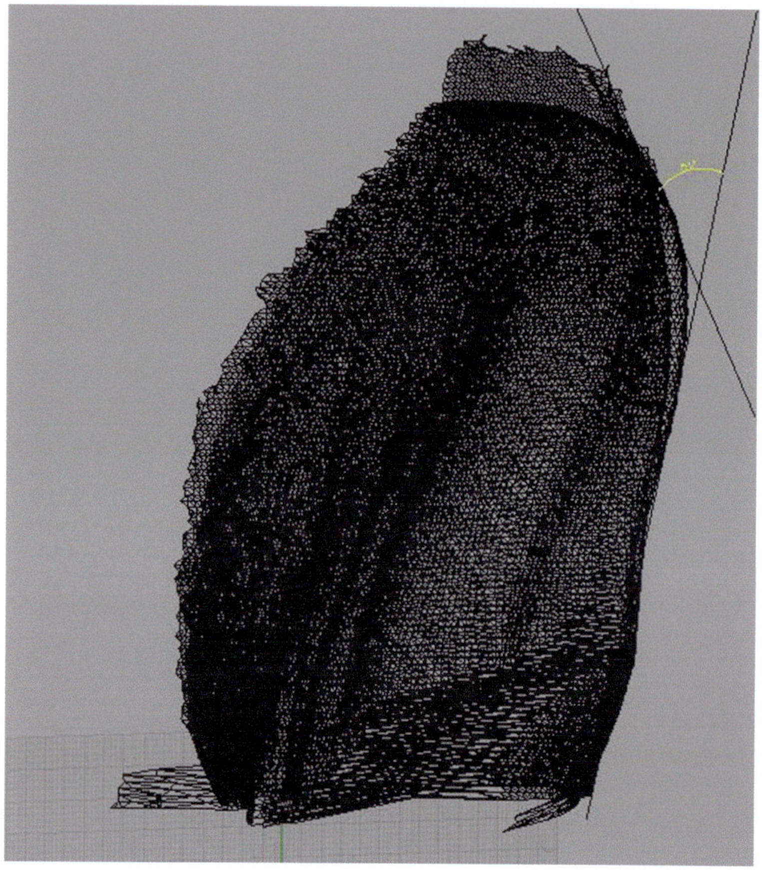

Fig. 29.14 *Yellow line* is angle of deflection

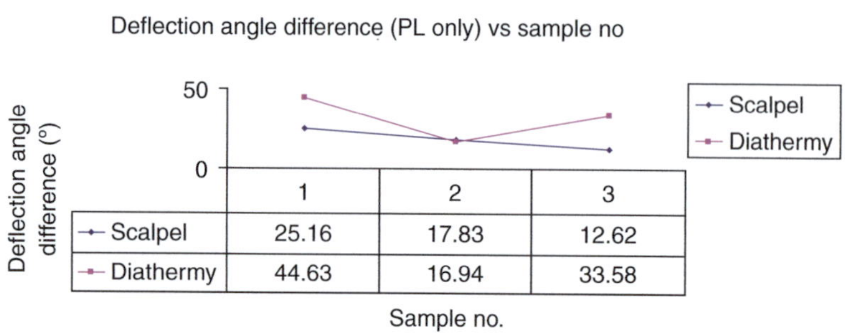

	1	2	3
Scalpel	25.16	17.83	12.62
Diathermy	44.63	16.94	33.58

Fig. 29.15 Graph to show deflection angle difference as distributed within the three samples in the scalpel and diathermy groups

References

1. Mustarde JC. The correction of prominent ears using simple mattress sutures. Br J Plast Surg. 1963;16:170–8.
2. Morestin PHM. De la reposition et du plissement cosmetiques due pavillon de l'oreille. Rev Orthop. 1903; 4:289.
3. Becker OJ. Correction of the protruding deformed ear. Br J Plast Surg. 1952;5(3):187–96.
4. McEvitt WG. The problem of the protruding ear. Plast Reconstr Surg. 1947;2:358–61.
5. Burningham AR, Stucker FJ. Otoplasty technique: how I do it. Facial Plast Surg Clin North Am. 2006; 14(2):73–7.
6. Stenstrom SJ, Heftner J. The Stenstrom otoplasty. Clin Plast Surg. 1978;5(3):465–70.
7. Bhatti AZ, Donovan DO. Sutureless otoplasty by scoring of the cartilage: a study in 34 patients. Br J Oral Maxillofac Surg. 2007;45(3):217–20.
8. Qureshi TR, Hurren JS, Gourlay T. The effectiveness of scoring and bipolar diathermy on ear cartilage behavior: ex vivo study. Ann Plast Surg. 2007; 58(3):321–7.

9. Bajaj Y, Rokade A, De PR. Otoplasty: experience with a modification using a drill, and literature review. J Laryngol Otol. 2007;121(1):61–4.
10. Janis JE, Rohrich RJ, Gutowski KA. Otoplasty. Plast Reconstr Surg. 2005;115(4):60e–72.
11. Adamson JE, Horton CE, Crawford HH. The growth pattern of the external ear. Plast Reconstr Surg. 1965;36(4):466–70.
12. Porter CJ, Tan ST. Congenital auricular anomalies: topographic anatomy, embryology, classification, and treatment strategies. Plast Reconstr Surg. 2005; 115(6):1701–12.
13. Tan ST, Abramson DL, MacDonald DM, Mulliken JB. Molding therapy for infants with deformational auricular anomalies. Ann Plast Surg. 1997;38(3):263–8.
14. Adamson PA, Strecker HD. Otoplasty techniques. Facial Plast Surg. 1995;11(4):284–300.
15. Furnas DW, Lin SJ. Ear, prominent ear. April 9, 2007. http://www.emedicine.com/plastic/topic454.htm. Accessed 27 Mar 2007.
16. Ballenger JJ, Snow JB. Otorhinolaryngology head and neck surgery. 15th ed. Philadelphia: Williams & Wilkins; 1996.

Diamond Burr Drill Use in Otoplasty

30

Yogesh Bajaj and Natasha Choudhury

Introduction

Prominent ears are the most common congenital deformity in the head and neck region [1], with an incidence of about 5 % in Caucasians [1]. Prominent ears are usually not associated with other abnormalities or syndromes but may be considered an aesthetic handicap [2].

The basic deformities present in different degrees and combinations are decreased definition or absence of the antihelical fold, presence of a large, deep conchal bowl or an inadequate definition of the helical rim. Due to these deformities, the helical rim separates more than 2 cm from the cranium. In addition, some other defects may be present such as excessive prominence of the tail of helix, excessive protrusion of the antitragus, or forward bending of the earlobe. The technique is easy to learn and master with minimal postoperative morbidity.

Prominent ears may cause considerable emotional disturbance as a youngster usually becomes a subject of ridicule by schoolmates. At that age when personality is developing, teasing may result in a tendency towards isolation or aggressiveness [3]. While the auricle continues to develop from birth throughout life, the majority of growth occurs at an early age. Eighty-five percent of the ultimate size of pinna is attained at the age of three, and seven-eighths of the total growth takes place before the age of seven [4]. After 9 years of age, no substantial growth takes place. The average difference in length of a fully developed ear and one at 9 years of age is about 5 mm [3]. Therefore, in order to avoid emotional disturbances which can lead to personality disorder, surgical correction of prominent ears should preferably be done at or before the start of schooling.

The goal of otoplasty is to achieve a normal antihelical fold with a scaphoconchal angle of about 90°, normally curved superior crus, and an adequate depth of the concha. After recession of the ear, neither the tail of the helix nor the antitragus should be abnormally prominent and the lobe should not bend forward. The vertical helical rim should be about 1.5 cm from the scalp, and the rim should have a curl [3].

Although Sushruta (seventh century BC, Indian surgeon) and Tagliacozzi (sixteenth century, Italian surgeon) described otoplasty techniques, the modern era of otoplasty can be traced to 1848, when the term "otoplastik" was first used by Dieffenbach in his description of the repair of microtia [1]. Ely performed and published otoplasty by an anterior approach in 1881 [4]. He removed a full thickness strip of the auricle, but this left a visible scar along the line of antihelix on either side of the pinna. Keen [1] modified the

Y. Bajaj, M.D. • N. Choudhury
Department of ENT,
Barts & Royal London Hospitals,
London, UK
e-mail: ybajaj@hotmail.co.uk;
natashamasood1@aol.com

M.A. Shiffman (ed.), *Advanced Cosmetic Otoplasty*,
DOI 10.1007/978-3-642-35431-1_30, © Springer-Verlag Berlin Heidelberg 2013

same technique by leaving the anterior skin bridge intact to prevent a noticeable scar.

A post-auricular incision was first published by Morestin in 1903 [4]. After this, many attempts were made to correct prominent ears by using various antihelical and conchal cartilage excisions using this posterior approach. In 1940s, attempts were made to weaken the cartilage by mechanically thinning or placing partial incisions in it. In 1947 McEvitt [5] made parallel incisions in the posterior cartilage plane, whereas Tanzer in 1962 [6], in addition to the parallel incisions, anchored the antihelical plica with permanent suture. In 1960s, Mustarde used permanent retention sutures in a combined technique with a fusiform skin excision to recreate the antihelical fold. In 1963, Stenstrom and Chongchet [7] scored the anterior part of the conchal cartilage to create an antihelix through a posterior incision. In 1968, Furnas [8] described a procedure, which consisted of securing the concha to the mastoid periosteum posteriorly, thereby decreasing the concha-scaphoid angle. In 1967, Kaye [9] used mattress sutures that were placed in the auricular cartilage through small anterior incisions, and Johnson [10] in 1994 emphasized obliquely placed sutures to control the final curve and shape of the antihelix, performed through a posterior approach. An ideal technique to correct protruding ears has not yet been established. This chapter describes another modification of otoplasty using a diamond burr drill to thin the cartilage and form the antihelix.

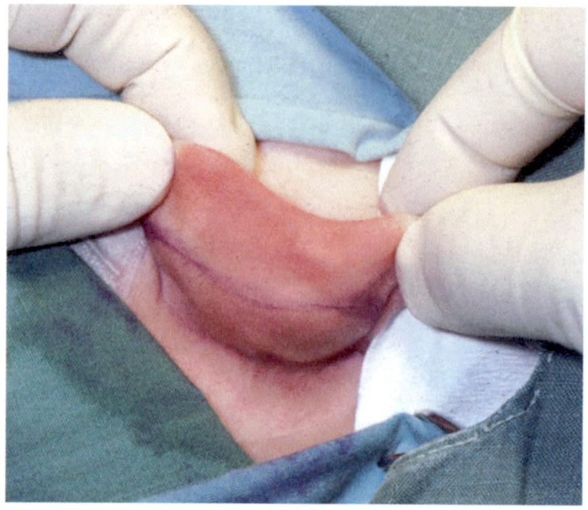

Fig. 30.1 Incision marked for skin excision

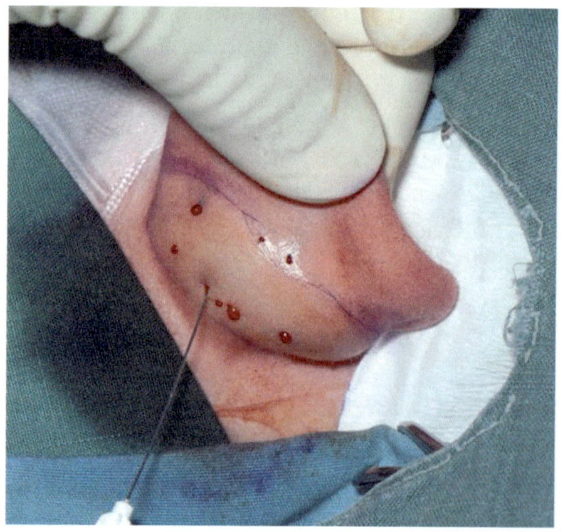

Fig. 30.2 Injecting lignocaine with adrenaline

Surgical Technique

The operation is performed under general anaesthesia. The line where the antihelix has to be created is marked with methylene blue. Three to four markings are made by passing a straight hypodermic needle through the skin and the cartilage; the tip is then dabbed with a cotton bud soaked in the dye and withdrawn. This helps to leave marks on the cartilage (Fig. 30.1). The cranial surface of the pinna is infiltrated with 2 % lignocaine with 1:80,000 adrenaline (Fig. 30.2). Keeping the methylene blue markings as the middle reference point, a spindle-shaped incision is marked (Fig. 30.1). This spindle-shaped skin is excised from the posterior surface of the pinna (Fig. 30.3). The perichondrium on the exposed posterior surface is incised along the markings made before with methylene blue (Fig. 30.4). The perichondrium is elevated off the cartilage for about 5 mm on either sides of the incision (Fig. 30.5). The exposed cartilage is thinned using a 2 mm diamond burr over a width of 5 mm along the markings for the antihelix (Fig. 30.6). The end point of the drilling is the pinkish hue of the lateral surface. The aim should be to leave a very thin layer of the cartilage over the perichondrium on the lateral side. Also care should be taken not to thin the superior crus too much to

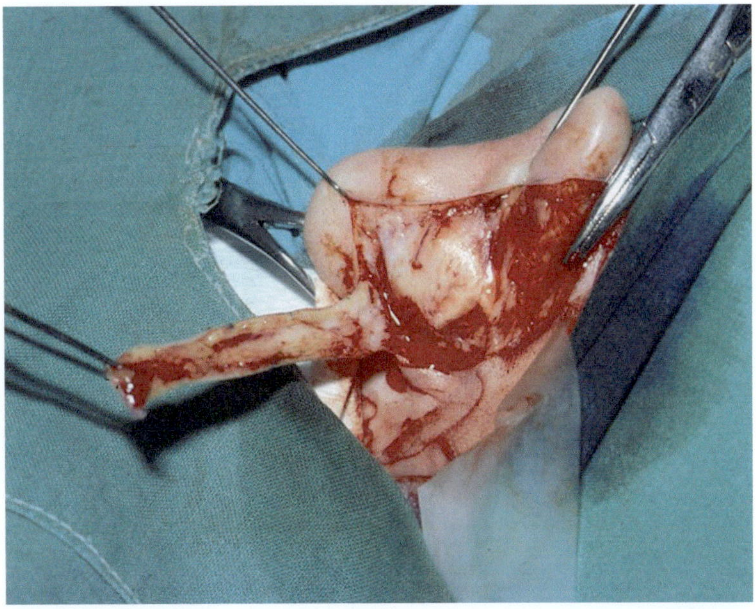

Fig. 30.3 Excising spindle-shaped skin from medial surface of pinna

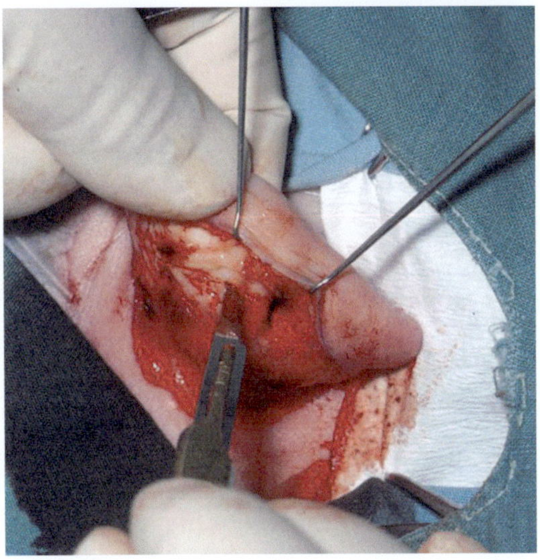

Fig. 30.4 Perichondrium incised over the previously marked antihelix

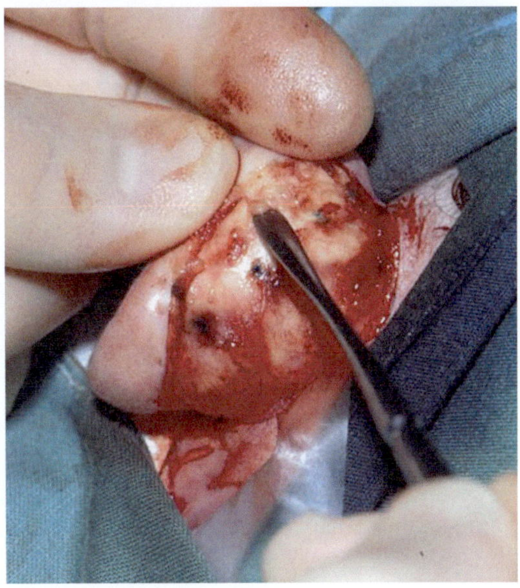

Fig. 30.5 Perichondrium elevated off the cartilage for 5 mm either side of the incision

avoid a sharp ridge. At this stage the perichondrial flaps on the posterior surface are sutured with 3.0 undyed Vicryl interrupted sutures to create the missing antihelix (Fig. 30.7). The contours are checked continuously while suturing. The skin edges are then sutured with 3.0 undyed Vicryl interrupted mattress sutures. Overcorrection of the deformity is desirable at the end of the operation (Fig. 30.8). Acriflavine-soaked cotton wool is molded into the contours on both surfaces of the pinna. A turban dressing is done after adequate padding to prevent hematoma formation. The dressing is removed after 1 week. After this the patients are advised to use bandage at night for 3 weeks.

Preoperative assessment included the state of the antihelical fold, the condition of the conchal

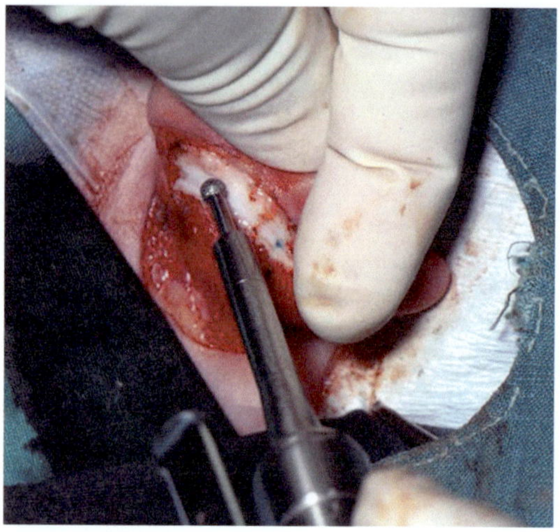

Fig. 30.6 Exposed cartilage is thinned using diamond burr drill

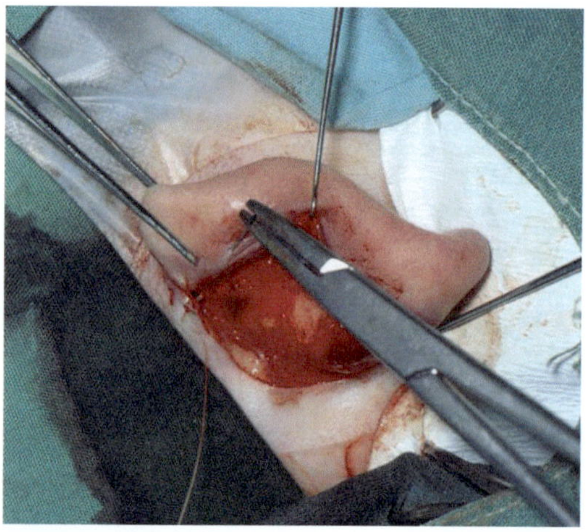

Fig. 30.7 Perichondrium flaps sutured to create antihelix

bowl, the plane of the lobule and the quality and spring of the auricular cartilage. Pre- and postoperative photographs should be taken for all patients (Fig. 30.9). The results using this technique have been published [11].

Discussion

Otoplasty is an artistic exercise in creating the proper form and dimension of the ear. The goal of otoplasty is to produce symmetrical, natural-looking ears with no obvious signs of surgery. The preoperative assessment should include

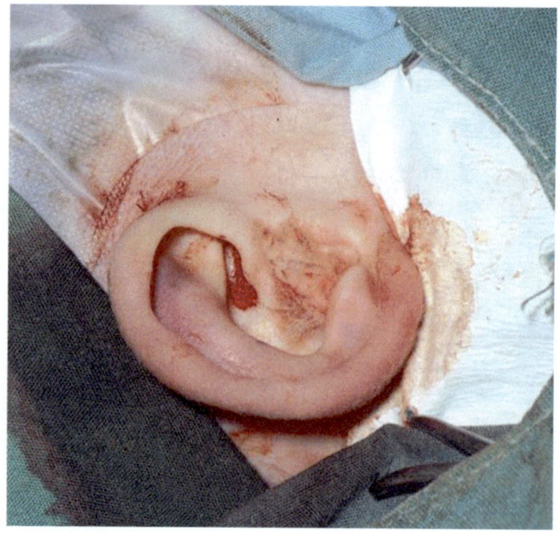

Fig. 30.8 End result after suturing

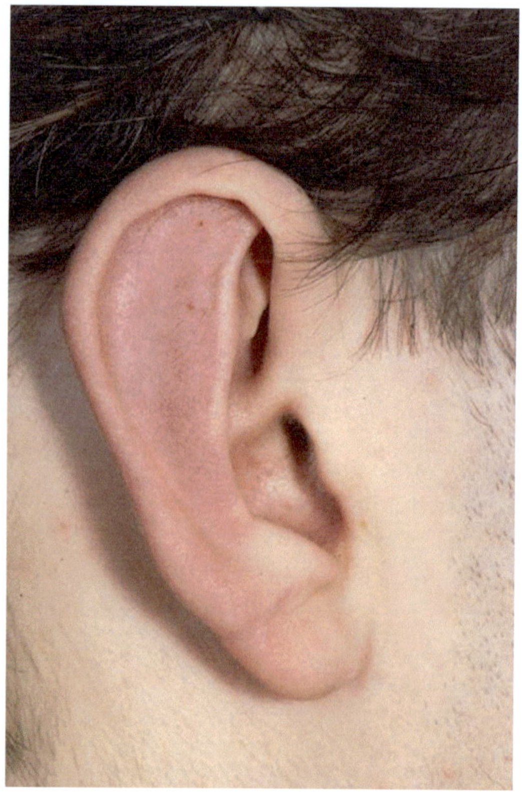

Fig. 30.9 Result 6 month postoperatively

detailed history including bleeding tendency and history of keloids.

A variety of techniques are available to shape the auricular cartilage that forms the framework of the ear. The basic requisite for good results is controlling the position and degree of folding of the antihelix. Otoplasty techniques can be divided, in general, into cartilage-sparing and cartilage-cutting techniques.

The cartilage-sparing techniques offer the surgeon the ability to do this without disrupting the structural integrity of the ear. Of these, Mustarde [12] and Furnas [13] concha-mastoid sutures are the most commonly described. The Mustarde technique is one of the most commonly used methods for creation of the antihelical fold in the prominent ear deformity. One part of this procedure that can be difficult to perform is precise tightening of the cartilage-conforming sutures. Because the surgeon's attention is directed laterally to achieve the desired antihelical shape, tightening the sutures medially generally is done without direct exposure. This manoeuver is awkward and creates a risk of undercorrection by tying the knots too loosely because of soft tissue entrapment and the tendency for the cartilage to unfold [14]. There may be pain from nonabsorbable sutures pricking the dermis from beneath [15]. Also, post-auricular suture extrusion may result [16]. Messner and Crysdale [17], observing patient's treated using Mustarde technique for at least 1 year after surgery, found that in up to 40 % of ears, the final position had returned to within 3 mm of the preoperative state. Tan [18] found that with placement of Mustarde suture alone, 24 % of patients required reoperation for recurrent deformities.

The other major group is cartilage-cutting techniques of which the anterior scoring method is most commonly used [19, 20]. Scoring facilitates the bending of the cartilage, but it may cause painful and unattractive ridging if performed too aggressively. Calder and Nassan [20] observed that 8 % of ears treated with anterior scoring retain some residual deformity. Cutting the auricular cartilage subjects the antihelix to irreversible, unpredictable distortion by wound contraction forces [1]. There has been increasing criticism of anterior scoring method because of unacceptably high complication rates (24 %), especially in training grade surgeons [21]. These complications arise from the anterior dissection causing anterior hematoma that may lead to anterior skin necrosis. Chondritis may follow secondary to hematoma and infection, and this may result in irreparable cartilage irregularities [22, 23].

This technique described using drill to thin the auricular cartilage posteriorly seems to be a more delicate approach. Thinning of the cartilage by drilling softens the cartilage spring and allows accurate shaping which can be held in a stable position by mattress sutures. It is a safe and controlled technique, and one can stop drilling when the desired result has been achieved. It is a middle path between cartilage-sparing and cartilage-cutting techniques and thus avoids the complications associated with both the techniques.

Conclusions

The technique of otoplasty described using the drill to thin the auricular cartilage is safe and easy to learn and perform. It has few complications and has reproducible cosmetic results. The long-term results are very good, and it can be used as a standard technique.

References

1. Yugueros P, Friedland JA. Otoplasty: the experience of 100 consecutive patients. Plast Reconstr Surg. 2001; 108(4):1045–51.
2. Vuyk HD. Cartilage sparing otoplasty: a review with long term results. J Laryngol Otol. 1997;111(5): 424–30.
3. Hinderer UT, Del Rio JL, Fregnal FJ. Otoplasty for prominent ears. Aesthetic Plast Surg. 1987;11(2):63–9.
4. Hell B, Garbea D, Heissler E, Klein M, Gath H, Langford A. Otoplasty: a combined approach to different structures of the auricle. Int J Oral Maxillofac Surg. 1997;26(6):408–13.
5. McEvitt WG. The problem of protruding ear. Plast Reconstr Surg (1946). 1947;2(5):481–96.
6. Tanzer RC. The correction of prominent ears. Plast Reconstr Surg. 1962;30:236–46.
7. Stenstroem SJ. A natural technique for correction of congenitally prominent ears. Plast Reconstr Surg. 1963; 32:509–18.
8. Furnas DW. Correction of prominent ears by conchamastoid sutures. Plast Reconstr Surg. 1968;42(3): 189–93.
9. Kaye BL. A simplified method for correcting the prominent ear. Plast Reconstr Surg. 1967;40(1):44–8.
10. Johnson PE. Otoplasty: shaping the antihelix. Aesthetic Plast Surg. 1994;18(1):71–4.

11. Bajaj Y, Rokade A, De PR. Otoplasty: experience with a modification using drill and review of literature. J Laryngol Otol. 2007;21(1):61–4.
12. Mustarde JC. Correction of prominent ears using buried mattress sutures. Clin Plast Surg. 1978;5(3):459–64.
13. Furnas DW. Correction of prominent ears with multiple sutures. Clin Plast Surg. 1978;5(3):491–5.
14. Hilger P, Khosh MM, Nishioka G, Larrabee WF. Modification of the Mustarde otoplasty technique using temporary contouring sutures. Plast Reconstr Surg. 1997;100(6):1585–6.
15. Rigg BM. Suture materials in otoplasty. Plast Reconstr Surg. 1979;63(3):409–10.
16. Horlock N, Misra A, Gault DG. The postauricular fascial flap as an adjunct to Mustarde and Furnas type otoplasty. Plast Reconstr Surg. 2001;108(6):1487–90.
17. Messner AH, Crysdale WS. Otoplasty: clinical protocol and long term results. Arch Otolaryngol Head Neck Surg. 1996;122(7):773–7.
18. Tan KH. Long term survey of prominent ear surgery: a comparison of two methods. Br J Plast Surg. 1986; 39(2):270–3.
19. Caouette-Laberge L, Guay N, Bortoluzzi P. Otoplasty: anterior scoring technique and results in 500 cases. Plast Reconstr Surg. 2000;105(2): 504–15.
20. Calder JC, Nassan A. Morbidity of otoplasty: a review of 562 cases. Br J Plast Surg. 1994;47(3): 170–4.
21. Jeffery SL. Complication following correction of prominent ears: an audit review of 122 cases. Br J Plast Surg. 1999;52(7):588–90.
22. Reynaud JP, Gary-Bobo A, Mateu J, Santoni A. Chondrites postopertoires de l'oreille externe: 2 cases from a series of 200 cases (387 otoplasties). Ann Chir Plast Esthet. 1986;31(2):170–3.
23. Adamson PA. Complications of otoplasty. Ear Nose Throat J. 1985;64(12):568–74.

Conchal Setback Without Resection in Prominent Ear Deformity

31

Naci Karacaoglan, Mustafa Keskin, and Bulent Cigsar

Introduction

Providing a natural-appearing ear contour has always been a key component of a successful prominent ear surgery. To achieve a natural-appearing ear, the surgical manipulations should be kept as simple as possible with little dissection and with minimum destruction. Another surgical philosophy we share is that no tissue should be removed from the body unless it is absolutely necessary. From this standpoint the authors feel that conchal cartilage hypertrophy can be and should be managed without removing the excess cartilage. To achieve a natural shape, a technique is presented that was reported by the senior author (NK) which is based on the conchal setback without resection combined with antihelical fold formation [1].

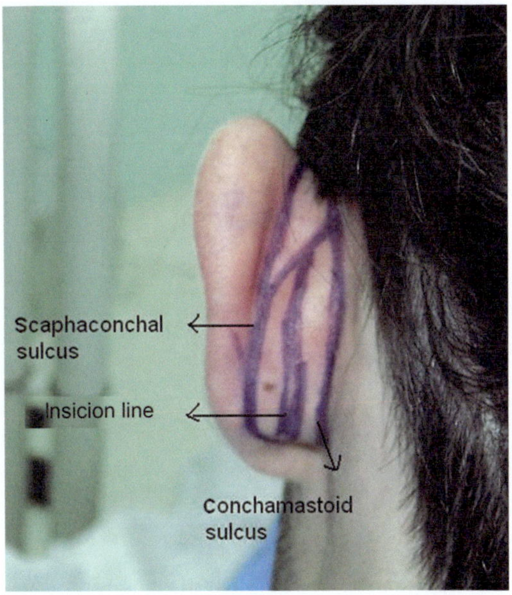

Fig. 31.1 Incision line is preoperatively marked between conchal-mastoid sulcus and conchal-scaphoid fold

Markings and Surgical Technique

The deformity is analyzed before surgery to determine the anatomical elements that are contributing to the abnormal appearance. Standardized photographs are obtained. Before the local anesthesia injection, a gentle setback of the antihelix with finger pressure will accurately estimate the severity of conchal hypertrophy and the amount of setback needed to restore balanced and aesthetically pleasing ears. Incision line is determined and marked with marker pen (Fig. 31.1).

N. Karacaoglan, M.D. (✉)
Istanbul Medipol Universitesi Tip Fakultesi, Ataturk Bulvari no 27 Unkapani, Fatih, Istanbul 34083, Turkey

Department of Plastic and Reconstructive Surgery, Medipol University, Kadikoy, Istanbul 34718, Turkey
e-mail: naci.karacaoglan@medipol.com.tr

M. Keskin, M.D. • B. Cigsar, M.D.
Istanbul Medipol Universitesi Tip Fakultesi, Ataturk Bulvari no 27 Unkapani, Fatih, Istanbul 34083, Turkey

Department of Plastic and Reconstructive Surgery, Medipol University Medical School Istanbul, Istanbul, Turkey
e-mail: mustafa.keskin@medipol.com.tr; bulent.cigsar@medipol.com.tr

M.A. Shiffman (ed.), *Advanced Cosmetic Otoplasty*, DOI 10.1007/978-3-642-35431-1_31, © Springer-Verlag Berlin Heidelberg 2013

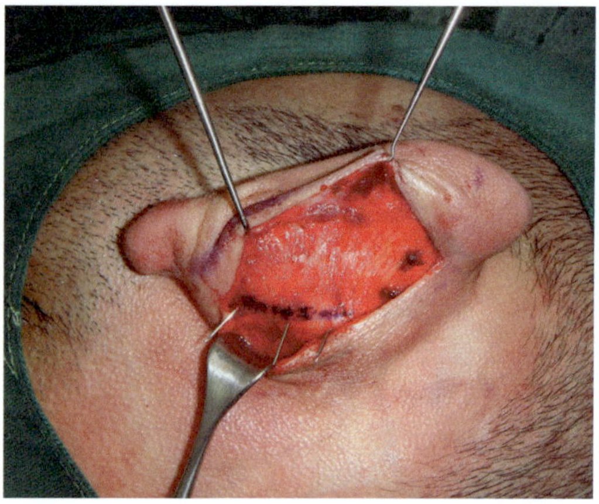

Fig. 31.2 Posterior ear skin is elevated up to helical rim and the conchal border is determined by the guidance of the needles inserted from anterior surface

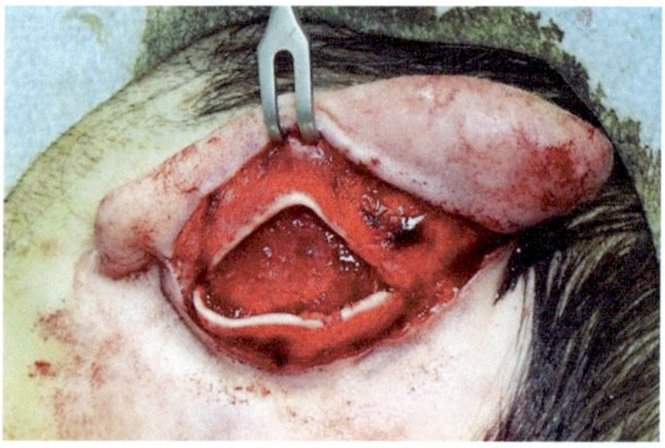

Fig. 31.3 Cartilage incision is done obliquely while the anterior skin is dissected to let the cartilage to override

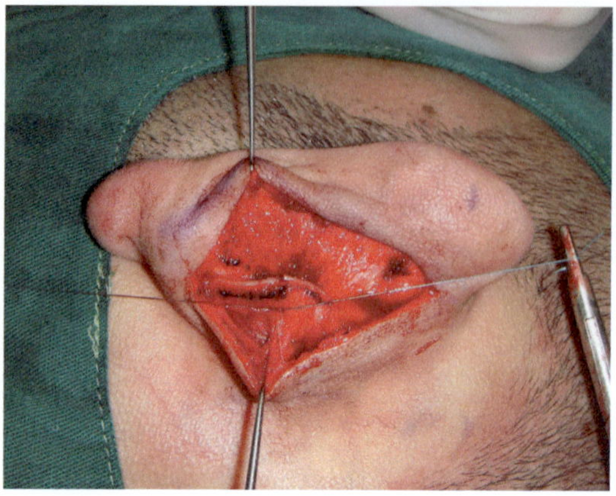

Fig. 31.4 The cartilages are held in their new position with nonabsorbable sutures

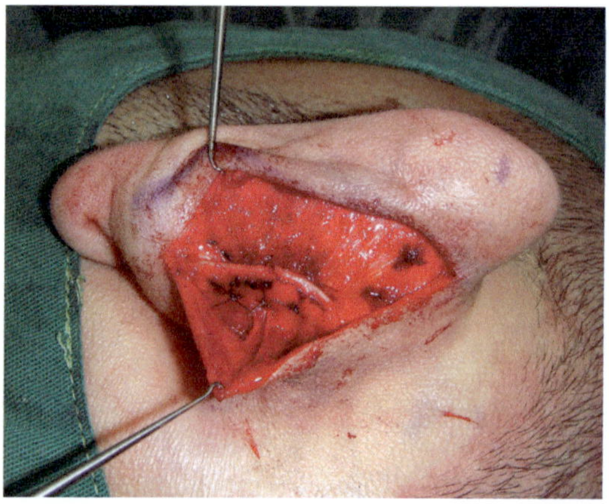

Fig. 31.5 Lateral cartilage segment overrides the lateral segment anteriorly to allow setback

After appropriate surgical cleaning and draping, the local anesthesia injection with a lidocaine and 1/100,000 adrenalin solution to block the ear sensation and minimize bleeding is performed. The skin incision reaches down to the cartilage. The posterior skin of the ear is undermined up to the conchal-mastoid sulcus medially and to the helical rim laterally. After exposing all the posterior side of the ear cartilage, the border of conchal cartilage is marked with pen according to guidance of the needles approaching from the anterior side (Fig. 31.2). Through the cartilage incision the anterior skin and conchal cavum are separated with dissection (Fig. 31.3). It is preferred to do the cartilage incision obliquely rather than perpendicularly. With gentle pressure on the helix, the amount of overriding required to produce the desired ear position can be determined. With a slight digital pressure over the conchal rim, the lateral conchal segment is positioned anteriorly and the medial segment posteriorly. If the upper and lower parts of the cartilage incision are impeding the medial movement of the cartilage, the incision can be lengthened upwards and downwards until impediment is overcome. Stabilization of the two overlapped edges of the cartilages is achieved by interrupted, inverted nonabsorbable, multifilament, white polyester 4/0 suture (with 16 mm ½ tapered needle) (Politer ® Doğsan, Trabzon, Turkey) (Figs. 31.4 and 31.5). After the conchal setback is performed the Mustardé's approach is utilized to create a soft, gentle antihelical

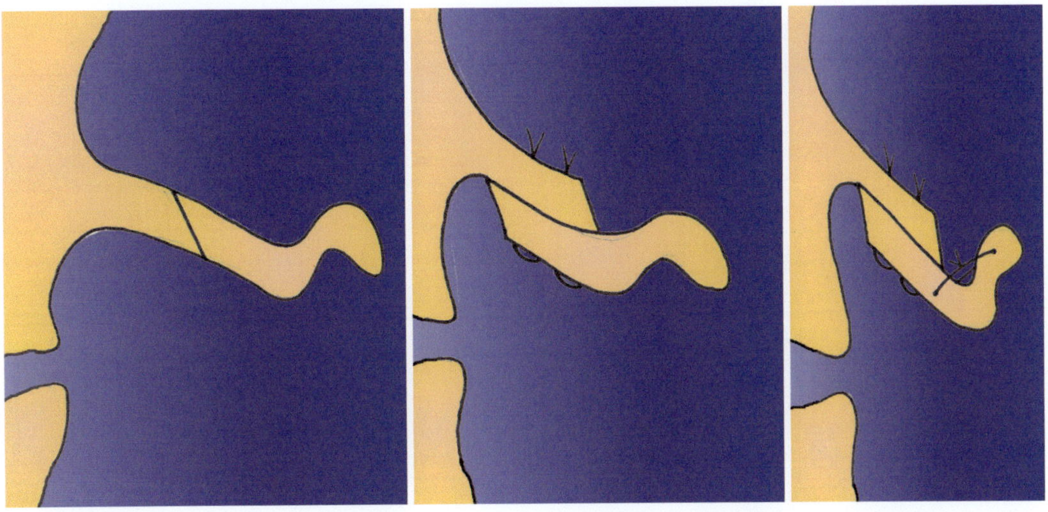

Fig. 31.6 Schematic design of the conchal setback without excision and formation of antihelical fold with Mustarde's technique

fold. The desired antihelical fold contour produced by exerting gentle digital pressure on the helix is marked on the skin. Three mattress sutures (Politer ® Doğsan, Trabzon, Turkey) are used for creating the antihelical fold (Fig. 31.6). After meticulous hemostasis, the postauricular skin incision is closed subcuticularly using an absorbable suture material. Drains should not be needed and are not routinely used (Figs. 31.7, 31.8 and 31.9).

Postoperative Care

The dressing is carried out as follows: an antibiotic ointment impregnated nonsticky gauze is placed over the postauricular suture line. Then a fluffed, cotton gauze dressing is wetted and carefully placed into the new antihelical folds and the concha. This gauze is continued to the posterior surface. Dry, fluffed, all-cotton gauze is then placed over the wet gauze. The gauzes are held in place with an Ace bandage. The dressings are removed on the third postoperative day and the patient is given a headband that is to be worn continuously for 3 weeks and at night for a minimum of 1 month to prevent accidental stresses on the ear during sleep. After the dressing is removed, showers and shampooing are allowed.

Complications

Regardless of the procedure used, the prominent ear surgery yields a high patient satisfaction rate with minimal complications. Complications such as hematoma, infection, and skin and cartilage necrosis are usually preventable with skillful surgery and not strictly related to the technique implemented. Depending on the technique used, recurrence can be a common complication and may be decreased by combining appropriate techniques. The technique described here has the potential to cause sharp edge deformity at the anterior conchal bowl. The sliding anterior segment edge can be visible if the cartilage has been cut perpendicular. To prevent this deformity the sliding anterior edge should be cut obliquely and should be smooth.

Discussion

Many methods have been described to correct prominent ears, but no single operation is currently capable of resolving all cases. A critical evaluation and planning is critical to accommodate the different etiologies. It is better to define the components of the problem for each case and plan the surgical correction rather than

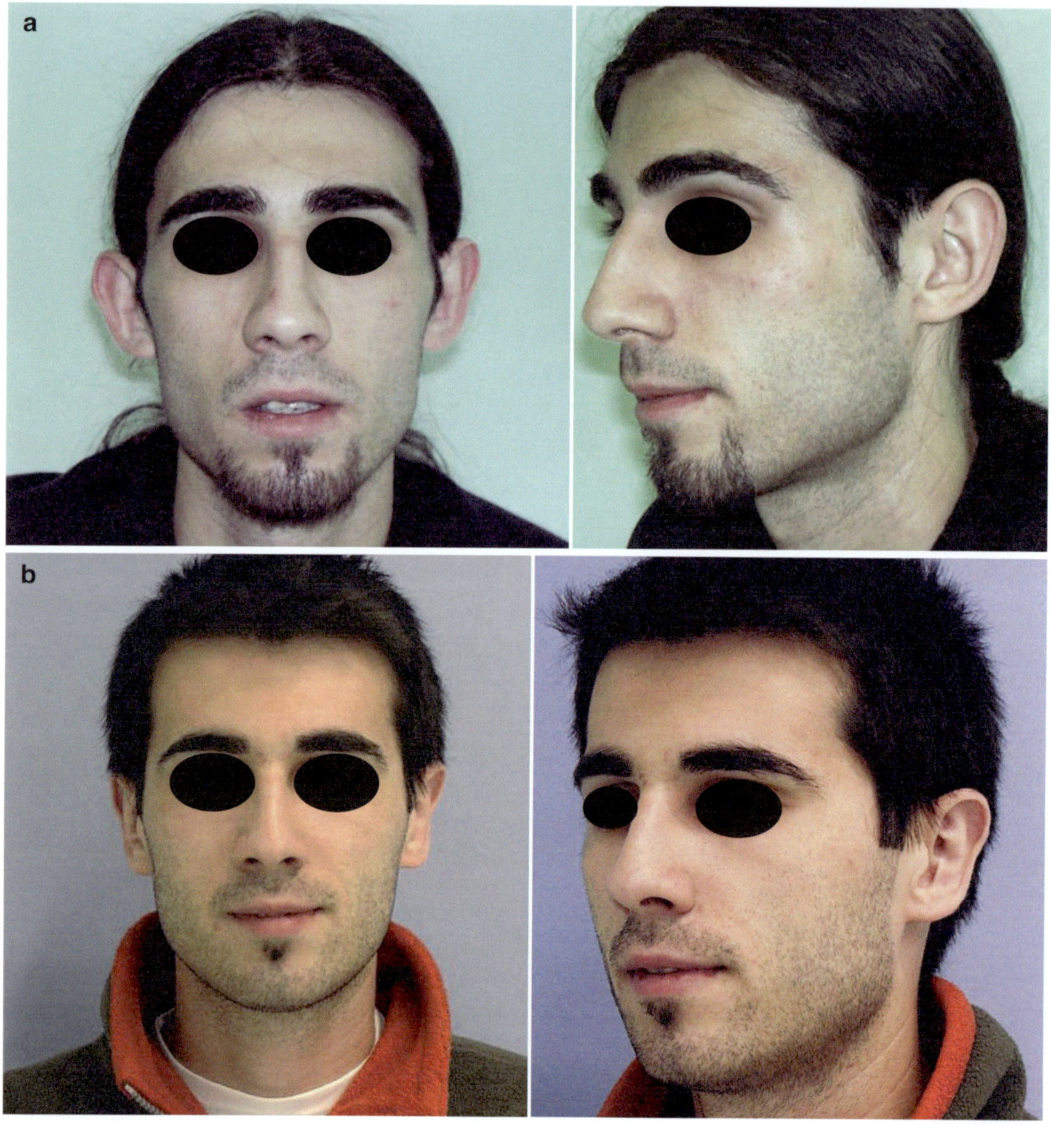

Fig. 31.7 (**a**) Preoperative. (**b**) Postoperative a year after the operation of a patient treated with described technique

performing a standard approach for each case. A prominent ear is characterized by either underdevelopment of the antihelical fold or an oversized concha alone or in combination of these two in varying degrees [2]. Most of the surgeries done for prominent ears are primarily focused on antihelical fold alone and conchal hypertrophy is ignored. The majority of patients seen for secondary otoplasty have been those whose conchal hypertrophy has been ignored, inadequately corrected, or missed [3].

Conchal deformity can be successfully addressed by several methods, including suturing techniques, excisional techniques, and posterior auricular muscle manipulations [4]. Conchal-mastoid sutures can be used to correct conchal excess of the ear. This is performed before correction of any antihelix defect. The main problem with conchal-mastoid suture is that medial repositioning of the cartilage causes narrowing of the acoustic meatus. If excessive medial rotation is required to achieve adequate setback, the tragus will be forced to rotate in a

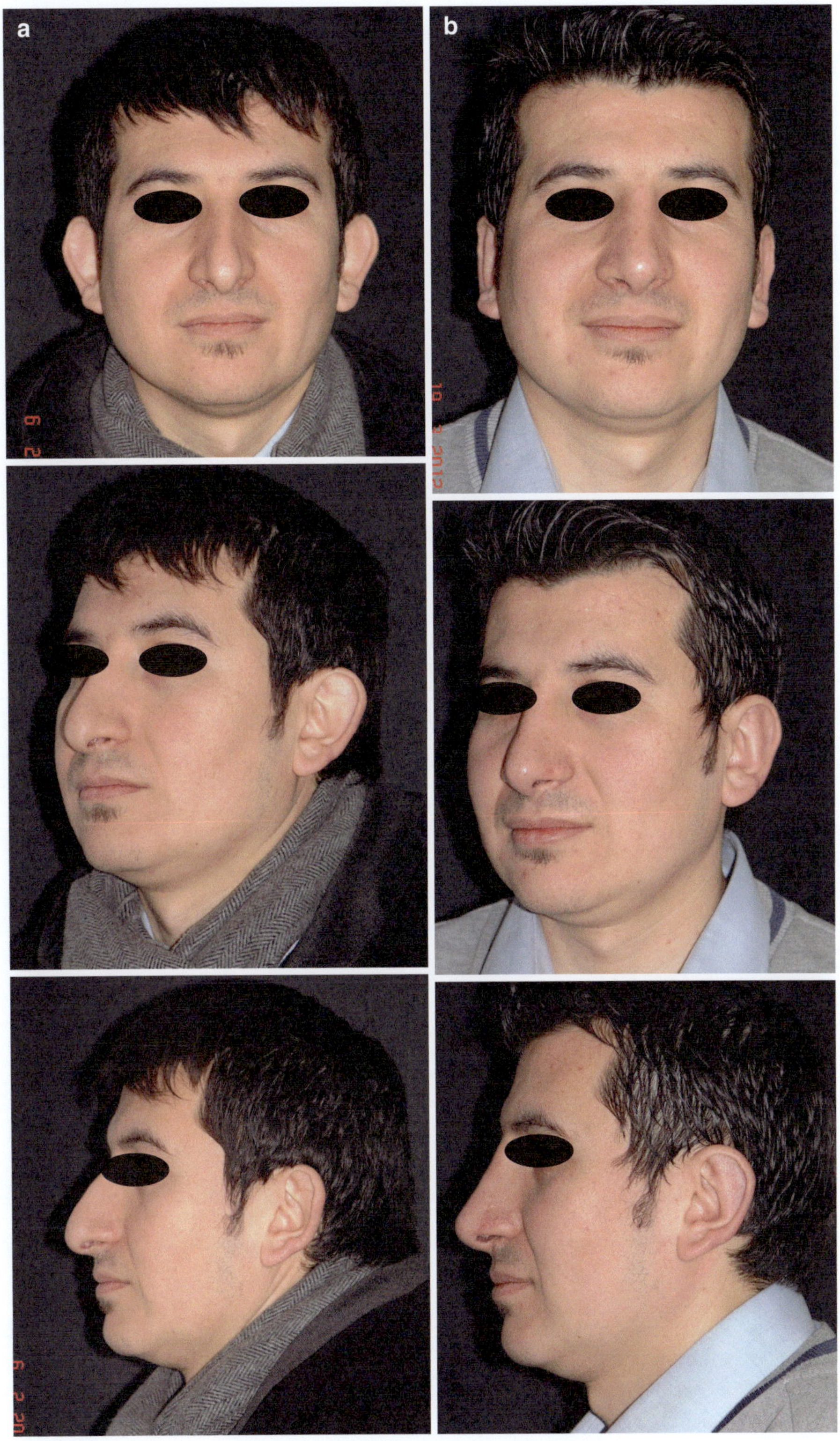

Fig. 31.8 (**a**) Preoperative. (**b**) Postoperative a month after the operation of a patient treated with described technique. Rhinoplasty was also performed

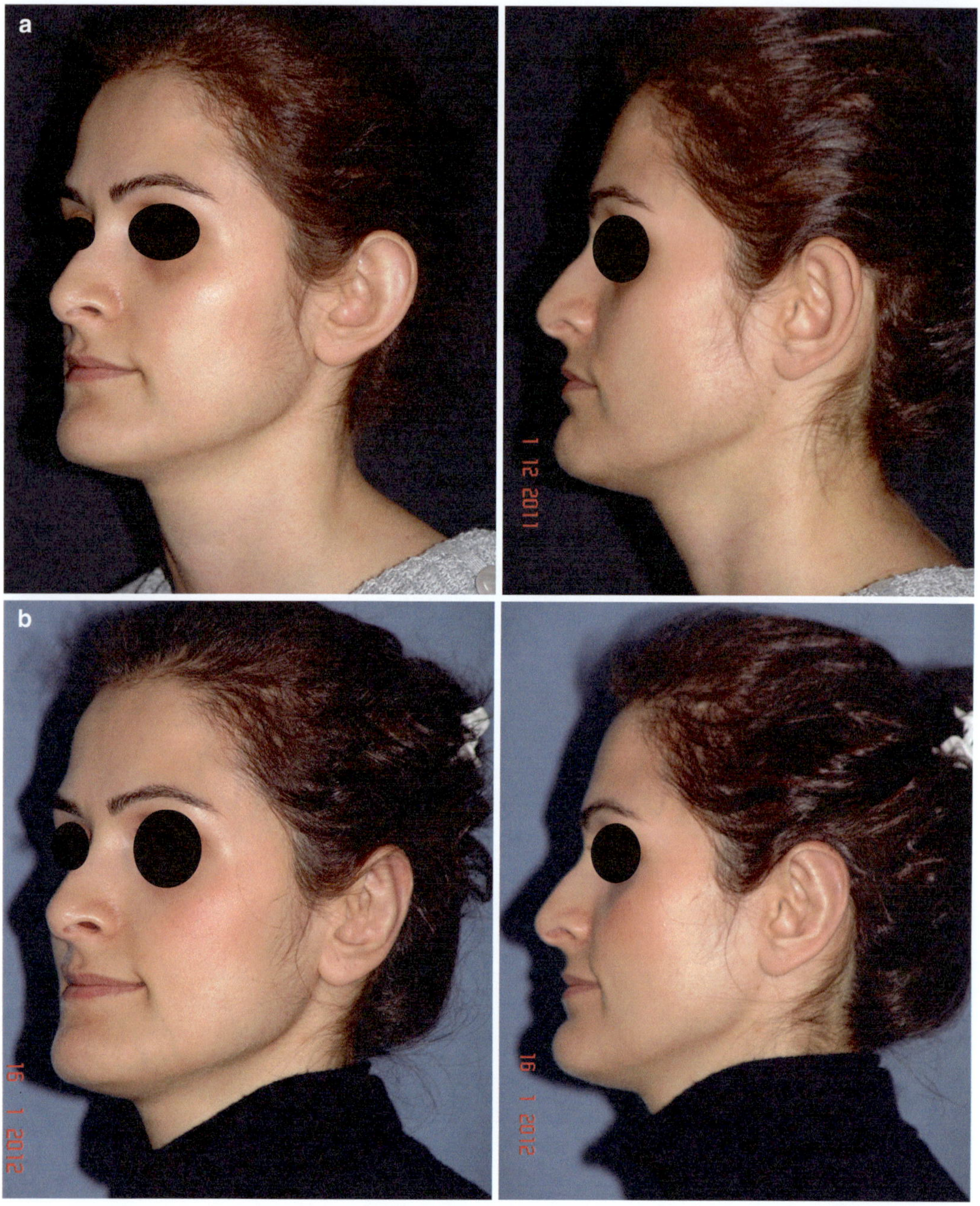

Fig. 31.9 (**a**) Preoperative. (**b**) Postoperative a month after the operation of a patient treated with described technique

lateral direction, which produces an unsightly prominence and deformity of the tragus [3]. If excessive dissection over the mastoid area is done, there is the risk of damaging posterior auricular muscle which pulls the auricle back toward the head and affecting its dynamics [5, 6].

The hypertrophied concha may be recalcitrant to conchal-mastoid suture repositioning techniques and may require cartilage excision. Cartilage can be excised alone or with anterior skin. The cartilage-only procedures are usually performed through a posterior approach, whereas the skin and cartilage techniques are usually performed through an anterior approach. Cartilage removal is an aggressive and complicated procedure and may cause cartilage destruction and irregularities. Scarring is also a problem if anterior approach to the concha is used. Furthermore, cartilage excision is irreversible so it should be done cautiously [7].

Cartilage-sparing techniques are gaining popularity in cosmetic surgeries [8]. They are preferred because of their safety and readjustability. To reposition the concha, we use the technique where the conchal hypertrophy is corrected without excising the conchal cartilage but by sliding the lateral conchal cartilage segment over the medial segment after a cartilage incision. As a consequence of this maneuver, the conchal-mastoid angle is restored again and the antihelical fold is formed up to some degree so lesser Mustarde's sutures are needed. For this reason the conchal hypertrophy must be corrected before creating the antihelical fold. The sliding of cartilage segments over each other reduces the risk of anterior skin redundancy, preserves cartilaginous support, and helps creating a softer conchal bowl contour when compared to conventional conchal excision. There is no need for wide posterior dissections over the mastoid bone so the posterior auricular muscle is not affected. The movement of the lateral conchal cartilage segment over the medial segment does not disturb the external auditory canal. On the other hand conchal sutures can be undone and symmetry can be provided again by reestablishing the setback. The reversible nature of suture placement allows adjustment. We believe it is this controllability and precision that allows us to achieve better form and symmetry. Finally as conchal cartilage is not excised, it is saved as a possible cartilage graft donor in further reconstructive operations especially considering rhinoplasty.

References

1. Karacaoglan N, Ciloglu SN. Conchal setback without resection in prominent ear deformity. Otolaryngol Head Neck Surg. 2011;145(6):930–1.
2. Salgarelli AC, Bellini P, Multinu A, Landini B, Broccaioli E, Consolo U. Combined technique for the correction of prominent ears: results in 140 patients. Br J Oral Maxillofac Surg. 2009;47(7):545–9.
3. Bauer BS, Song DH, Aitken ME. Combined otoplasty technique: chondrocutaneous conchal resection as the cornerstone to correction of the prominent ear. Plast Reconstr Surg. 2002;110(4):1033–40.
4. Janis JE, Rohrich RJ, Gutowski KA. Otoplasty. Plast Reconstr Surg. 2005;115(4):60e–72.
5. Guyuron B, DeLuca L. Ear projection and the posterior auricular muscle insertion. Plast Reconstr Surg. 1997;100:457–60.
6. Yazici I, Findikçioğlu F, Ozmen S, Noyan N, Yavuzer R. Posterior auricular muscle flap as an adjunct to otoplasty. Aesthetic Plast Surg. 2009;33(4):527–32.
7. Bauer BS, Margulis A, Song DH. The importance of conchal resection in correcting the prominent ear. Aesthet Surg J. 2005;25(1):72–9.
8. Keskin M, Tosun Z, Savaci N. The importance of maintaining the structural integrity of the lateral crus in tip rhinoplasty. Aesthetic Plast Surg. 2009;33(6): 803–8.

32 Cartilage Folding Technique in Otoplasty

Cristina Isac and Aurelia Isac

Introduction

Few if any other features as prominent ears can elicit such negative reactions and lead to serious psychosocial disturbances beginning with childhood. They may be a major cause of distress and frustration for the patient. Prominent ears have a frequency of 5 % in Caucasians and their hereditary component is well known. The surgery is recommended beginning with the age of 5 before the child is school-aged, considering that at age 3 the ear has achieved 85 % of its total growth [1] and at 5–6 years of age, the growth is almost completed [2].

Prominent ears have a normal chondrocutaneous structure which is abnormally shaped. Thus, they differ from other congenital malformations, such as cup ear, lop ear, Stahl's ear, cryptotia, or microtia. Their main feature is an increased cephaloauricular angle (greater than 35°), conchoscaphal angle greater than the normal 90°, and an increased distance of the auricle from the temporal scalp greater than the normal range of 17–21 mm. The goal of any otoplasty procedure is achieving a natural, symmetric result with minimal complications and short recovery.

Perhaps more than 200 procedures have been described over the years for correction of protruding ears. There is no single technique applicable in every case, rather the surgeon should posses an armamentarium of techniques and apply different procedures according to each deformity. These techniques are roughly categorized as either those using sutures or those using cartilage incision or excision. Nowadays, most of the techniques are a combination of cartilage incision and suturing and the innumerable variations of the techniques attest to the fact that in pursuit of the "holy grail" in otoplasty there is still a long way.

This chapter will deal mainly with protruding ears, although they are many times associated with other malformations, such as constricted ear or macrotia which are treated separately in other chapters. The authors will describe in detail their preferred technique consisting of cartilage incision and folding described in 1955 by Converse [3] and modified in 1963 by Chongchet [4]. The authors also tried to briefly summarize in comparison the other techniques used; also this is rather difficult considering their impressive number.

C. Isac, M.D., Ph.D. (✉)
Department of Plastic Surgery,
University of Medicine and Pharmacy "Carol Davila",
Bucharest, Romania

Department of Plastic Surgery,
University Hospital for Plastic Surgery and Burns,
Calea Grivitei 218, Sector 1, Bucharest, Romania
e-mail: ina@drisac.ro, inaisaac@yahoo.com

A. Isac, M.D., Ph.D.
Department of Plastic Surgery,
University Hospital for Plastic Surgery and Burns,
Calea Grivitei 218, Bucharest, Romania
e-mail: ireliflorin@yahoo.com

M.A. Shiffman (ed.), *Advanced Cosmetic Otoplasty*,
DOI 10.1007/978-3-642-35431-1_32, © Springer-Verlag Berlin Heidelberg 2013

Preoperative Assessment

Preoperatively the ear is assessed in terms of:

1. Antihelical fold development (superior and inferior crus) (Fig. 32.1)
2. Conchal depth (Fig. 32.2)
3. Earlobe protrusion (Fig. 32.3)
4. Cartilage stiffness
5. Degree of auricular protrusion assessed by the cephaloauricular angle, conchoscaphal angle, and the distance from the auricle to the temporal scalp
6. Symmetry [5]

Full-face anterior and posterior photographs are taken as well as close-up views of both ears.

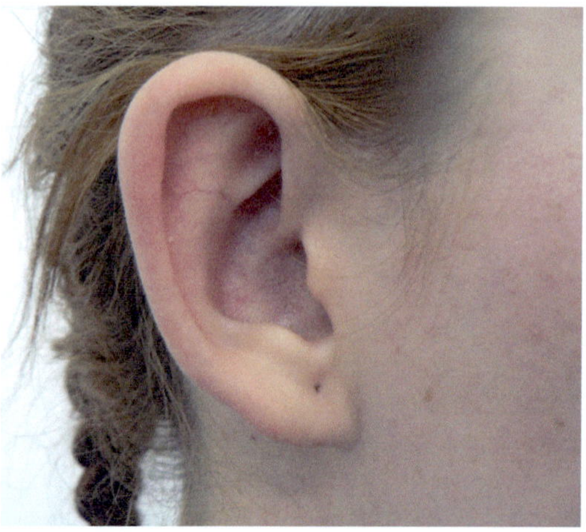

Fig. 32.1 Antihelical fold underdeveloped

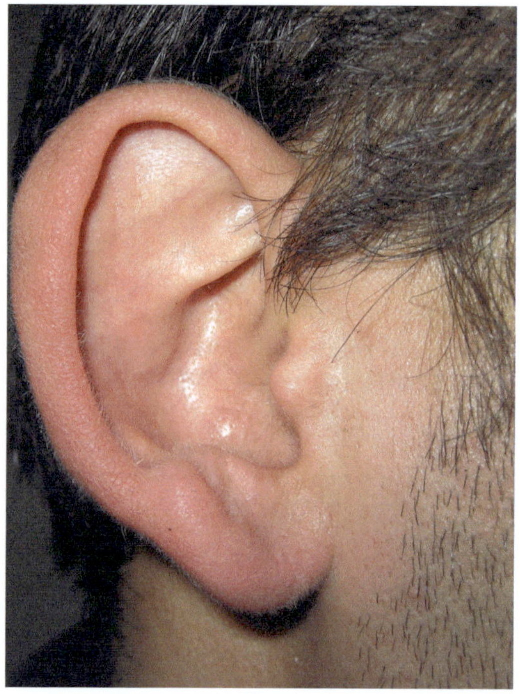

Fig. 32.3 Lack of antihelical fold, deep conchal bowl, and protrusion of the earlobe

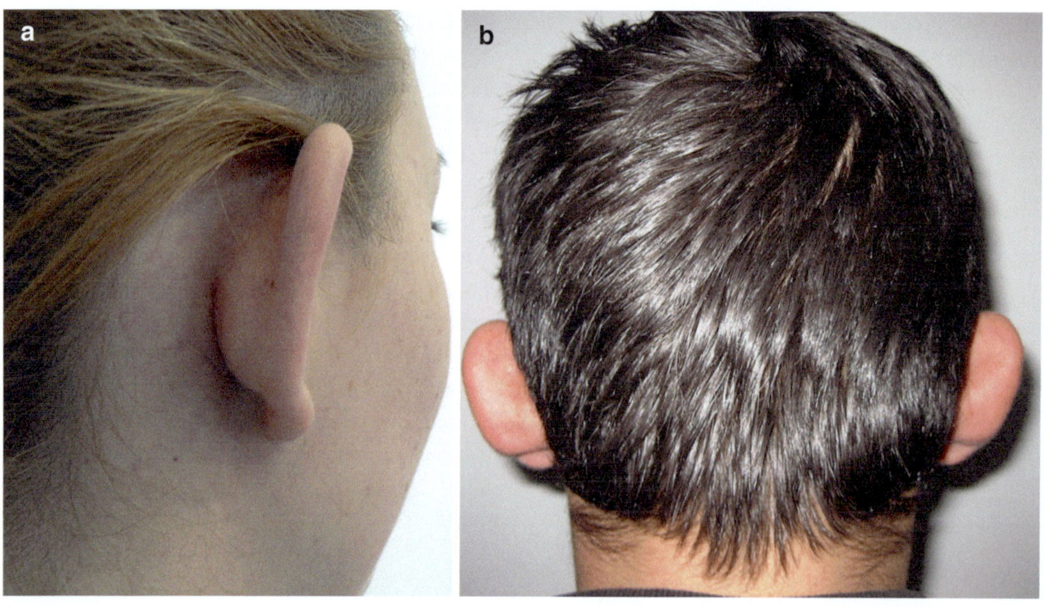

Fig. 32.2 (**a**, **b**) Excessive conchal depth

Technique of Cartilage Folding

The auricular and periauricular region are cleaned and the area is draped. The location of the new antihelical fold is established by gently pressing on the helical rim toward the mastoid region (Fig. 32.4). The ear will be bent backward and an antihelix with a natural appearance will be formed. The degree of conchal hypertrophy can also be estimated using this maneuver. The location of the antihelix is marked. The marking begins at the upper part of the triangular fossa and crosses over the future superior crus, parallel to the helical rim, in the deepest part of the scapha. Then it follows the lateral part of the future antihelix and reaches the helical tail (Fig. 32.5).

If the patient is a child, the surgery is performed under general anesthesia; if the patient is adult, it may be performed under local anesthesia potentially combined with sedation. The local anesthesia is composed of 1 % lidocaine, 1:100,000 epinephrine, and bicarbonate. Ten minutes should be awaited before beginning the surgery.

An elliptical shape of skin is excised from the posterior part of the auricle (Fig. 32.6). The skin incision extends from the upper corner of the fossa triangularis to the antitragus and is placed close to the postauricular sulcus. The width of the ellipse is about 1–2 cm. In the caudal part, the ellipse is widened in a rhomboid shape to correct the protruding lobule. The

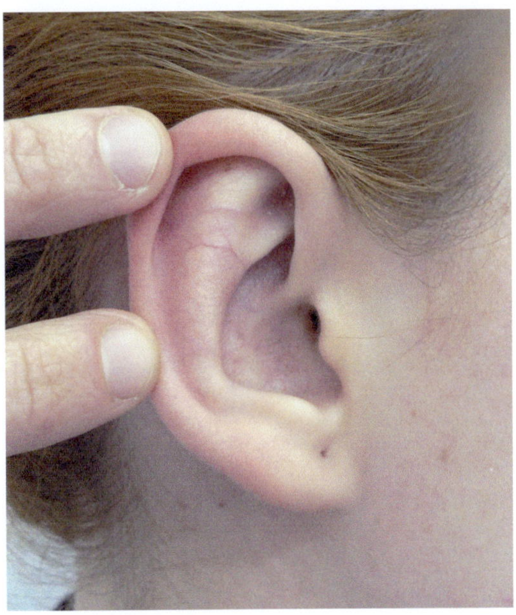

Fig. 32.4 The new antihelical fold is established by gently pressing the helical rim toward the mastoid region

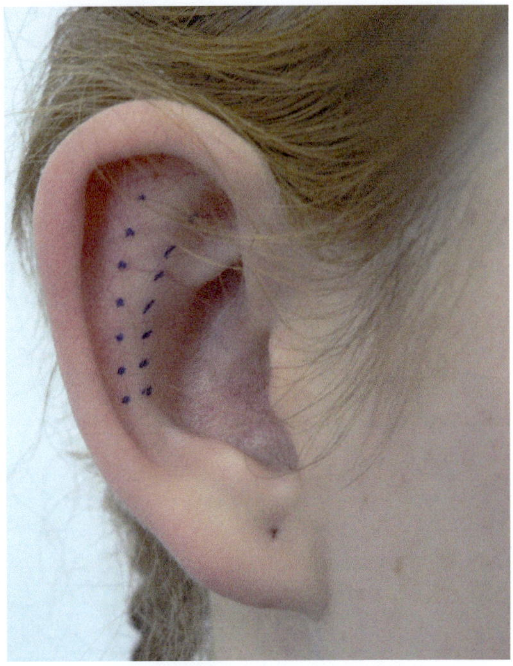

Fig. 32.5 The new antihelical fold marked

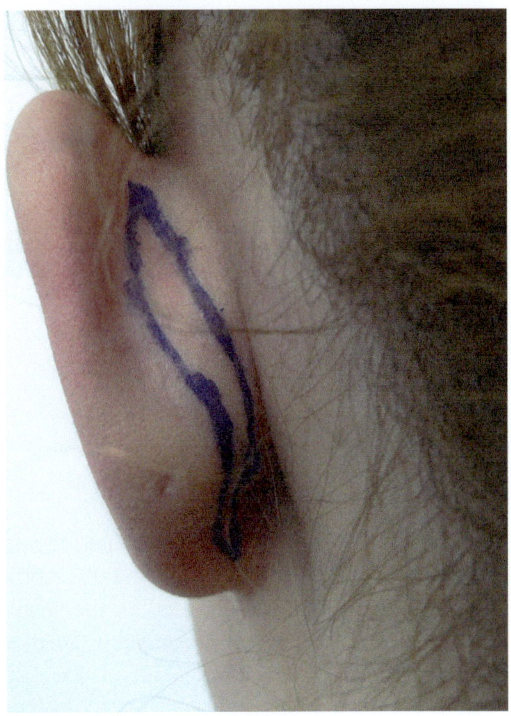

Fig. 32.6 The skin excision marked

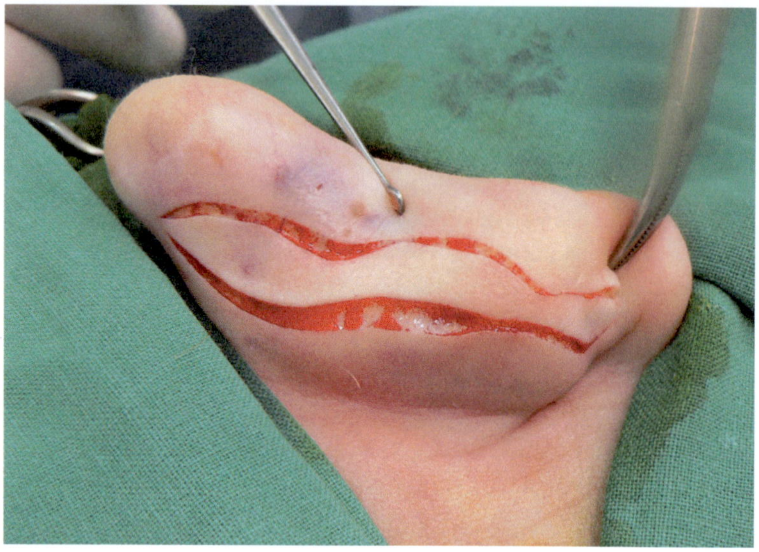

Fig. 32.7 Skin incision

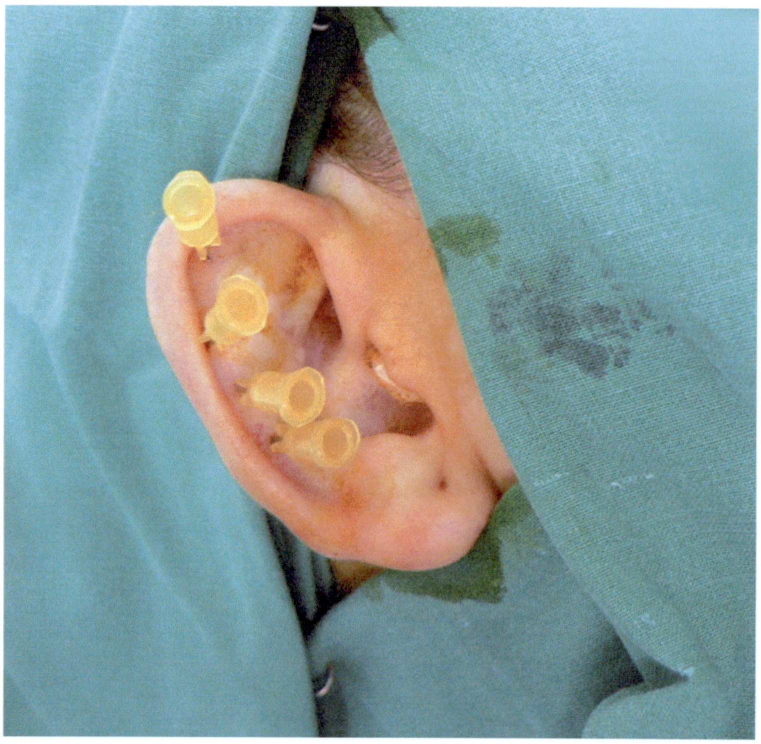

Fig. 32.8 The anterior markings are transposed on the posterior surface using transcutaneous needles

incision stops 1 cm short of the superior and inferior poles of the auricle (Fig. 32.7). The previously marked line is transposed on the posterior side of the ear using transcutaneous needles (Fig. 32.8).

After the skin is excised (Fig. 32.9), the undermining is performed in the loose areolar plane toward the helical margin and the cartilage is incised parallel to the helical rim. The cartilage incision is guided by the corresponding needles

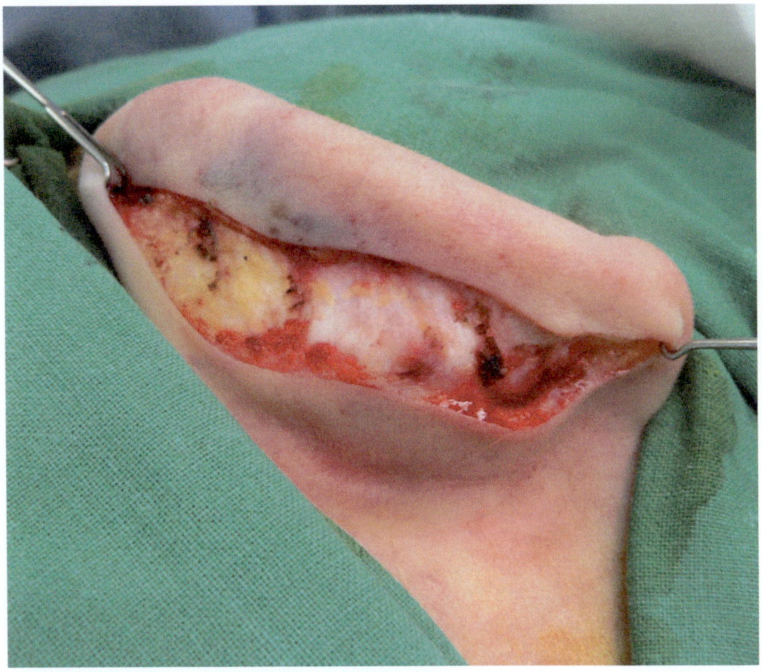

Fig. 32.9 Skin excised and the supraperichondrial plane exposed

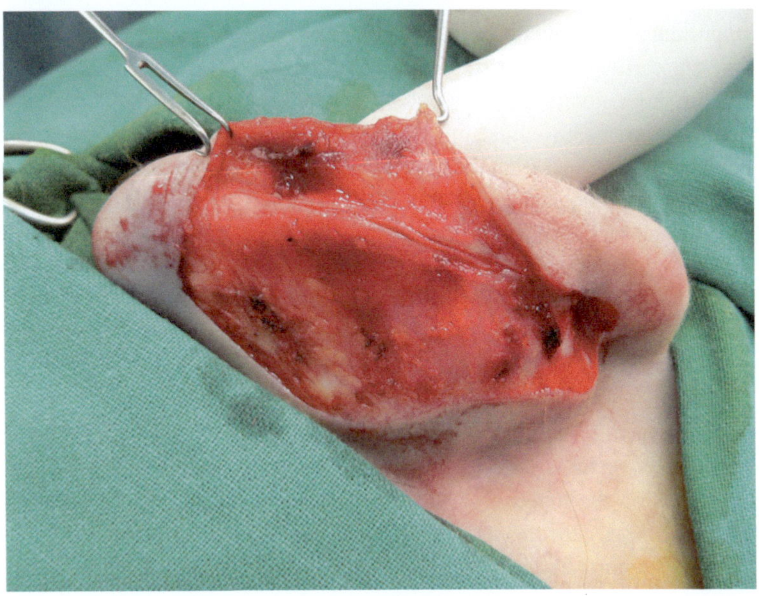

Fig. 32.10 Skin undermining in the supraperichondrial plane and cartilage incision parallel to the helical margin, leaving a strip of 0.4 cm of helix

and should leave a strip of helix of at least 0.4 cm (Fig. 32.10). The dissection is supraperichondrial so that the perichondrium on the posterior surface is carefully preserved. The upper cartilage incision follows the markings and it starts as far up as possible, anteriorly beyond the superior crus, separating the scapha from the helical rim. At the caudal end of the helix, the incision is full thickness, separating completely the helical tail from the new antihelical fold (Fig. 32.11). This will break the cartilaginous spring and will allow the cartilage to be folded back 180°. The undermining is continued on the anterior surface of the cartilage in the subperichondrial plane. It is

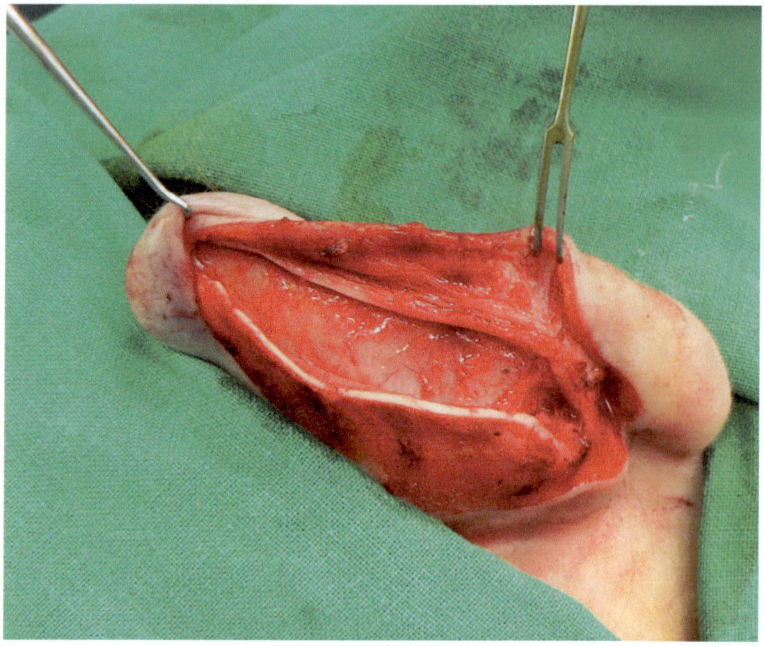

Fig. 32.11 The cartilage is incised from the scapha to the helical tail and the anterior undermining is performed in the subperichondrial plane. Note the full-thickness incision which completely separates the helical tail from the newly formed antihelix. This allows the cartilage to be folded back, by weakening its spring, and diminishes the size of the scapha and the protrusion of the earlobe

important to manipulate the cartilage very gently (the ear cartilage is very fragile and brittles easily) in order not to injure it which may cause abnormal visible irregularities. The skin on the anterior side is freed from the cartilage surface all over the antihelical area and continued down on the surface of the conchal bowl as much as the surgeon feels that, by folding the cartilage on itself, he/she can achieve the appropriate shape and dimension of the auricle as well as the appropriate distance from the helical rim to the mastoid. It is important that the anterior perichondrium be left intact to camouflage any irregularities. When the concha is very deep, the undermining continues on the anterior side of the concha so that when the cartilage is folded, much of the concha is diminished in size.

The anterior part of the cartilage which has been rolled can be gently scored (only partial-thickness incisions and only at the periphery at the newly formed antihelix, not on the top of it) with the knife but with great care so that no fracture of the cartilage should occur which can lead to visible and palpable irregularities.

At the superior end of the rolled cartilage, a triangular wedge can be excised to facilitate the folding. At the helical tail-antitragus junction there usually is a double layer of resistant cartilage that is completely removed in order for the antihelix to roll backward.

The rolled cartilage is sutured on itself with 4-0 PDS or clear nylon horizontal mattress sutures (Fig. 32.12). If the free edge of the folded cartilage seems excessive, it can be trimmed in order to avoid a protruding edge which would allow wound dehiscence (Fig. 32.13). The prominent lobule is set back with different methods. The authors prefer to use a single suture from the helical tail to the most inferior part of the concha to set back the lobule (Figs. 32.14 and 32.15). If the helical root is also prominent, then it is fixed to the temporoparietal fascia with a fossa-fascia suture in order to avoid a telephone ear deformity.

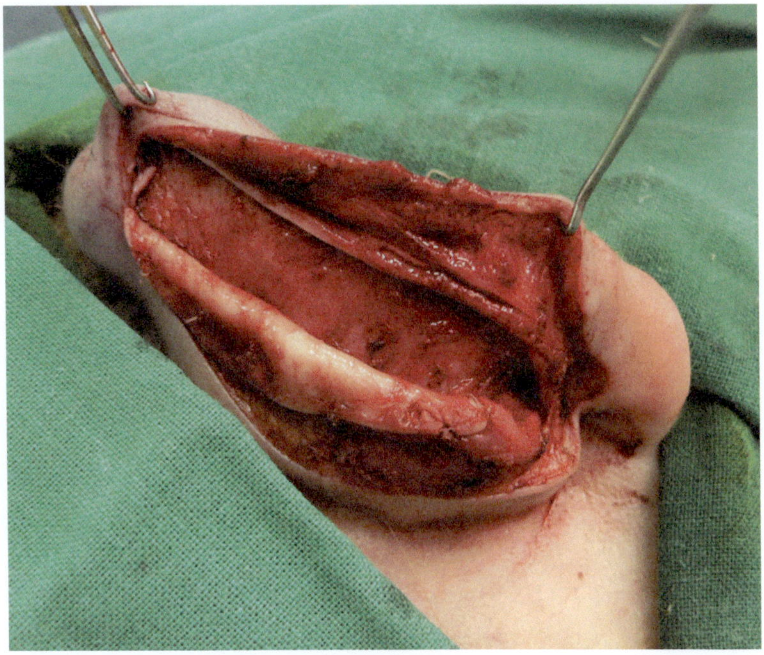

Fig. 32.12 The cartilage is folded back and sutured with 4-0 clear PDS horizontal mattress sutures

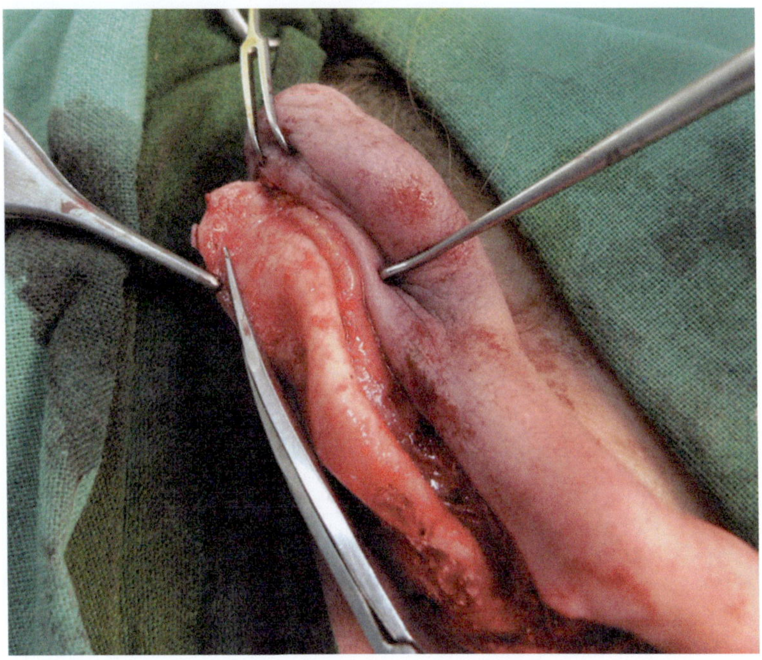

Fig. 32.13 The excessive free edge of the folded cartilage is trimmed

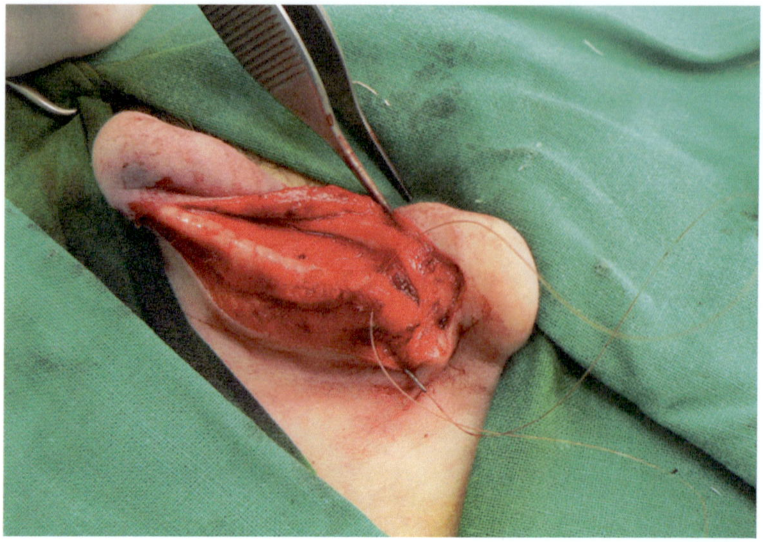

Fig. 32.14 A single suture is used from the helical tail to the concha in order to set back the lobule which forms a unit with the helix being attached to it

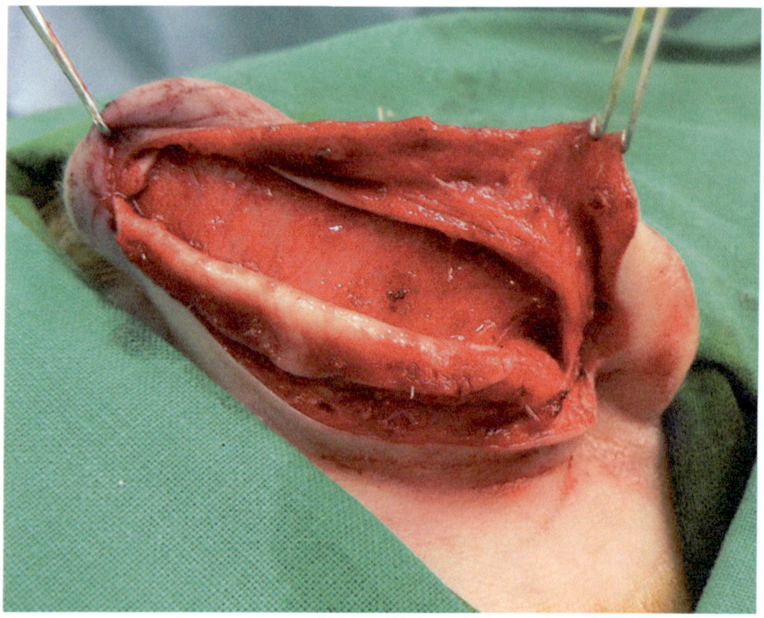

Fig. 32.15 The folded cartilage and the helical tail-concha suture in place

Hemostasis is achieved throughout the procedure using fine-tipped electrocautery.

Most patients develop significant swelling and marked ecchymosis after the procedure (Figs. 32.16 and 32.17). The dressing consists of rolls of Betadine-impregnated cotton which fill the various depressions of the ear, and an elastic bandage is applied externally (Fig. 32.18). One

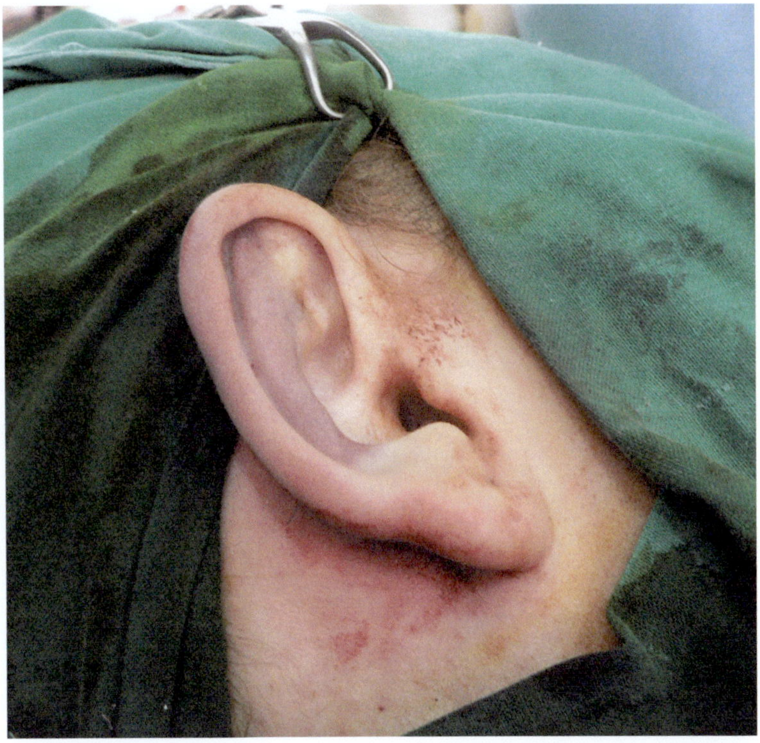

Fig. 32.16 Appearance of the auricle immediate after skin suture

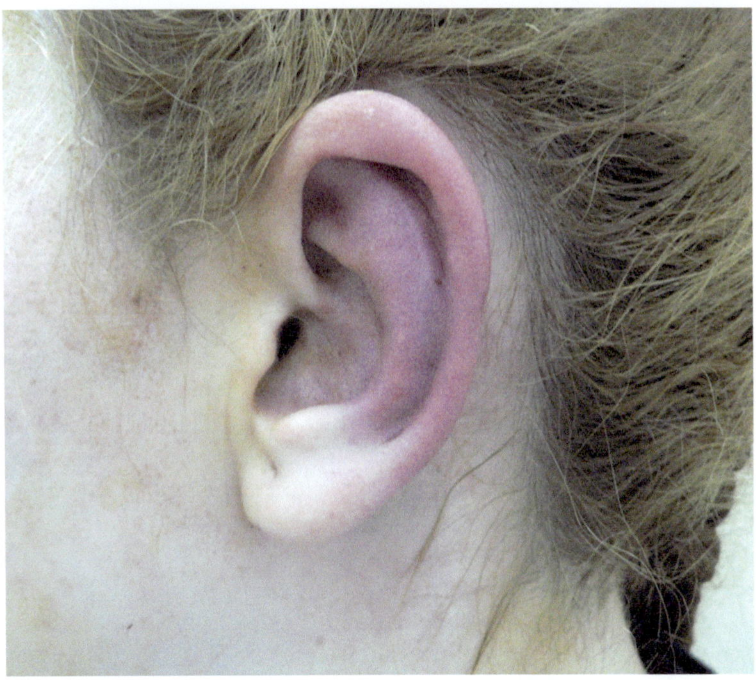

Fig. 32.17 Appearance of the auricle 24 h after surgery

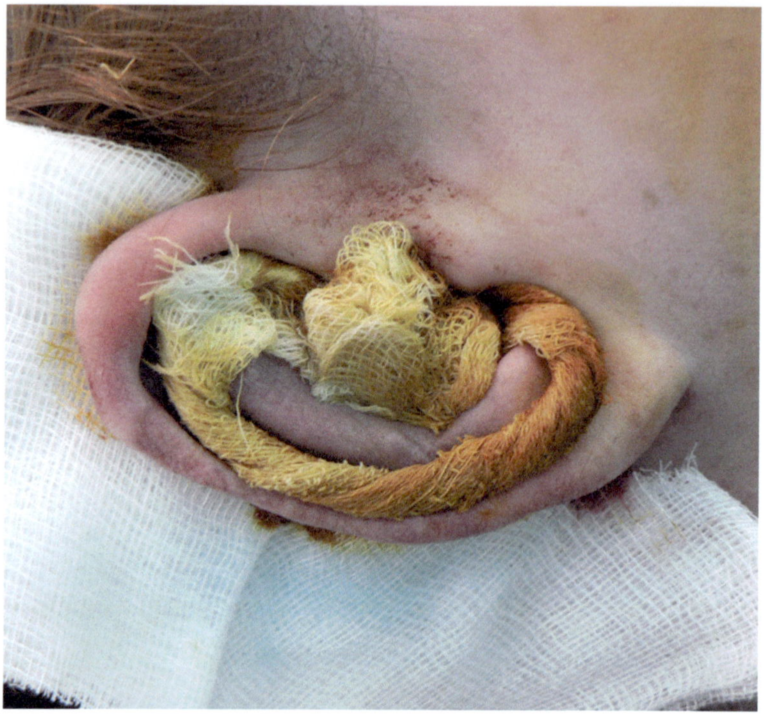

Fig. 32.18 The dressing consists of rolls of Betadine-impregnated cotton which fill the various depressions of the ear

dose of intravenous antibiotic is administered before the procedure and then is continued orally for 5 days. The patient wears the elastic headband for 1 month.

Some results using the technique described above are illustrated in Figs. 32.19, 32.20, 32.21, 32.22, 32.23, and 32.24.

Complications

Hematoma is usually due to insufficient hemostasis and warrants reintervention and evacuation.

Infection is rare in ear surgery because of the luxuriant blood supply of the pinna; when it appears, however, it necessitates aggressive intravenous antibiotic therapy to prevent permanent cartilage damage.

Skin necrosis is rare because of the rich bold supply of the ear which allows wide undermining; it is usually due to tight dressings which obstruct the venous return.

Recurrence of the deformity is rare with the cartilage folding technique compared with sutures-only techniques due to suture fatigue or knot looseness.

Irregular helix with sharp edges produced mainly by aggressive scoring of the anterior part of the antihelix or full-thickness cartilage incisions.

Overcorrection (pinned-back look)/under correction.

Telephone ear deformity – the upper and lower third of the ear remain protruded and the middle third is closer to the mastoid area.

Other complications are keloid formation, suture extrusion, asymmetry, abnormal helical shape, and helix behind the antihelix.

Discussion

The two main causes of prominent ears are an unfolded antihelix with a flat scapha and a deep conchal bowl. These two features may be isolated

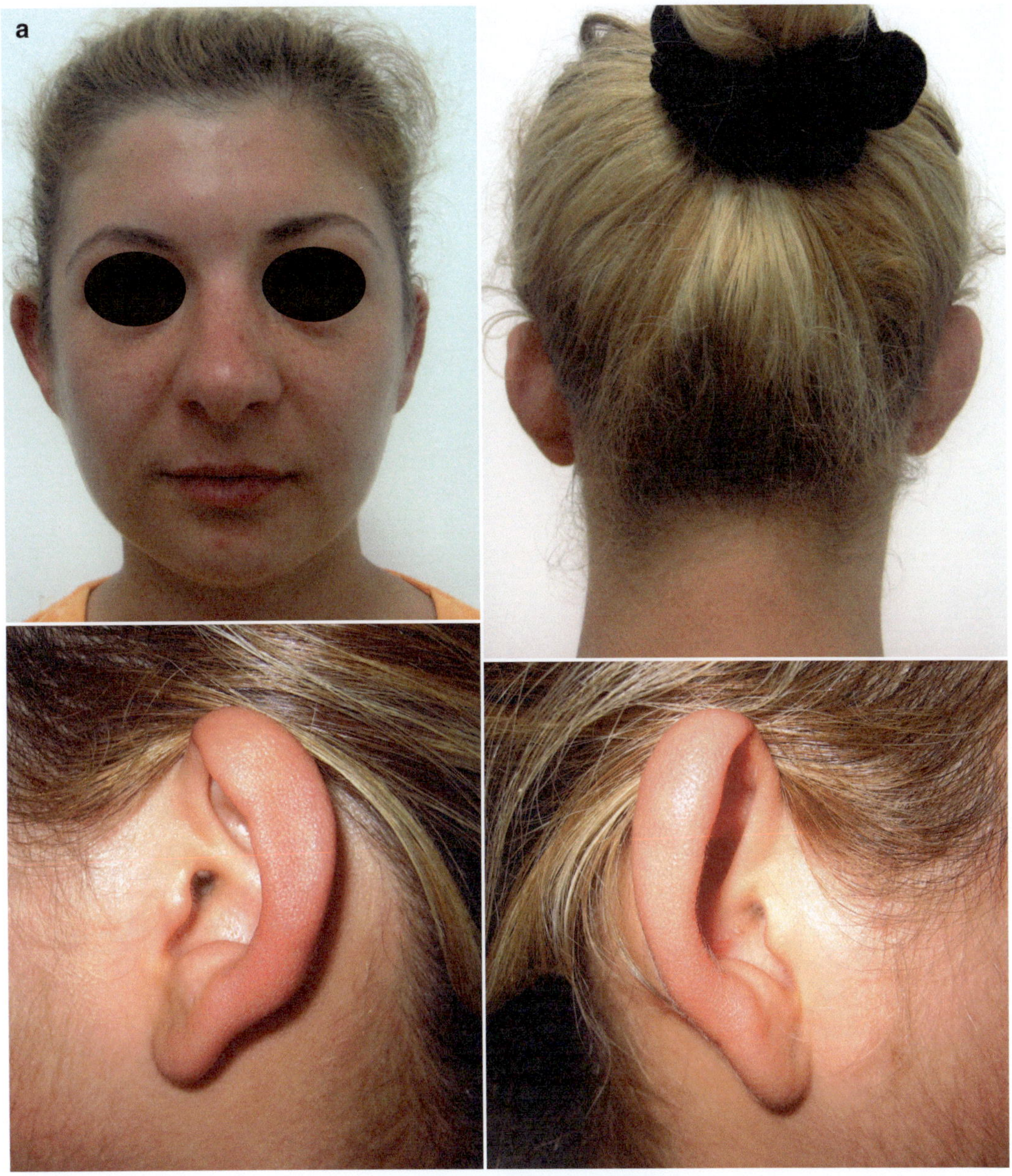

Fig. 32.19 (**a**) Preoperative 25-year-old girl with protruding ears, abnormal shape of the helix, and very stiff cartilage. (**b**) Four months postoperative after using the cartilage folding technique

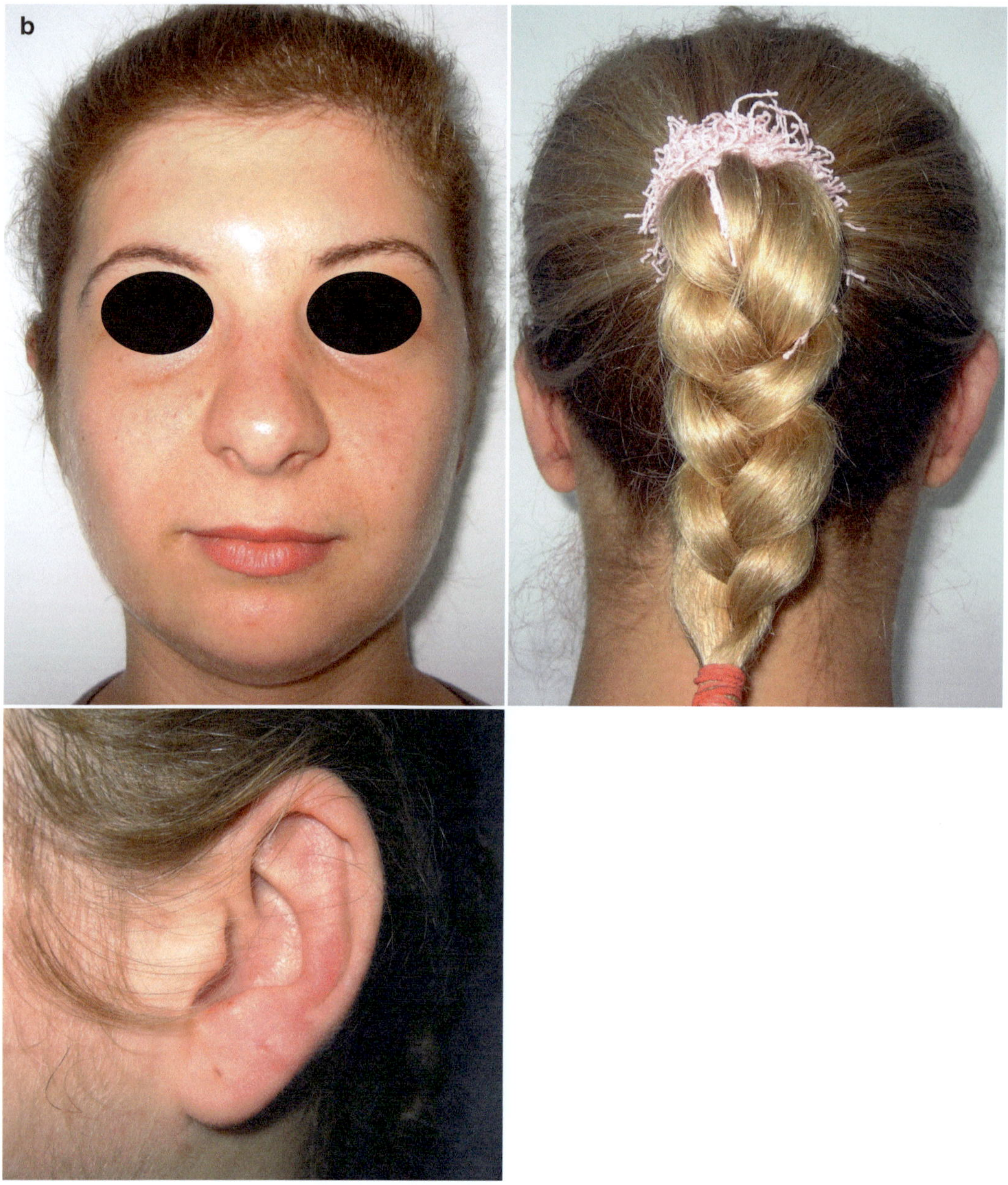

Fig. 32.19 (continued)

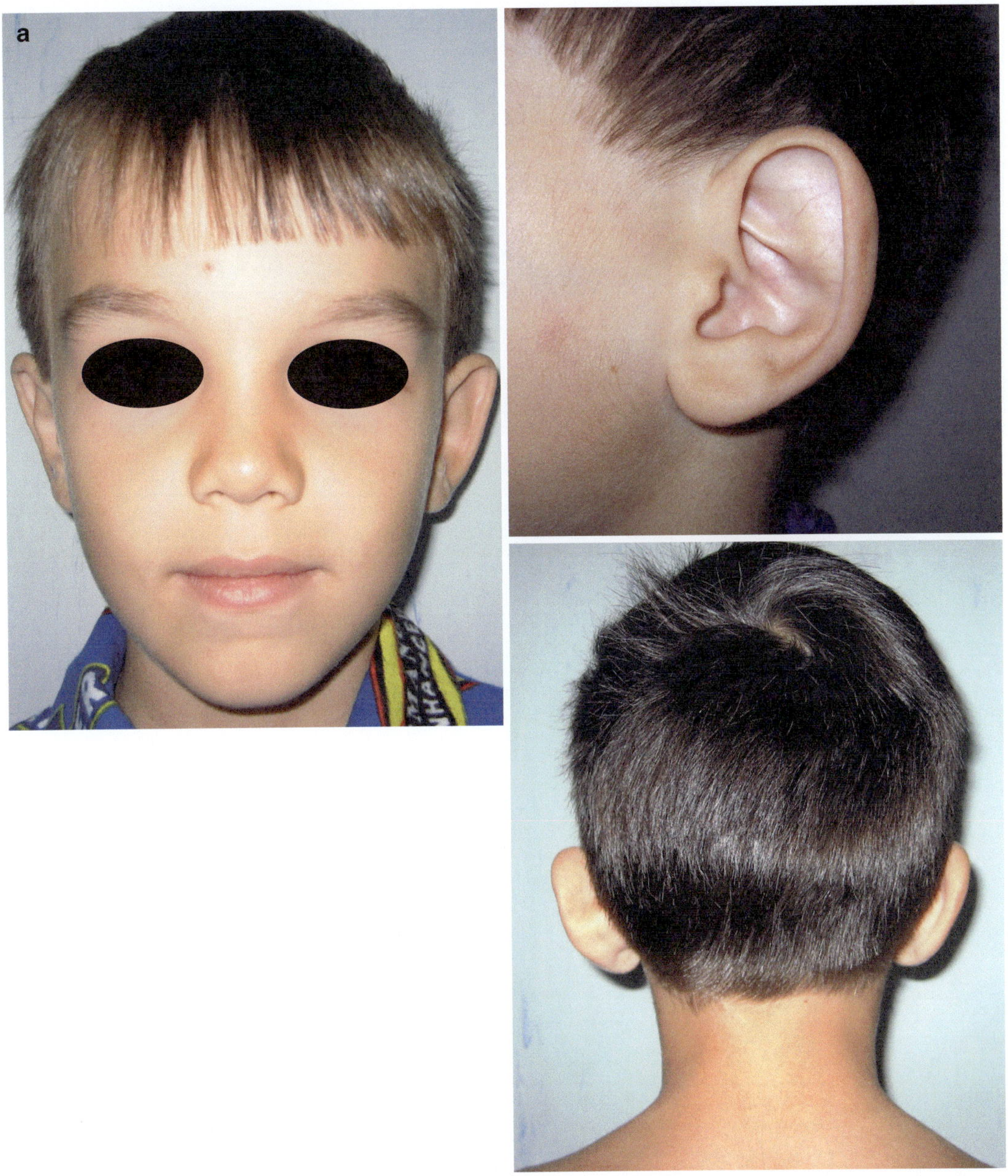

Fig. 32.20 (**a**) Preoperative 6-year-old boy with left prominent ear. (**b**) Two weeks postoperative after using the cartilage folding technique

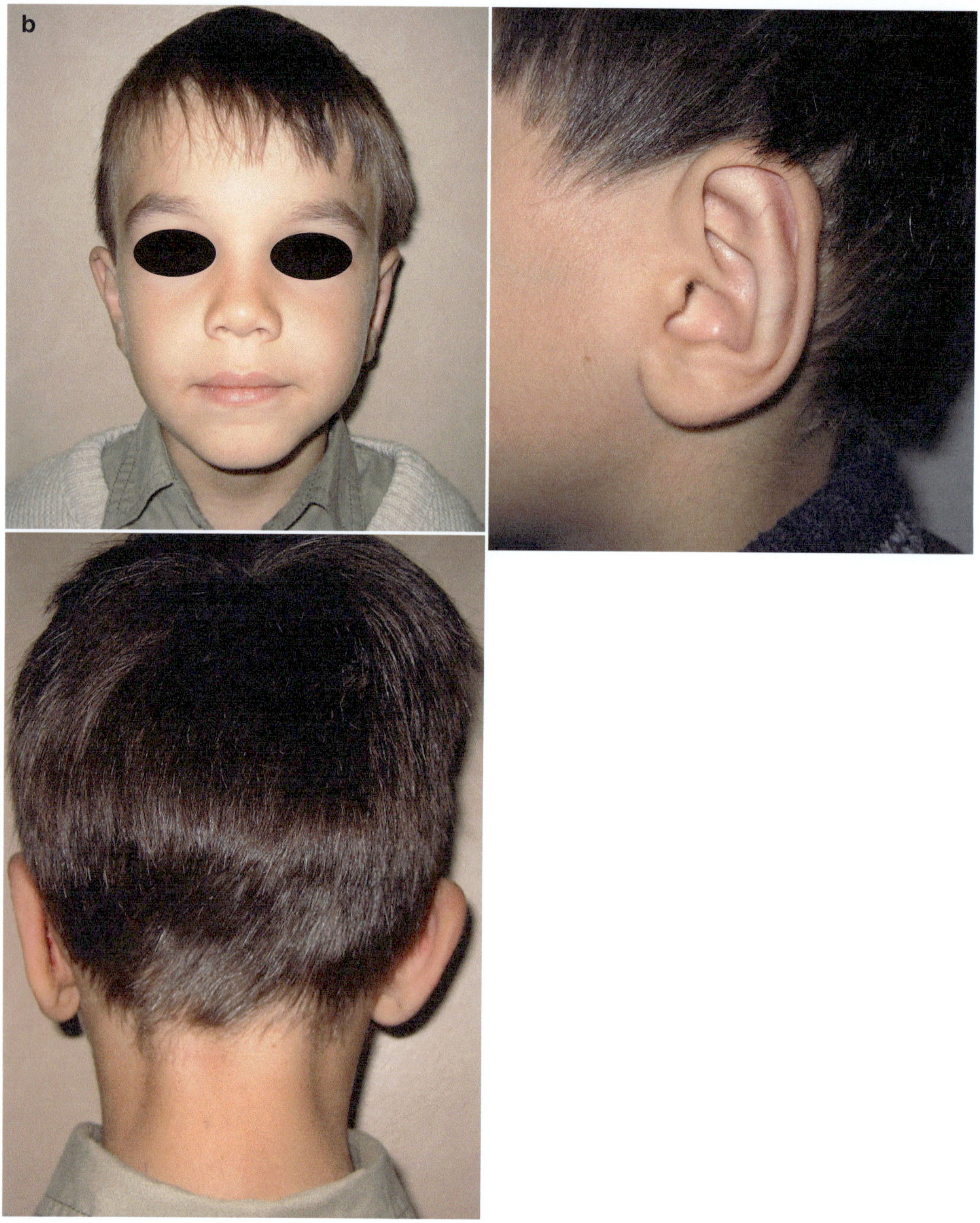

Fig. 32.20 (continued)

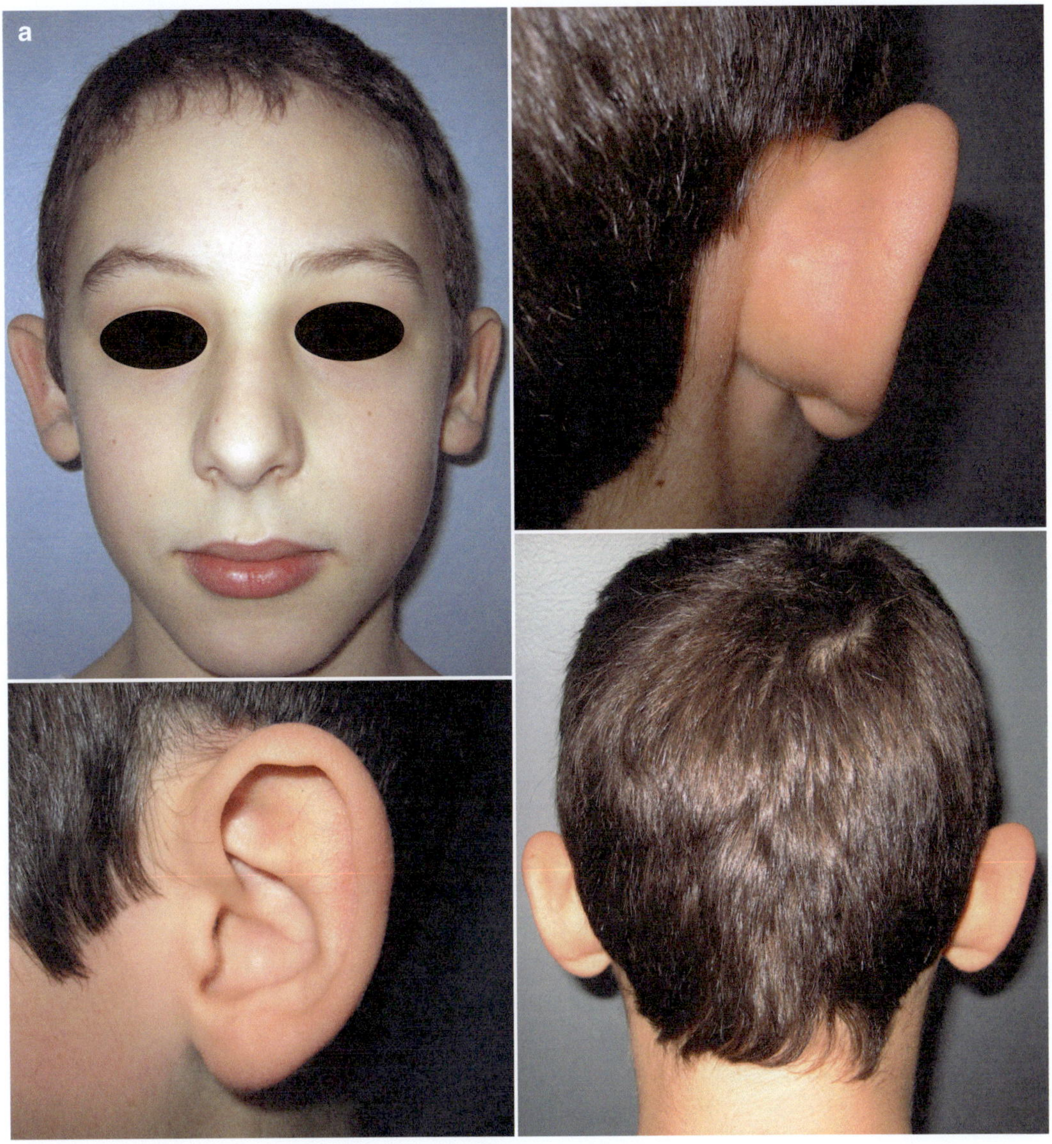

Fig. 32.21 (**a**) Preoperative 13-year-old boy with protruding ears, lack of antihelical fold, deep concha, and stiff cartilage. (**b**) Six months postoperative following use of the cartilage folding technique

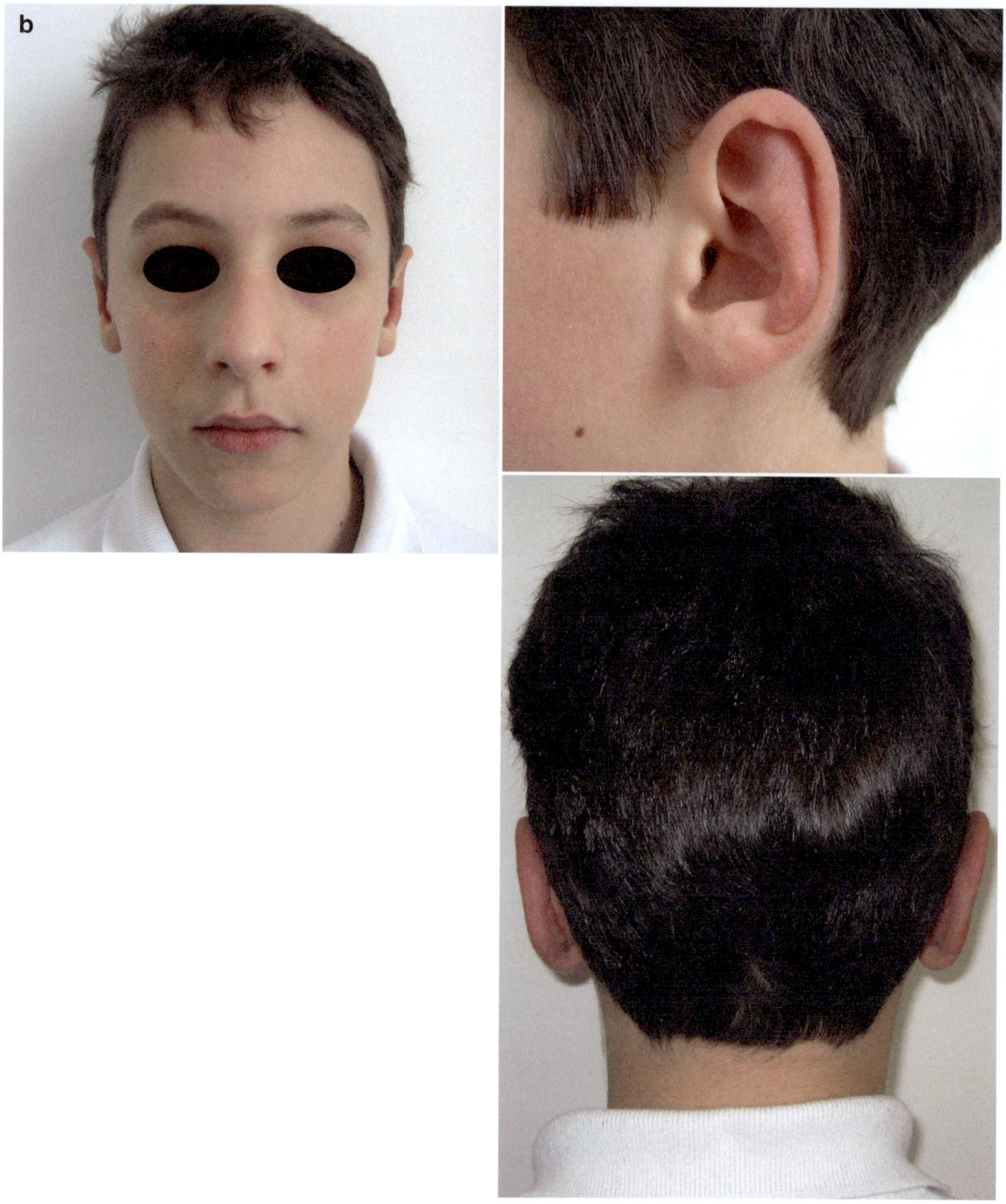

Fig. 32.21 (continued)

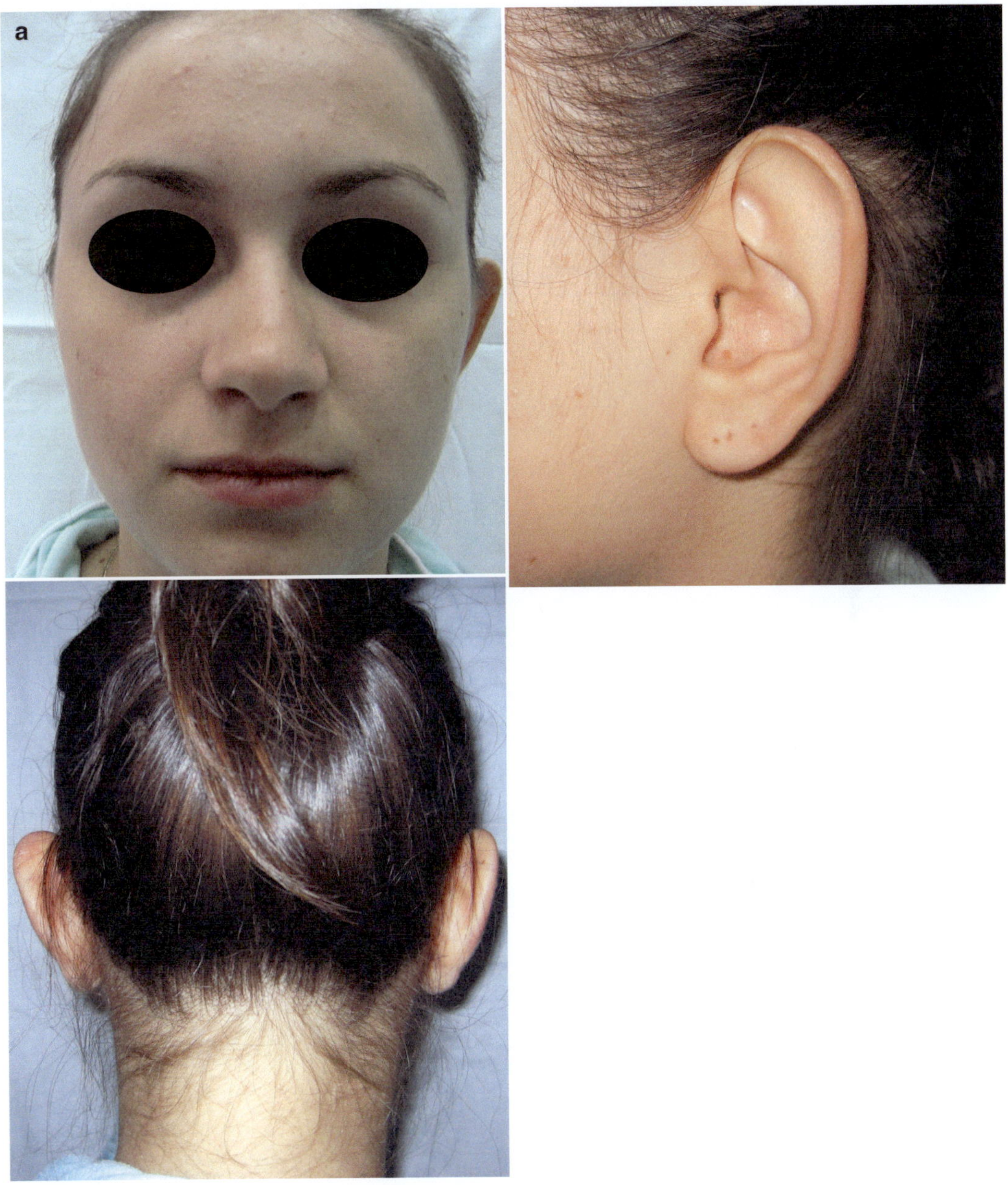

Fig. 32.22 (**a**) Preoperative 21-year-old girl with left prominent ear. (**b**) Four months postoperative after treated with the cartilage folding technique. The technique allows decreasing the size of the auricle at the same time with the creation of the antihelical fold

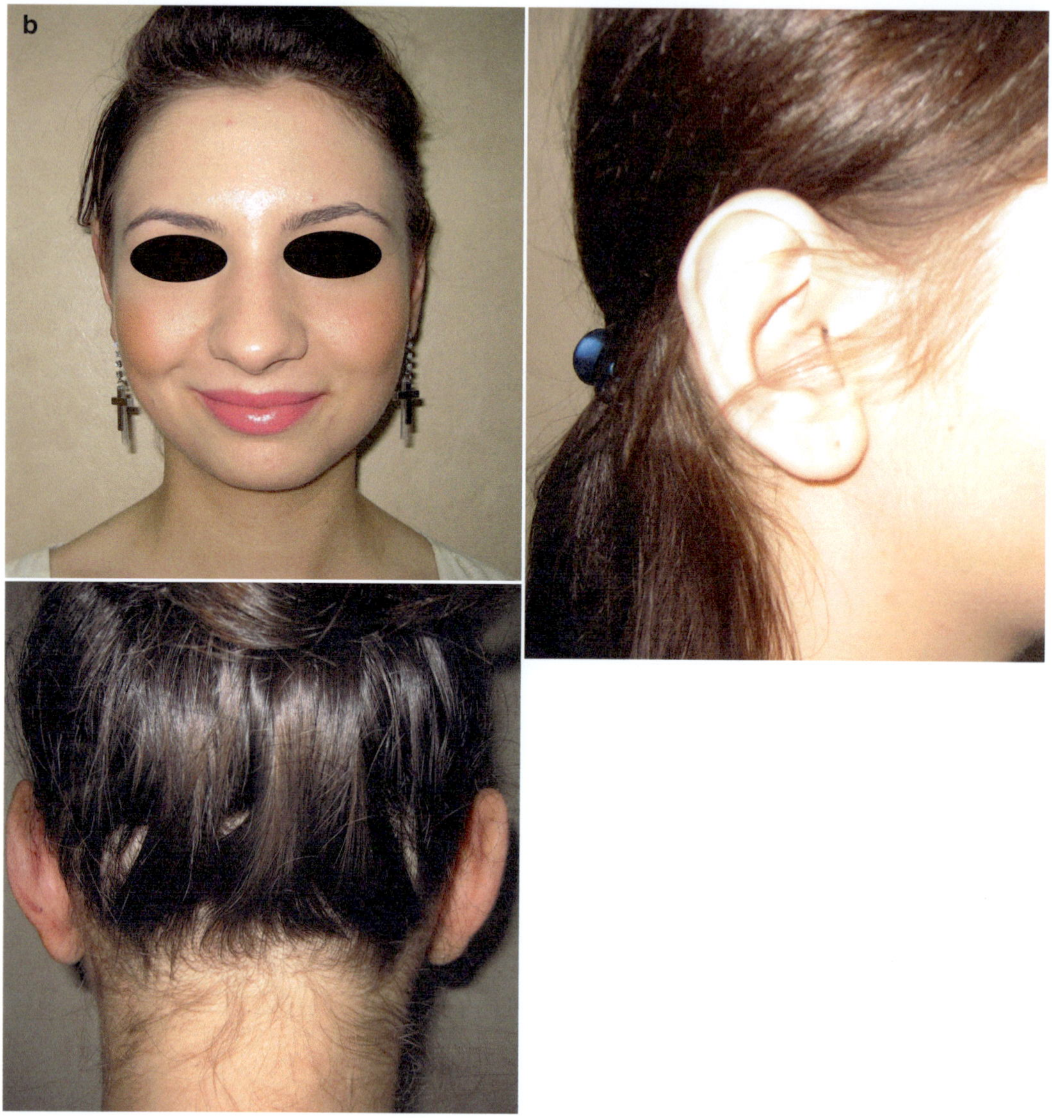

Fig. 32.22 (continued)

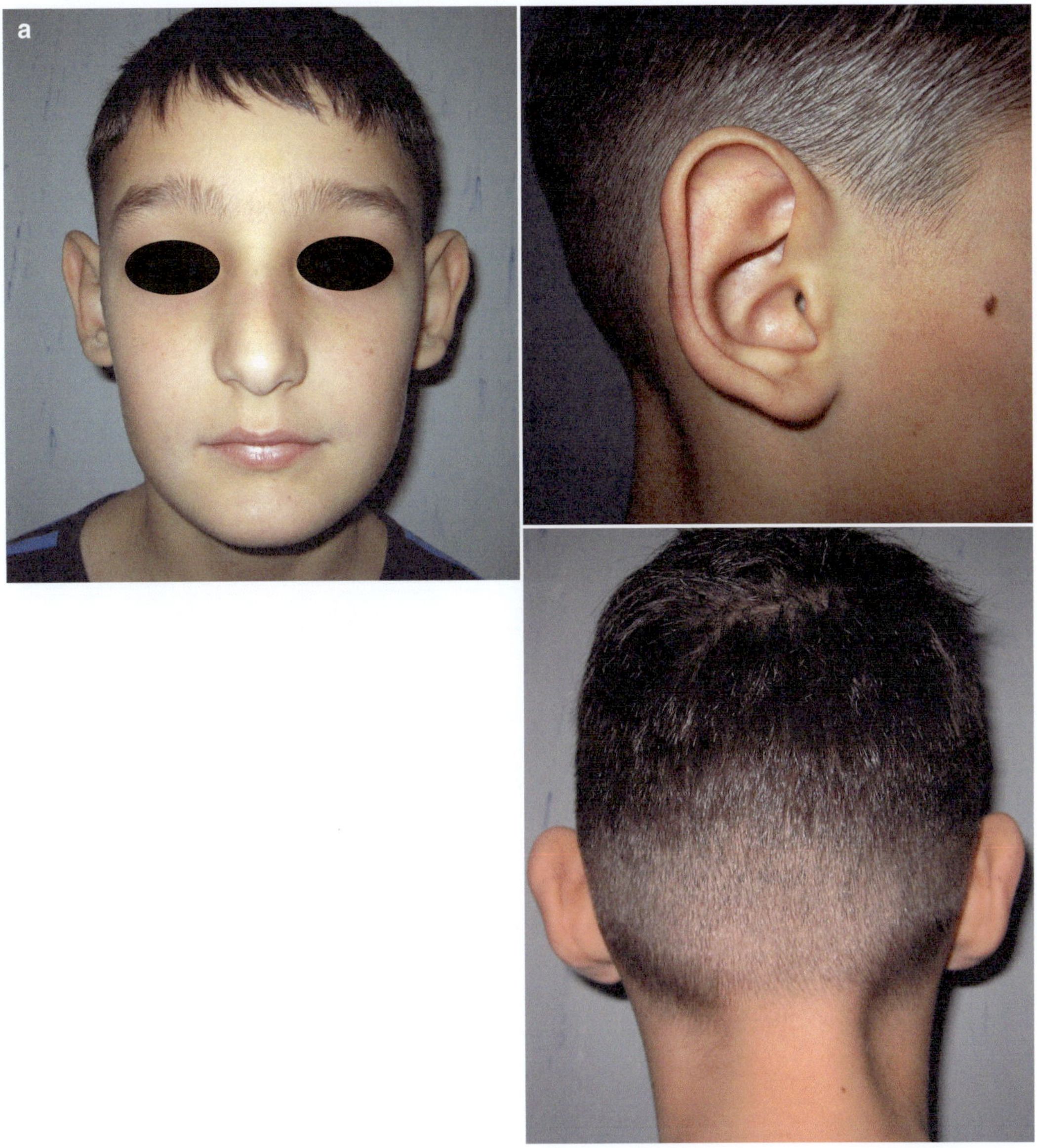

Fig. 32.23 (**a**) Preoperative 12-year-old boy with effaced antihelical fold and conchal hypertrophy. (**b**) Four months postoperative after cartilage folding technique demonstrating clearly visible helical rims on frontal view, smooth antihelical folds, and excellent symmetrical, undisturbed postauricular sulcus

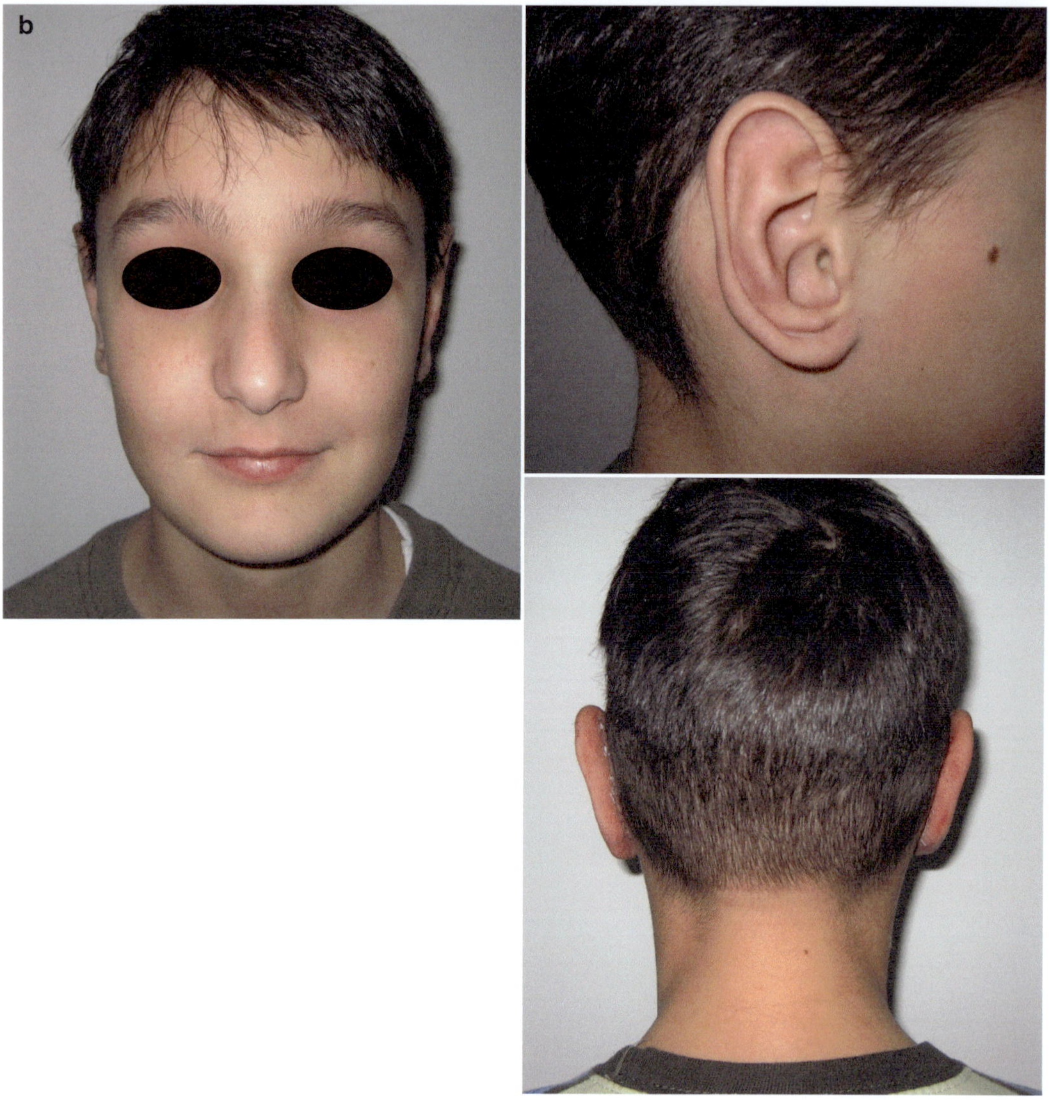

Fig. 32.23 (continued)

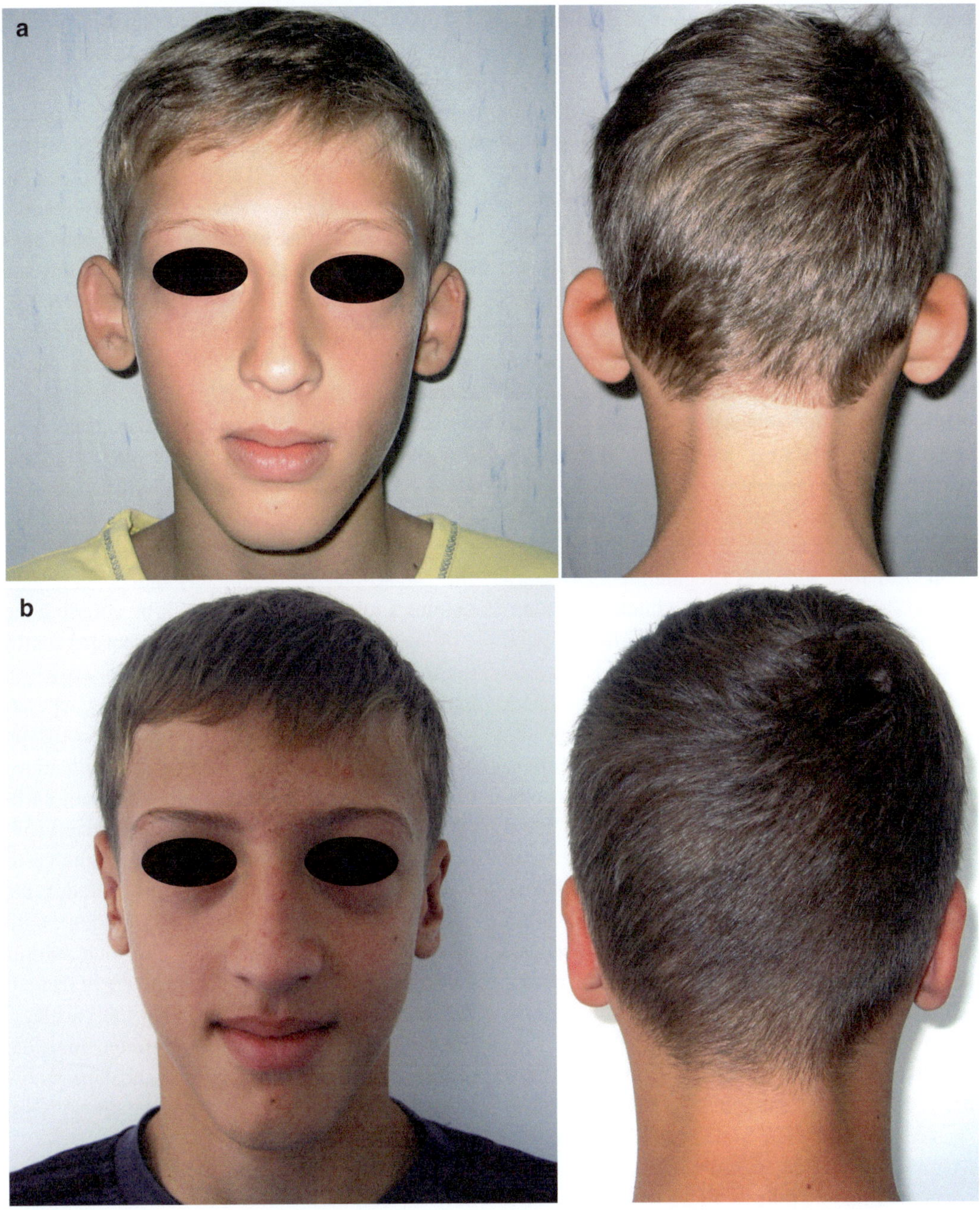

Fig. 32.24 (**a**) Preoperative 9-year-old boy with important conchal hypertrophy. (**b**) Fourteen months postoperative

or found together and they may be associated in some cases with lobular protrusion. The main challenge in otoplasty is achieving a natural appearance of the antihelical fold, i.e., nicely rounded with no sharp edges. Different methods of cartilage excision, incision, scoring, and suturing have been proposed. They can be grouped in cartilage-cutting and cartilage-suturing techniques. No consensus has been reached, however, and no method has been declared superior than the other. The ideal method should be simple, fast, and applicable to many anatomical variations of the auricle, with minimal complications, quick recovery, and minimal recurrence rate.

Cartilage-cutting (incisions combined with excisions of the cartilage) techniques have been proposed over time by Ely [6] (1881), Morestin [7] (1903), Luckett [8] (1910), Becker [9] (1952), Straith [10], Converse [11] (1963), Cloutier [12], and Pitanguy [13] (1961). After Mustarde [14] and Furnas [15] promoted their suturing techniques, many surgeons adopted their cartilage-sparing maneuvers which, in their opinion, avoided the unsightly cartilage irregularities and sharpness of the antihelical fold induced by cartilage scoring and incision. Different techniques of cartilage shaping without incision or excision of the cartilage have also been proposed. Rasping seems to be safer than scoring in terms of producing a smoother antihelical fold with less irregularities and sharp edges. Stenstroem [16] (1963) abraded the anterior side of the cartilage with a specially designed rasp to form a new antihelix. Scoring may be achieved through partial-thickness incisions with knife, electrocautery [17], hypodermic needle [18], rasp, Adson-Brown forceps [19], or mechanical abrader [20]. Cartilage scoring has been combined with different suturing and incisions method in order to obtain satisfactory results. The main problem with all these techniques is the unnatural, sharp-edged antihelical fold that may result if the cartilage is excessively thinned or cut full thickness. Scoring or abrasion of the cartilage runs the potential risk of visible cartilage irregularities and a sharp antihelical fold.

Although cartilage-suturing techniques have been shown to be safer and to give a more natural shape to the antihelical fold than cartilage-cutting techniques [21, 22], many studies in literature concluded that cartilage-cutting techniques have lower recurrence rates [23, 24]. Cartilage-cutting techniques result in good stability over time because they break the cartilage spring, but sometimes, if used too aggressively, they may lead to an excessively sharp, irregular, and unnatural antihelix with an operated look. On the other hand, cartilage-sparing techniques by means of sutures, when used alone, carry a high risk of undercorrection or recurrence of the deformity [5] up to 25 % or stitch extrusion up to 15 % [24, 25]. This is especially true when the concha is very deep or the cartilage is very stiff. That is why lately many authors adopted a mixture of techniques, combining some kind of cartilage splitting or scoring [26] techniques that break the cartilaginous spring with suture stabilization. Thus, most of the techniques used nowadays derive from their original descriptions of Converse [3] and Chongchet [4] involving some type of cartilage incision between the helix and antihelix, folding the cartilage with or without scoring or rasping followed or not followed by suturing.

The cartilage folding technique was first described by Davis [27], Converse [3], and Chongchet [4] and modified by others [28–31]. Davis [27] uses an anterior approach, incises the cartilage in the helical sulcus, so that the helical rim and scapha are completely independent, and obtains a folding of the antihelix by abrading the cartilage with a sandpaper. Chongchet [4] scores the anterior surface of the cartilage to weaken it and obtains a natural bending, again by separating completely the helix and antihelix through an incision. Technical refinements and modifications of Converse and Chongchet's technique of cartilage incision have been proposed. Nordzell [32] (1965) exposes the anterior surface of the cartilage through a posterior incision, abrades the anterior surface of the scapha and antihelix until the cartilage bends backward, and then sutures the medial edge of the incised cartilage in front of the lateral edge. He does not fold the cartilage. Colpaert [33] uses the same cartilage incision, scores the anterior surface of the cartilage with a scalpel, and sutures the folded cartilage with 4-0 Vicryl.

All proposed methods of cartilage incision have in common some kind of helix-antihelix separation so that the folded cartilage which will induce the new antihelical formed formation should not affect the shape of the helix. Folding the cartilage allows an important reduction in the conchal height which contributes a lot to the prominence of the ear. In this way, conchal excision is not needed anymore. A large concha can be significantly reduced by a greater degree of folding of the cartilage. In our technique we preserve the perichondrium on the posterior surface of the cartilage which will determine the cartilage to bend toward the side with the intact perichondrium when it is incised on one side only, according to Gibson and Davis' principle [34]. The preserved perichondrium on the posterior surface also helps in keeping the blood supply for the cartilage.

The excised skin should not be excessive to prevent a telephone ear deformity and preserve a good retroauricular sulcus. Lack of tension will also prevent a keloid scar. Most of the authors using cartilage folding technique design a skin excision on the posterior surface of the auricle with the anterior limit of skin excision corresponding 1 cm medial to the helical margin [28] or 5 mm anterior to the tattoo marks [29]. The authors prefer designing the skin ellipse closer to the postauricular sulcus to avoid superimposing the incision line with the lateral edge of the folded cartilage which may predispose to suture extrusion or excessive tension on the scar and keloid formation. The skin incision is usually widened inferiorly in a fishtail or rhomboid shape because after setting back the auricle, the lobule almost always appears protruding. In these cases methods for setting back the lobule should be added. If the antitragus is excessive, it can be partially resected.

When the cartilage is folded, the incision should completely separate the scapha from the helix in order for the helix to preserve its rounded shape. If the helix is not separated from the scapha, then the folded antihelix will induce a deformed, angled helix [27, 35]. The tail of the helix should be resected in some cases. It is also very important to extend the caudal part of the incision through the tail of the newly formed antihelix. This full-thickness incision allows the cartilage to fully fold backward, creates a less prominent antitragus, and thus, sets back the lobule and also diminishes the size of the concha.

The rim of helix that is left behind should be of sufficient width to avoid buckling [33] but at the same time should not be too wide as this will hamper the setback of the scapha.

The cartilage folding technique is very useful in cases with very thick and sturdy cartilage, in children or male adults especially, where the sutures-only methods cannot be trust because they may not have enough strength to keep the cartilage folded. In these cases it is necessary to break the cartilage spring in order to achieve a long-lasting result, and this can be achieved only by means of cartilage incisions and folding. The method prevents superior pole recurrence deformity compared to cartilage-suturing techniques [36]. Apart from floding the cartilage and forming the antihelical fold, another main advantage of the technique is that it results in a smaller size of the auricle, which in many cases is very useful.

In order to avoid the sharp, noticeable edges of the newly formed antihelix that may be induced by cartilage incision and scoring, we preserve the perichondrium on the anterior surface of the cartilage. Horlock [24] uses a postauricular fascial flap to reduce stitch extrusion and recurrence in association with Mustardé and Furnas sutures.

Bauer [37] states that the vast majority of prominent ears demonstrate some degree of conchal hypertrophy and the concha may be the cornerstone of its treatment. He excises a crescent chondrocutaneous segment from the concha via an anterior approach and combines the conchal excision with suture placement via a posterior approach in almost all cases. Elliott [38] excises only conchal cartilage through an anterior approach. In the cartilage folding technique, there is no need for conchal excision, as the concha is reduced in height as much as the surgeon feels by simply folding the cartilage more.

Conclusions

Cartilage-cutting techniques have been much criticized for the possible distortions created if used by the novice. However, they can be very reliable and can lead to stable and satisfying results in experienced hands. The advantages of the cartilage folding method are multiple. Because no cartilage is excised, there are no excess skin folds on the anterior part of the concha. The shape of the antihelix is a very natural one. The height of the concha can be reduced as much as desired by folding the cartilage. The method is simple and quick. It is a very safe and reliable method, delivering satisfactory results with minor complications. The folded and sutured cartilage is very stable over time so that the rate of recurrence is very low. It is the method of choice both in children and adults with strong, stiff, and unyielding cartilage where sutures alone cannot fold enough the cartilage and sustain it in time. Also scoring techniques alone in these cases are not enough either. Weakening the spring of the cartilage helps in stabilizing the results over time.

Some improvements of the method (such as covering the folded cartilage with various perichondrial flaps) may allow obtaining even better results with more natural shape of the antihelical fold.

References

1. Adamson P, McGraw B, Troppeer GJ. Otoplasty: critical review of clinical results. Laryngoscope. 1991;101(8):883–8.
2. Preuss S, Eriksson E. Prominent ears. In: Achauer B, Eriksson E, Guyuron B, Coleman III JJ, Russell RC, Vander Kolk CA, editors. Plastic surgery- indications, operations and outcomes. Philadelphia: Mosby; 2000. p. 1057–65.
3. Converse JM, Nigro A, Wilson FA, Johnson N. A technique for surgical correction of lop ears. Plast Reconstr Surg. 1955;15(5):411–8.
4. Chongchet V. A method of antihelix reconstruction. Br J Plast Surg. 1963;16:268–72.
5. Foda H. Otoplasty: a graduated approach. Aesthetic Plast Surg. 1999;23(6):407–12.
6. Ely ET. An operation for the prominence of the auricles. Arch Otolaryngol. 1881;10:97.
7. Morestin MH. De la reposition et du plissement cosmetique du pavillion de l'oreille. Rev Orthop. 1903;4:289–303.
8. Luckett WH. The classic reprint: a new operation for the prominent ears based on the anatomy of the deformity. Surg Gynecol Obstet. 1910;10:635–7.
9. Becker OJ. Correction of the protruding deformed ear. Br J Plast Surg. 1952;5(3):187–96.
10. Straith RE. Correction of the protruding ear. Plast Reconstr Surg. 1959;24:277–85.
11. Converse JM, Wood-Smith D. Technical details in the surgical correction of the lop ear deformity. Plast Reconstr Surg. 1963;31:118–28.
12. Cloutier AM. Correction of outstanding ears. Plast Reconstr Surg. 1961;28:412–6.
13. Pitanguy I, Müller P, Piccolo N, Ramalho E, Solinas R. The treatment of prominent ears: a 25-year survey of the island technique. Aesthetic Plast Surg. 1987;11:87–93.
14. Mustarde JC. The treatment of prominent ears by buried mattress sutures: a ten year survey. Plast Reconstr Surg. 1967;39(4):382–6.
15. Furnas DW. Correction of prominent ears by conchomastoid sutures. Plast Reconstr Surg. 1968; 42:189–93.
16. Stenstroem SJ. A "natural" technique for correction of congenitally prominent ears. Plast Reconstr Surg. 1963;32:509–18.
17. Epstein JS, Kabaker SS, Swerdloff J. The "electric" otoplasty. Arch Facial Plast Surg. 1999;1(3): 204–7.
18. Bulstrode NW, Huang S, Martin DL. Otoplasty by percutaneous anterior scoring. Another twist of the story: a long-term study of 114 patients. Br J Plast Surg. 2003;56(2):145–9.
19. Tan O, Atik B, Karaca C, Barutcu A. A new instrument as cartilage scorer for otoplasty and septoplasty: Adson-Brown forceps. Plast Reconstr Surg. 2005;115(2):671–2.
20. Di Mascio D, Castagnetti F, Baldassarre S. Otoplasty: anterior abrasion of ear cartilage with dermabrader. Aesthetic Plast Surg. 2003;27(6):466–71.
21. Kompatscher P, Schuler CH, Clemens S, Seifert B, Beer GM. The cartilage-sparing versus cartilage-cutting technique: a retrospective quality control comparison of the Francesconi and Converse otoplasties. Aesthetic Plast Surg. 2003;27(6):446–53.
22. Panettiere P, Marchetti L, Accorsi D, Del Gaudio GA. Otoplasty: a comparison of techniques for antihelical defects treatment. Aesthetic Plast Surg. 2003;27(6): 462–5.
23. Fatih P, Bahattin C. Otoplasty: anterior scoring and posterior rolling technique in adults. Aesthetic Plast Surg. 2002;26:267–73.
24. Horlock N, Misra A, Gault DT. The postauricular fascial flap as an adjunct to Mustardé and Furnas type otoplasty. Plast Reconstr Surg. 2001;108(6):1487–90.
25. Nuara M, Mobley SR. Nuances of otoplasty: a comprehensive review of the past 20 years. Facial Plast Surg Clin North Am. 2006;14(2):89–102.
26. Hoehn J, Ashruf S. Otoplasty: sequencing the operation for improved results. Plast Reconstr Surg. 2005;115(1):5e–16.
27. Davis J. Prominent ear. In: Davis J, editor. Aesthetic and reconstructive otoplasty. New York: Springer; 1987. p. 129–87.
28. Mattheis SS, Siegert RR. The modified converse technique in combination with cavum rotation. Facial Plast Surg. 2004;20(4):271–5.
29. Nachlas NE, Duncan D. Otoplasty. Arch Otolaryngol. 1970;91(1):44–9.
30. Walter C. Reconstructive procedures on the auricle. Trans Am Acad Ophthalmol Otolaryngol. 1969; 73(2):266–73.

31. Heppt WJ. The incision-excision technique in minor auricular deformities. Facial Plast Surg. 2004;20(4): 287–92.
32. Nordzell B. Open otoplasty. Plast Reconstr Surg. 2000;106(7):1466–72.
33. Colpaert SDM, Missotten FEM. Otoplasty for prominent ears: personal technique and review of 150 consecutive cases. Eur J Plast Surg. 2005;28(3):179–84.
34. Gibson T, Davis W. The distortion of autogenous cartilage grafts: its cause and prevention. Br J Plast Surg. 1958;10:257–74.
35. Caouette-Laberge L, Guay N, Bortoluzzi P. Otoplasty: anterior scoring technique and results in 500 cases (review). Plast Reconstr Surg. 2000;105(2):504–15.
36. Adamson P, Litner J. Selected cartilage-cutting otoplasty techniques. In: Adamson P, editor. Aesthetic otoplasty (Thomas procedures in facial plastic surgery). Shelton: People's Medical Publishing House USA Ltd; 2011. p. 63–71.
37. Bauer B. Evolution and refinements in otoplasty techniques. In: Nahai F, editor. The Art of aesthetic surgery- principles and techniques. St Louis: Quality Medical Publishing; 2005. p. 1463–95.
38. Elliott Jr RA. Otoplasty for prominent ears: a combined approach. Clin Plast Surg. 1990;17(2):373–81.

Cartilage-Sparing Aesthetic Otoplasty

33

Fernando D. Burstein

Introduction

Otoplasty is one of the most frequently performed aesthetic surgical procedures in children and adolescents. Many techniques have been described that can give satisfactory results in experienced hands [1–10]. Some of these techniques are difficult to learn and consistent results may be hard to achieve. The author reports on the evolution and application of a cartilage-sparing otoplasty technique that addresses all the components of the typical prominent ear deformity [6]. This technique has given good, reproducible results in 180 patients treated over a 20-year period. An 8 % revision rate and minimal complications were encountered.

Aesthetic otoplasty is one of the most frequently performed procedures in children and teenagers. Several different otoplasty procedures have been described over the years. The plethora of techniques reflects the fact that no single technique has been deemed superior. In general the goals of aesthetic otoplasty are decreasing the prominence and protrusion of the ear, producing the antihelical fold and superior crus, if absent or effaced, and making the lobule proportionate to the rest of the ear. More subtle technical points include a "natural look," avoiding a pinned-back appearance, and achieving maximal symmetry. Accepted techniques include variations on the Stenstroem [3] cartilage scoring technique, the Mustardé [2] suture technique, and the Furnas [4] technique. Bauer et al. [8] have emphasized the concha as the key anatomical feature in correction of the prominent ear and have reported excellent overall results.

To avoid an unfavorable result in otoplasty, the author has endeavored to develop a technique that is not technically demanding and gives easily reproducible and consistent results with minimal complications. This technique has been refined over the last 20 years. Initially a conchal takeout technique was used in over 30 patients. This technique led to several modifications, which culminated in the technique presented here. This technique borrows elements from many previous reports, including those of Stenstroem, Mustardé, Tanzer, Furnas, and Bauer [1–9]. The current technique has been applied to 180 consecutive patients with prominent ears over a 20-year period. Follow-up has been at least 24 months in all cases.

Technique

Figures 33.1, 33.2, 33.3, 33.4, and 33.5 present the key steps in performing this technique. The deformity is analyzed before surgery to determine the anatomic elements that are contributing

F.D. Burstein, M.D.
Center for Craniofacial Disorders
Children's Healthcare of Atlanta,
975 Johnson Ferry Road, Suite 100,
Atlanta, GA 30342, USA

Department of Plastic and Reconstructive Surgery,
Emory University, Atlanta, GA, USA
e-mail: fburstein@aol.com,
fernandoburstein@yahoo.com

M.A. Shiffman (ed.), *Advanced Cosmetic Otoplasty*,
DOI 10.1007/978-3-642-35431-1_33, © Springer-Verlag Berlin Heidelberg 2013

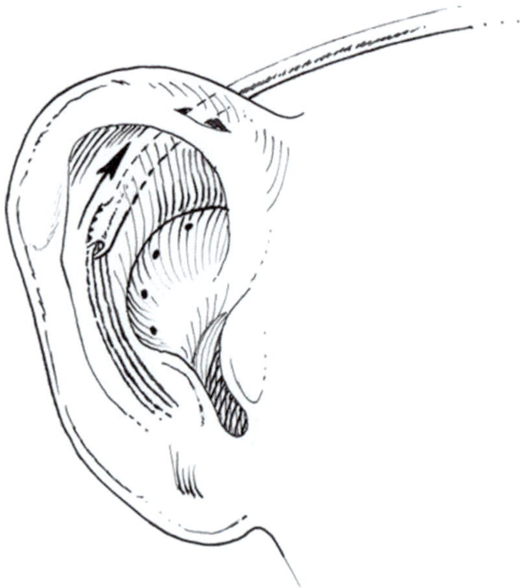

Fig. 33.1 Dingman otoabrader has been inserted through the scapha incision. The anterior perichondrium and cartilage are scored along the line of the proposed antihelical fold. Note the tattoo markings on the lateral edge of the concha

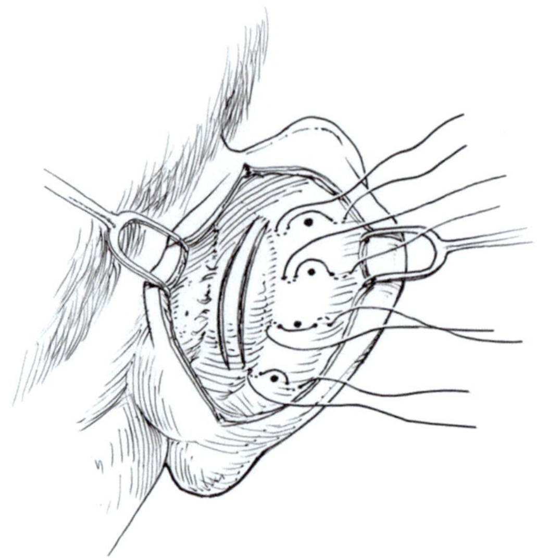

Fig. 33.3 Sutures for creation of the antihelical fold are placed partial thickness through the cartilage and full thickness through the perichondrium. Once tightened they will create the antihelical fold

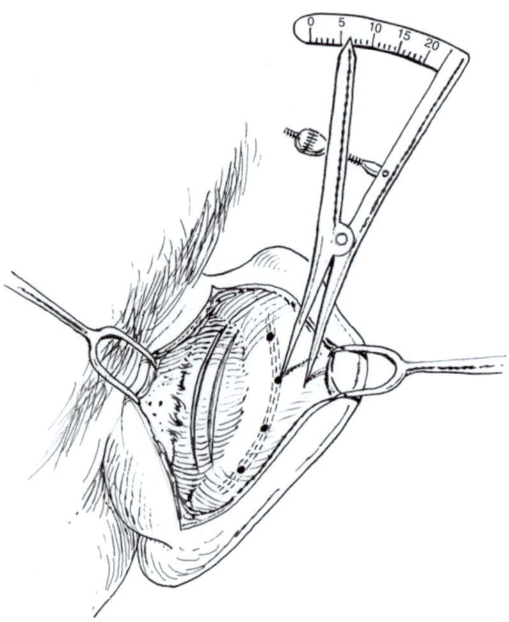

Fig. 33.2 Measurements for placement of the antihelix sutures are made with calipers behind the area of the scapha. One or two parallel conchal incisions are carried out, separated by approximately 6.0 mm. The mastoid periosteum has been exposed

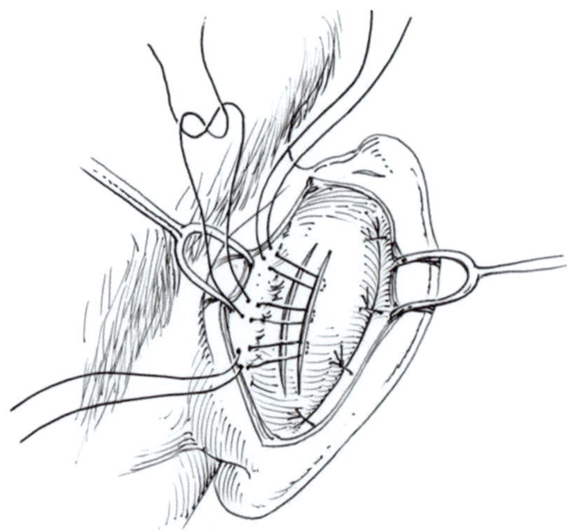

Fig. 33.4 After the antihelix is created, sutures are placed from the lateral conchal incision to the mastoid periosteum and tightened. The sutures are placed on the lateral conchal incision for more setback and on the medial conchal incision for less setback

to the abnormal appearance of the ear. Particular attention is paid to the concha-scapha angle, presence or absence of the antihelical fold and superior crus, lobular size and position, asymmetries caused by the size or position of the auricle, and

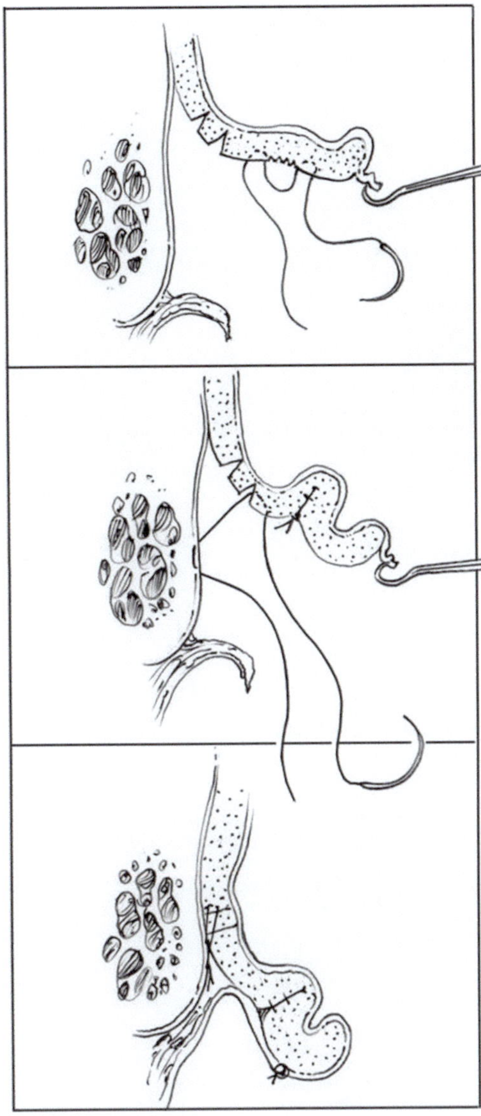

Fig. 33.5 Sequential effects of surgical maneuvers on ear protrusion. (*Bottom*) Partial-thickness scoring of the scapha with suture placement to create the antihelical fold. Full-thickness incisions in the concha to break the spring of the cartilage are indicated. (*Middle*) Sutures placed from the lateral conchal cut to the mastoid periosteum to bring the concha closer to the head. (*Top*) Final result with scapha position after creation of antihelical fold and correction of the conchal hypertrophy. The most lateral point of the helix should be 1.8–2.0 cm from the mastoid

conchal depth. Standardized photographs are obtained – most importantly, anterior/posterior and front to back (Figs. 33.6, 33.7, and 33.8).

The procedure is performed under general anesthesia; usually an LMA technique is sufficient. A first-generation cephalosporin is given at the beginning of the case, along with a single dose of intravenous steroids. Methylene Blue and a 22-gauge needle are used to mark the proposed antihelical fold, superior crus, and anatomic borders of the concha.

The postauricular skin is injected with 0.25 % bupivacaine with 100,000–400,000 epinephrine, whereas the anterior surface is injected with bupivacaine alone. An S-shaped postauricular incision is carried out from the highest point of the proposed antihelical fold to the lobule. If a lobule reduction is desired, a small triangle is added to the end of the incision for debulking. Dissection to the mastoid periosteum and helical rim is carried out using a microcautery needle. The posterior perichondrium is left intact for suture retention. The scapha is pierced at the level of the superior crus under the helix rim. The anterior skin is undermined with small tenotomy scissors and a tunnel created with a small septal elevator along the proposed antihelical fold. A Dingman otoabrader is used to create multiple microabrasions along the course of the proposed antihelix and superior crus onto the anterior scapha surface. Care is taken to only weaken and not transect the scapha cartilage. In the younger patients or those with thin pliable cartilage, the scissor and elevator dissection may suffice to weaken the cartilage enough to create the desired fold without scoring. Clear nylon mattress 4/0 sutures are placed along the proposed crus and the antihelix forms an antihelical fold and superior crus. Tapered sutures are recommended. The placement of the sutures is determined by the markings made with the Methylene Blue tattoo. A caliper is used to measure approximately 6.0 mm from the center of the tattoo for placement of each bite of the horizontal mattress suture. Fairly small bites are taken to prevent bunching of the cartilage. The perichondrium should be included in each bite for strength. This suture determines the height of the antihelical fold, approximately 6.0 mm above the plane of the scapha. This can be modified as required so that the antihelical fold height is slightly lower than that of the helix on frontal view. If the fold is too low, the distance from the central tattoo can be increased, whereas

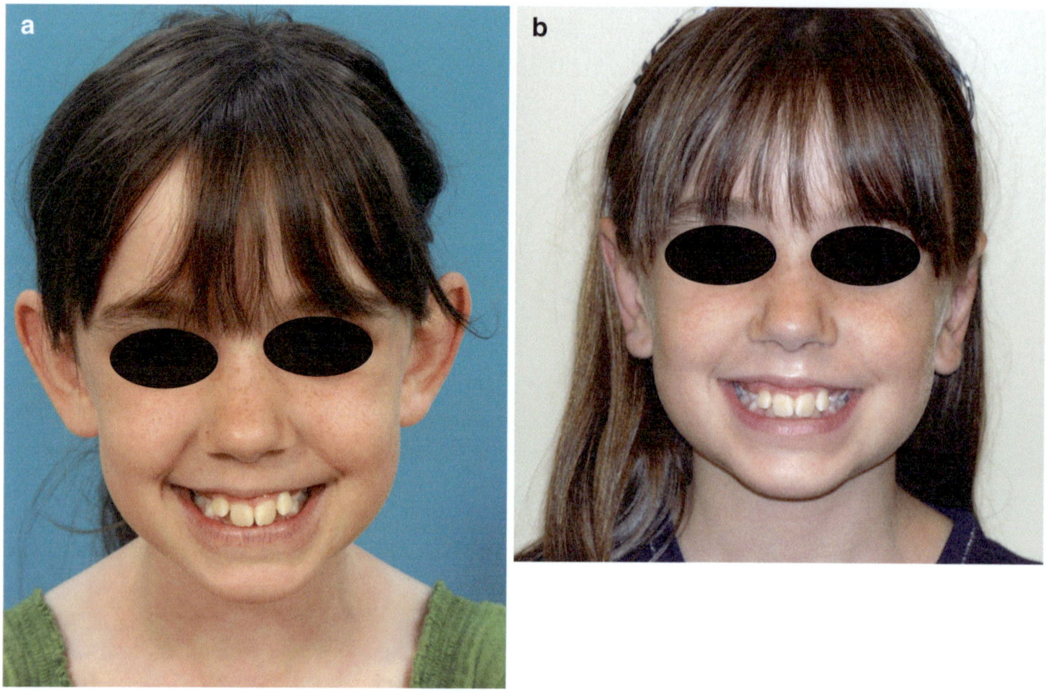

Fig. 33.6 (**a**) Preoperative female with prominent ears. (**b**) Following surgical correction

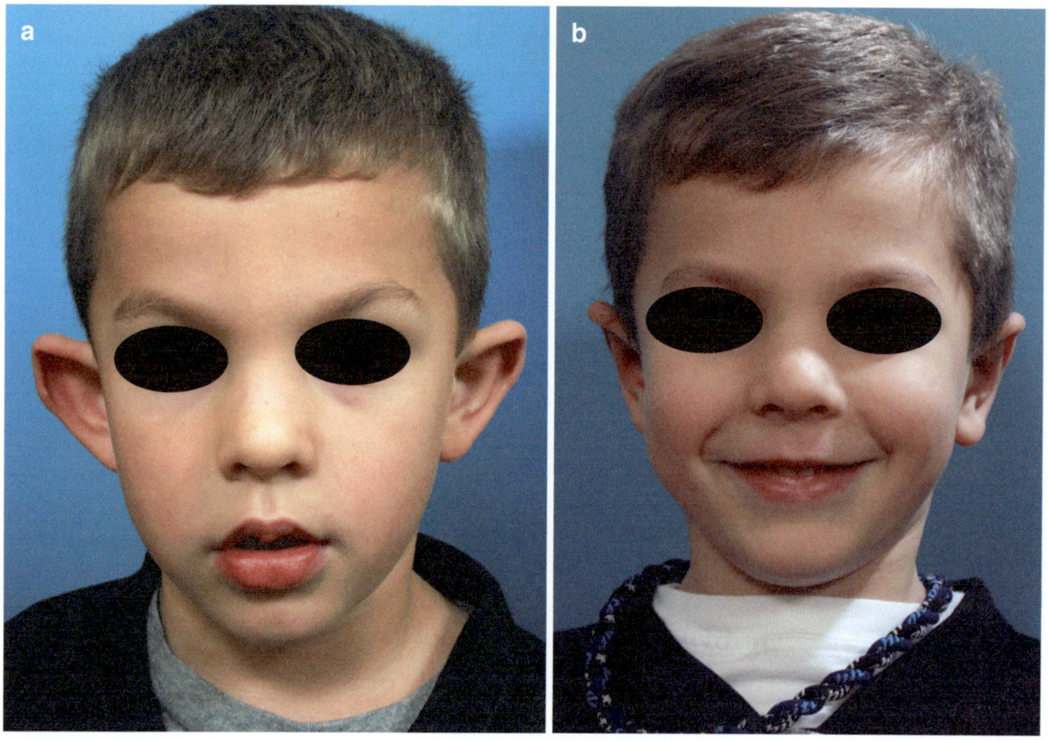

Fig. 33.7 (**a**) Preoperative male with prominent ears and marked superior pole protrusion. (**b**) Postoperative

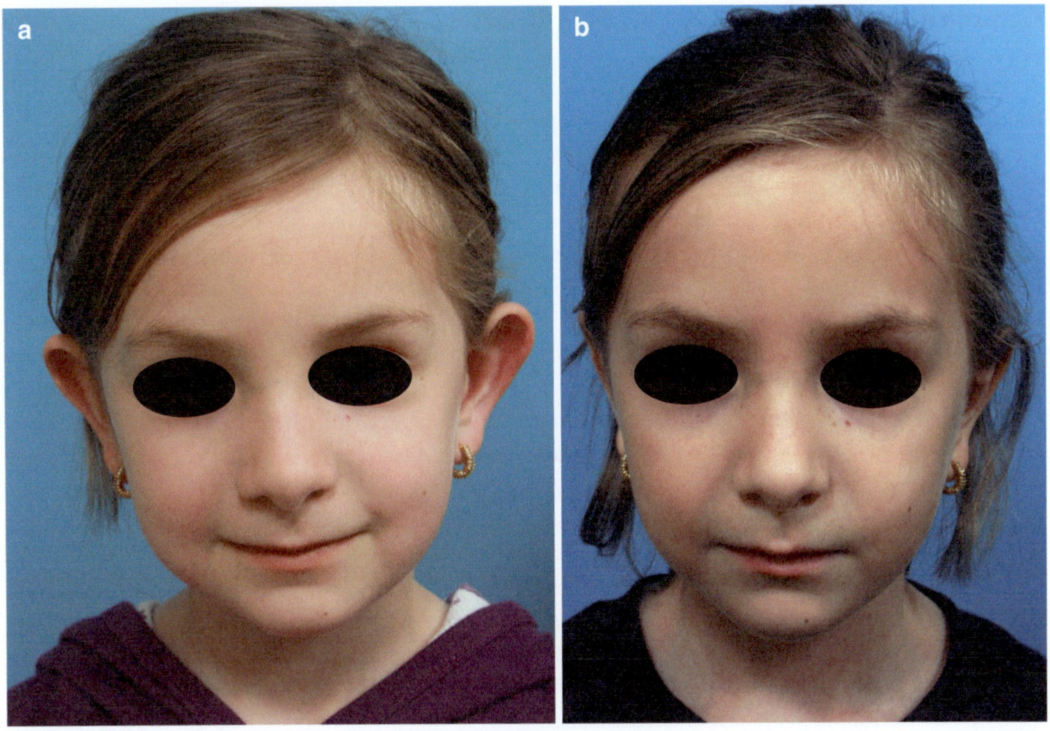

Fig. 33.8 (**a**) Preoperative female with asymmetric ear deformity. (**b**) Postoperative

if it is too high the distance can be decreased before placing an additional three sutures.

The conchal protrusion component of the deformity is then addressed. The previously marked conchal limits are used to mark the proposed conchal scoring incisions, which parallel the access of the ear. The first mark is made at the lateral limit of the conchal bowl in the cymba conchae. If there is an extreme amount of protrusion, a parallel conchal incision is made approximately 6.0 mm medial to the first. The perichondrium is cut with the microcautery needle and the cartilage is cut with a scalpel, taking care to preserve the anterior skin. In most cases only the lateral incision is necessary. This maneuver breaks the skin of the conchal bowl. Three to four 4-0 clear nylon mattress sutures are then placed 6.0 mm apart between the distal edge of the most lateral conchal scoring incision and the mastoid periosteum. This brings the scapha posteriorly against the concha and closer to the mastoid, correcting the central ear prominence. It is important that the conchal setback sutures be placed along the entire length of the conchal release incisions to prevent tethering of the central ear. The wounds are then irrigated with antibiotic solution, all bleeding points are hemocoagulated, and symmetry is confirmed. The most lateral point of the helix should be no closer than 18.0 mm from the mastoid to prevent a pinned-back appearance. Redundant skin is then trimmed in an hourglass pattern, avoiding tension. Care must be taken to avoid over-resection of the skin in the central part of the wound to prevent a telephone ear deformity. At this point if the lobule is excessive, the previously marked wedge of soft tissue can be completely removed perpendicular to the long access incision. The wounds are closed with a running 4-0 chromic gut suture and coated with antibiotic ointment.

A pressure dressing consisting of Dacron fluffs and gauze is applied for 36 h only. Oral acetaminophen with codeine is given, along with oral cephalosporin for 4 days. Patients are asked to sleep with a headband on for 4 weeks and can shower and shampoo within 36 h.

Complications

A total of 180 patients (360 ears) underwent otoplasty surgery over a 20-year period. There were no major complications. There were no infections. A total of 15 minor complications were recorded. These include: three minor postauricular hematomas, which were evacuated under local anesthesia; 12 patients required unilateral revision for a variety of problems; six ears had slightly recurrence of the superior pole prominence, which was corrected by simple postauricular skin excision under local anesthesia in the office; four ears required replacement of one or more sutures at the superior third of the antihelical fold for recurrent deformities; two developed small hypertrophic postauricular scars, which were excised at the time of antihelical fold correction and injected with steroid; and one of these patients also developed a small hypertrophic scar along the anterior aspect of the newly created antihelical fold, which responded to topical steroids.

Discussion

Previous authors have documented a plethora of technical pitfalls that can occur in otoplasty surgery [11–14]. Common iatrogenic problems include telephone ear deformity, caused by overly enthusiastic central conchal resection or excessive skin resection in the central portion of the incision. Scoring the cartilage of the proposed antihelical fold too deeply or completely cutting it can create an edge effect that can be visible from anterior view. The pinned ear can be caused by overly tight suturing of the concha to the mastoid or by over-resection of the postauricular skin. The conchal skin folding deformity may be caused by aggressive conchal resection with insufficient skin undermining. In the previously described technique, the concha is not removed, which has greatly reduced any type of visible conchal deformity after setback. Other less common problems include gross asymmetry or an antihelical fold that is far higher than the helical rim, giving an odd appearance. Damage to the anterior auricular skin and hypertrophic scars or keloid formation of the postauricular scars is rare but reported [11–14].

Any surgical technique and especially any aesthetic surgical technique must be judged by its simplicity, reproducibility, and overall safety. The technique described in this chapter has been applied to 180 consecutive patients over a 20-year period. The results have been consistently good, with a minimum of complications and an overall 8 % revision rate. All of the minor complications were easily corrected; most required only minor office surgery or a brief anesthetic. All the recurrent deformities of this series occurred in the superior part of the antihelical fold and were easily corrected. All were the results of suture failure or sutures pulling through the cartilage. These problems have become less frequent and most occurred early in the series. These are attributed to insufficient cartilage scoring, superficial placement of the antihelical sutures, and failure to preserve the perichondrium to add strength to the repair. All of the recognized components of the prominent ear deformity, including lack of the antihelical fold and superior crus, conchal hypertrophy, and a prominent lobule, are addressed with this technique. A combination of mattress sutures that describe a Mustardé technique [2] and cartilage scoring similar to that described by Stenstroem [3] are used for forming the antihelical fold as well as the superior crus. Unlike the Mustardé technique, the mattress sutures are completely tightened down rather than adjusted individually, which can be difficult to reproduce from side to side. When the conchal-mastoid sutures are fully tightened and are placed the same distance on each side, reproducible results can be easily obtained. Measuring the proposed peak of the antihelical fold has been helpful in achieving symmetrical results as well as in avoiding the hidden helix. To avoid sharp ridges along the antihelix, gentle partial-thickness abrasion of the anterior surface of the scapha is used to weaken the cartilage. Unlike the Stenstroem technique in which the entire scapha is exposed, limited skin undermining of the anterior scapha is advocated to avoid potential subcutaneous hematoma and resulting secondary deformity.

Bauer et al. [8] reported the role of conchal hypertrophy as a central component of the prominent ear deformity, which must be addressed to prevent undesirable results. Certainly, this is a key component in successful repair. They perform an anterior chondrocutaneous dissection with a postauricular approach used to create the antihelical fold. Other authors have also advocated addressing the concha through excision from the anterior-posterior approach. Bauer et al. point out that failure to resect the skin with the conchal cartilage can result in visible skin wrinkling. The author prefers to approach both the scapha and the concha through a postauricular incision because of the small but finite possibility of hypertrophic scar formation, which would be visible from the anterior approach. Rather than resect the concha with or without skin, I prefer to weaken the spring by making parallel incisions through the postauricular perichondrium and full thickness through the conchal cartilage, leaving the anterior perichondrium intact. This is similar to the scapha incision described by Tanzer [9], for creation of the antihelical fold. Currently, most conchal hypertrophy can be addressed with a single incision at the juncture of the concha and scapha. If necessary a second incision can be placed approximately 6.0 mm medially. The amount of conchal resection can then be adjusted. If less conchal resection is desired, the sutures can be placed more medially along the concha, which has the effect of allowing greater concha-scapha angle. If more conchal setback is desired, the sutures are placed more laterally. This method is a powerful tool for complete correction of the conchal hypertrophy component of the deformity and avoids potential visible anterior scars as well as conchal skin deformities. Anterior skin wrinkling has not been observed with this technique. The final skin and lobule tapering have been well described by others [1–9]. The surgeon must not rely on the final skin excision to correct any significant residual cartilage deformities because the stretching of the skin will eventually result in recurrence. The simplified and shortened postoperative care regimen with minimal bandaging has resulted in excellent patient and parental acceptance. Both the patient and the parents must be committed and motivated for optimal postoperative results.

This technique combines cartilage-sparing and scoring techniques of Stenstroem and portions of the Mustardé and Furnas technique, also addressing the conchal hypertrophy as advocated by Bauer et al. [2, 3, 8]. It allows for symmetric aesthetic improvement of the prominent ear. The author suggested guidelines for the height of the antihelical fold, conchal setback, and concha-scapha distance, which can be measured from side to side to insure a reproducible result.

References

1. Luckett WH. A new operation for prominent ears based on the anatomical deformity. Surg Gynecol Obstet. 1910;10:635–7.
2. Mustarde JC. The correction of prominent ears using simple mattress sutures. Br J Plast Surg. 1963;16: 170–8.
3. Stenstroem SJ. A “natural” technique for correction of congenitally prominent ears. Plast Reconstr Surg. 1963;33:509–18.
4. Furnas DW. Correction of prominent ears by conchamastoid sutures. Plast Reconstr Surg. 1968;42: 189–93.
5. Kaye BL. A simplified method for correcting the prominent ear. Plast Reconstr Surg. 1967;40(1):44–8.
6. Burstein FD. Cartilage sparing complete otoplasty technique: a 10 year experience in 100 patients. J Craniofac Surg. 2003;14(4):521–5.
7. McDovell AJ. Goals in otoplasty for protruding ears. Plast Reconstr Surg. 1968;41(1):17–27.
8. Bauer BS, Song DH, Aitken ME. Combined otoplasty technique: chondrocutaneous resection as the cornerstone to correction of the prominent ear. Plast Reconstr Surg. 2002;110(4):1033–40.
9. Tanzer RC. The correction of prominent ears. Plast Reconstr Surg. 1962;30:236–46.
10. Cohen SR, Burstein FD. Protruding ear. In: Spitz L, Coran AG, editors. Rob and Smith’s operative surgery. London: Chapman and Hall Medical; 1995. p. 76–85.
11. Elliott Jr RA. Complications in the treatment of prominent ears. Clin Plast Surg. 1978;5(3):479–90.
12. Spira M. Otoplasty: what I do now: a 10 year perspective. Plast Reconstr Surg. 1999;104(3):834–40.
13. Spira M. Reduction otoplasty. In: Goldwyn R, editor. The unfavorable result in plastic surgery. Boston: Little, Brown and Company; 1972. p. 168–9.
14. Spira M, Stal S. The conchal flap: an adjunct in otoplasty. Ann Plast Surg. 1983;11(4):291–8.

34 Posterior Suturing with Postauricular Fascial Flap Otoplasty

Mark V. Schaverien and Kenneth J. Stewart

Introduction

Prominent ear correction was first described over 150 years ago [1] and since then a myriad of techniques have been described. Of these the anterior scoring methods of Stenströem [2] and Chongchet [3] and the posterior suturing technique of Mustardé [4–10] have become the most popular. There is currently no universally favored technique and long-term results of the various techniques are lacking in the literature.

The posterior suturing with postauricular fascial flap otoplasty technique was first described by Horlock et al. [11]. The innovative technique was designed to address the high rate of postauricular suture extrusion and recurrence with the cartilage-sparing techniques of Mustardé and Furnas. It utilizes conchoscaphoid and conchomastoid suturing with permanent sutures as described by Mustardé with the addition of a postauricular superficial muscular aponeurotic system (SMAS) flap sutured to the helical rim to cover the permanent sutures. Inherent in the technique is the versatility and control of the posterior suturing techniques that are not usually a feature of the anterior scoring otoplasty techniques. At our institution this is the favored technique following our outcome studies that have demonstrated superiority in long-term aesthetic outcome and recurrence rate when compared with posterior suturing alone or anterior scoring otoplasty techniques, with improved appearance and symmetry with time since surgery [12, 13].

M.V. Schaverien, MBChB, MRCS, MSc, MEd, M.D. (✉)
K.J. Stewart, MBChB, M.D., FRCS(Ed)(Plast)
Department of Plastic Surgery, Royal Hospital for Sick Children, 9 Sciennes Road, Edinburgh EH9 1LF, UK
e-mail: markschaverien@fastmail.fm; ken.stewart@luht.scot.nhs.uk

Surgical Technique

Surgery can be performed under general or local anesthesia, with local anesthetic with 1:200,000 adrenaline infiltration as a ring block and into the anterior and posterior surfaces of the ear in all cases. A posterior approach is utilized with excision of a narrow skin ellipse, leaving the subcutaneous layers intact on the posterior aspect of the auricle (Fig. 34.1). The remaining anterior skin on the back of the ear is reflected anteriorly in a subdermal plane as far forward as the helical rim, as dissecting anterior to this point can lead to distortion of the helical rim. A composite flap of postauricular SMAS and perichondrium is reflected from this point posteriorly, with care not to score the cartilage. Dissection is continued posteriorly until the mastoid periosteum is reached using scissors to create a pocket of adequate size to house the conchal bowl without distortion. A row of four 4/0 undyed Ethibond (Ethicon) sutures are inserted with a round-bodied needle to create the new antihelical fold, starting caudally. The round-bodied needle avoids the tendency of the suture material to cut through the

M.A. Shiffman (ed.), *Advanced Cosmetic Otoplasty*,
DOI 10.1007/978-3-642-35431-1_34, © Springer-Verlag Berlin Heidelberg 2013

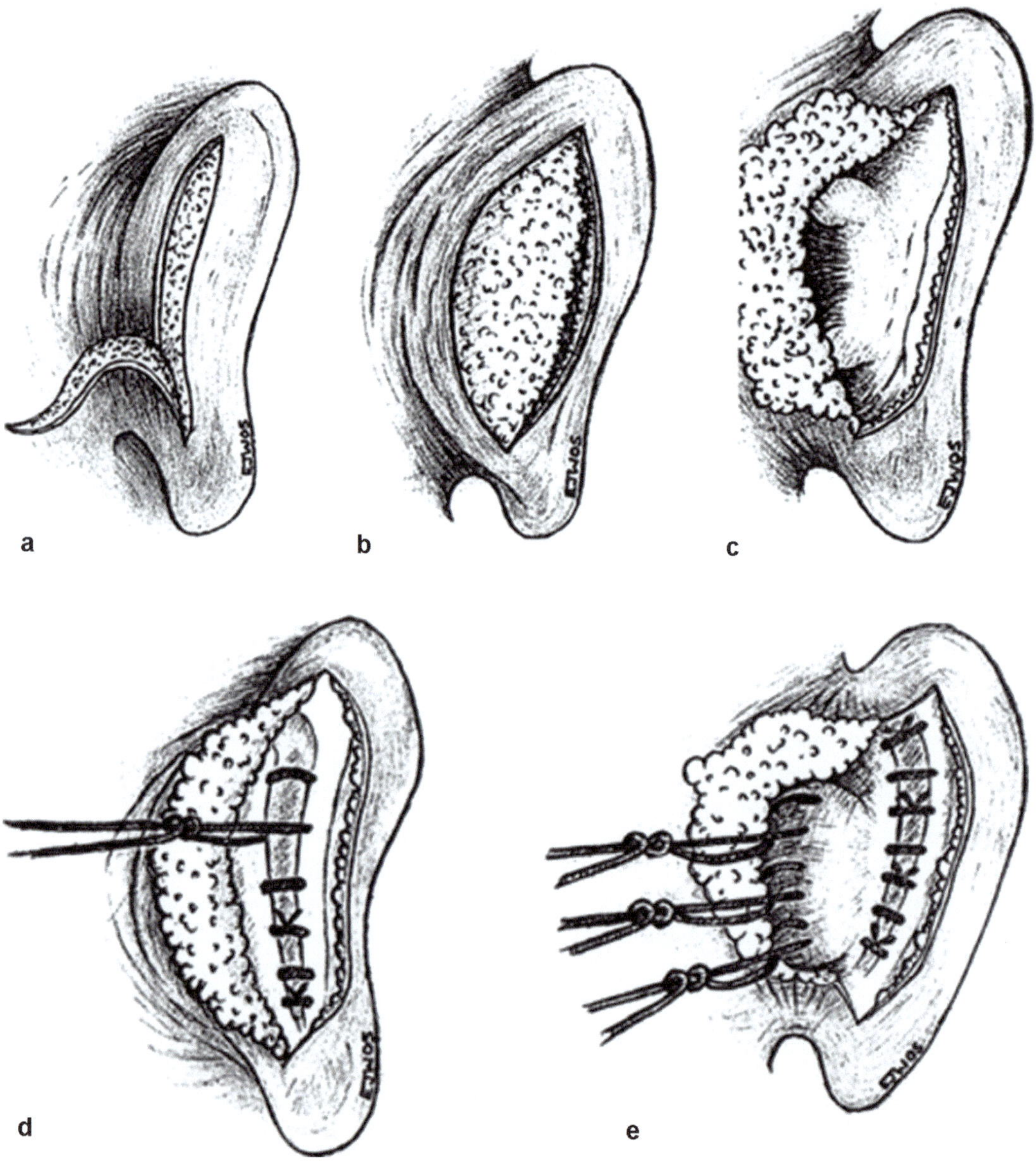

Fig. 34.1 (**a**) Postauricular incision. (**b**) Postauricular ellipse of skin excised with preservation of the underlying fascial layer. (**c**) Raising postauricular composite flap of postauricular SMAS and perichondrium. (**d**) Conchoscaphoid sutures. (**e**) Conchomastoid sutures

delicate cartilage. A second row of sutures is then placed between the mastoid periosteum and the rim of the conchal bowl (Fig. 34.1). The auricularis posterior muscle is not divided and the first of the conchomastoid sutures is passed under the auricularis posterior muscle to ensure good anchorage. To facilitate access to the mastoid pocket, all sutures are inserted and held with a clip prior to tying, and care must be taken not to inadvertently include the fascial flap when tightening the sutures. In all of our cases, we do not overcorrect at surgery, but we try to achieve the appearance we are looking for. The posterior fascial flap is then replaced over the cartilage and sutured to the posterior aspect of the helical rim with 5/0 Vicryl rapide without tension to cover

Table 34.1 Complications of posterior suturing with postauricular fascial flap otoplasty (n=82 ears), posterior suturing otoplasty alone (n=188 ears), and anterior scoring otoplasty (n=136 ears) techniques

		Posterior suturing with postauricular fascial flap	Posterior suturing	Anterior scoring
Early complications	Delayed healing	0	2.1	1.5
	Infection	0	0.5	0.7
	Bleeding/ haematoma	1.2	2.7	0.7
Late complications	Anterior skin necrosis	0	0	0.7
	Residual pain	0	0	1.4
	Cartilage spur	0	0	0.7
	Scarred notch	0	0	0.7
	Stitch granuloma	0	1.1	0
	Extrusion	1.2	2.1	0
	Prominent scars/ keloids	0	2.1	1.4
	Recurrence	4.8	8	11
	Reoperation for recurrence	3.6	6	8.8

Figures given as percentages of number of ears (Adapted from Mandal et al. [12])

all Ethibond sutures. Skin is closed using 4/0 Prolene subcuticular sutures that are removed at 1 week postoperatively. A standard head bandage is applied for 1 week that is replaced with a headband worn at night for 6 weeks following removal of sutures.

Preoperatively, on the table following surgical correction, and at all follow-up points, the authors measure and record the perpendicular distance from the mastoid to the helical rim at the middle third of the pinna at level of Frankfort line, a standardized cephalometric line connecting the infraorbital rim and the superior aspect of the external auditory meatus. With the same person taking this measurement, there may be a difference of 1–2 mm if the measurement is repeated twice on the same ear, and therefore, this can be considered a standardized measurement of correction [9].

Surgical and Aesthetic Outcomes

The surgical and aesthetic outcomes of the posterior suturing with postauricular fascial flap otoplasty technique were studied and comparison of cartilage scoring and cartilage-sparing otoplasty was done in 203 cases [12]. The authors performed bilateral otoplasty by either posterior suturing with postauricular fascial flap otoplasty (n=41 patients), posterior suturing alone (n=94 patients), and anterior scoring otoplasty (n=68 patients) techniques. The median patient age was 9 years (range 5–16 years) and the median follow-up was 11 months (range 9–36 months). The study found that the overall complication rate, recurrence rate, and rate of reoperation for recurrence was lowest in the posterior suturing with postauricular fascial flap otoplasty group (Table 34.1). The overall appearance and symmetry scores on a visual analogue scale (VAS) as assessed by a blinded physician and blinded lay observer demonstrate consistently better scores for the posterior suturing with postauricular fascial flap technique (Figs. 34.2 and 34.3).

A study was done [13], which evaluated long-term outcomes of the posterior suturing with postauricular fascial flap otoplasty technique. Sixty patients (112 ears) who had their surgery performed by a single surgeon (KJS) were included in the study. Patients were invited on a single episode to a follow-up clinic where detailed evaluation was performed and further measurements taken by two separate observers. Photographs taken preoperatively, at 6 weeks postop-

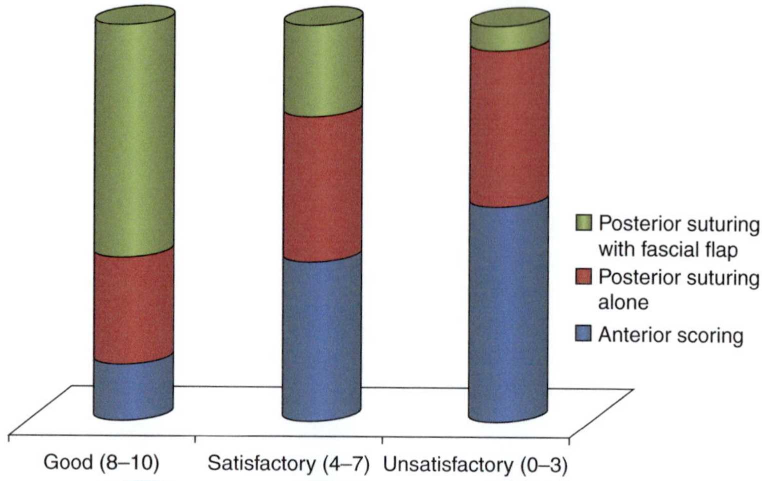

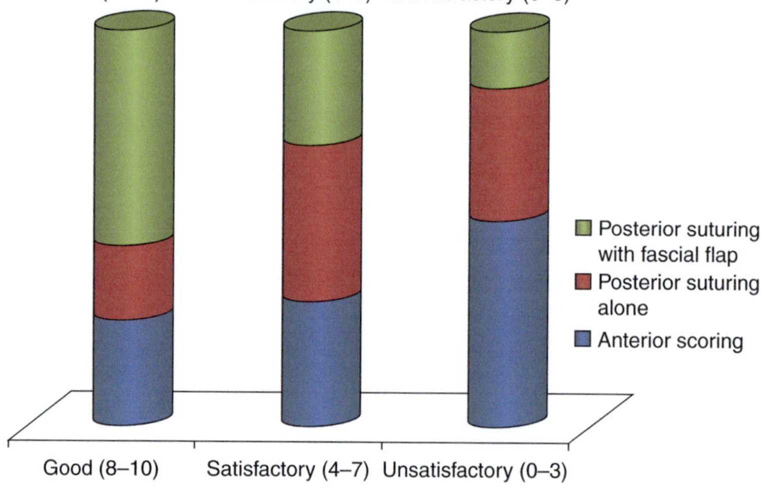

Figs. 34.2 and 34.3 Overall appearance and symmetry score based on pre- and postoperative photographs (Adapted from Mandal et al. [12])

eratively, and at the follow-up clinic were evaluated by an independent blinded consultant plastic surgeon observer for overall appearance and symmetry using a VAS. The mean age at surgery was 8.5 years (range 4–14) and the mean postoperative follow-up period was 3.9 years (range 1.5–7.8). Overall five patients (five ears) had clinical recurrence (4.5 %), three of which had undergone revisional surgery. Clinical recurrence occurred at a mean of 2.5 years following surgery (range 1–5.8 years). The immediate postoperative measurements were 20 mm or less for all ears except two.

Thirty patients attended follow-up clinic following a single invitation (57 ears). The mean immediate postoperative correction was 11.3 mm and the mean correction found at follow-up was 10.6 mm, with a mean loss of correction of 0.7 mm (6.2 %) at the Frankfort line. The number of ears where there was a loss of correction of 1 mm or more was 26 (46 %). In 15 ears (26 %), there was improvement in correction from that found immediately postoperatively of 1 mm or more. There was no relationship between the mastoid-to-helical rim measurement and duration since surgery, and there was also no relationship between the amount of initial correction and the loss of correction at long-term follow-up.

Patients were generally satisfied with the results in terms of size, shape, and symmetry (Figs. 34.4, 34.5, and 34.6). All patients that were dissatisfied with their outcome had an obvious clinical recurrence except for one. The mean VAS scores given by the blinded observer at late postoperative review were higher than those given for photographs taken at 6 weeks postoperatively (Table 34.2). The blinded observer gave better

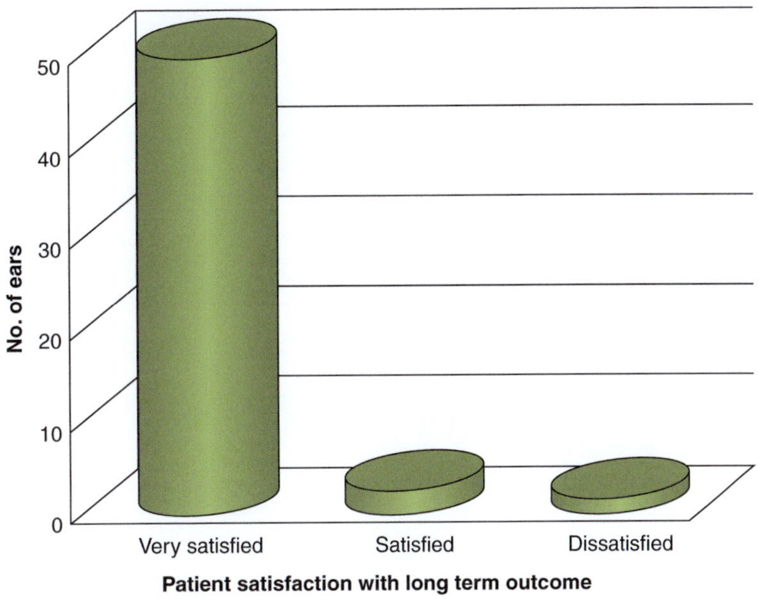

Fig. 34.4 Patient satisfaction with outcome at late postoperative follow-up (Adapted from Schaverien et al. [13])

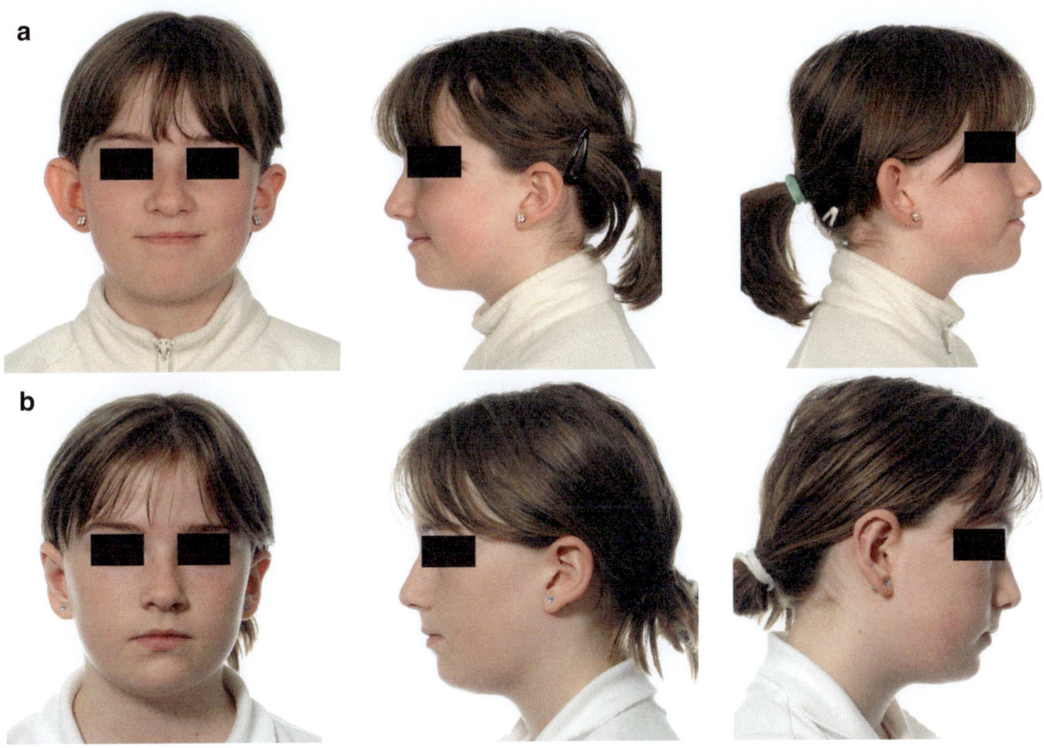

Fig. 34.5 (**a**) Preoperative. (**b**) Six weeks postoperative. (**c**) Four years postoperative

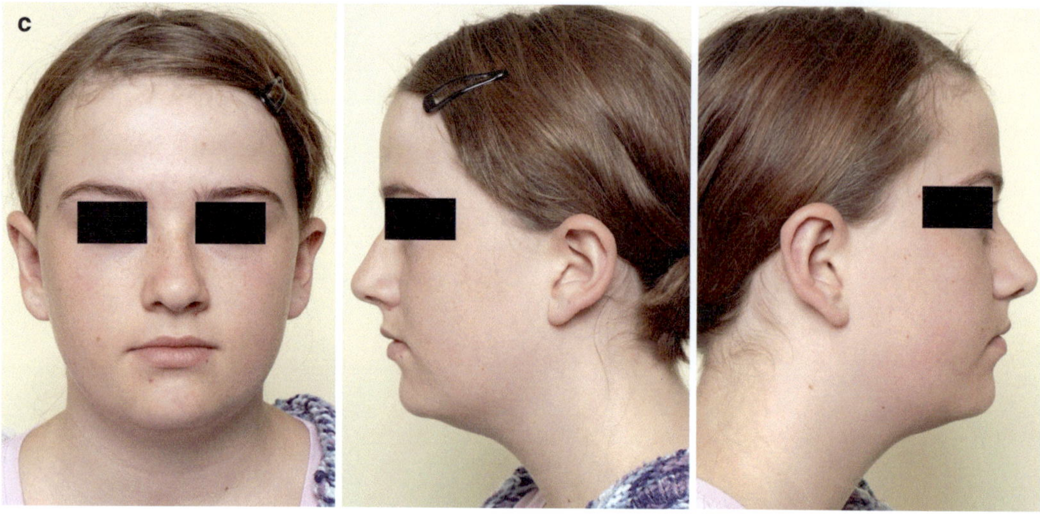

Fig. 34.5 (continued)

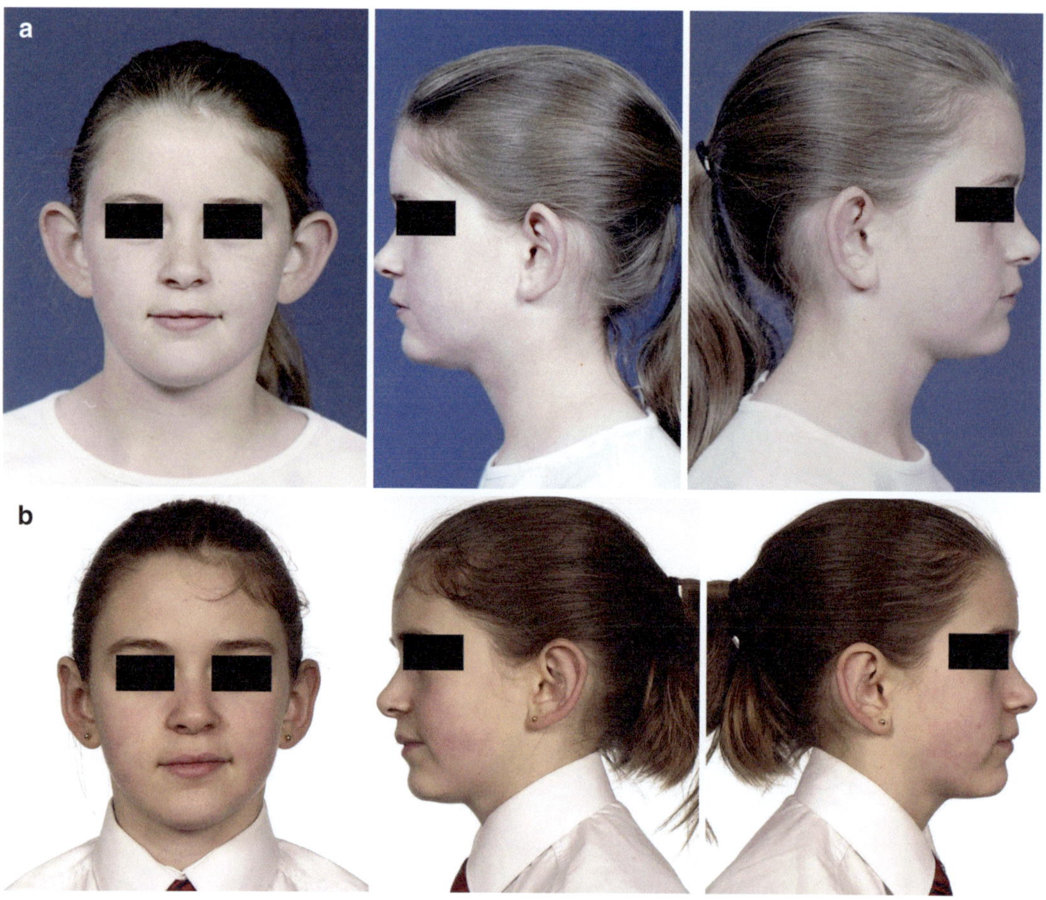

Fig. 34.6 (**a**) Preoperative. (**b**) Six weeks postoperative. (**c**) Five and three fourths years postoperative

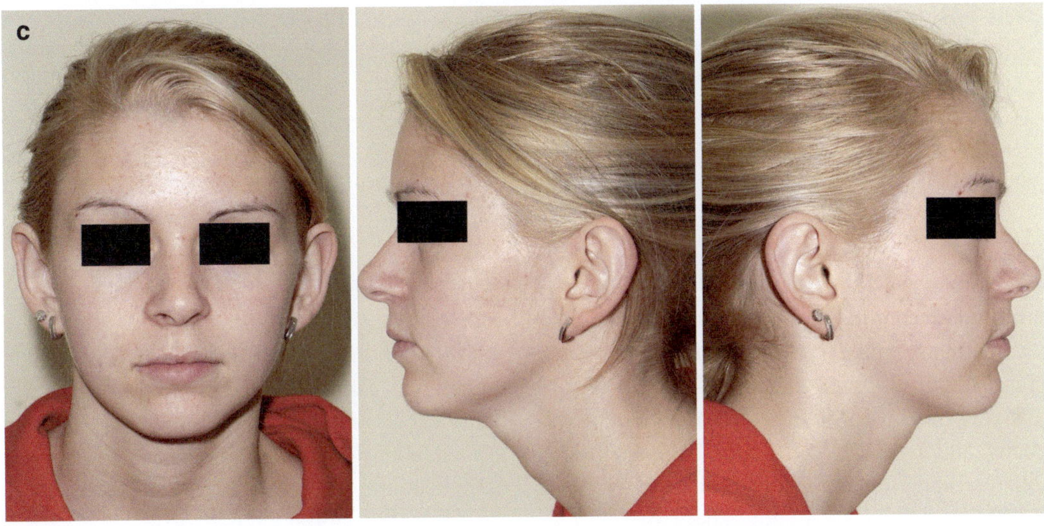

Fig. 34.6 (continued)

Table 34.2 Blinded observer visual analogue scale scores

Appearance	Mean	Range	*P*-value
Preoperative overall appearance	32.3	16–60	
Immediate postoperative overall appearance	62.7	32–91	
Late postoperative overall appearance	70	48–91	$P=0.01$
Symmetry			
Preoperative symmetry	44.1	15–80	
Immediate postoperative symmetry	58.9	33–93	
Late postoperative symmetry	64.1	40–92	

Adapted from Schaverien et al. [13]

scores at late compared with 6-week postoperative follow-up for 11 patients. There was a statistically significant improvement in appearance between the 6-week postoperative photographs and those taken at late follow-up ($P=0.01$). There was no relationship between VAS scores and duration since surgery.

Minor complications occurred in six ears (5.4 %). Suture extrusion occurred in one ear, and three ears developed painful and palpable permanent sutures, two of which required local anesthetic procedures for removal of sutures.

Discussion

Otoplasty is an effective procedure in alleviating psychosocial distress in the vast majority of children that undergo the operation [14]. The ultimate goal for the procedure is the production of ears with a natural and symmetrical appearance with minimal complications or recurrence. Unfortunately all pinnaplasty techniques have a clinical recurrence rate and little is known about the long-term stability of the technique [4, 8, 9, 15].

At our institution posterior suturing combined with a postauricular fascial flap as described by Horlock et al. [11] is our favored technique. The literature is supportive of the excellent outcomes that are achievable with this technique (Table 34.3). In their original study Horlock et al. evaluated their results in 51 patients (96 ears). The patients ranged in age from 4 to 72 years, with a median of 10 years of age, and median follow-up was 11 months. There were no hematomas and no patients developed suture extrusion or granuloma. Recurrence of deformity occurred with eight ears in six patients (8.3 % of ears, 11.8 % of patients), two of whom requested further surgery (4 %)

Table 34.3 Outcomes from studies of the posterior suturing with postauricular fascial flap otoplasty technique

	No. of patients	No. of ears	Suture extrusion	Recurrence (%)
Horlock et al. [11]	51	96	0	8.3
Mandal et al. [12]	41	82	1.2 %	4.8
Schaverien et al. [13]	60	112	0.9 %	4.5
Sinha and Richards [16]	227	435	2.6 %	3.7

[11]. Sinha and Richard reported their outcomes using the technique in 435 ears in 227 consecutive patients, with age range from 6 to 16 years. Ten patients (14 ears) had complications (4.4 % patients, 3.2 % ears), 6 of which had suture extrusions, and 1 patient had a head bandage-related bilateral anterior skin necrosis that fully healed with conservative treatment. There were 6 unilateral and 5 bilateral recurrences representing 4.8 % patients and 3.7 % ears, and all but one of these required redo of the original technique with a satisfactory outcome. Ninety-seven percent of patients had a good or excellent outcome noted at the time of final review by the clinician [16].

The authors feel that conchoscaphoid suturing leads to greater control and predictability in contouring of the antihelix than with cartilage scoring or cutting techniques, creating a natural-looking antihelical fold and helical rim (Figs. 34.5 and 34.6). The avoidance of anterior skin dissection leads to an inherently safer procedure than cartilage-cutting otoplasty, where anterior skin or cartilage necrosis has been reported.

The addition of the postauricular fascial flap to cover the internal permanent sutures, which is fast and easy to raise, appears to provide a supplementary vascularized layer to reduce the risk of suture extrusion [4, 5, 7]. The flap is repositioned without tension and therefore is unlikely to contribute postauricular support to prevent recurrence. The reasons for improved aesthetic appearance with time since surgery as assessed by a blinded observer, however, are unclear [13]. The authors' long-term results suggest that it is unnecessary to overcorrect during surgery, as the correction is stable or improves with time. Any recurrence that does occur can be addressed relatively simply by revisional surgery. The authors prefer to use undyed Ethibond sutures (Ethicon) as the extrusion rate is lower when compared with Prolene (Ethicon) sutures.

Although during these studies a posterior skin ellipse was excised, it is currently our practice not to excise any skin as it does not play any part in maintenance of correction. Reconstruction for complications is also much more difficult when there is a skin shortage posteriorly.

The authors' studies have demonstrated a low suture extrusion and other complication rate and a low rate of recurrence, with an excellent long-term aesthetic outcome that may improve further with time since surgery. These results are limited to children since adults tend to have stiffer cartilage and therefore perhaps a higher predisposition to recurrence due to higher constant strain on the permanent fixation sutures. For this reason although our usual method for revision is further simple suturing in children, we have a low threshold for simultaneous conchal reduction in adults where the cartilage is stiff.

Conclusions

The addition of the postauricular fascial flap to Mustardé and Furnas otoplasty as described by Horlock et al. [11] is a valuable refinement that reduces suture extrusion and recurrence rates. The refinement maintains a relatively simple, controllable, and intrinsically safe otoplasty that avoids irreparable complications and has become our technique of choice.

Acknowledgements The authors are indebted to the Department of Medical Photography at the Royal Hospital for Sick Children for production of the photographs; Mr. Patrick Addison, consultant plastic surgeon, for his help with this study; Miss Elizabeth Whallett, consultant plastic surgeon, for illustrative figures; and above all the patients involved in the study and their parents.

References

1. Dieffenbach JF. Die operative Chirurgie. Leipzig: FA Brockhause; 1845.
2. Stenstroem SJ. A "natural" technique for correction of congenitally prominent ears. Plast Reconstr Surg. 1963;32:509–18.
3. Chongchet V. A method of antihelix reconstruction. Br J Plast Surg. 1963;16:268–72.
4. Mustardé JC. The correction of prominent ears using simple mattress sutures. Br J Plast Surg. 1963;16:170–8.
5. Mustarde JC. Results of otoplasty by the author's method. In: Goldwyn RM, editor. Long-term results in plastic and reconstructive surgery. Boston: Little Brown & Co; 1980. p. 138–44.
6. Furnas DW. Correction of prominent ears by conchal mastoid sutures. Plast Reconstr Surg. 1968;42(3):189–93.
7. Minderjahn A, Hüttl WR, Hildmann H. Mustardé's otoplasty–evaluation of correlation between clinical and statistical findings. J Maxillofac Surg. 1980;8(3):241–50.
8. Adamson PA, McGraw BL, Tropper GJ. Otoplasty: critical review of clinical results. Laryngoscope. 1991;101(8):883–8.
9. Messner AH, Crysdale WS. Otoplasty. Clinical protocol and long-term results. Arch Otolaryngol Head Neck Surg. 1996;122(7):773–7.
10. Ellis D, Keohane J. A simplified approach to otoplasty. J Otolaryngol. 1992;21(1):66–9.
11. Horlock N, Misra A, Gault DT. The postauricular fascial flap as an adjunct to Mustardé and Furnas type otoplasty. Plast Reconstr Surg. 2001;108(6): 1487–90.
12. Mandal A, Bahia H, Ahmad T, Stewart KJ. Comparison of cartilage scoring and cartilage sparing otoplasty – a study of 203 cases. J Plast Reconstr Aesthet Surg. 2006;59(11):1170–6.
13. Schaverien MV, Al-Busaidi S, Stewart KJ. Long-term results of posterior suturing with postauricular fascial flap otoplasty. J Plast Reconstr Aesthet Surg. 2010; 63(9):1447–51.
14. Cooper-Hobson G, Jaffe W. The benefits of otoplasty for children: further evidence to satisfy the modern NHS. J Plast Reconstr Aesthet Surg. 2009;62(2): 190–4.
15. Webster RC, Smith RC. Otoplasty for prominent ears. In: Goldwyn RM, editor. Long-term results in plastic and reconstructive surgery. Boston: Little Brown & Co.; 1980. p. 146–86.
16. Sinha M, Richard B. Postauricular fascial flap and suture otoplasty: a prospective outcome study of 227 patients. J Plast Reconstr Aesthet Surg. 2012;65(3): 367–71.

The Role of the Postauricular Fascia in Otoplasty: A Complete System for Otoplasty

35

Kayvan Shokrollahi

Introduction

The ultimate goal for otoplasty is to provide a simple operative procedure that produces a natural correction of deformity, with the least degree of tissue trauma and the lowest rates of recurrence and complications. While numerous techniques exist, a number of outcome measures are not routinely examined by surgeons. Therefore, of the numerous techniques which may yield equivalent technical results in the correct hands, they may do so in a way that does not take into account factors such as patient comfort, postoperative inconvenience, necessity for postoperative head bandages, and requirement for patients to attend appointments to deal with dressings.

There has been a resurgence of interest in suture-based techniques. There is a perception by some that while cartilage scoring techniques [1, 2] can achieve consistent and favorable results in the majority of patients, when complications do occur they can be significant and difficult to correct without residual deformity. It has been suggested but not proven without doubt that scoring techniques have a higher hematoma rate. Moreover, patients undergoing anterior scoring otoplasty usually need dressings and head bandages and at least one appointment in a dressing clinic. The head bandages themselves can be a cause of a number of problems including a need to re-attend the ward or clinic if they have slipped off, over-tight dressings leading to necrosis of part of the skin, the negative effect on hearing while they are worn, the cosmetic issues of wearing a head bandage, and the inability to shower or wash the hair because of the head bandage. Therefore, while anterior scoring can give good results, the occasional severe complications, and all the listed problems with discomfort and dressings, lead the author to favor an alternative approach which means that the aesthetic outcome is better and complications are minimal and if they occur they are easy to correct. Patients do not need head bandages and can shower the day after surgery while not requiring attendance for dressings, and especially in females with long hair, there are no stigmata of surgery at all.

Nevertheless, suture techniques such as originally described by Mustardé [3] have their own complications, the main ones being recurrence or suture extrusion. If undertaken incorrectly, they can also cause an overly angulated appearance at the antihelical fold and an unnatural form with a greater chance of "overcorrection."

K. Shokrollahi, MD, BSc, MB ChB, MSc, LLM, MRCS(Eng), FRCS(Plast)
Mersey Regional Burns and Plastic Surgery Unit, Ward 4D, Whiston Hospital, Warrington Rd, Liverpool L35 5DR, UK
e-mail: kshokrollahi@hotmail.com

Electronic supplementary materialThe online version of this chapter (doi:10.1007/978-3-642-35431-1_35) contains supplementary material, which is available to authorized users.

M.A. Shiffman (ed.), *Advanced Cosmetic Otoplasty*,
DOI 10.1007/978-3-642-35431-1_35, © Springer-Verlag Berlin Heidelberg 2013

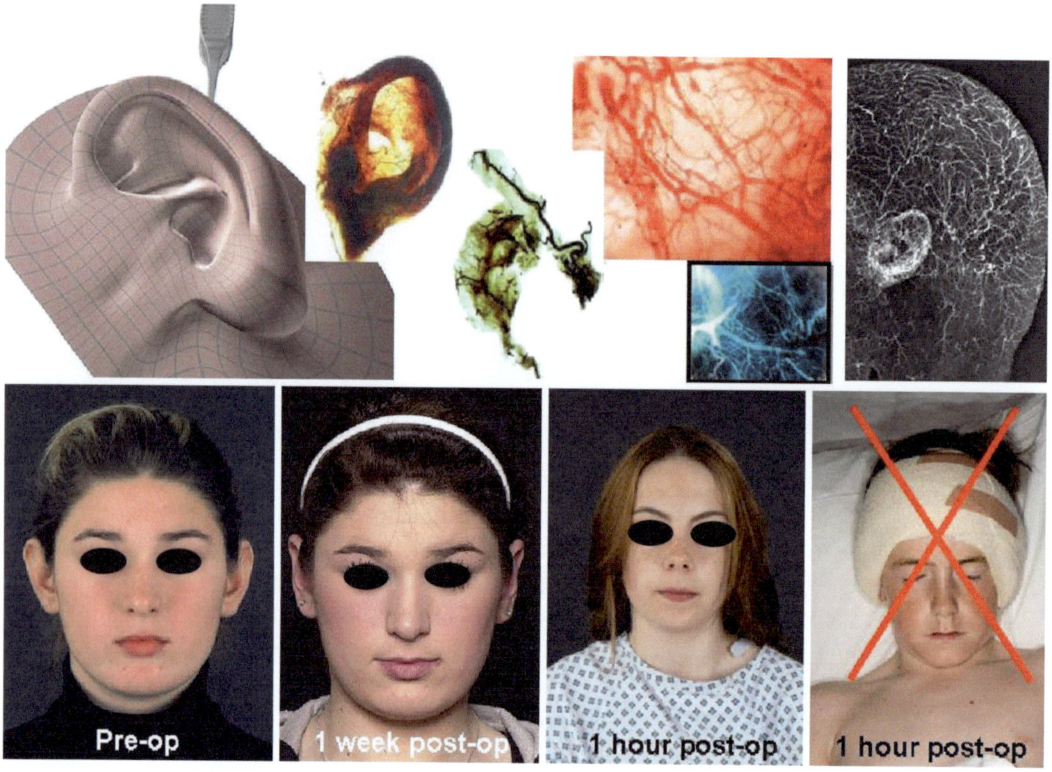

Fig. 35.1 Advantages of using an anteriorly based (helix-based) postauricular fascial flap in otoplasty: a natural symmetrical result, minimal bruising and discomfort post-operatively, hiding of the stigmata of surgery beneath long hair by avoiding head bandages, and using skin glue as both a dressing and splint which also allows showering the day after surgery

Horlock et al. [4] raised a flap of fascia on the posterior surface of the pinna, under which the sutures/suture knots could be placed for the purpose of reducing extrusion. This posteriorly (proximally) based fascial flap is raised and then sutured back into place over the Mustardé repair. The subsequent advance in using the postauricular fascia was the concept that the fascia itself can play an integral role in the structural and aesthetic otoplasty technique with the following advantages [5]:

1. Minimal recurrence rates due to removal of all tension on the Mustardé sutures.
2. A natural aesthetic without angularity.
3. Removing the need for head bandages.
4. Maintaining cover of sutures and knots.
5. A "nothing to lose" approach – raising the flap does not interfere with a surgeon's usual technique, as a starting point for learning/experimenting with the flap.

These superior endpoints using the fascial flap are achieved by raising an anteriorly/distally based flap, based on the helical rim, instead of a posteriorly based flap. The advantages of this strategy are summarized in Fig. 35.1.

Flap Anatomy and Vascular Supply

The fascia on the posterior aspect of the pinna – which the author calls the intrinsic postauricular fascia (IPF) – receives its blood supply from branches of the posterior auricular and superficial temporal branches of the external carotid artery (Fig. 35.1). The auricular branch of the posterior auricular artery and the posterior branch of the superficial temporal artery provide a dense and prosperous anastomotic arcade [5, 6], which subsequently allows a fascial flap to be raised with a distal base. The fascia itself is less fibrous and tough than the fascia overlying the region of the head posterior to the auriculocephalic sulcus which we refer to as the extrinsic postauricular fascia (EPF); however, its elastic properties and presence of perichondrium enable it to act as an excellent strong supportive framework.

Surgical Technique

Raising the Anteriorly/Distally Based Fascial Flap

After infiltration of local anesthetic with epinephrine, excision of a postauricular skin ellipse is undertaken (Fig. 35.2), which instead of being positioned over the auriculocephalic sulcus, is undertaken closer to the helical rim – about halfway between the sulcus and the rim. As well as providing mechanical advantage for a fascial flap, this positions the eventual scar to be less visible from the back as we have demonstrated in a provisional study. The excision should be skin only, such as when harvesting a full-thickness skin graft to maintain a thick and robust layer of fascia. The underlying fascia is then incised at its inferior border down to the chondral surface (Fig. 35.3) and elevated distally (Fig. 35.4). The most appropriate instrument to utilize is a pair of sharp tenotomy scissors, as the curve aids with dissection. The flap should be raised until the

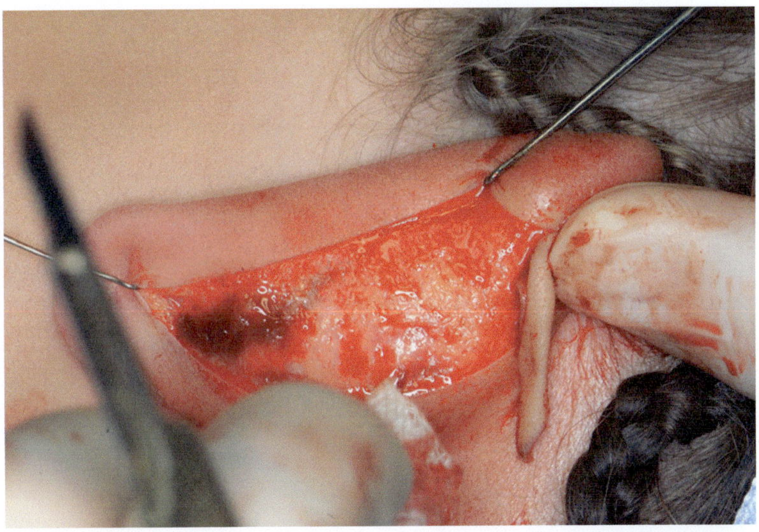

Fig. 35.2 Excise a thin postauricular skin ellipse

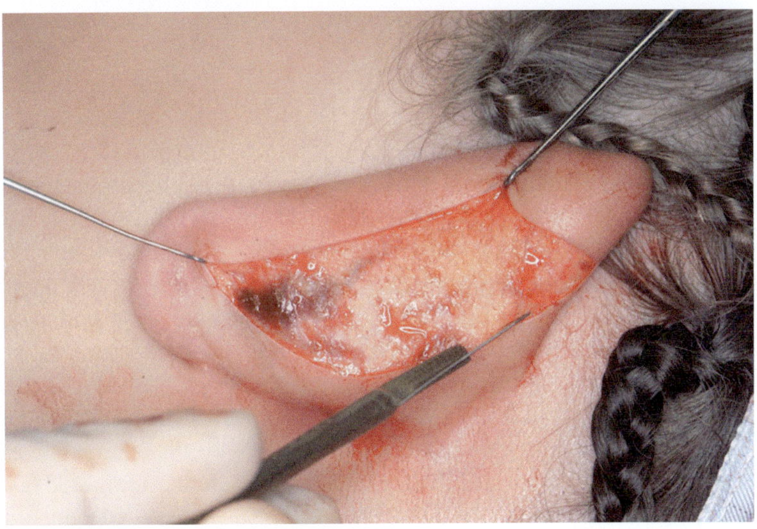

Fig. 35.3 Incise the inferior border of the fascia

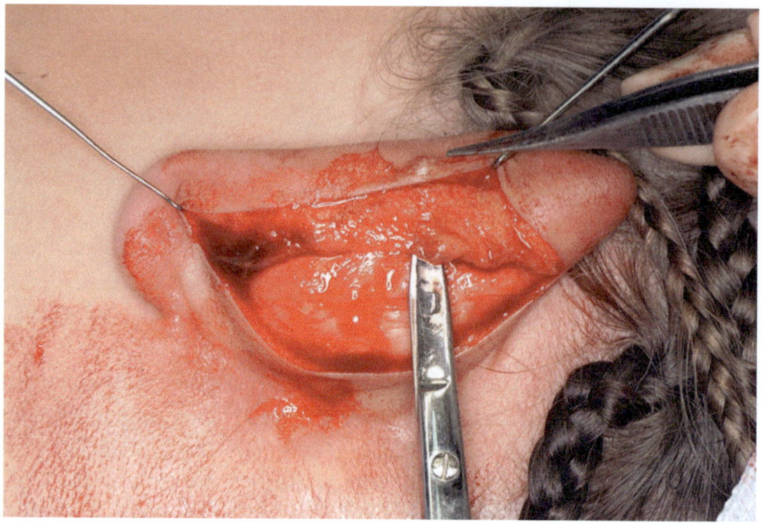

Fig. 35.4 Raise the fascial flap to the sulcus of the helical rim

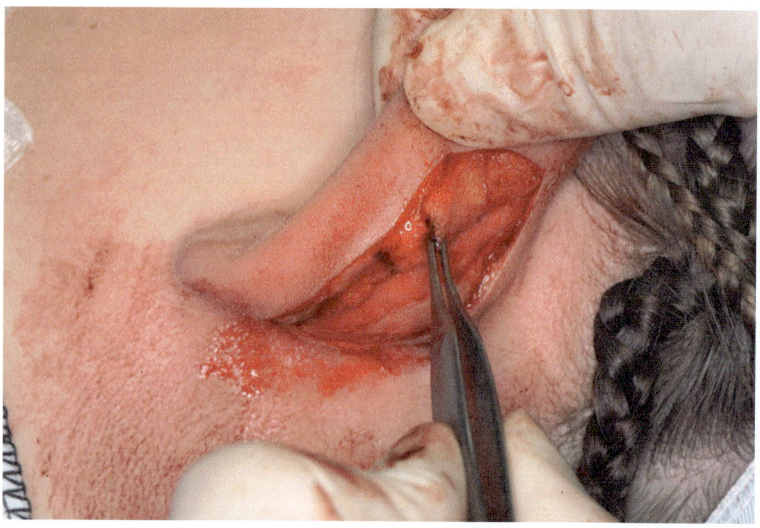

Fig. 35.5 Grasp the fascia

sulcus of the helical rim is reached. The fascia is adherent to the cartilage along the entire length of the helical rim. This results in a good level of exposure for positioning of Mustardé sutures near the rim. It also provides good exposure around the mastoid area for suture positioning for the fascia-to-mastoid suture which is a key part of the procedure.

Suturing the flap to the mastoid once the fascial flap is raised, it can be held in a forceps (Fig. 35.5) and moved around such that the entire ear will move and can be positioned in such a way as to correct the prominence of the ear. A natural antihelical fold can be created by grasping the fascia and approximating it to the appropriate location in the mastoid area, which has the same effect as numerous sutures and without the possibility of an artificially angular appearance. A location on the mastoid should be found such that the correction of the ear prominence and correction of the antihelical fold are ideal (Fig. 35.6). It is important to keep this location medial to reduce any potential to obliterate the postauricular sulcus. The simplest method is to approximate the fascia to the appropriate area on the mastoid using the forceps (Figs. 35.6, 35.7, 35.8, and 35.9).

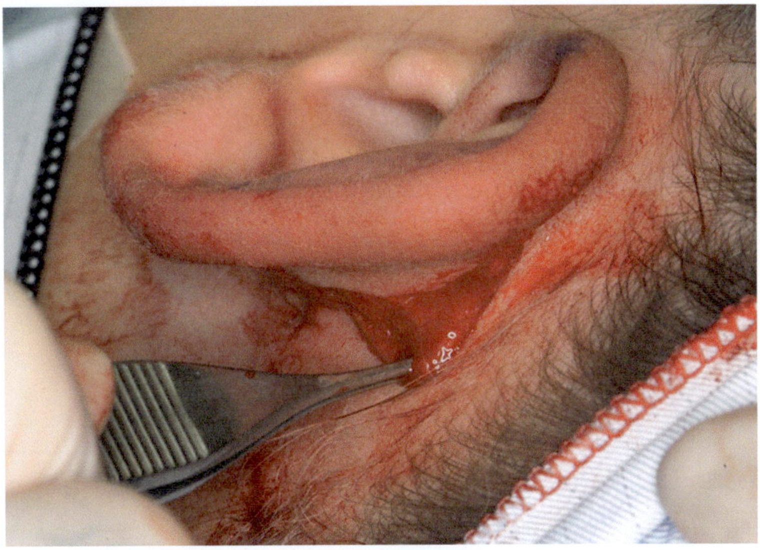

Fig. 35.6 Manipulate the ear

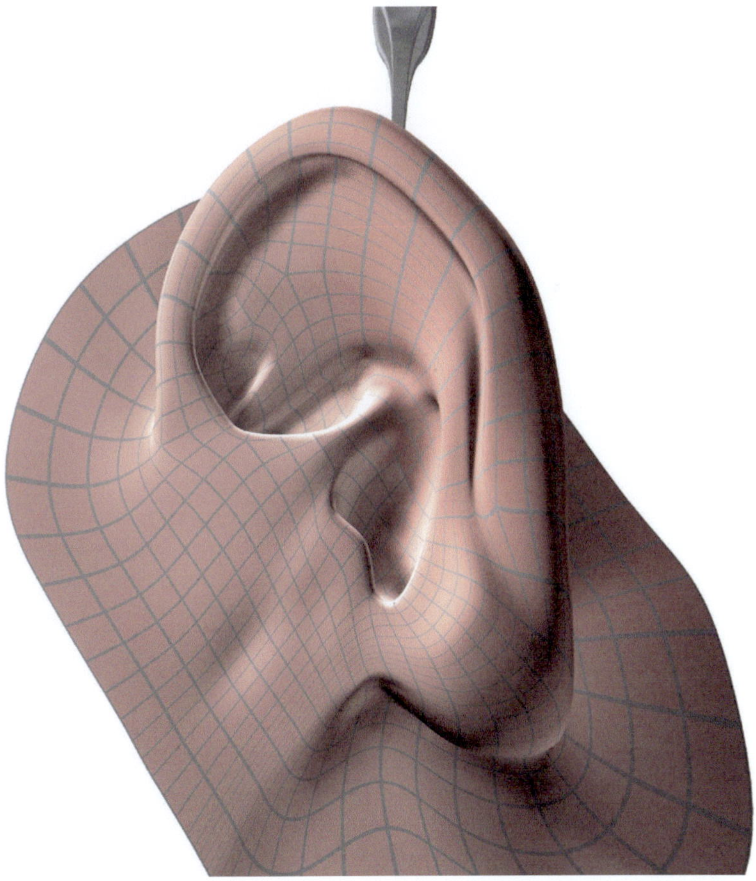

Fig. 35.7 Best location for fascial manipulation

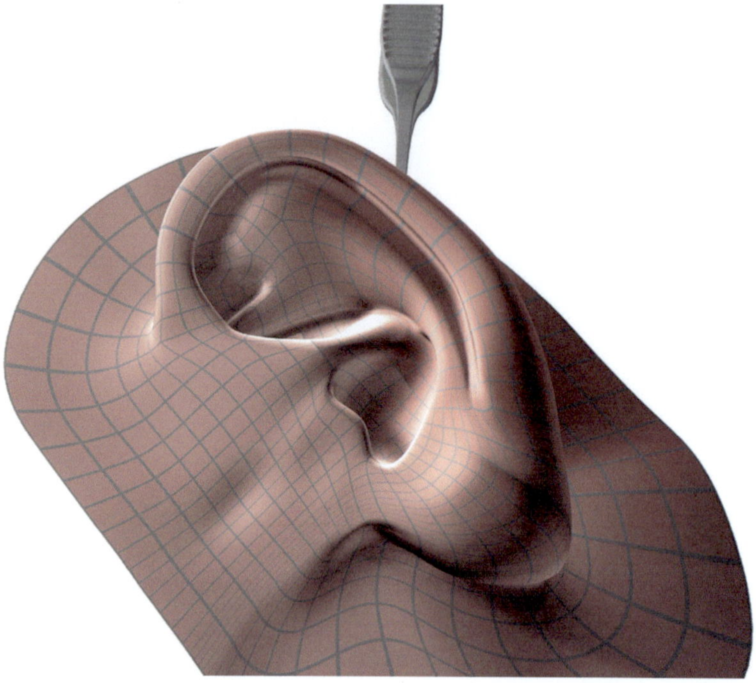

Fig. 35.8 The antihelix is created when the fascia is approximated to the mastoid

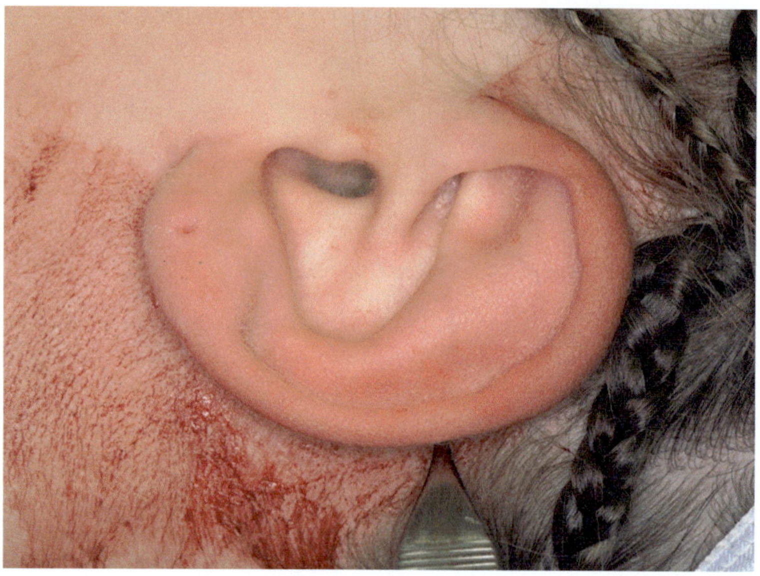

Fig. 35.9 The prominence of the ear is corrected with this maneuver

Mark the area on the skin, dissect down to the mastoid (Figs. 35.10, 35.11, and 35.12), and place a 4/0 braided suture such as Ethibond or Ticron at the periosteal level (Fig. 35.13). Next take a bite of the fascia (Fig. 35.14) where it was previously gripped in the forceps (Fig. 35.10), and tie the fascia-to-mastoid suture with a single non-locking throw as a trial (Figs. 35.15, 35.16, and 35.17), thereby correcting the prominence of the ear. Experiment with the ideal position for the fascial bite suture position – after a shallow learning curve, the ideal position will come naturally at the first attempt and be confirmed by tying the suture. When the ideal location is chosen, release the suture from the fascia (Fig. 35.18) and position Mustardé sutures between the concha and the scapha to create a gentle antihelical curve (Figs. 35.19 and 35.20). Mustardé sutures should

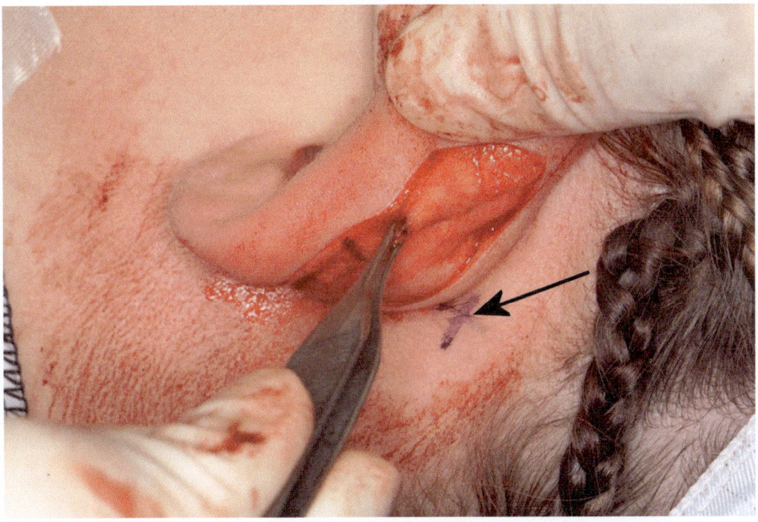

Fig. 35.10 Mark the skin over the mastoid at the location where correction is optimum

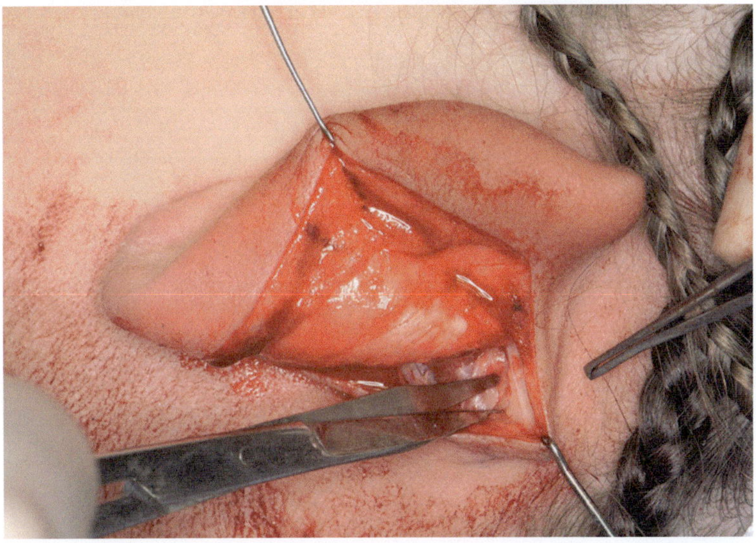

Fig. 35.11 Dissect down to the mastoid beneath the mark

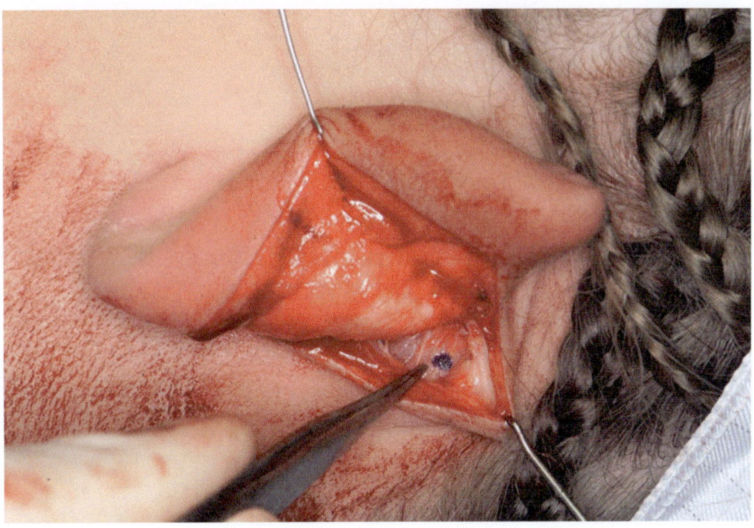

Fig. 35.12 Identify the suture position

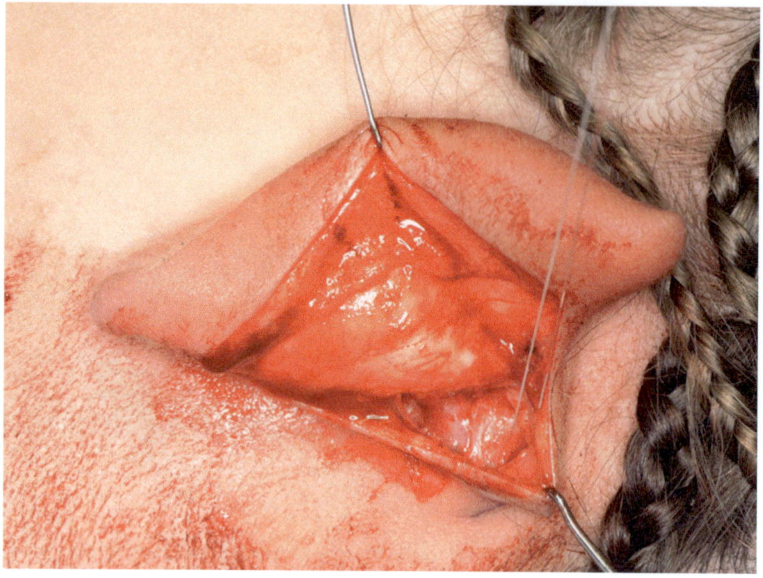

Fig. 35.13 Place a 4/0 Ethibond or Ticron at the periosteal level

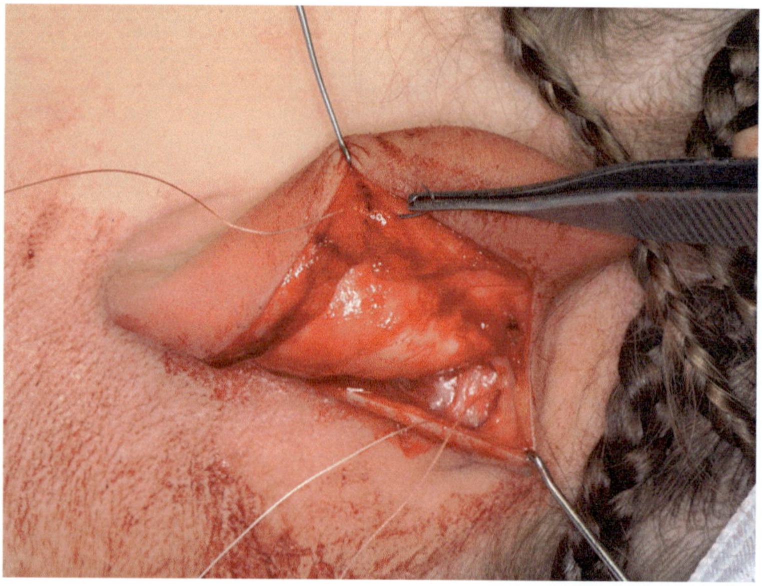

Fig. 35.14 Take a bite of the fascia in the appropriate location as a "test"

always be tied, inferior suture first and superior suture last. This is so that the critical superior suture is tied with the greatest degree of accuracy leaving the superior pole at exactly the correct distance from the head and avoiding angularity. Once the Mustardé sutures are tied, the mastoid-fascia suture is finally tied over the top as judged in the initial "trial and error" (Figs. 35.15, 35.16, and 35.17). This results in the following advantages:

1. The tension on the mastoid sutures is completely released, reducing the likelihood of knots slipping, tearing out, and recurrence.
2. The sutures and knots are covered with vascular tissue, reducing the possibility of suture extrusion.

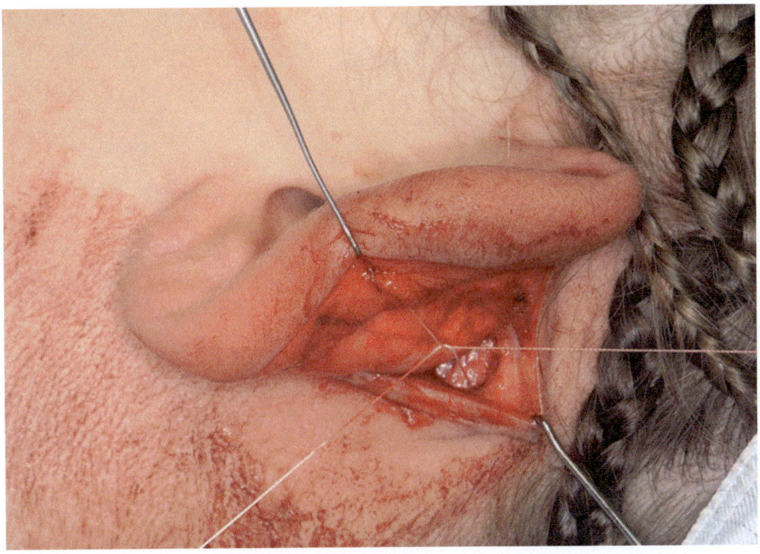

Fig. 35.15 Tie the test suture with only one non-locking throw on the suture, for easy release

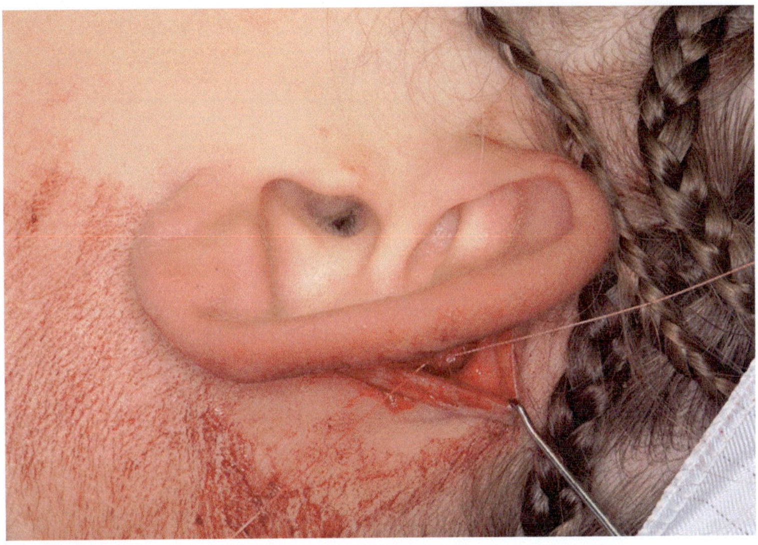

Fig. 35.16 The ear begins to correct

3. An "internal corset" for support of the ear is created which reduces the need for head bandages.
4. A fine-tuning and "naturalization" of the contour of the ear is created.
5. A rotational effect is created, similar to a conchamastoid suture (Furnas suture [6]).

If the lower pole of the ear, or the earlobe itself, requires a greater degree of correction, a second suture can be sited. The fascia can also be partially divided centrally to create separate superior and inferior fascial flaps, with different vectors acting upon them dependent upon suture positioning. Learning this technique is simple as the surgeon does not have to commit to using the fascial suture after raising the fascia unless, and until such time as, he or she is convinced that it will provide a suitable result. The procedure can continue as a simple suture-based technique once the fascial flap has been raised, with the fascia simply taking on the role as a cover and reinforcement for the sutures once they have been placed.

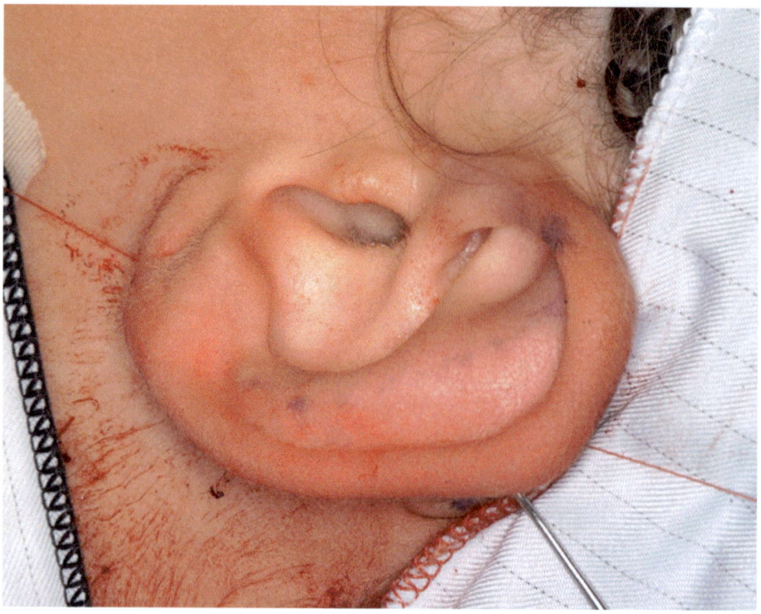

Fig. 35.17 The prominence of the ear is corrected, and a natural antihelix is formed

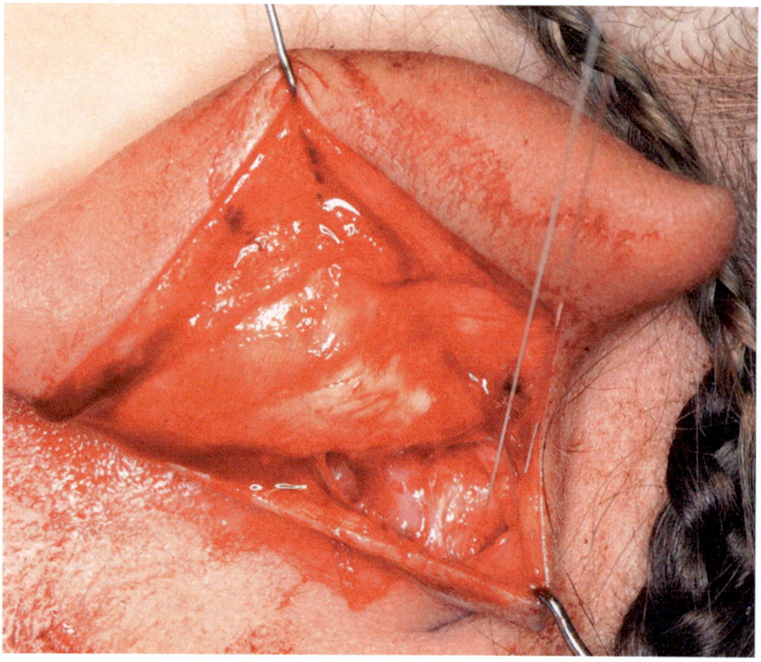

Fig. 35.18 Loosen the suture and remove the bite from the fascia, keeping the deep mastoid suture in place. Place a clip on this suture so it can be tied towards the end of the procedure

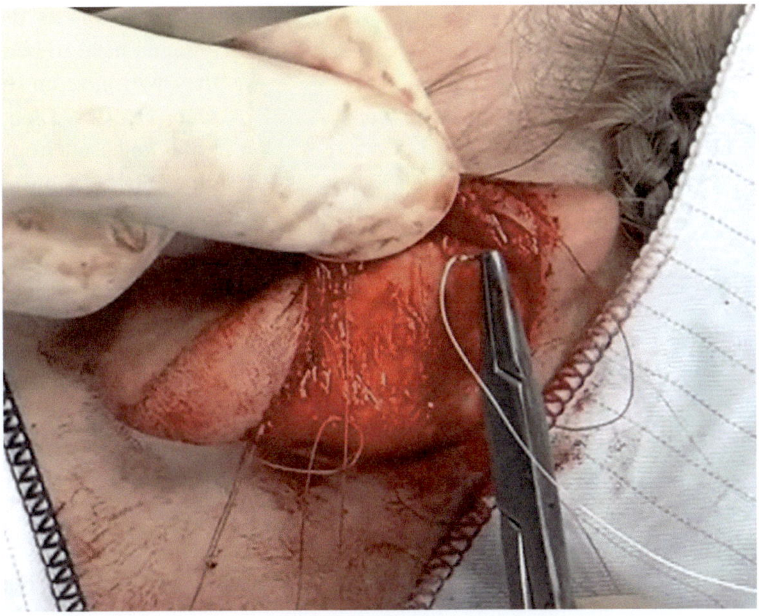

Fig. 35.19 Place Mustardé sutures between the scapha and the concha

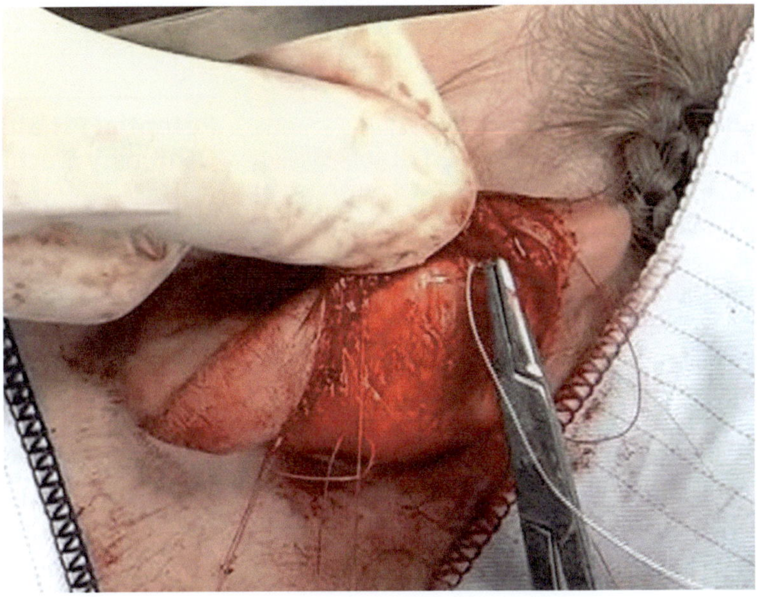

Fig. 35.20 Use three Mustardé sutures and tie them in the order inferior to superior

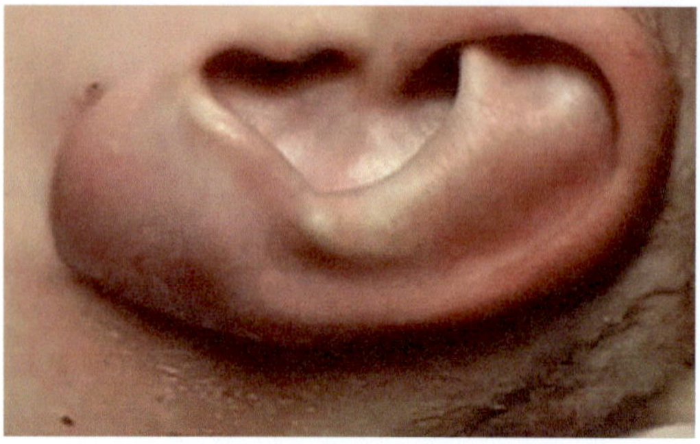

Fig. 35.21 Close the skin, glue the suture line, and glue the ear to the side of the head for splintage

Completing the Surgery and Avoiding Head Bandages

To complete the procedure, the skin is closed with 4/0 Vicryl or Monocryl as per surgeon preference. The wound is sealed with skin glue, and finally the ear is glued to the side of the head with more skin glue (Fig. 35.21). This was first described by Shokrollahi et al. in the context of the fascial flap otoplasty technique in 2008 [5] and by Shokrollahi and Tanner [7] as a separate short paper in the same year and subsequently recommended by other authors in 2010 [8, 9]. These and other papers regarding the role of glue in otoplasty were reviewed by Patel and Price in 2011 [10]. The fascial flap is already supporting the ear internally, reducing the requirement for external support. Skin glue, depending on brand, will last for up to 2 weeks, but averages about a week. Those with long hair will therefore exhibit no stigmata of surgery, and all patients can shower the next day (Fig. 35.22). One less appointment is needed in clinic for removal of head bandages and dressings as there are no dressings at all. Patients need to be informed preoperatively that they will have an overcorrected look due to the glue (Fig. 35.23) and that often one ear is sometimes released from the adhesive effects of the glue earlier than the other. Some brands of glue create more crusting than others, and patients should be reassured regarding the robustness of their ear correction such that they feel comfortable washing gently in the shower to clean the ears and residual glue if necessary. All patients should be photographed preoperatively and postoperatively. Patients should be given access to a dressing clinic appointment in case of any problems but not as routine, and a routine appointment in outpatients at 6–10 weeks is appropriate. Postoperative results of patients who have had fascial flap combined with Mustardé sutures show good symmetry with very natural shape to the ears without an "operated" look (Figs. 35.24, 35.25, 35.26, and 35.27).

Potential Pitfalls of the Fascial Flap Otoplasty Technique

The first few attempts at raising the flap may result in the surgeon believing that the fascia is not strong or robust enough to undertake the procedure. It is essential to ensure that the skin excision is extremely thin and relatively wide, in order to preserve as much of the fascia as possible. Perseverance will lead to the raising of a substantial flap on a consistent basis. It is not uncommon at first to raise flaps with holes in, especially on the inferior aspect. This rarely has

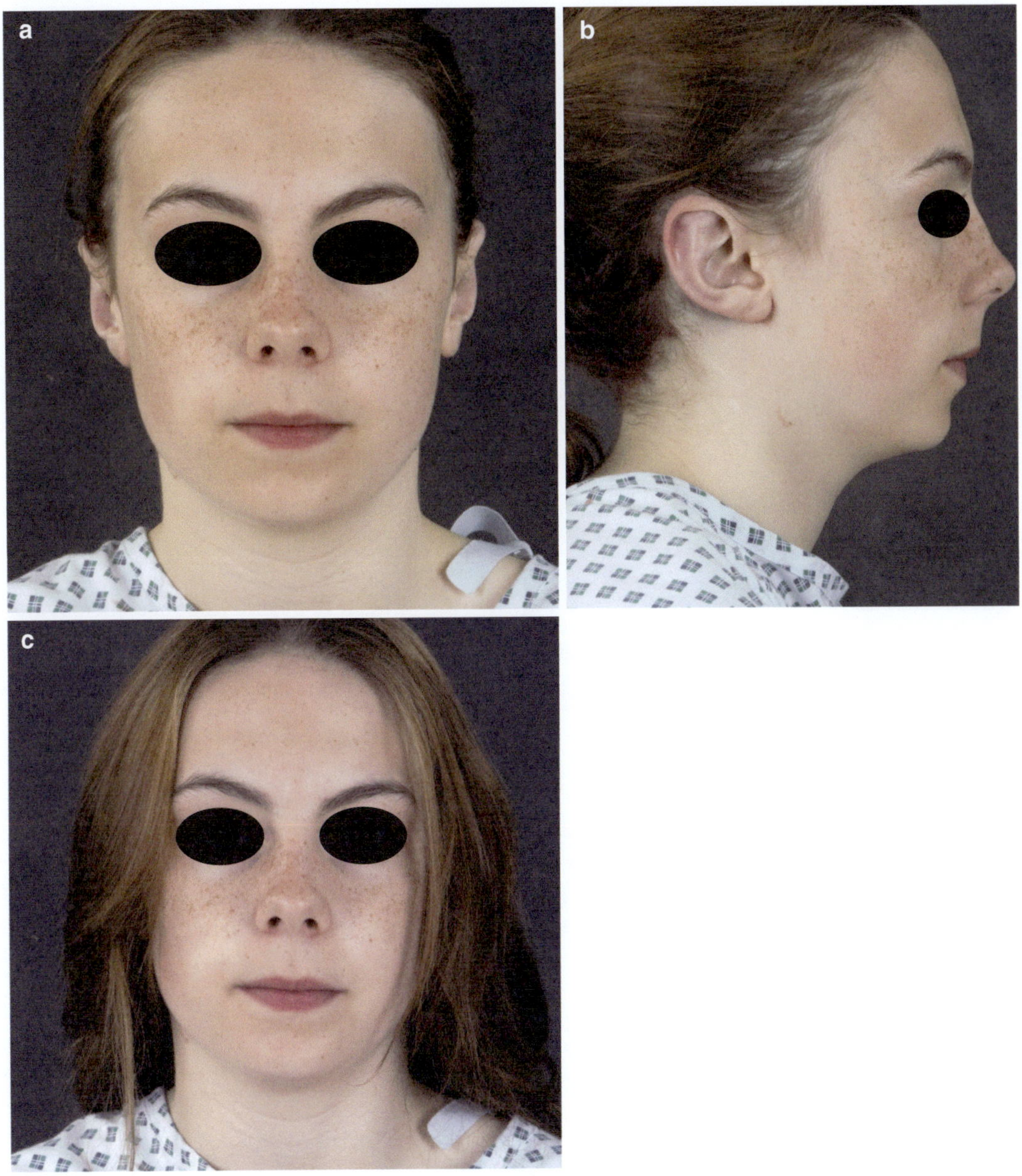

Fig. 35.22 (**a–c**) Two hours postoperative with glue as splint. No stigmata of surgery and she is able to hear without difficulty. Furthermore, she will have a shower tomorrow the following day

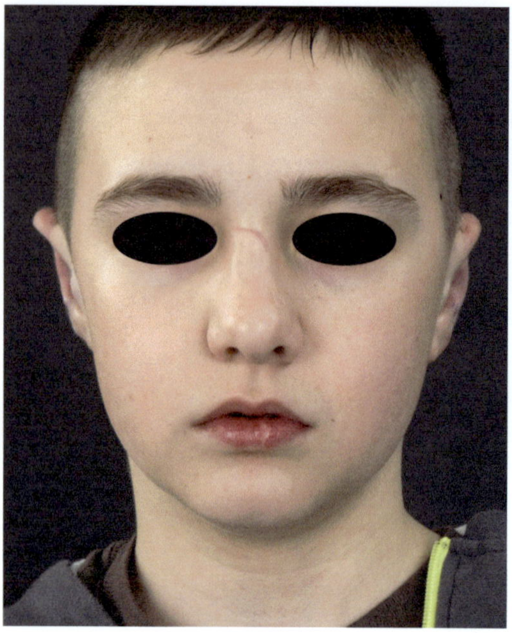

Fig. 35.23 Two hours postoperative with glue as splint. Those with short hair must be warned about the overcorrected look for some days after surgery. Nursing staff and other staff need to be educated about the technique which they may not have encountered before

any significant effect on its suitability for use or on the force of the correction vectors, and the issue will be eliminated with practice. It is also important to ensure the lower pole of the ear is assessed accurately to determine if a second suture may be necessary. It is worth realizing that historically when skin was excised, both the fascia and skin were often excised and discarded.

Postoperative Results

In the first series of otoplasties utilizing the fascial flap adjunctively, performed on 15 patients (age range 8–16 years) by a single surgeon (KS), there were no significant complications over an 11-month period [5]. To date, over 40 such surgeries have been performed without significant complications with reliable results and symmetry. "Soft" outcome measures such as patient comfort, ability to shower, and others are difficult to quantify but become obvious after a few surgeries.

Conclusions

The raising of a distally based fascial flap can act as an adjunct to suture-based otoplasty techniques and offers numerous advantages for both patients and surgeons aiming for the ultimate goals in otoplasty: satisfied patients and simple and stress-free surgery with consistent results.

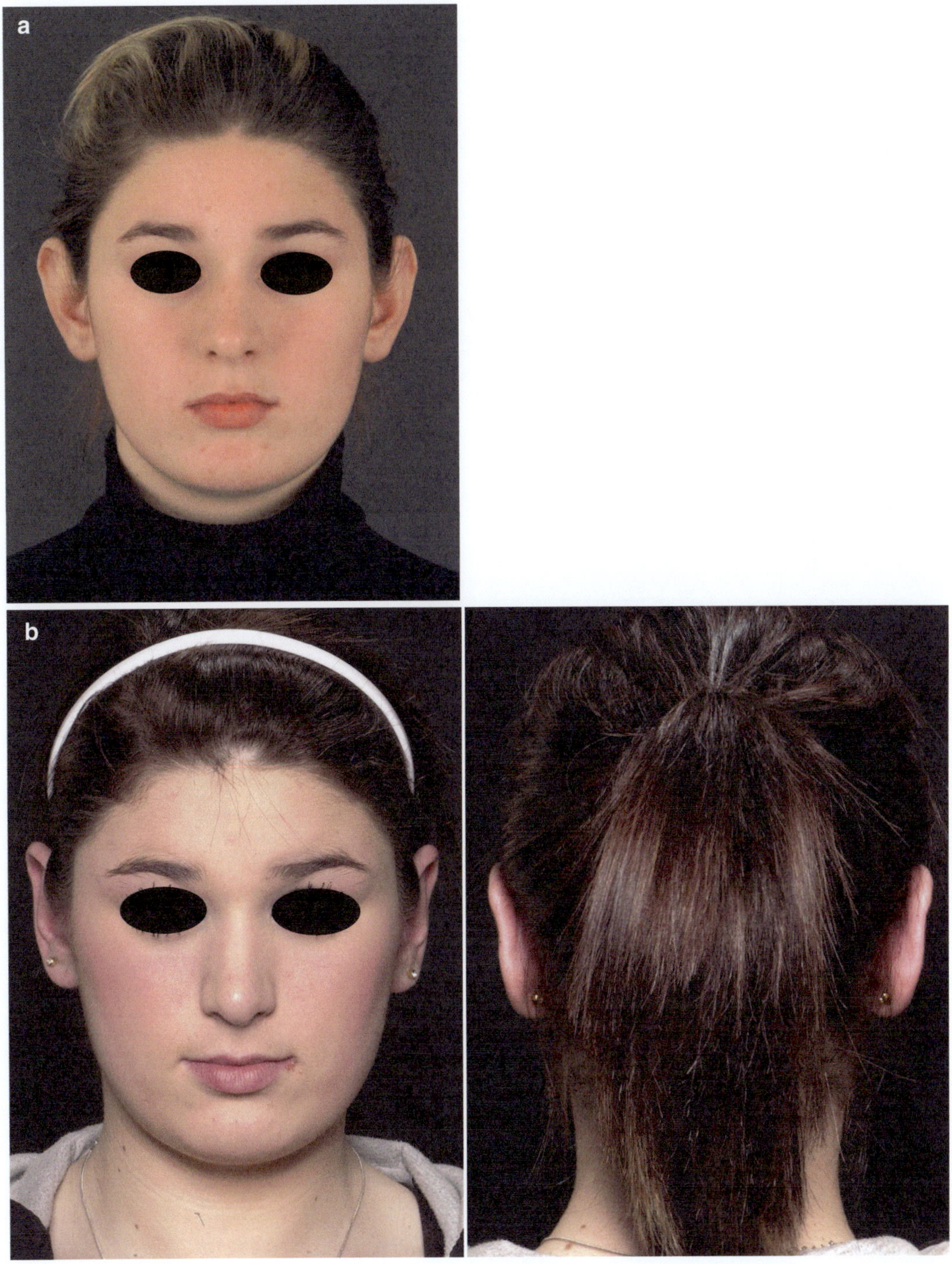

Fig. 35.24 (**a**) Preoperative teenage female. (**b**) Postoperative with a natural “unoperated” and symmetrical look without overcorrection. Well-hidden scar

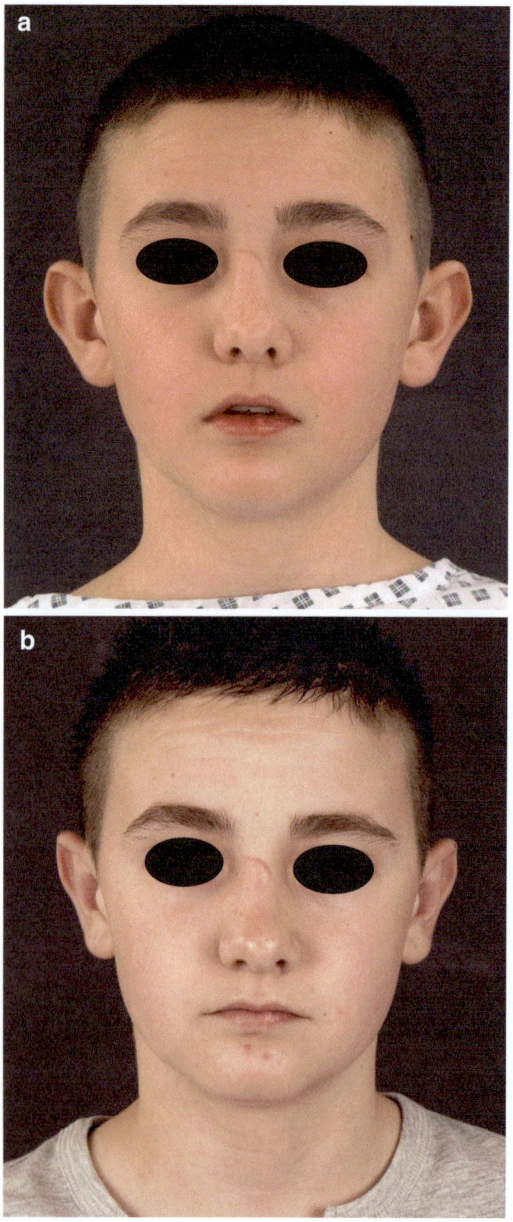

Fig. 35.25 (**a**) Preoperative teenage male. (**b**) Four-month postoperative with a natural "unoperated" and symmetrical appearance without overcorrection

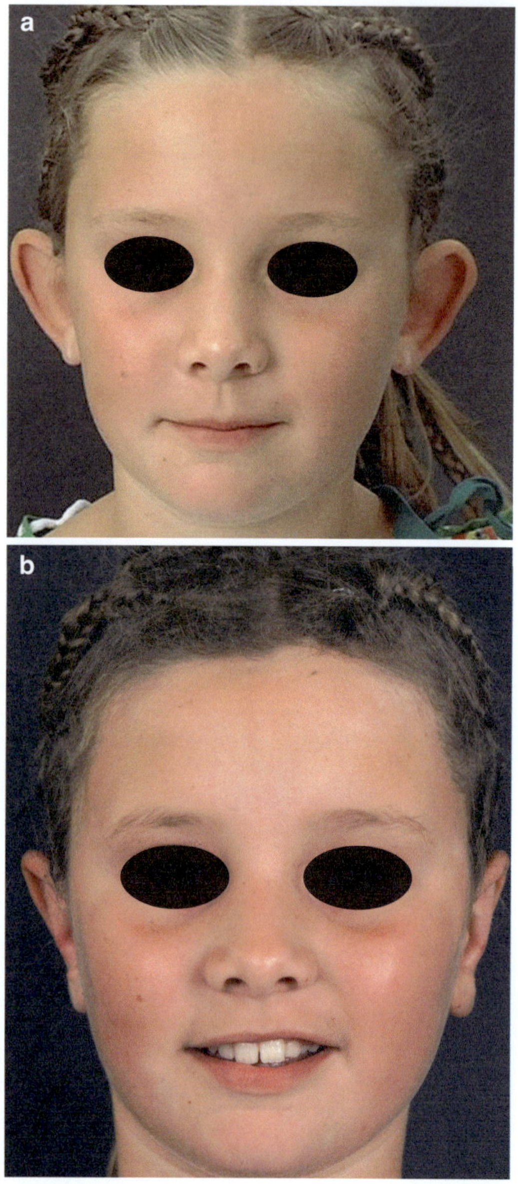

Fig. 35.26 (**a**) Preoperative young female (the first patient to have had this procedure). (**b**) Postoperative with some mild asymmetry but a good result in light of the severity of presenting deformity. Demonstrates the natural shape of the antihelical fold

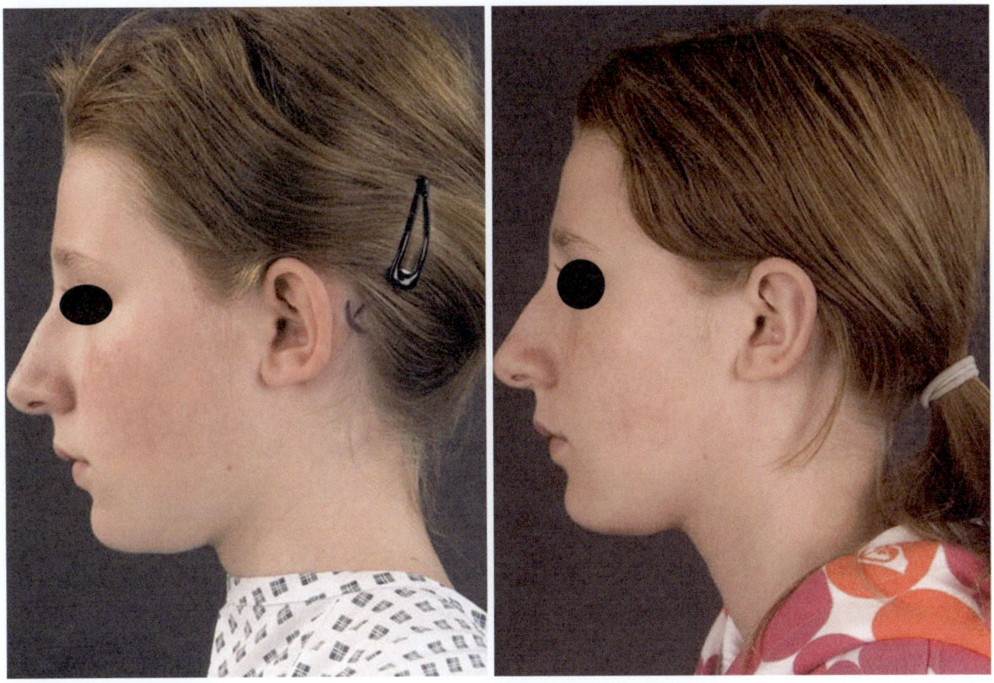

Fig. 35.27 (*Left*) preoperative young girl. (*Right*) postoperative

References

1. Chongchet V. A method of antihelix reconstruction. Br J Plast Surg. 1963;16:268–72.
2. Thomas SS, Fatah F. Closed anterior scoring for prominent-ear correction revisited. Br J Plast Surg. 2001;54:581–7.
3. Mustardé JC. The correction of prominent ears using simple mattress sutures. Br J Plast Surg. 1963;16:170–8.
4. Horlock N, Misra A, Gault DT. The postauricular fascial flap as an adjunct to Mustardé and Furnas type otoplasty. Plast Reconstr Surg. 2001;108:1487–90.
5. Shokrollahi K, Cooper MA, Hiew LY. A new strategy for otoplasty. J Plast Reconstr Aesthet Surg. 2009;62(6):774–81.
6. Furnas DW. Correction of prominent ears by conchamastoid sutures. Plast Reconstr Surg. 1968;42:189–93.
7. Shokrollahi K, Tanner B. "Glue Ear": beginning of the end for head bandages after prominent ear correction? J Plast Reconstr Aesthet Surg. 2008;61:1077.
8. Vetter M, Foehn M, Wedler V. A new postoperative otoplasty dressing technique using cyanoacrylate tissue adhesives. Aesthetic Plast Surg. 2010;34(2):212–3.
9. Bovill ES, Boulton R, Wharton S. Use of dermabond as a dressing for prominent ear correction: a sound alternative to head dressings. J Plast Reconstr Aesthet Surg. 2010;63(6):1065–6.
10. Patel AJ, Price RD. The use of tissue glue in prominent ear correction surgery. Aesthetic Plast Surg. 2011;35(2):245–7.

Posterior Auricular Muscle Flap with Otoplasty

36

Ilker Yazici

Introduction

Commonly accepted anatomical components of prominent ear deformity are (1) antihelical fold deficit or poor definition, (2) conchal hypertrophy, (3) a "wider-than-normal" angle between helical root and scalp, and (4) prominent lobule [1]. These deformities may have variable expression or combinations among patients. Although less stressed and mentioned in the definition of prominent ear deformity, some other concerns shall also be taken care of during surgical correction such as (1) the nature (stiffness-elasticity) of the ear cartilage, (2) patient cooperation and expectation, and (3) combination of variable deformities with variable phenotypic expression such as macrotia, cup ear, constricted ear, and Stahl's ear. These combinations make prominent ear surgery demanding and comprehensive. Underestimation of these components may lead to failure.

Although components of prominent ear deformities were defined clearly in many textbooks, prominent ear correction techniques reveal a heterogeneous strategical spectrum. Precise choice of surgical technique, when combined with comprehensive clinical experience, reveals the fact that each prominent ear patient needs serious preoperative evaluation prior to tailoring of individualized surgical procedure combinations. In other words, "one-size-fits-all" approach commonly leads to disappointment.

In order to define a position for posterior auricular muscle flap otoplasty techniques, there is a necessity to classify surgical techniques of prominent ear correction. A systematic classification for this purpose can be found in Table 36.1 including: (1) excisional techniques, (2) suture techniques with or without cartilage scoring, (3) using anatomical structures in order to obtain anatomical correction, and (4) molding techniques.

Posterior Auricular Muscle

From everyday perspective, we see domestic dogs retract their ears as a gesture of gratitude and joy. An entertaining artifact from evolution, some people can also selectively move their ears posteriorly. The muscle which its function is mentioned above (pulling ear posteriorly) is known as "posterior auricular muscle," a member of extrinsic auricular muscles. Extrinsic ear muscles consist of superior auricular, anterior auricular, and posterior auricular muscles (Fig. 36.1). Most functional of all, posterior auricular muscle origins from mastoid process and inserts to ponticulus innervated by facial nerve and receiving perfusion from posterior auricular artery. Because of its more superior insertion and position, the amount of posterior excursion during ear retraction is more on upper pole than lower parts of the ear (Fig. 36.2).

I. Yazici, M.D.
Department of Plastic Reconstructive and Aesthetic Surgery, Kirikkale University Medical Faculty, Sağlık Sok. Fabrikalar Mah, Kirikkale 71100, Turkey
e-mail: ilkeryazici@gmail.com

M.A. Shiffman (ed.), *Advanced Cosmetic Otoplasty*,
DOI 10.1007/978-3-642-35431-1_36, © Springer-Verlag Berlin Heidelberg 2013

Table 36.1 Classification of otoplasty techniques including some instances and the qualitative position of posterior auricular muscle flap techniques among them

Target tissue	Excisional techniques	Suture techniques with or without cartilage scoring	Using anatomical structures in order to obtain correction	Molding techniques
Cartilage – antihelix	Luckett Converse Pitanguy	Mustarde Stenström Fritsch (minimal invasive)	Karacaoglan et al. Scuderi et al.	Matsuo et al. Lindford et al.
Cartilage – concha	Conchal excision	Furnas (concha-mastoid suture)	Karacaoglan et al. Scuderi et al.	Matsuo et al. Lindford et al.
Posterior auricular muscle and/or fascia	Elliot	Furnas (concha-mastoid suture) Posterior auricular muscle flaps Horlock et al. (fascial flap)	Posterior auricular muscle flaps Horlock et al. (fascial flap)	NA

Note that some instances may not be included. Majority of these techniques were referenced by Patterson and Friedman [2]

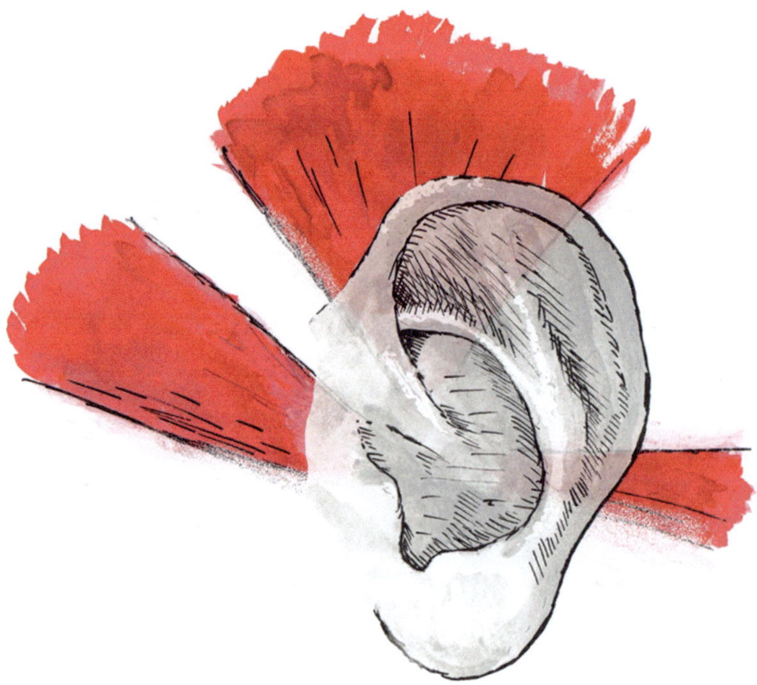

Fig. 36.1 Anatomy of the extrinsic ear muscles which are temporal area extensions of galea aponeurosis, resembling frontalis and occipitalis muscles anatomically, sharing the same anatomical plane

The posterior auricular muscle plays an important role on prominency of the ear and prominent ear deformity pathogenesis. Smith and Takashima [3] worked on the ears of anencephalic births and found that absence or hypoplasia of this muscle is associated with prominency of the ear. They also present ear prominency as a neuromuscular sign. As a part of facial nerve innervated mimic muscles inserting on ear cartilage, dysfunction or hypoplasia of posterior auricular muscle eventually leads to ear prominency. Another study regarding the role of posterior auricular muscle on prominent ear pathogenesis was performed by Guyuron and DeLuca [4] in 1997. They observed a linear relationship between posterior auricular muscle insertion site and projection of ear, based on their measurements during surgeries of 30 prominent ear cases. They also worked on the usage of this muscle for correction of prominent ear deformity. It is obvious that there is a rising attention

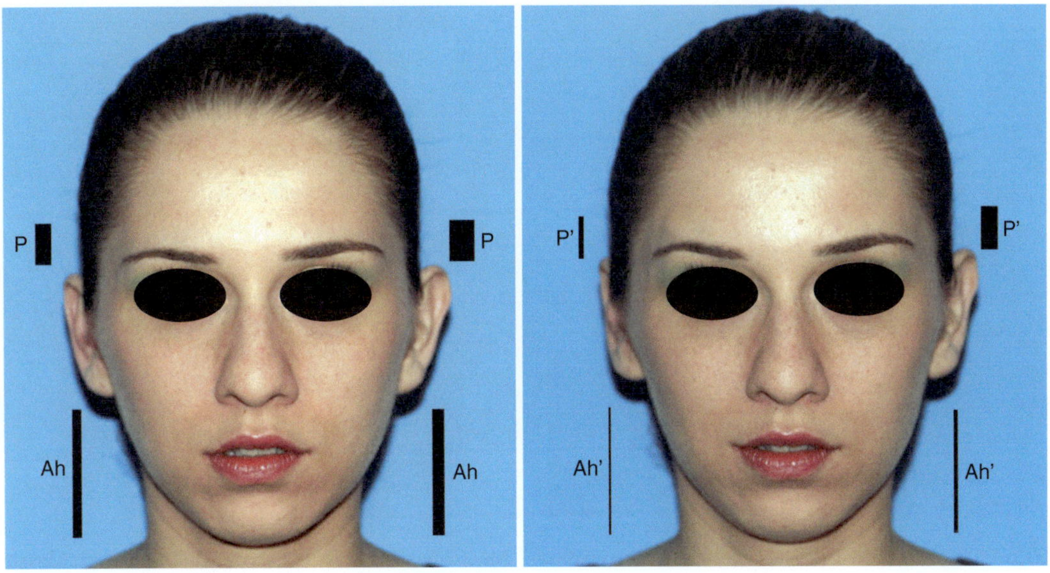

Fig. 36.2 The function of the posterior auricular muscle on human. The *bars* adjacent to the ears show the projection of upper pole (*P*) and antihelix to helical border distance (*Ah*). Please note the excursion amounts before P,Ah and after P′,Ah′ posterior auricular muscle contraction. The upper pole excursion is more than antihelix to helix distance as well as lobule. (*Left*) before contraction. (*Right*) after contraction

to prominent ear deformity pathogenesis and the role of posterior auricular muscle [3, 4]. The primary effect of posterior auricular muscle anatomical variation or failure is the valgus deformity of the ear. Cranio-auricular angles of 25 for men and 21 for women are regarded normal [5]. Generally, valgus deformity denotes the increased angle between helix and scalp. Cranio-auricular angle greater than 40° is named as auricular valgus deformity [4, 5]. Although this deformity may be originated from conchal hypertrophy, conchal anterior displacement, and less defined antihelical fold; the principle deformity dedicated to the failure of the posterior auricular muscle is the abductory slide of the ear.

Posterior Auricular Muscle Flap Utilized in Otoplasty

Nicoletis and Guerin-Surville [6] published the first report on the utilization of posterior auricular muscle for otoplasty in 1978. They transposed the posterior auricular muscle to scapha combined with cartilage incision. They have obtained correction of valgus deformity and enhancement of antihelical fold with no recurrence. In contrast to Mustarde sutures and Stenstrom technique, in which the primary target is to create an antihelical fold transferring the tension of cartilage fold on the cartilage and sutures, using posterior auricular muscle enables a well-vascularized and a more durable repair in order to fold the cartilage. Additionally enabling posterior relocation of the whole ear, addressing valgus deformity. Although perichondrioplasty (perichondrial flap tacked posteriorly which has the effect of creating antihelical fold and posterior setback) procedure can also provide these, muscular repair seems to be more durable and relapse-free. Azad et al. [7] have also transferred posterior auricular muscle to scapha in 2003. Scuderi et al. [8] published the largest series consisting of 103 patients. They have refined the technique and transferred the muscle flap to scapha by including conchal cartilage insertion on the tip of the flap. This approach addresses conchal hypertrophy and antihelix by including a reliable muscle flap. Additionally repair site was reinforced by the cartilage graft/flap. Patients with stiff auricular

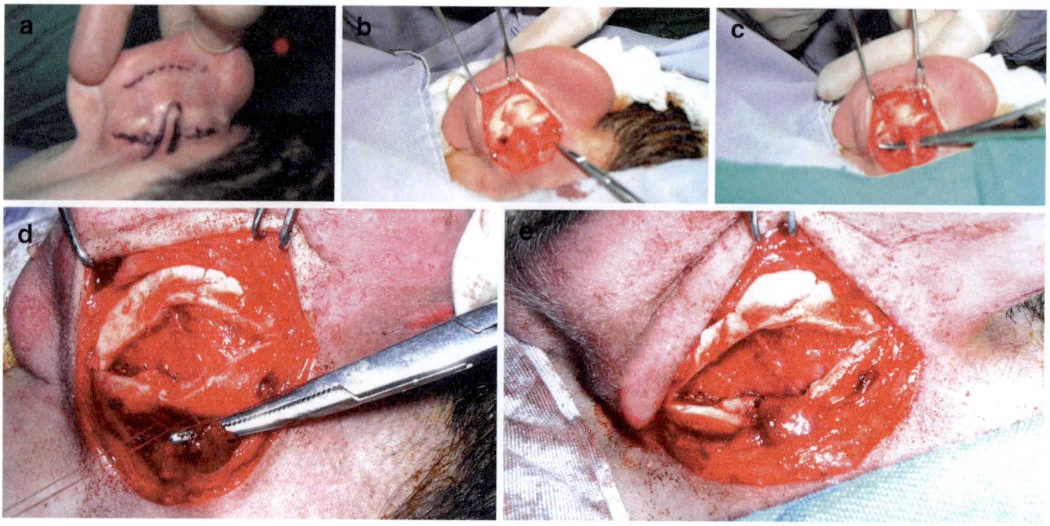

Fig. 36.3 (**a**) Posterior auricular muscle outlined before surgery using a simple manipulation, anterior traction of ear. It is easy to see the size of the muscle after traction. (**b**) Posterior auricular muscle inserted to ponticulus. (**c**) Muscle flap is dissected and ready to transfer. (**d**) Muscle flap is detached from ponticulus and conchal excision performed. (**e**) Transfer of the muscle flap to conchal base as published by Yazici et al. [13]

cartilage and excessive valgus deformity may benefit from this technique provided to the armamentarium of prominent ear surgery.

Conchal reduction surgery is another field for the usage of posterior auricular muscle. Bauer et al. [9] stress the importance of conchal hypertrophy in prominent ear deformity. Blindly focusing to correct scapha-conchal angle "antihelix" is a common mistake. Well-established cornerstone procedures for conchal correction were presented and appreciated as follows: Concha-mastoid suture, described by Furnas [10], and excision of conchal cartilage are among the mostly performed ones. As routinely performed by Elliot [11], excision of postauricular muscle and posterior fibrofatty tissue is another adjunctive method for correction of valgus deformity. Deep concha (>2.5 cm) combined with stiff auricular cartilage grants conchal reduction. Concha-mastoid sutures and conchal excision are respectively prone to recurrence and meatal narrowing. Spira's posterior conchal flap was designed to decrease meatal complications of conchal reduction. Redundant anterior skin after conchal reduction is another complication to prevent. Anterior approach for conchal reduction may be used, a gamble for the price of keloid formation. Conchal angulation and irregularities may also be a problem to be encountered associated to conchal excision. In order to accomplish a smooth conchal curve during conchal reduction, Karacaoglan and Ciloglu [12] have used excised conchal cartilage as an onlay graft.

In order to overcome some of the drawbacks of conchal reduction and to present another reliable prominent ear correction technique, Yazici et al. [13] have used posterior auricular muscle as a flap. The purpose was to overcome the risks of conchal reduction surgery by using posterior auricular muscle flap combined with perichondrioplasty (perichondrial flap tacked posteriorly) for better results with repositioning (Figs. 36.3 and 36.4). This approach enables (1) better posterior replacement by positioning conchal floor posteriorly by the help of muscle tonus and placing helical rim posteriorly by the virtue of additional perichondrioplasty (this maneuver also increases antihelix definition) (Fig. 36.5), (2) to hide knots and provide a better healing environment, and (3) creating a softer conchal bowl, preventing anterior skin redundancy (Fig. 36.6). This approach can relieve the necessity of anterior approach for conchal excision and utilizes posterior auricular muscle rather than excising, enabling two lines of repair site serving to correct valgus deformity.

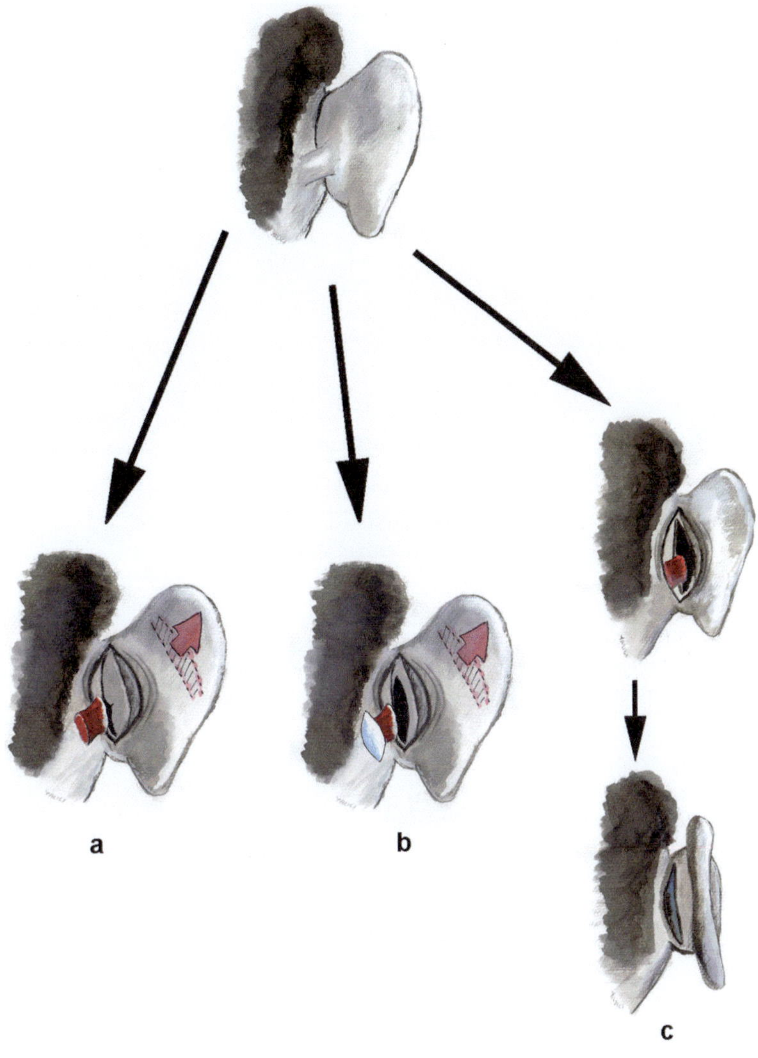

Fig. 36.4 Different surgical procedures utilizing posterior auricular muscle flap used up to date. (**a**) Transposition of the flap to scapha as first performed by Nicoletis and Guerin-Surville [6]. *Dotted area* represents antihelical fold area. (**b**) Conchal cartilage on the tip of the graft prior to transposition to scapha as performed by Scuderi et al. [8]. (**c**) Posterior auricular muscle flap transfer to conchal base with conchal excision and perichondrioplasty as published by Yazici et al. [13]

All surgical procedures which use posterior auricular muscle flap transposition for the service of prominent ear correction share the same technical point: "the preparation of posterior auricular muscle flap." In order to prepare the flap, sequential to postauricular incision, 1–2 cm of posterior undermining is enough after visualizing ponticulus and the base of concha (Fig. 36.3). Blunt dissection is enough to dissect the muscle. Next the surgeon can detach the muscle from ear cartilage or can include the conchal resection portion cartilage on the flap. After dissection of the flap, it is possible to use it for prominent ear correction as stated above with combination of conventional techniques (Fig. 36.4). Regarding the existence and size of the muscle, variations may exist. Posterior auricular muscle may be too weak for use in some cases, and this risk should be kept in mind while planning the procedure. Preoperative examination of the ear by anterior traction can be helpful to check the muscle "whether usable or not." The author has encountered only two cases of very thin and unusable posterior auricular muscles in around 50 otoplasty cases (sequential cases having prominent ear in which mustarde, perichondrioplasty and posterior auricular muscle flap techniques were used for correction). These techniques using posterior auricular muscle are needed to be evalu-

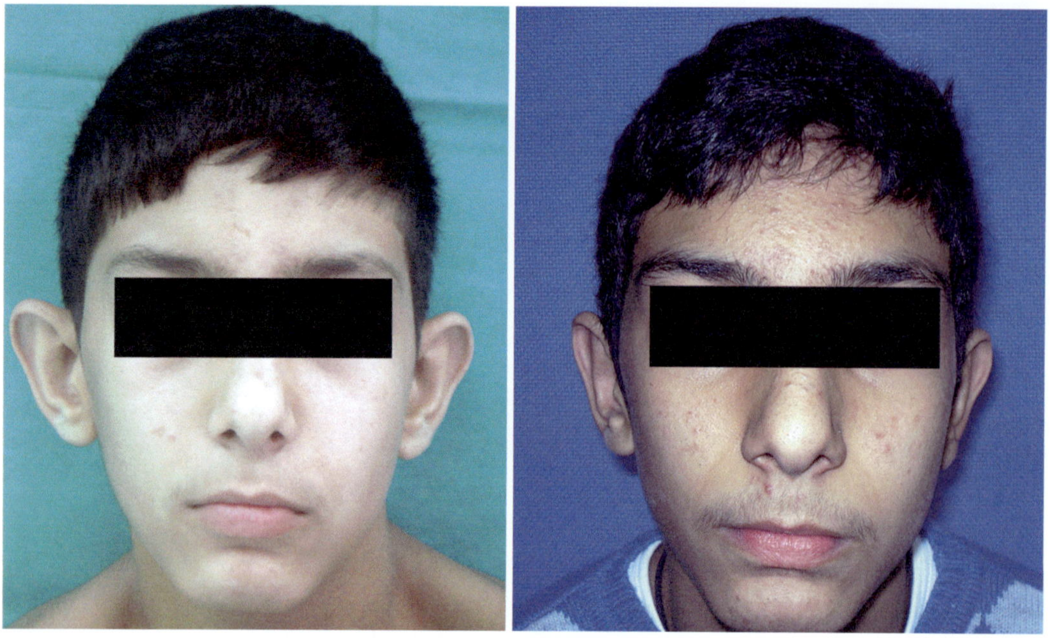

Fig. 36.5 (*Left*) Preoperative. (*Right*) Postoperative patient after conchal reduction and perichondrioplasty combined with postauricular muscle flap as published by Yazici et al. [13]

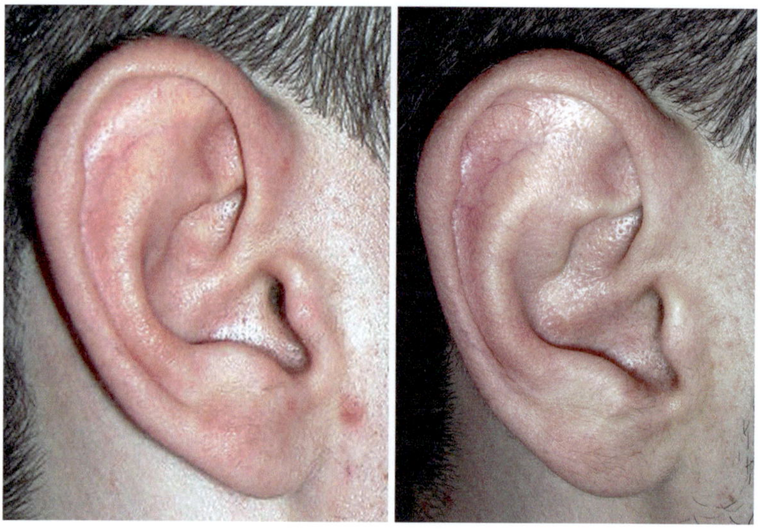

Fig. 36.6 (*Left*) Preoperative. (*Right*) Note the natural conchal bowl contour 6 months postoperatively after transfer of posterior auricular muscle flap combined with conchal excision

ated with further clinical studies, involving a much bigger patient population.

Posterior auricular muscle is a good adjunct in antihelix creation, conchal hypertrophy, and associated valgus deformity correction. The author has not used this flap for isolated antihelix creation. According to our experience, posterior auricular muscle flap-indicated cases were approximately 15 % of all prominent ear cases.

According to reports of techniques and our experience, utilization of posterior auricular muscle in conchal reduction and auricular valgus deformity enables good results. Using posterior auricular muscle as mentioned above or any other way will provide at least a vascular healing environment and eventually increase the durability of the correction. Alternative transposition procedures of this muscle may also be possible in the future. Using anatomical structures rather than excising is an important reconstructive virtue. Posterior auricular muscle is a good instance for this.

References

1. Spira M. Otoplasty: what do I do now- a 30-year perspective. Plast Reconstr Surg. 1999;104(3):834–40.
2. Petersson RS, Friedman O. Current trends in otoplasty. Curr Opin Otolaryngol Head Neck Surg. 2008; 16(4):352–8.
3. Smith DW, Takashima H. Ear muscles and ear form. Birth Defects Orig Artic Ser. 1980;16(4):299–302.
4. Guyuron B, DeLuca L. Ear projection and posterior auricular muscle insertion. Plast Reconstr Surg. 1997;100(2):457–60.
5. Kelley P, Hollier L, Stal S. Otoplasty: evaluation, technique, and review. J Craniofac Surg. 2003;14(5): 643–53.
6. Nicoletis C, Guerin-Surville H. Prominent ears. Transposition of the posterior auricular muscle on the scapha: a new technique. Aesthetic Plast Surg. 1978;2:295.
7. Azad S, Edwin A, Kumar PV. Posterior auricular muscle – a useful adjunct in otoplasty. Br J Plast Surg. 2003;56(7):722–3.
8. Scuderi N, Tenna S, Bitonti A, Vonella M. Repositioning of posterior auricular muscle combined with conventional otoplasty: a personal technique. J Plast Reconstr Aesthet Surg. 2007;60(2):201–4.
9. Bauer BS, Song DS, Aitken ME. Combined otoplasty technique: condrocutaneous conchal resection as the cornerstone to correction of the prominent ear. Plast Reconstr Surg. 2002;110(4):1033–41.
10. Furnas DW. Correction of prominent ears by conchamastoid sutures. Plast Reconstr Surg. 1968;42(3): 189–93.
11. Elliot Jr RA. Complications in the treatment of prominent ears. Clin Plast Surg. 1978;5(3):479–90.
12. Karacaoglan N, Ciloglu SN. Conchal setback without resection in prominent ear deformity. Otolaryngol Head Neck Surg. 2011;145(6):930–1.
13. Yazici I, Findikçioğlu F, Ozmen S, Noyan N, Yavuzer R. Posterior auricular muscle flap as an adjunct to otoplasty. Aesthetic Plast Surg. 2009;33(4):527–32.

Various Applications of Retroauricular Advancement Skin Flap to Treat the Surgical Defect of the Ear

37

Peter Kim

Introduction

Surgical defect of the ear, whether due to removal of a skin cancer or due to other trauma, is relatively common, and it is frequently managed in the office-based setting [1]. Limited availability of skin is one of the main challenges in the cosmetically satisfying reconstruction of the anterior surface and helix of the ear following a skin cancer excision. Various surgical options are available to repair the surgical defects of the ear [2]: wedge excision, local flap surgery (using skin from same anatomical unit), and skin grafting. They do produce a successful outcome, but they invariably cause ears that are smaller postoperatively (Fig. 37.1). In majority of cases, the size discrepancy between the two ears is well accepted, but the avoidance of this complication is cosmetically desirable especially if a procedure is not associated with a significant morbidity. Distant flap, by filling the surgical defect using the soft tissue outside the ear (e.g., retroauricular area [3–5]), does provide a solution to this postsurgical miniaturization of the ears.

This chapter presents various applications of retroauricular cutaneous advancement flap, a versatile flap, to successfully repair the surgical defects of the ear in its different locations, following a skin cancer excision.

P. Kim, M.D., MBBS, FACCS, FIBCS
Simply Beautiful Cosmetic Surgery
& Laser Clinic, 4 Farnell Street, West Ryde,
Sidney, NSW 2114, Australia
e-mail: drpeterkim@yahoo.com,
dr.peterkim@yahoo.com.au

Technique

Advancement flap is a well recognized and a popular skin flap technique in skin cancer surgery. It is a sliding type of flap where the surgical defect is filled by the flap of skin that is slid/advanced towards it (Fig. 37.2). In retroauricular area, a flap of retroauricular soft tissue can be advanced towards and fill the surgical defects of the anterior surface and the helical rim of the ear. This flap can be placed over the helical rim, through the cartilage to fill the defect of the deeper anterior conchal surface, or be rolled up to recreate the helical rim defect (Fig. 37.3). Although the mechanism of this flap is that of advancement, as the flap is skipping over a bridge of normal skin to fill the surgical defect of the ear, it is by definition termed interpolation flap. This flap needs to be divided at a later date to free the ear from the retroauricular area, hence making this a two-staged procedure.

Design and Creating the Flap (Fig. 37.4)

Markings

Basal cell carcinoma (BCC) and its appropriate margins are preoperatively marked (Fig. 37.4a). Tunnel through which the flap will be pulled through (from posterior auricular surface anteriorly)

M.A. Shiffman (ed.), *Advanced Cosmetic Otoplasty*,
DOI 10.1007/978-3-642-35431-1_37, © Springer-Verlag Berlin Heidelberg 2013

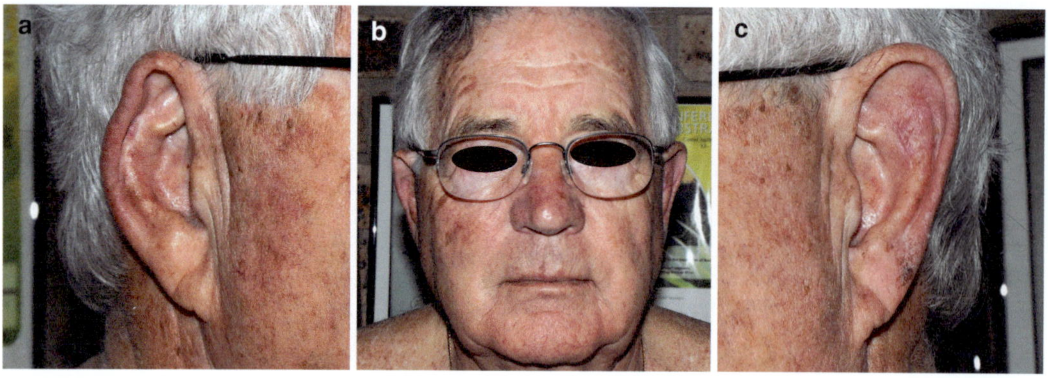

Fig. 37.1 Ears from the same patient. (**a**) Right ear following skin cancer excision using local flap surgery, (**b**) anterior view, (**c**) left ear following skin cancer excision using distant flap. The right ear is noticeably smaller and distorted compared to the left ear

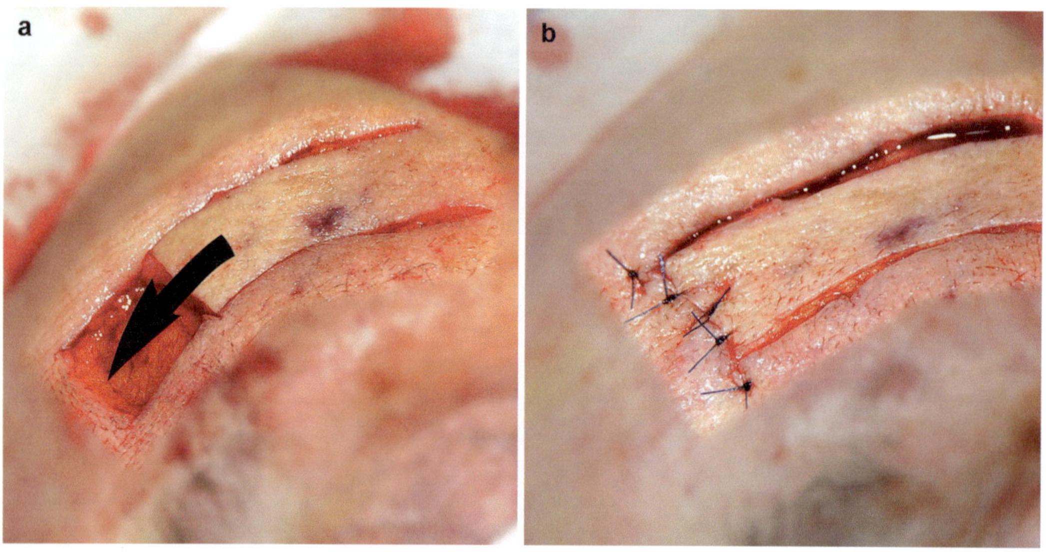

Fig. 37.2 (**a**) Advancement skin flap with *arrow* showing the direction of advancement. (**b**) Flap advanced to fill the surgical defect

is marked (corresponding to the posterior border of the surgical margin) and the length of the retroauricular skin flap marked (Fig. 37.4). Retroauricular skin is marked posterior to the retroauricular skin crease and a few mm longer than the length of the surgical defect. Ensure that the flap length is not more than 1:2.5 ratio to maximize the flap survival.

Procedure

The skin cancer is excised (Fig. 37.4c primary defect). Cartilage slit is made to allow the skin flap to be pulled through on the anterior auricular surface (Fig. 37.4d). Retroauricular skin flap is incised (Fig. 37.4e), and it is then undermined to its base (Fig. 37.4f, secondary defect). Undermine to enhance the flap mobility but only as required to minimize the damage to the flap vascularity. Elevated skin flap is then grasped (Fig 37.4g) and pulled through the cartilage tunnel and placed on the anterior surface of the ear (Fig. 37.4h). At this point, the flap should be comfortably filling the surgical defect and under minimal tension. Base of the flap is sutured to the postauricular sulcus

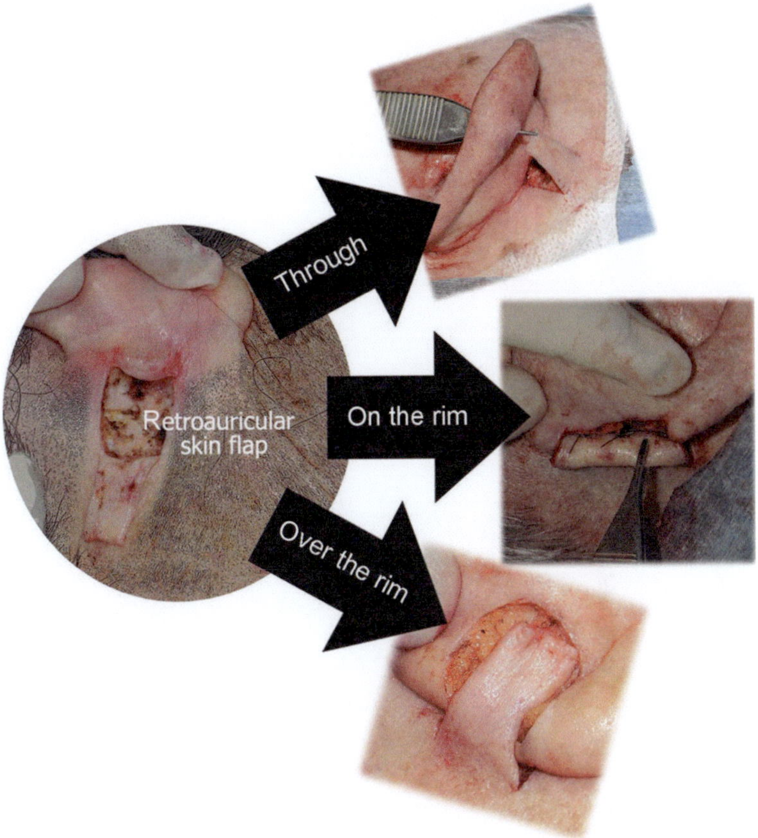

Fig. 37.3 Various applications of retroauricular advancement flap to fill the surgical defects of the anterior surface and helix of the ear

(Fig 37.4i). Skin flap is then sutured into place (Fig 37.4j). The ear is immobilized by suturing it down to the mastoid process by using deep periosteal sutures (Fig 37.4k, l). This suture reduces the resting tension and prevents the flap from inadvertent and accidental tension.

Dividing the Flap (Fig. 37.5)

The skin flap heals well, and it is ready for detachment in 2 weeks (Fig. 37.5a). The flap is now divided from the anterior surface (Fig. 37.5b), at a point where there is adequate posterior primary defect coverage. The divided flap is then suture approximated with the posterior margin of primary defect (Fig. 37.5c). Incision in the posterior surface of the ear (Fig. 37.5d) is then sutured (Fig. 37.5e). For a small cartilage defect such as this, repair is not required. Healing of small secondary defect is well advanced by secondary intention in this case (Fig. 37.5e), and only a trimming of the flap stump (Fig. 37.5f) and a precise suture approximation of its edges (Fig. 37.5g) were required. Sutures were removed after 1 week. Final result is usually satisfactory after 3 months, and there were no miniaturizations of the ear.

Applications

Repairing Anterior Surface Defect of the Lobule (Fig. 37.6)

This 63-year-old woman presented with a biopsy-proven BCC of the anterior surface of the right lower ear lobule. BCC and the surgical margin were marked, and the appropriate retroauricular advancement flap was designed. BCC was excised and the flap elevated. In this case, the flap was advanced over the helical rim to fill the surgical defect of the anterior surface of the lower ear

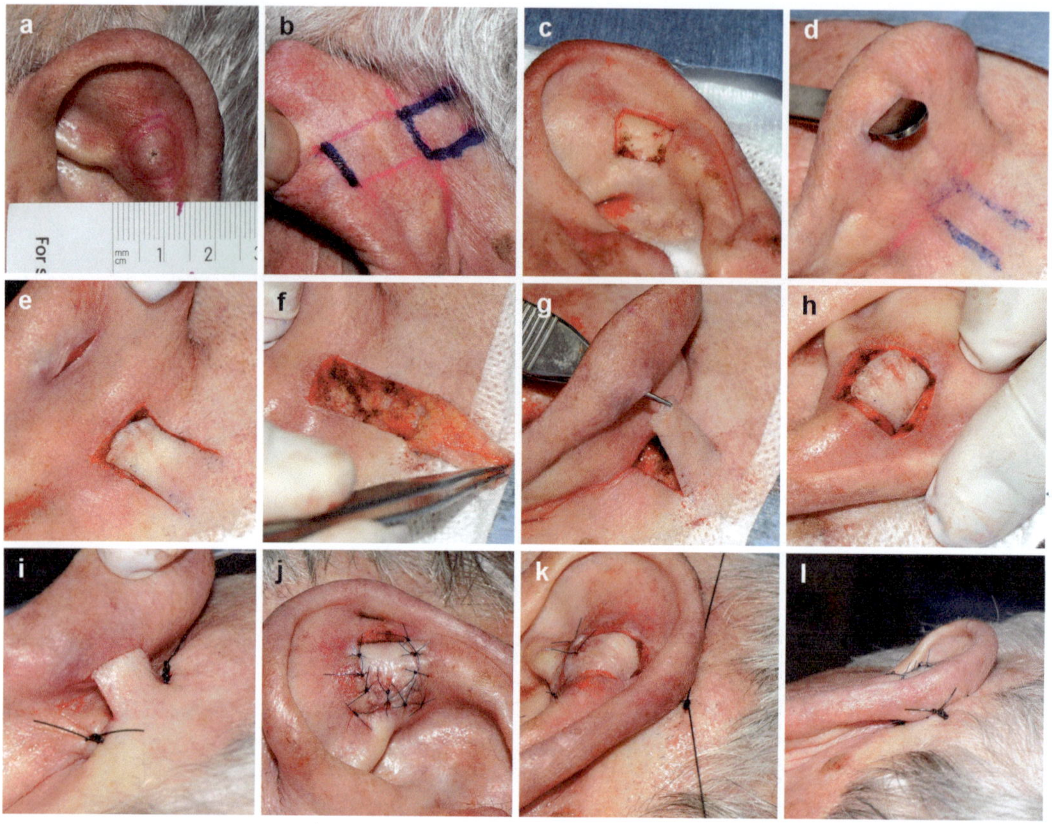

Fig. 37.4 Stage one of the retroauricular advancement flap. (**a**) Basal cell carcinoma (BCC). (**b**) Appropriate margins around BCC are preoperatively marked. (**b**) Tunnel through which the flap will be pulled through (from posterior auricular surface anteriorly) is marked (corresponding to the posterior border of the surgical margin) and the length of the retroauricular skin flap marked. (**c**) The skin cancer is excised – primary defect. (**d**) Cartilage slit is made to allow the skin flap to be pulled through on the anterior auricular surface. (**e**) Retroauricular skin flap is incised, and (**f**) it is then undermined to its base – secondary defect. (**g**) Undermine to enhance the flap mobility but only as required to minimize the damage to the flap vascularity. Elevated skin flap is then grasped and (**h**) pulled through the cartilage tunnel and placed on the anterior surface of the ear. (**i**) Base of the flap is sutured to the postauricular sulcus. (**j**) Skin flap is sutured into place. (**k, l**) The ear is immobilized by suturing it down to the mastoid process by using deep periosteal sutures

lobule. Flap was sutured and it was stabilized by pinning the ear down to the mastoid process. After 2 weeks, the flap was divided and the ear released. Patient was reviewed after 3 months, and both the recipient and the donor site have healed well, and there was no miniaturization of the ear.

Repairing the Inner Ear Defect, Anterior Conchal Surface (Fig. 37.7)

This 63-year-old male presented with squamous cell carcinoma (SCC) of the anterior conchal surface of the right ear. SCC was surgically excised and the margins deemed clear from the review of its frozen section. Appropriate amount of retroauricular skin flap was created. Shortest distance in which the skin flap needs to be advanced to fill the surgical defect was through the conchal cartilage. For this reason, cartilage tunnel was created. The retroauricular skin flap was tunneled through the cartilage to place it on the anterior surface of concha. Flap was sutured into place. Usual flap division took place after 2 weeks, and further 1 week later, those sutures were removed.

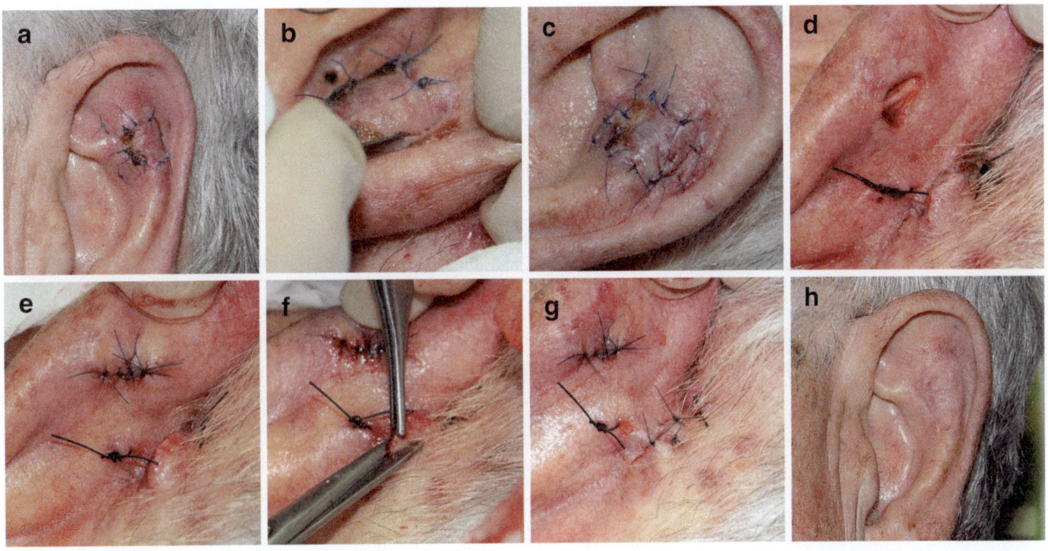

Fig. 37.5 Stage 2 of retroauricular skin flap. (**a**) The skin flap heals well, and it is ready for detachment in 2 weeks. (**b**) The flap is now divided from the anterior surface, at a point where there is adequate posterior primary defect coverage. (**c**) The divided flap is then suture approximated with the posterior margin of primary defect. (**d**) Incision in the posterior surface of the ear (**e**) is then sutured. (**e**) Healing of small secondary defect is well advanced by secondary intention in this case, and (**f**) only a trimming of the flap stump and (**g**) precise suture approximation of its edges were required (**h**) Final result

Repairing Full-Thickness Helical Rim Defect (Fig. 37.8)

This 73-year-old male presented with helical rim defect following excision of melanoma in situ. Scar was excised. Retroauricular skin flap was created to fill the helical rim defect. In order to create a rolled appearance of the helical rim, the skin flap was doubled up into a roll. This roll of flap was then sutured into the surgical defect. The ear was pinned back to the retroauricular area to avoid inadvertent pulling of the ear that can damage the flap. Flap has healed well after 2 weeks, and it was divided. The retroauricular skin was slow to granulate; hence S-plasty [2] was performed for a direct closure. Cosmetic outcome after 3 months appears satisfactory.

Discussion

Surgical defect of the ear following a skin cancer excision, when repaired using the soft tissue of the same ear (wedge excision and local flap surgery), often produces miniaturization of that ear, and this is particularly noticeable when the defect is on the helical rim. Using skin or composite graft to fill these defects can avoid smaller ear postoperatively, but especially when the surgical defect involves the helical rim, the resulting cosmetic outcome may be unsatisfactory. Distant flap does emerge as an attractive option in filling the surgical defects of the ear without miniaturizing it, as it does not require the use of the soft tissue of an already limited soft tissue reserve of the ear.

Retroauricular soft tissue is geographically located in close proximity to the ear; thus, a skin flap of this region can easily be advanced to fill its soft tissue defects. Due to its close proximity to the ear flap, length and mobilization can be minimized which reduces the vascular burden of that flap. Its other attractions are that there is an abundant supply of well-vascularized soft tissue for ear reconstruction [6], flap donor site scar can be easily concealed behind the ear, and the miniaturization of the ear can be avoided.

There are several essential factors that need to be taken into consideration and be customized for

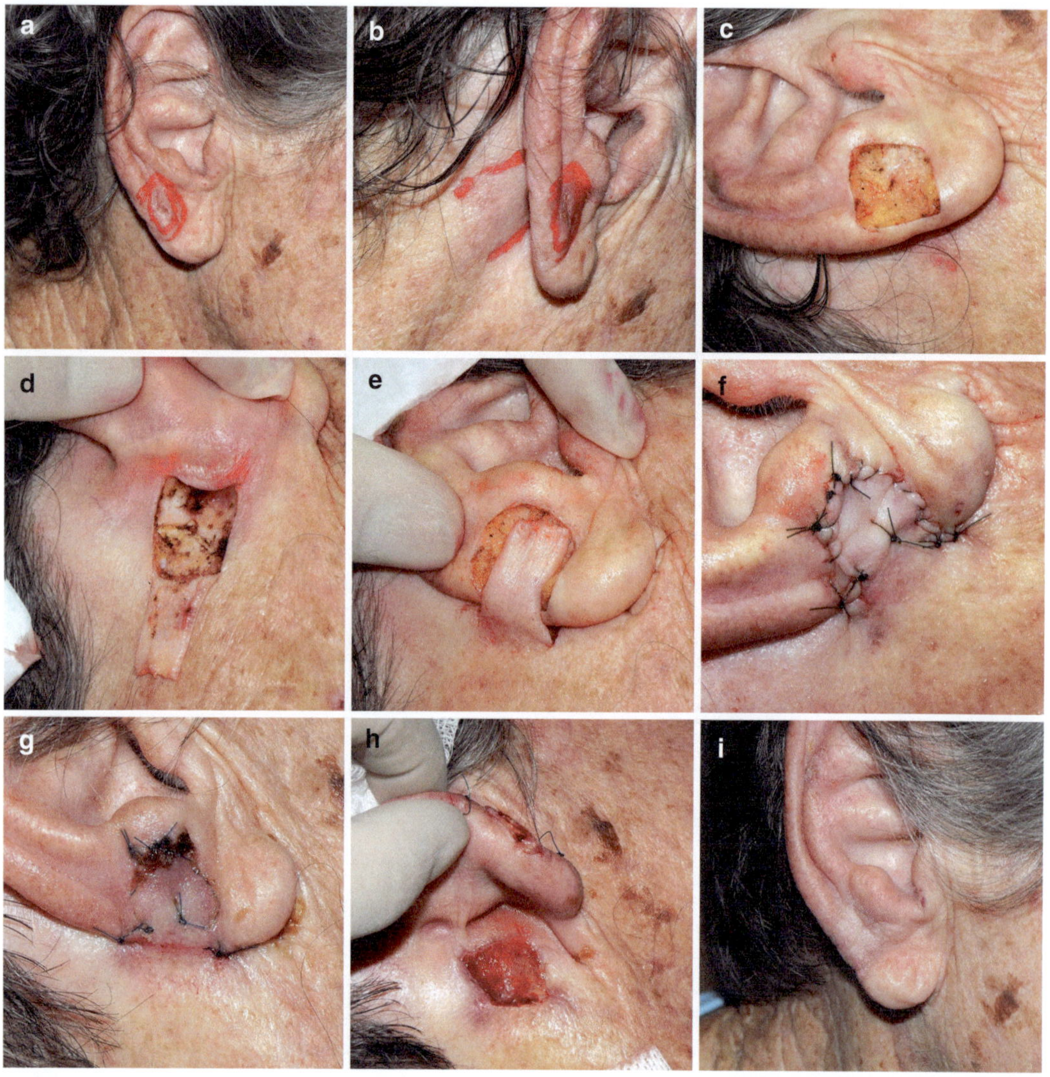

Fig. 37.6 Repairing anterior surface defect of the lobule. (**a**) Basal cell carcinoma (BBC) surgical margin is marked. (**b**) The appropriate retroauricular advancement flap was designed. (**c**) BCC is excised. (**d**) The flap is elevated. (**e**) The flap is advanced over the helical rim to fill the surgical defect of the anterior surface of the lower ear lobule. (**f**) The flap is sutured and stabilized by pinning the ear down to the mastoid process. (**g**) Flap after two weeks. (**h**) The flap is divided and the ear released. (**i**) Three months post-operative and both the recipient and the donor site have healed well, and there was no miniaturization of the ear

a successful retroauricular advancement skin flap surgery. And these factors are:

Flap Length

Correct approximation of the length of the skin flap and by creating the flap that is approximately 2 mm longer than the surgical defect to be filled but not to overlengthen the flap as to create devascularization. When the flap is intended to be rolled up to reconstruct the helical rim defect, flap length should be approximately 4 mm longer than the anticipated length.

Flap Thickness

Thick retroauricular soft tissue enables the operator to produce a variable thickness of flap to

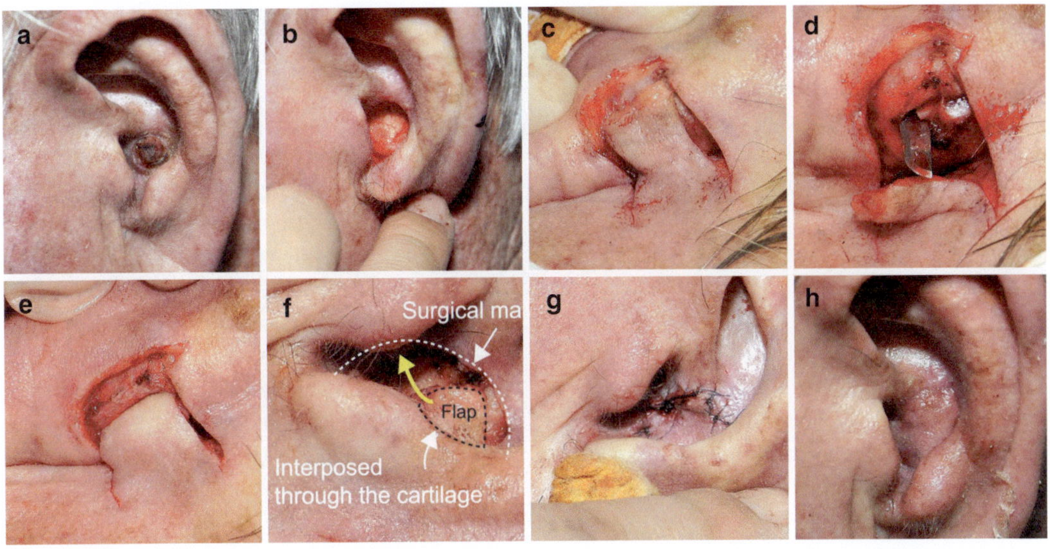

Fig. 37.7 Repairing the inner ear defect, anterior conchal surface. (**a**) This 63-year-old male presented with squamous cell carcinoma (SCC) of the anterior conchal surface of the right ear. (**b**) SCC was surgically excised and the margins deemed clear from the review of its frozen section. (**c**) Appropriate amount of retroauricular skin flap was created. (**d**) Since the shortest distance in which the skin flap needs to be advanced to fill the surgical defect was through the conchal cartilage, a cartilage tunnel was created. (**e**) The retroauricular skin flap was tunneled (**f**) through the cartilage to place it on the anterior surface of concha. Flap was sutured into place. (**g**) Usual flap division took place after 2 weeks, and 1 week later, those sutures were removed. (**h**) Final result

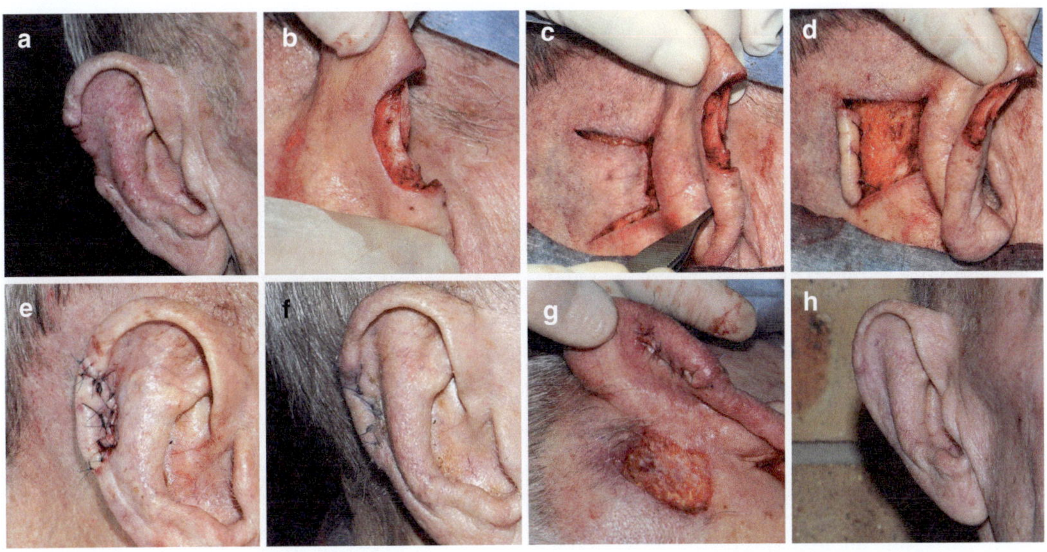

Fig. 37.8 Repairing full-thickness helical rim defect. (**a**) This 73-year-old male presented with helical rim defect following excision of melanoma in situ. (**b**) The scar was excised. (**c**) Retroauricular skin flap was created to fill the helical rim defect. (**d**) In order to create a rolled appearance of the helical rim, the skin flap was doubled up into a roll. (**e**) This roll of flap was then sutured into the surgical defect. (**f**) Flap has healed well after 2 weeks, and it was divided. (**g**) The retroauricular skin was slow to granulate, hence S-plasty. (**h**) Final result

reconstruct the surgical defect of the ear. It can be rolled up and thickened to recreate helical rim, or its distal end can be thinned to avoid step deformity. Wide-based pedicle of this type of flap and the rich random-pattern blood supply of retroauricular skin do facilitate this.

Flap Tension

Reduce the tension placed along the flap by immobilizing the ear to the mastoid process by suture fixation. By pinning the ear back onto the retroauricular region, inadvertent pulling of the flap can be prevented.

Hemostasis

Meticulous hemostasis is essential in any surgery, but it is particularly important in the ear and the periauricular region as the hematoma and delayed hemorrhage can cause a significant patient distress.

Postoperative

Compression dressing is applied, and the dressing is left intact for 1 week. After 1 week, the wound can be showered and cleansed daily.

Timing: Leave the flap for at least 2 weeks before dividing it and detaching it from the retroauricular skin. This allows an adequate collateral revascularization which is essential in preventing flap loss.

Secondary Defect

The longer you leave the second procedure, there is a more significant granulation of the secondary defect. Smaller secondary defects (2 cm) close completely in 2–4 weeks. The delay between the first and second procedure of greater than 2 weeks is advantageous as the second stage procedure can then be performed relatively quickly and easily. If the secondary defect is large and or if the wound bed is slow to granulate, then this defect should be closed with primary intention.

Obvious downside of this procedure is that it is a 2-staged procedure: first to create flap and second to divide the flap at a later date. Also there is a donor site wound that may require repairing. However, it is a relatively simple procedure of skin advancement flap with numerous advantages: good match of skin color and texture, better ear profile, and no miniaturization of the ear.

Conclusions

Excisional surgery of the ear often produces a smaller ear postoperatively. Soft tissue of retroauricular region is well vascularized, and the advancement flap of retroauricular skin can be used for a successful and cosmetically satisfying reconstruction of the ear without miniaturizing it.

References

1. Kim P, Kim HJ. S-plasty: less is more. Aust Fam Physician. 2011;40(4):224–5.
2. Kim P. Prophylactic Z-plasty – correcting helical rim deformity from wedge excision. Aust Fam Physician. 2010;39(9):649–50.
3. Cordova A, D'Arpa S, Pirrello R, Giambona C, Moschella F. Retroauricular skin: a flaps bank for ear. J Plast Reconstr Aesthet Surg. 2008;61 Suppl 1:S44–51.
4. Johnson TM, Fader DJ. The staged retroauricular to auricular direct pedicle (interpolation) flap for helical ear reconstruction. J Am Acad Dermatol. 1997;37(6):975–8.
5. Koopmann C, Couthard SW. "How I do it" – otology and neurotology. A specific issue and its solution. A postauricular muscle-skin flap for conchal defects. Laryngoscope. 1982;92(5):596–600.
6. Yang D, Morris SF. Vascular basis of the retroauricular flap. Ann Plast Surg. 1998;40(1):28–33.

The Tubular Technique in Otoplasty 38

Vladimir Kljajic, Ljiljana Vlaski, Jovan Radmanovic, and Slobodan Savovic

Introduction

The earlobe size corresponds to the middle third of the face, just like the nasal pyramid, or one-fifth of the facial height. Proportionate relationship between ears creates a balanced and beautiful look of the whole face and head. If the earlobes are too large or protruding, the facial harmony is impaired, often causing embarrassment. Even young children with protruding ears are often teased by their peers. This is the reason why parents often insist on correcting this issue at a young age. Most authors agree that otoplasty should be done after the age of 7. Padovan considers that otoplasty should be performed by the age of 6 and Weerda by the age of 5 years [1, 2].

Protruding ears are diagnosed if the auriculocephalic angle, determined by the line from the root of the helix to its most lateral edge and the mastoid plane, is over 25°. However, some authors believe that in patients with prominent ears, the angle of protrusion is at least 30° [2]. The most common causes of ear protrusion are underdeveloped or poorly developed antihelix. According to Potter, protruding ears are transmitted as a dominant characteristic, with an incidence of 5 %, and most authors agree with his opinion [3–5].

Dieffenbach [6] was the first to describe his technique of otoplasty in 1845, to correct a post-traumatic prominent auricle. He excised the retroauricular skin and used a conchomastoidal suture for the fixation of the ear. After him, numerous authors have applied partial removal of cartilage. This surgical concept provided unsatisfactory results, especially in the profile view. A new concept of protruding ear surgery was created by Luckett [7], who pointed to the importance of antihelical fold in shaping the earlobe. He also analyzed the primary deformity in most protruding ears as either the absence or underdevelopment of the antihelical fold. Converse et al. [8] created a new tubular procedure with a formation of antihelix in the lower part of the earlobe by tabulation. Converse performed incomplete cartilage

V. Kljajic, M.D. (✉)
Medical Faculty of Novi Sad, ENT Clinic, Clinical Center of Vojvodina, Hajduk Veljkova 1, Novi Sad, Serbia

Medical Faculty of Novi Sad, ENT Clinic, Clinical Center of Vojvodina, Turgenjeva 15, Novi Sad 21000, Serbia
e-mail: kljaja@eunet.rs

L. Vlaski, M.D.
Medical Faculty of Novi Sad, ENT Clinic, Clinical Center of Vojvodina, Branimira Ćosića 10, Novi Sad 21000, Serbia
e-mail: vlaskilj@eunet.rs

J. Radmanovic, M.D.
ENT Department, Hospital of Sremska Mitrovica Severni, Bedem 52/4, Sremska Mitrovica 22000, Serbia
e-mail: niki05@open.telekom.rs

S. Savovic, M.D.
Medical Faculty of Novi Sad, ENT Clinic, Clinical Center of Vojvodina, Dalmatinska 24, Veternik 21203, Serbia
e-mail: savovics@yahoo.com

M.A. Shiffman (ed.), *Advanced Cosmetic Otoplasty*,
DOI 10.1007/978-3-642-35431-1_38,

incisions from the posterior side in combination with fixation sutures. Weerda [2] classified all types of otoplasty procedures in regard to the incision site into two great groups, those with retroauricular and those with auricular incision.

Preoperative Patient Preparation

Preoperative patient preparation comprises providing patient's photographs and general preoperative care. Two photographs are necessary, 10×15 cm in size, of the front and back view. Male patients should have short haircut in order to evaluate the degree of ear protrusion, and female patients should wear their hair up to reveal their ears (Fig. 38.1).

Preoperative laboratory testing includes basic analyses and hemostasis. If the patient is undergoing general anesthesia, pulmonary and cardiac functions should be checked by a pediatrician or an internist.

Otoplasty: Step-by-Step

Tubular techniques are recommended for managing ears without a formed antihelix. Converse is considered the creator of these techniques. The main difference between his techniques and the technique we use today is that he performs cartilage thinning and then folds it, while our technique is characterized by full-thickness incisions of cartilage and folding of the edges to form a tube corresponding with the antihelix.

The surgery can be performed under general or local anesthesia. Local anesthesia is usually performed in adult patients. Local anesthesia is performed using a local anesthetic solution containing adrenaline 1: 200,000. Adrenaline is used to suppress intraoperative bleeding. General anesthesia is performed using total intravenous anesthesia. Retroauricular infiltration is done using 0.9 % NaCl and adrenaline 1: 200,000 to prevent intraoperative bleeding.

After preoperative cleansing and isolation of the surgical site, retroauricular infiltration of the region with a diluted adrenaline solution is done, either with a local anesthetic or with 0.9 % NaCl. Marking an elliptical incision line 0.5 cm from the retroauricular fold is then done. A symmetrical semiellipse is drawn in the retroauricular region on the mastoid plane. When the incision of the skin and subcutaneous tissue is made, a surface of an elongated ellipse is obtained (Fig. 38.2).

Hemostasis is provided by a bipolar cautery to minimize injury. After that, soft tissues of the posterior earlobe are lifted by fine scissors up to the edge of the cartilage. It is recommended that the posterior auricular ligament be removed as well, if it is too prominent, in order to provide a better layer for the earlobe cavum (Fig. 38.3).

When the posterior part is exposed, future antihelix is marked. This is done using eight to ten insulin needles on the anterior part of the earlobe, marking the future antihelix (Fig. 38.4). During formation of the antihelix, the surgeon may decrease the depth of the conchal cavum in order to create an acceptable and natural ear shape. Half of the needles are placed along one side of the newly formed antihelix, while the left are placed on the other side. A retroauricular cartilage incision is then made between the needle tips. When the needles are removed, the incisions are put together to form two semiellipses, which are nearly parallel. Fine-pointed dissecting scissors are used in cutting cartilage edges. The suture material of choice is 5-0 Prolene, which is used to fold the newly formed antihelix. Thus, a tubular form is made, and the antihelix is reconstructed (Fig. 38.5).

4-0 Prolene is recommended for the conchal mastoid to pull the perichondrium of the conchal cavum cartilage to the mastoid periosteum. Individual stitches using Vicryl 4-0 close the subcutaneous and Prolene 4-0 to close the skin layer. The newly created antihelix is then protected by a cotton dressing soaked in Rivanol antiseptic and Hepathrombin ointment to prevent hematoma. The same dressing material is used retroauricularly as well.

The same procedure is repeated on the other ear. After the surgery of both ears is finished, a bulky bandage dressing is wrapped around the patient's head, while the elastic band should not be too tight.

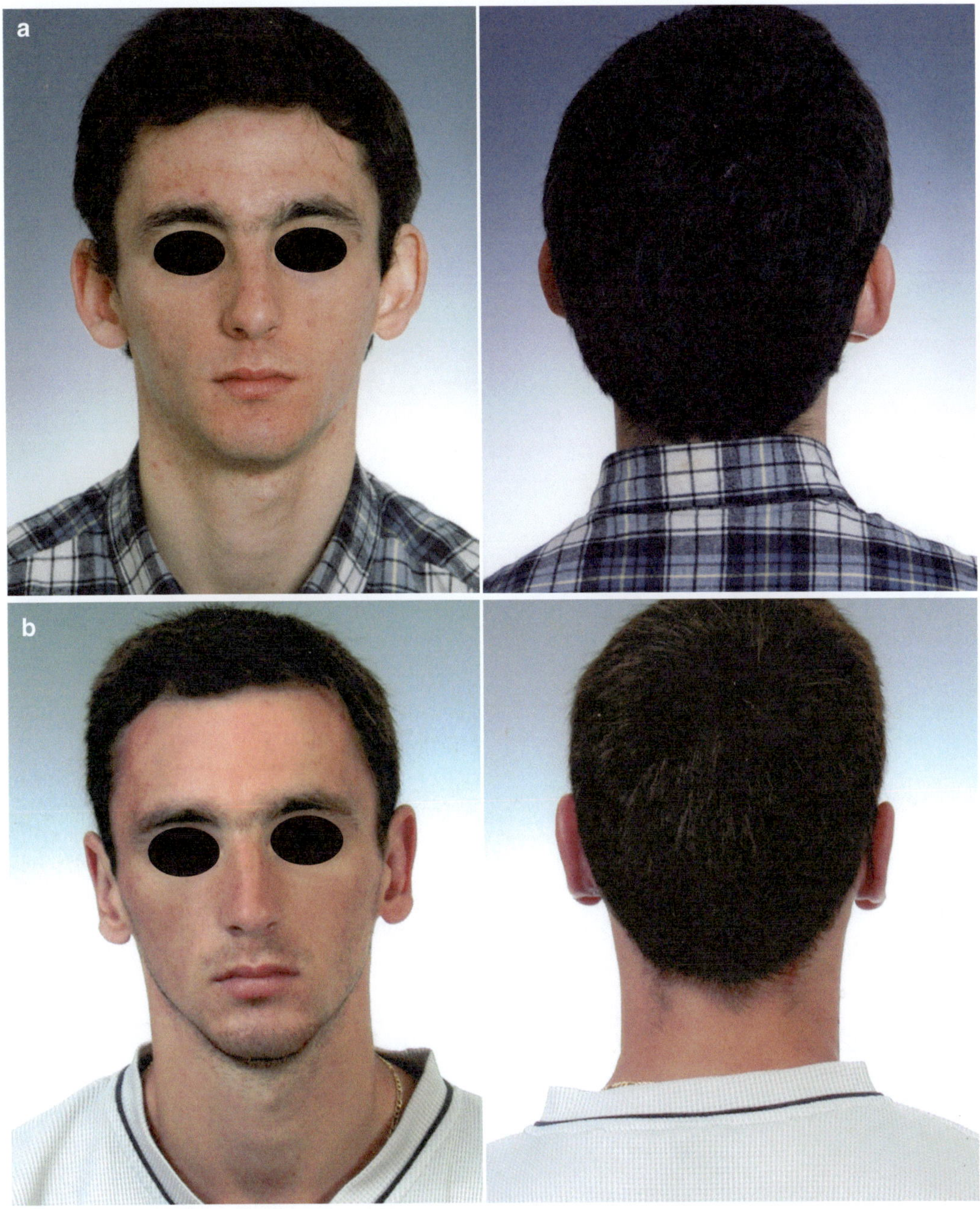

Fig. 38.1 (**a**) Preoperative patient. (**b**) Postoperative

Postoperative Care

In the early postoperative period, the patient receives analgesics. In our opinion, re-bandaging is not necessary until the seventh postoperative day, when the stitches are usually removed. On the seventh postoperative day, bandages are carefully removed from both ears. The treated area is disinfected, usually by Octenisept, and then retroauricular stitches are removed. After that,

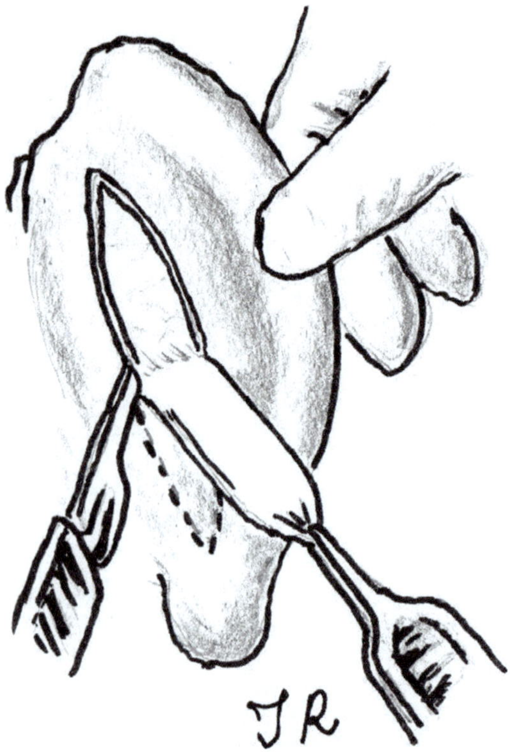

Fig. 38.2 Skin excision

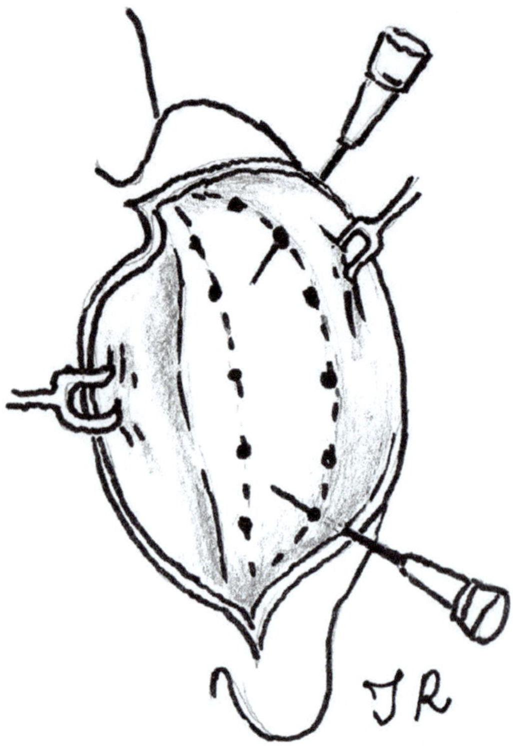

Fig. 38.4 Marking the future antihelix

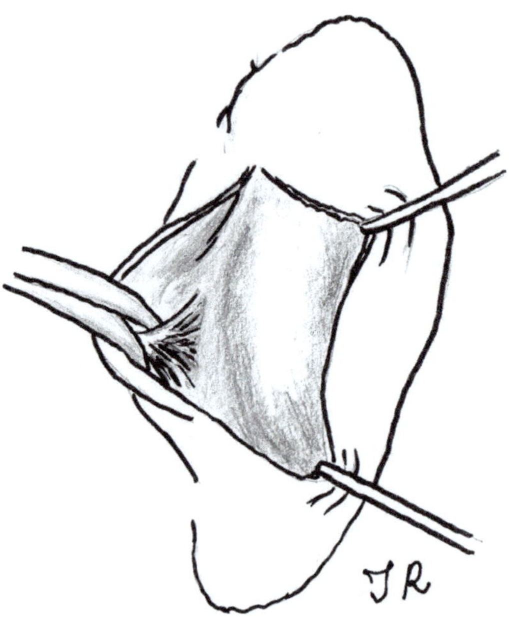

Fig. 38.3 Resection of the posterior auricular ligament

a smaller quantity of folded gauze is placed over both ears, and the elastic band remains for another 5 days. On the 12th postoperative day, the bandages are removed, and the patient is recommended to wear the elastic band during the night. Three months after the surgery, the patient brings two pictures (10×15 cm in size), his front and back view.

Complications

Complications can be divided into intraoperative and postoperative, whereas postoperative may be early and late.

Intraoperative complications include allergic reactions to the local anesthetic, or in case of general anesthesia, allergic reaction to anesthetic agents used for general anesthesia. During surgery and cartilage incision, the skin may also be involved. If the skin lesion is small, it can be stitched using Prolene 5-0 after final cartilage incision, which is usually treated with an antibiotic ointment. These skin lesions, if primarily carefully stitched, result with minimal scarring. Intraoperative bleeding is usually minimal, and it is managed with cauterization.

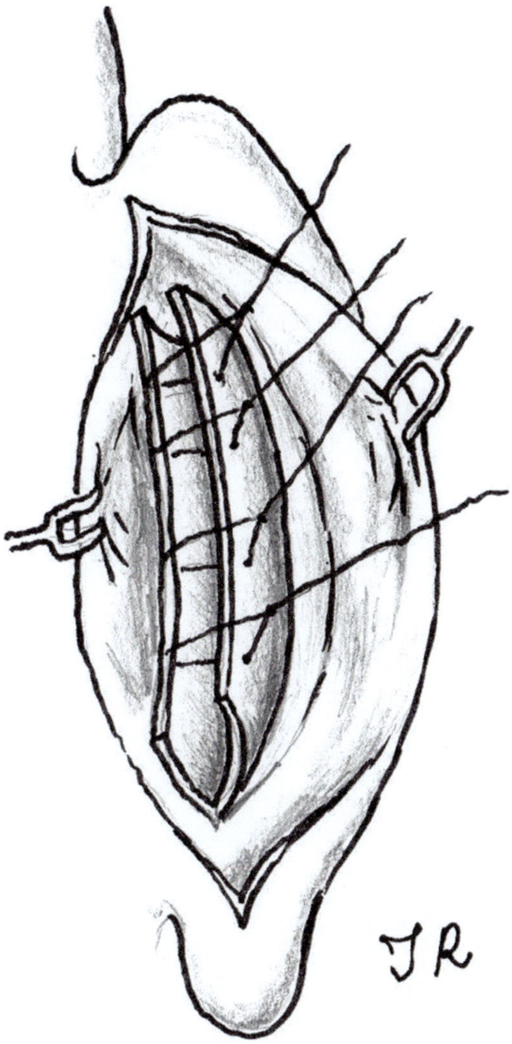

Fig. 38.5 Formation of the tubular structure

Early postoperative complications include bleeding, when revision surgery is required. Postoperative bleeding is never life threatening, but if it is not managed, it may cause hematoma in the earlobe area, leading to sterile cartilage necrosis, or if inflammation takes place, to perichondritis (abscess). Proper ear cavity tamponade and placement of an elastic band on ears is a very important factor in preventing postoperative hematoma and abscess.

Late postoperative complications include development of keloid scars (Fig. 38.6); earlobe deformities, especially "telephone ear"; and sharp cartilage edge on the anterior part of the auricle.

The authors have not had any postoperative complications in the last 10 years, except in one case of a retroauricular wound dehiscence after stitch removal. The problem was managed by secondary sutures. After removal of stitches, the earlobe was of pleasing appearance, without prominent scarring.

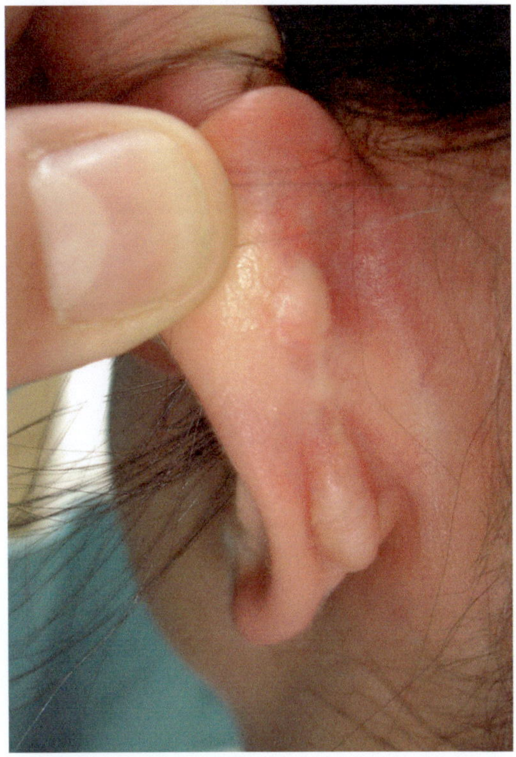

Fig. 38.6 Retroauricular keloid

Conclusions

1. In the management of protruding ears, tubular techniques are suitable for cases without formed antihelix.
2. A modified Converse technique is successfully used in patients with poorly formed antihelix, but with a deep conchal cavity.
3. When using this surgical procedure, complications are extremely rare.
4. The basic advantage of this procedure is that the anterior auricular surface is spared of damage.

References

1. Padovan I. Otorinolaringologija. Kirurgija uha. Zagreb: Školska klnjiga; 1982. p. 255–70.
2. Weerda H. Surgery of the auriculae: tumors. Trauma. Defects. Abnormalities. New York: Georg Thieme Verlag; 2007.
3. Potter EI. A hereditary ear malformation transmitted through five generations. J Hered. 1937;28:255–8.

4. Janis JE, Rohrich RJ, Gutowsky KA. Otoplasty. Plast Reconstr Surg. 2005;115(4):60e–72.
5. Kompatscher P, Schuler CH, Clemens S, Seifert B, Beer GM. The cartilage-sparing versus the cartilage-cutting technique: a retrospective quality control comparison of the Francesconi and Converse otoplasties. Aesthetic Plast Surg. 2003;27(6):446–53.
6. Dieffenbach JF. Die Operative Chirurgie. Leipzig: FA Bruckhaus; 1845.
7. Luckett WH. A new operation for prominent ears based on the anatomy of the deformity. Surg Gynecol Obstet. 1910;10:635–7.
8. Converse JM, Nigro A, Wilson FA, Johnson N. A technique for surgical correction of lop ears. Trans Am Acad Ophthalmol Otolaryngol. 1956;60(4):551–6.

The Deep Conchal Bowl: Accentuation of the Helical Crus

39

Sapna Patel and Kathleen C.Y. Sie

Introduction

Otoplasty surgical techniques continue to evolve since the original description in 1845. As newer techniques are introduced, it is important to realize that the basis of management arises from careful evaluation of the ear. There are four general categories of abnormalities that contribute to prominent ear deformity: absent or poorly formed antihelix, deep conchal bowl, inadequate helical rim, and an abnormal lobule, with the first two being most common [1]. It is important for the surgeon performing otoplasty to critically assess the prominent ear and to understand different approaches to optimize its appearance. We will focus on a novel approach to address the deep conchal bowl.

The conchal bowl is embryologically derived from the first Branchial groove. The conchal bowl is a concavity separated by the helical crus into the concha cymba superiorly and concha cavum inferiorly. It is also important to assess the relationship of the conchal bowl with the scapha and the mastoid cortex. A deep conchal bowl, generally defined as deeper than 1.5 cm, can be present in isolation or in combination with other anomalies, most notably involving the antihelical fold.

There have been many techniques described to address the deep conchal bowl. In 1845 Dieffenbach described conchomastoid fixation through a postauricular incision with the goal of minimizing the appearance of the deep concha bowl; this was also the focus of techniques popularized by Furnas [2] and Morestin [3], with the latter excessive conchal cartilage.

Some of the commonly used procedures can be categorized based on technique: suturing, conchal cartilage flap, and cartilage scoring [4–6]. Placement of conchomastoid sutures requires a great deal of precision, as placement more anterior on the mastoid or more posterior on the concha will result in anterior rotation of the conchal bowl. This has been associated with narrowing of the external auditory meatus resulting in cerumen retention and difficulty with otoscopic examination. Spira and Stal [7] modified this by anchoring a lateral cartilage flap to the mastoid periosteum helping to decrease the potential for external auditory meatus narrowing and creating a strong anchor for suturing. Excisional techniques in which a strip of cartilage with or without skin is excised to help minimize conchal prominence have been proposed [4]. The third popular technique is cartilage scoring, with attempts to create

S. Patel, M.D.
Department of Dermatology, Dermatologists & Dermatologic Surgeons, Morristown, NJ
e-mail: sapnap@uw.edu

K.C.Y. Sie, M.D. (✉)
Department of Otolaryngology, Childhood Communication Center, Seattle Children's Hospital, 4800 Sand Point Way, Seattle, WA 98105, USA

Department of Otolaryngology
Head and Neck Surgery, University of Washington, Seattle, WA, USA
e-mail: kathysie@uw.edu; kathleen.sie@seattlechildrens.org

M.A. Shiffman (ed.), *Advanced Cosmetic Otoplasty*,
DOI 10.1007/978-3-642-35431-1_39, © Springer-Verlag Berlin Heidelberg 2013

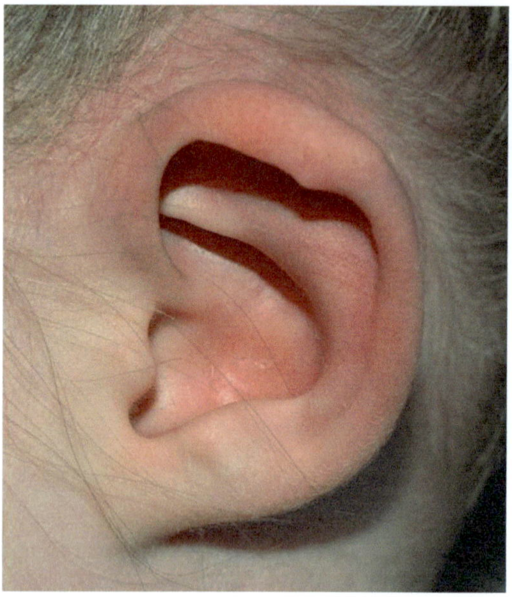

Fig. 39.1 Poorly formed helical crus contributes to the appearance of the deep conchal bowl

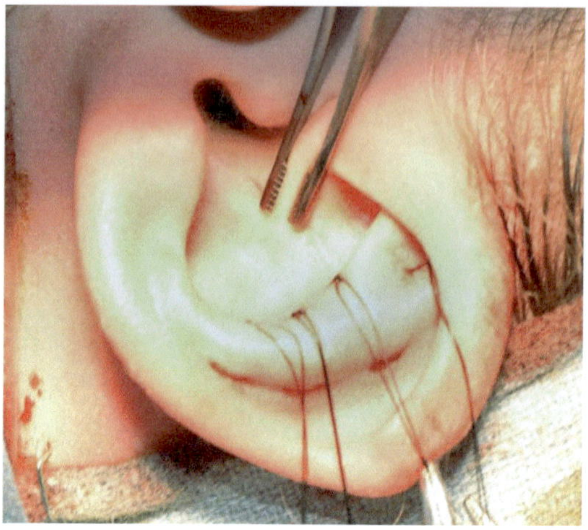

Fig. 39.2 Use of forceps to define the helical root after the antihelical fold has been accentuated. The laterally placed black sutures will be removed

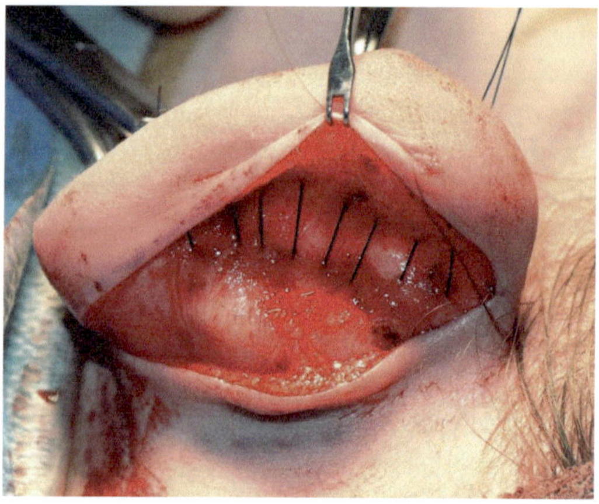

Fig. 39.3 Placement of the black nylon sutures that are used to define the position and tension of the permanent 4-0 clear nylon mattress sutures

striations in the cartilage to weaken its natural spring.

With the understanding that patients with prominent ear deformity typically have poorly defined convexities of the ear, as opposed to excessive cartilage, the senior author recognized that the deep conchal bowl deformity is commonly associated with an absent or poorly formed helical crus (Fig. 39.1). This observation is analogous to the role of the poorly defined antihelical fold in the appearance of prominent ears. The techniques used to emphasize the antihelical fold [8, 9] have been applied to the helical crus [10].

After definition of the antihelical fold with cartilage scoring and mattress sutures, the helical crus is created using similar techniques. A postauricular incision is created to expose the perichondrium of the posterior conchal bowl. This is left intact and the antihelical fold is addressed. Then the helical crus width is estimated using forceps (Fig. 39.2). Black nylon sutures are placed to define the position of the clear nylon sutures that are placed on the deep aspect of the conchal cartilage (Fig. 39.3). The deep aspect of the conchal cartilage between the sutures is scored using a 5910 Beaver blade. Care is taken to preserve the integrity of the cartilage that will accommodate the sutures. Once the clear nylon sutures have been placed, the black nylon sutures are removed. Accentuation of the helical crus is used in conjunction with other otoplasty techniques depending upon the issues that need to be addressed for any particular ear (Figs. 39.4 and 39.5).

In addition to managing the helical crus, shaving any eminentia on the deep surface of the conchal bowl can be helpful in cosmetic otoplasty.

Postoperative management follows with an antibiotic-ointment-coated cotton ball in the

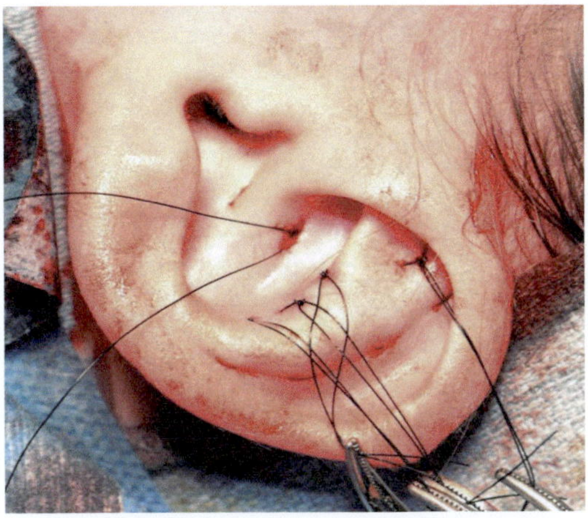

Fig. 39.4 Suture placed to create the helical crus

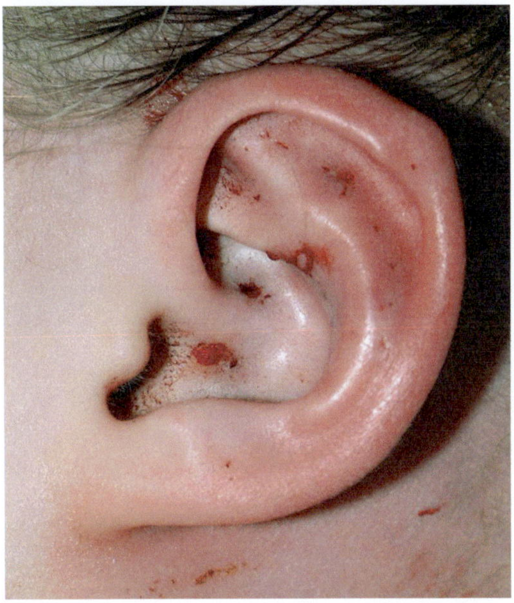

Fig. 39.5 Appearance of the reconstructed ear after removal of the black nylon positioning sutures. Note the accentuated helical crus

concavities of ear with an eye pad or folded gauze pad overlying it. Patients are instructed to wear a neoprene headband dressing day and night for 1 week and then nighttime only for an additional week.

This technique addresses the deep conchal bowl when the helical crus is underdeveloped. The creation or accentuation of the crus is flexible and can be performed, using one many of the previously described techniques from excision of cartilage to scoring. Moreover, this technique avoids any potential narrowing of the cartilaginous external auditory meatus. Conversely, this approach pulls the anterior edge of the conchal cartilage posterior superiorly, thereby opening the external auditory meatus. Also by avoiding placement of conchomastoid sutures, the postauricular sulcus remains well preserved.

There are a variety of potential causes of prominent ear deformity. A majority of the time, there are several etiologies. One must recognize the abnormalities of the ear and use appropriate surgical techniques to address each abnormality. The absent or poorly defined helical crus is a cause of the "deep" conchal bowl. Presence of small cartilaginous prominences, or eminentia, on the deep surface of the conchal cartilage can also affect the position of the conchal cartilage. These should be shaved at the time of otoplasty. Creation of the helical crus and shaving of eminentia should be considered for surgical management of the deep conchal bowl.

References

1. Janis JE, Rohrich RJ, Gutowski KA. Otoplasty. Plast Reconstr Surg. 2005;115(4):60e–72.
2. Furnas DW. Correction of prominent ears by conchamastoid sutures. Plast Reconstr Surg. 1968;42(3):189–93.
3. Morestin H. De la reposition et du plissement cosmétiques du pavillon de l'oreille. Rev Orthop. 1903;|4:394.
4. Beasley NJ, Jones NS. Otoplasty: the problem of the deep conchal bowl. J Laryngol Otol. 1996;110(9):864–8.
5. Bhatti A, Donovan D. Sutureless otoplasty by scoring of the cartilage: a study in 34 patients. Br J Oral Maxillofac Surg. 2007;45(3):217–20.
6. Bulstrode N. Otoplasty by percutaneous anterior scoring. Another twist to the story: a long-term study of 114 patients. Br J Plast Surg. 2003;56(2):145–9.
7. Spira M, Stal S. The conchal flap: an adjunct in otoplasty. Ann Plast Surg. 1983;11(4):291–8.
8. Luckett WH. A new operation for prominent ears base on the anatomy of the deformity. Surg Gynecol Obstet. 1910;10:365–7.
9. Mustarde JC. The correction of different types of prominent ears. Aesthetic Plast Surg. 1983;7(3):163–8.
10. Sie KC, Ou H. Otoplasty: an alternative approach to management of the deep conchal bowl. Laryngoscope. 2006;116(11):2092–4.

Otoplasty for the Treatment of Protuberant Ears

40

Payal Patel, Emil Bisaccia, and Dwight A. Scarborough

Introduction

Otoplasty is a common procedure for the treatment of protuberant ears [1]. The term prominent ears can be defined as ears that "stick out" regardless of size [2]. Prominent ear deformities occur in approximately 5 % of the population and can cause significant psychological stress on patients [3]. The goal of otoplasty is to make the protuberant ears less apparent by restoring them to a normal form and position while maintaining symmetry.

P. Patel, D.O. (✉)
Department of Dermatology,
Affiliated Dermatologists and Dermatologic Surgeons,
182 South Street, Morristown 07960, NJ, USA
e-mail: ppatel702@gmail.com

E. Bisaccia, M.D.
Department of Dermatology,
Affiliated Dermatologists and Dermatologic Surgeons,
182 South Street, Morristown 07960, NJ, USA

Department of Dermatology,
Columbia University of Physicians and Surgeons,
New York, NY, USA
e-mail: ebisaccia@gmail.com

D.A. Scarborough, M.D.
Department of Dermatology,
Affiliated Dermatologists and Dermatologic Surgeons,
650 Shawan Falls Drive, Dublin 43017, OH, USA

Department of Dermatology,
Ohio State University Hospital, Columbus, OH, USA
e-mail: das989sa@gmail.com

Historical Background

In 1845, Dieffenbach [4] reported the first surgical approach to correction of protuberant ears. His method involved simple excision from the posterior sulcus with sutures fixing the cartilage to the mastoid periosteum. This is known today as the posterior approach. In 1881, Ely [5] was credited for the first description of surgical alteration of the cartilage to treat prominent ears. Since that time, over 170 techniques and modifications have been reported in the literature for treatment of this condition.

The techniques can be categorized into three groups: (1) leaving the auricular cartilage intact and using only sutures to treat the prominent ears, a technique created by Mustarde [6, 7]; (2) incising the cartilage without resection in an effort to make it more pliable [8–10]; and (3) excising of cartilage to reduce protrusion [11]. The application of tape to the ears for several months while in infancy has even been described to successfully treat prominent ears, although many may find this to be a controversial method [12–14].

Anatomy and Development of the Ear

The ear of a newborn measures approximately 66 % of the length and 76 % of the width of an adult ear. By the age of 3, the ear has achieved approximately 85 % of its final size, and by the age of 7, the ear has nearly completely achieved its final, adult size. Interestingly, between the

M.A. Shiffman (ed.), *Advanced Cosmetic Otoplasty*,
DOI 10.1007/978-3-642-35431-1_40, © Springer-Verlag Berlin Heidelberg 2013

ages of 30 and 80 years, the length of the auricle may actually increase up to 1 cm due to lengthening of the cartilage and the cutaneous lobe. A thorough knowledge of the intricate anatomy of the ear is essential to perform a safe and successful otoplasty [15, 16].

The external ear consists of the auricle and the external auditory canal. The helix arises anteriorly and inferiorly from a crus extending horizontally above the external auditory meatus, thus creating the outer frame of the auricle. The helix merges inferiorly into the cauda helicis and connects to the lobule. The antihelical fold lies between the antihelical crus and is also known as the scapha. The antihelix extends upward from the cauda helicis medially to the helix until it bifurcates into the anterior superior and anterior inferior crura. The antihelix borders medically to the rim of the concha and the concha proper. The concha is composed of the conchal cymba superiorly and the conchal cavum inferiorly. These are separated by the helical crus and meet the antihelix at the antihelical rim. The conchal cavum anteriorly extends to the tragus and the external auditory meatus; inferiorly and posteriorly, it borders to the antitragus, which connects laterally with the antihelix. The tragus and antitragus are separated by the intertragal notch. The lobule does not contain cartilage and displays a variety of shapes and attachments to the adjacent cheek and scalp.

The ear consists of six clinically insignificant intrinsic muscles, which include the major and minor helices, tragus, antitragus, transverse, and oblique muscles. There are three extrinsic muscles of the ear, which include the anterior auricularis, posterior auricularis, and superior auricularis. These muscles provide minor structural support to the ear [3].

The arterial supply to the auricle and external auditory meatus is derived from the external carotid artery through the superficial temporal artery, which supplies most of the external ear canal and parts of the anterior auricle; the posterior auricular arteries provide blood flow to the posterior parts of the ear.

The sensory innervation of the ear involves several different nerves. They include the greater auricular nerve and the lesser occipital nerve, which are branches of the cervical plexus, and the auricular temporal nerve, a branch of the mandibular division of the trigeminal nerve. A portion of the posterior wall of the external meatus is innervated by the auricular branch of the vagus nerve [17]. Motor innervation to the external ear is supplied by the facial nerve, although this varies among individuals [3].

Indications for Otoplasty of Protuberant Ears

One important indication for otoplasty for prominent ears is in the case of psychological illness induced from the condition, especially in children. Children with protuberant ears are often the subject of verbal and even physical abuse by their peers, causing adverse, long-term psychological effects. It has been reported that 10 % of children on the National Health Service (NHS) waiting list for surgical correction of prominent ears had been evaluated by a psychiatrist at some point [18]. Sixty-seven percentage of children with condition reported social distress from the condition, reported by some to start as early as the age of 4. This psychological impact often leads to high parental concern, which then leads to their search for a surgical correction. It is very important, however, that the child also desires the surgical correction and voices it him or herself. Without the child's individual wish for correction, he or she is not a good candidate.

Another important consideration for otoplasty is the patient's age. As stated previously, 85 % of the final ear size is achieved by age 3. Therefore, many physicians choose to perform otoplasty at 4 or 5 years of age or prior to school age [19]. Some physicians choose to wait until the patient is 6 years of age to allow for children to participate in their own postoperative care [3]. Even still, other physicians prefer to restrict otoplasty to adolescence or adulthood, as this age group is more capable than young children to describe the auricular features of concern to them and their desire for correction [1].

Once the patient and parents agree upon the desire for surgical correction, the surgeon should then perform a thorough physical examination and review of medical history to assess the degree of surgical risk, if any, to the patient. If the surgical risk outweighs the benefit of treatment of the deformity, surgery should not be performed.

Anatomical Causes of Protuberant Ears

The average Caucasian female ear is 59.0 mm in height and 32.5 mm in width. The average Caucasian male ear is 63.5 mm in height and 35.5 mm in width. Asians tend to have longer ears, while Africans typically possess slightly shorter lengths of ears. The ear's width should be about 50–60 % of the length in an aesthetically ideal ear. The superior aspect of the ear should rest at the level of the brow. On lateral view, the slope of the ear approximates the nasal dorsum to within 15° or lies approximately 20° posterior to the vertical plane.

In the aesthetically ideal ear, the distance from the helix to the mastoid is 10–12 mm in the upper third of the ear, 16–18 mm in the middle third of the ear, and 20–22 mm in the lower third of the ear. The helix lies 2–5 mm laterally of the antihelix on frontal view. Conchal protrusion from the mastoid is about 12–16 mm, and the angle between the superior helix and mastoid is 20–30° [3]. The surgeon should keep these general proportions in mind while trying to create an aesthetic external ear with otoplasty.

Generally, there are four main anatomical malformations leading to ear prominence. In order to correct protuberant ears, it is important to understand the anatomical defects leading to this deformity:

1. *Underdeveloped antihelical fold*. The underdeveloped antihelical fold causes the scapha and helical rim to protrude. This commonly affects the upper and/or middle thirds of the ear and presents as a winglike defect.
2. *Conchal prominence and/or anterolateral rotation*. The concha may be excessively deep and/or the auriculomastoid angle may exceed 30°–40°. This defect would cause prominence of the middle third of the auricle.
3. *Prominent helix*. Excessive superior outer helical rim cartilage can cause "elf ears" or "spock ears," and excessive superior helical fold cartilage can cause "lop ears."
4. *Protruding earlobe*. This defect causes prominence of the lower third of the ear and can even occur with the aging earlobe as the skin's elasticity decreases over time [20–23].

Preoperative Considerations

A careful evaluation of the defect to determine the type of auricular anomaly or anomalies present is the first step. Only after a surgeon correctly identifies the specific cause of the auricular prominence can they establish an appropriate surgical plan. Most commonly, protuberant ears result from a combination of an underdeveloped antihelical rim and conchal prominence and/or anterolateral rotation [3]. However, a patient may present with all four deformities, in which case the order of correction should be creation of the antihelical fold first, followed by conchal reduction, then helical reduction, and, finally, earlobe reduction [1].

The physical exam should also note the degree of symmetry between the ears as well. These findings must be clearly documented in written form and with standard photography showing right and left lateral views, close-up right and left lateral views, right and left oblique views, and frontal views. Next, it is vital to set realistic expectations for the procedure. The surgeon must discuss with the patient what can and cannot be achieved with surgery, and the patient must understand and have appropriate expectations of the results.

Potential complications should be outlined verbally and in a written consent signed by the patient. Once the patient understands the surgery and its potential complications, has realistic expectations for improvement, and consents to the surgical correction, preoperative clearance can be obtained. This should include a thorough physical examination, as well as a normal electrocardiogram (EKG), chest X-ray, and standard laboratory tests. The patient's age, as discussed in depth previously, should be part of the preoperative considerations as determined by each individual surgeon.

Finally, the patient should be told to avoid nonsteroidal anti-inflammatory agents for 2 weeks prior to surgery to minimize bleeding and to wash the hair the day before surgery, as this cannot be done for several days after the procedure. A surgeon may consider prescribing the patient an oral benzodiazepine to take 1 h prior the procedure to decrease anxiety.

Surgical Techniques for Correction of Protuberant Ears

Many of the surgical subspecialties prefer general anesthesia in performing otoplasty, and others may choose to utilize conscious sedation. However, if the patient proves to be highly motivated, otoplasty can easily be performed with local anesthesia alone. Local anesthesia with a mixture of 1 % lidocaine and 1:100,000 epinephrine produces adequate anesthesia while also aiding in hemostasis. The age of the patient may also dictate the type of anesthesia used, as it is rare that a child under 10 years of age can tolerate local anesthesia. Therefore, in younger patients, it may become necessary to use general anesthesia or conscious sedation [1, 2].

The surgical technique for correct of the four most common anatomical defects will be described below.

Underdeveloped Antihelical Fold

An antihelical fold is created by lightly pressing the scapha onto the concha. The position of the fold is then marked on the anterior ear skin with a row of ink spots running just lateral to the antihelix from the superior pole of the superior crus down to the merging point between the antihelix and helix. Two ink spots are placed within the triangular fossa to mark the site of suture placement for reshaping the superior crus. The last set of ink marks run in the lateral concha just lateral to the newly created antihelical fold, noting the location of the placement of horizontal mattress sutures to keep the reshaped antihelix in place.

Next, these ink marks are transferred from the anterior to the posterior skin of the ear and its underlying cartilage with the help of an abraded 25-gauge needle. This is done by passing the needle through the ink marks in order and, each time, applying methylene blue at its distal end before withdrawing it. Next, a dumbbell-shaped piece of skin is removed from the posterior surface of the concha. The larger the protrusion of the upper third of the ear and/or the earlobe, the wider the excision must be at the corresponding end and the further up and/or down along the concha should it be placed.

Next, the posterior skin of the ear is dissected laterally, close to the helical rim, and medially to the postauricular sulcus and then the mastoid periosteum. Finally, 4-0 Mersilene on a noncutting needle is used to initially place and, thereafter, tie a number of horizontal mattress sutures: one from the triangular fossa to the upper scapha and at least four between the scapha and the lateral portion of the conchal cartilage, as described by Mustarde [24, 25]. Careful attention must be paid to tie the sutures with enough tension so that both the antihelical fold is more defined and the helical rim and scapha are moved posteriorly. The surgeon must also be careful to place the horizontal mattress sutures through the cartilage and not through helical skin.

It may be necessary to slightly overcorrect the defect, as studies have shown that up to 40 % of the loss of correction may occur in the first year postoperatively [3]. The dumbbell-shaped skin incision is then closed using absorbable 4-0 Vicryl subcutaneous sutures and nonabsorbable 5-0 Prolene running sutures on the skin.

Conchal Prominence and/or Anterolateral Rotation

The conchal enlargement and/or anterolateral rotation is addressed by excising an adequate piece of cartilage from the midportion of the concha, either from the posterior or anterior approach.

A crescent-shaped conchal strip is removed, approximately 3–6 mm wide and 2.0–3.0 cm long, extending from the midchoncha cymba down to the incisura terminalis auris. The surgeon should design the crescent-shaped conchal excision so that the incision closure line will fall at the junction of the floor and posterior wall of the concha so as to avoid distortion of the ear's normal contours [2]. This technique serves to reduce the height of the concha. The conchal defect should then be closed with 4-0 Vicryl sutures.

Conchal setback is then completed. A fusiform excision is made in the posterior auricular area. The width of this excision is estimated by pushing the concha toward the mastoid and marking the desired correction. The surgeon should excise the minimal amount of skin needed, as overexcision can lead to excessive tension on the wound and hypertrophic scarring. The skin of the concha, helix, and antihelix is then undermined using blunt scissors.

Conchal setback is then performed by placing multiple horizontal mattress sutures of 4-0 Mersilene between the conchal perichondrium and the mastoid periosteum, as described by Furnas. More specifically, the horizontal mattress sutures should be placed at the lateral third of the conchal cavum and conchal cymba, parallel to the natural curves of the auricle [3]. Finally, the skin is closed with several 4-0 Vicryl subcutaneous sutures and a running 5-0 Prolene suture on the skin [26]

Prominent Helix

Helical prominences can be divided into "spock ears" or "elf ears," caused by excess of the superior outer helical rim cartilage, or "lop ears," created by excess of the superior helical fold cartilage. "Spock ears" or "elf ears" are treated by excising a fusiform-shaped area on the outer helical rim, while "lop ears" are treated by excising a fusiform-shaped area under the helical rim.

Once the fusiform-shaped skin excision is performed, the surgeon should then excise any excess underlying cartilage with a scalpel blade. The skin is closed with nonabsorbable suture, such as 6-0 Prolene [3].

Protruding Earlobe

The protruding earlobe can be corrected by marking the new earlobe with a marker before local anesthesia is injected. Then, the surgeon should perform a fusiform incision anteriorly and posteriorly, and a wedge excision of the prominent lobe is performed. The skin is closed with nonabsorbable suture, such as 6-0 Prolene. The incision line should be hidden in the inferior border of the lobule so that it is not visible on frontal or posterior view.

Postoperative Care

After the surgical site has been cleansed, the corrected ear or ears should be properly dressed. The surgeon may create a molded bolster to effectively stabilize the positioning of the surgically corrected ears and avert hematoma formation. This is created using cotton balls soaked in povidone-iodine and shaped to fit the conchal bowl, scapha, and postauricular space. The mold is held in place with a light compression bandage. One must be careful to avoid too much pressure from the dressing, as this can lead to increased swelling, pain, abrasion, or even necrosis of the skin.

The patient returns one day postoperatively to have the dressing removed, and the surgeon should examine the area for hematoma formation. If there is no hematoma and the wound appears otherwise unremarkable, the dressing is reapplied and fixed with a standard head wrap for one more week. At this time, the nonabsorbable sutures may be removed, and the dressing may also be permanently removed. Following dressing removal, the patient must wear an elastic headband nightly for 3–6 weeks, depending on the scope of the corrective procedure. The purpose of this headband is to inhibit the corrected ear from being pulled forward when the patient rolls over in bed. The patient should be informed that the headband should only be tight enough so that it does not fall off; too tight a headband can erode the lateral surface of the ear and create an open wound. Postoperatively, follow-up is scheduled according to the procedure performed to allow for the early recognition of complications and their appropriate management.

Despite lack of evidence for the use of prophylactic antibiotics in otoplasty, patients may be treated with cephalexin, a first-generation cephalosporin. Typically, the antibiotic is given as a one-time dose intravenously at the time of surgery as a part of the general anesthesia or conscious sedation protocol. If the procedure is done with local anesthesia only, a 1-week course of cephalexin postoperatively is recommended. Alternatively, ciprofloxacin may be used in the patient allergic to penicillin and/or cephalosporins.

Results of the authors otoplasty techniques for the correction of protuberant ears are can be seen in Figs. 40.1, 40.2, 40.3, 40.4, and 40.5.

Complications

Overall, the satisfaction rate for patients undergoing otoplasty for treatment of protuberant ears is very high. However, the most common complication in otoplasty is unsatisfactory aesthetic outcomes for the patient involving inadequate correction, contour distortion, or an asymmetric correction. Overcorrection or unnatural contours is also a common complication of otoplasty. This can result from an incomplete estimation of the number and types of malformations contributing to the patient's protuberant ears or a lack of proper postoperative care. Contours of the corrected ear should be soft, round, and natural [1, 2].

Even though some retroprotrusion can be expected with most otoplasty techniques, it appears to be more common with Mustarde's technique, which uses permanent sutures alone to restructure the ear. In one study of prominent ears treated with Mustarde's technique, 40 % of patients revealed a return of the ear's position to within 3 mm of the preoperative state at 1 year [27]. These findings support the use of cartilage removal or incising techniques aimed at a slight overcorrection to achieve more permanent results. Other causes of recurrence of the original ear deformity include insufficient removal or incision of cartilage to break the cartilage spring, failure to choose a noncutting needle to avoid small cuts in the cartilage that make it more likely for sutures to tear through, and patient noncompliance with postoperative care.

The "telephone ear" deformity results from overcorrection of the middle third of the ear. It is characterized by protuberance of the inferior and superior poles of the ear relative to its middle portion. The use of a doughnut- or dumbbell-shaped excision on the posterior aspect of the ear can prevent this complication. "Reverse telephone ear" deformities can occur with overcorrection of the superior pole and ear lobe, causing a protrusion of the midauricle. Inadequate conchal setback may also produce this deformity. The "hidden helix" deformity is created by overcorrection of the antihelix, producing the incorrect positioning of the helix medial to the antihelix on frontal view. The above deformities may require revision surgery to correct if the patient desires [2].

In the immediate postoperative period, hemorrhage or hematoma formation is the most common complication, occurring about 2 % of the time according to one extensive review of the morbidity of otoplasty [28]. Studies have shown that this complication is one of the few early complications of otoplasty and occurs more commonly when cartilage is disrupted though incision or excision. Symptoms usually include unilateral or bilateral ear pain or tightness within the first 48 h postoperatively. The dressing should be removed, followed by careful inspection of the ear. A hematoma will usually present as a tense, violet-bluish swelling in the retroauricular space, often accompanied by ecchymosis of the surrounding tissue. Evacuation of the hematoma should be performed immediately to prevent perichondritis and the severe ear disfigurement as a result of cartilage necrosis. The patient should also be started on antibiotic therapy to prevent perichondritis [1].

Infection is rare after otoplasty but should be treated aggressively with antibiotic therapy targeting *Staphylococcus*, *Streptococcus*, and *Pseudomonas aeruginosa* to prevent perichondritis. Infection usually presents on day 3 or 4 postoperatively. Pain and tenderness of the ears following the surgery but unrelated to a specific treatable cause may occur up to 1 year postoperatively [29].

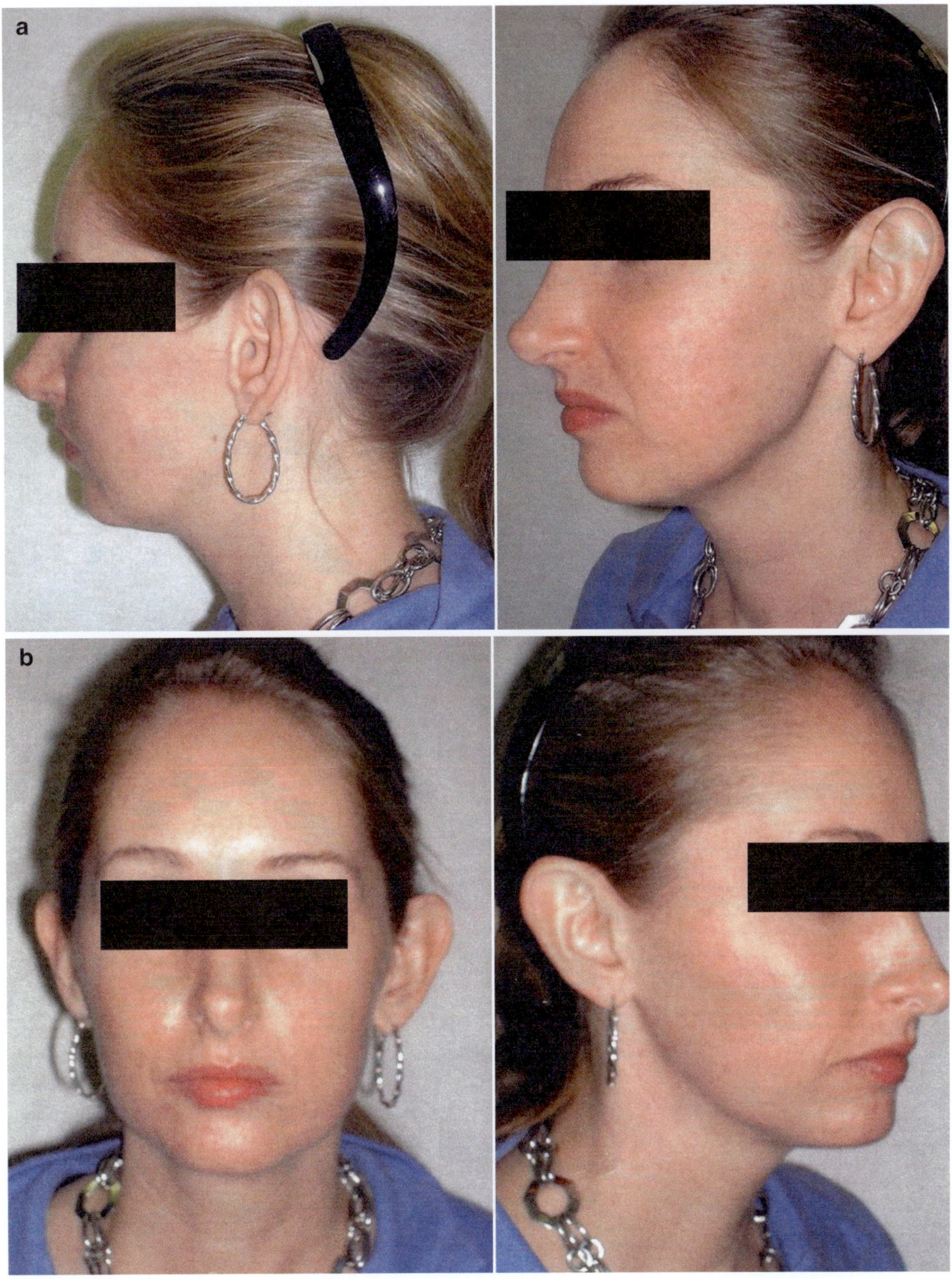

Fig. 40.1 (**a**, **b**) Preoperative patient with prominent ears

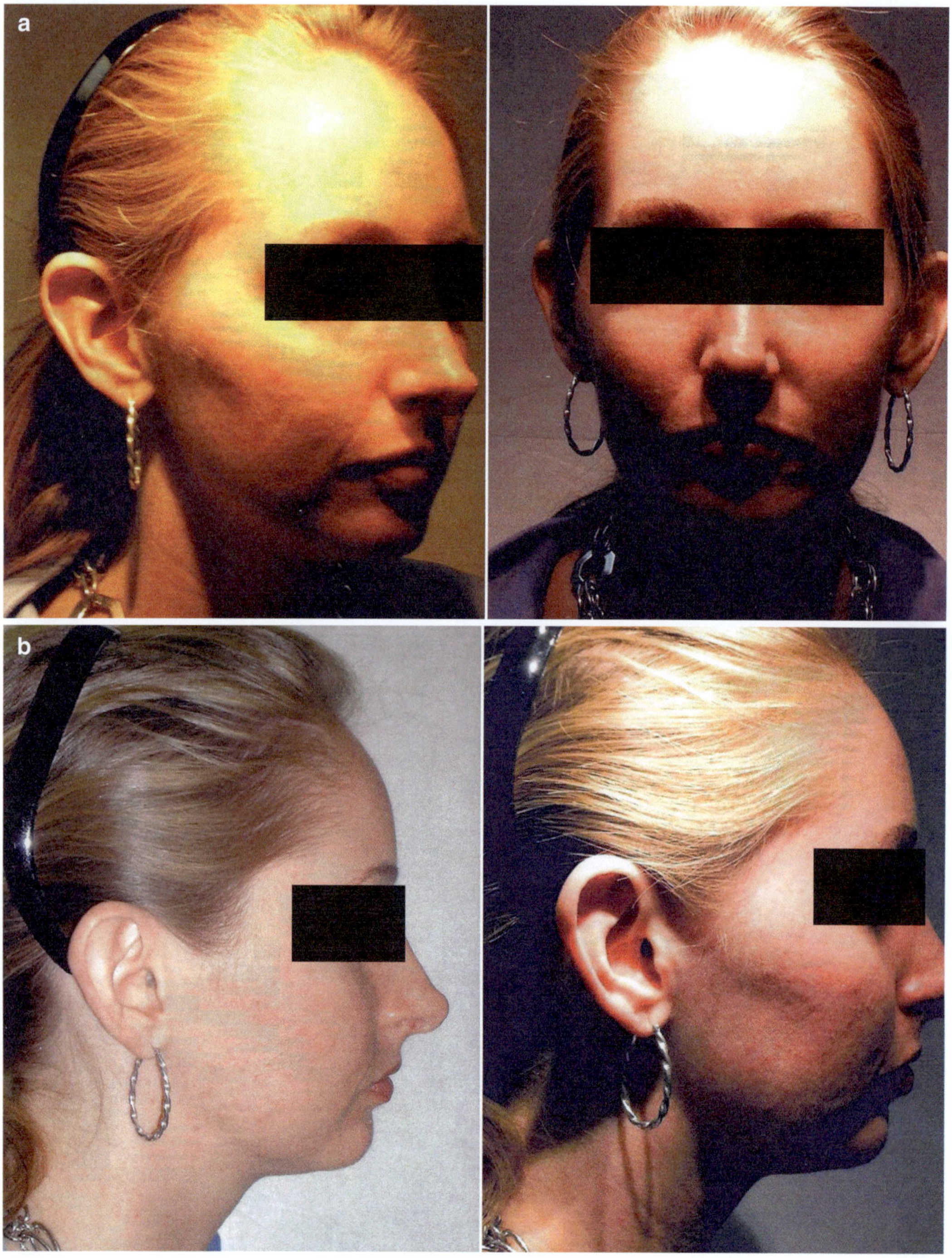

Fig. 40.2 (a, b) Preoperative patient with prominent ears

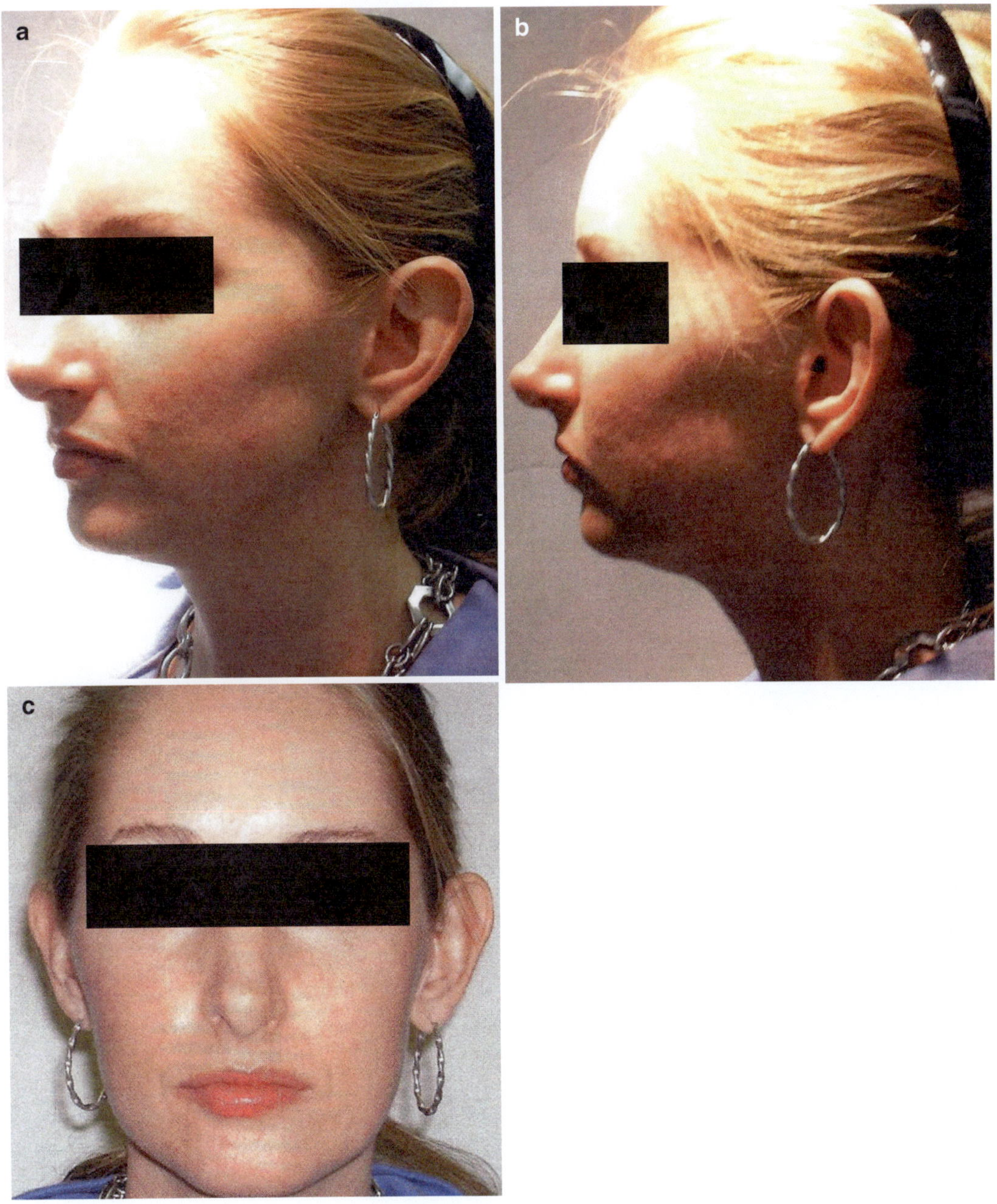

Fig. 40.3 (**a–c**) Preoperative patient with prominent ears

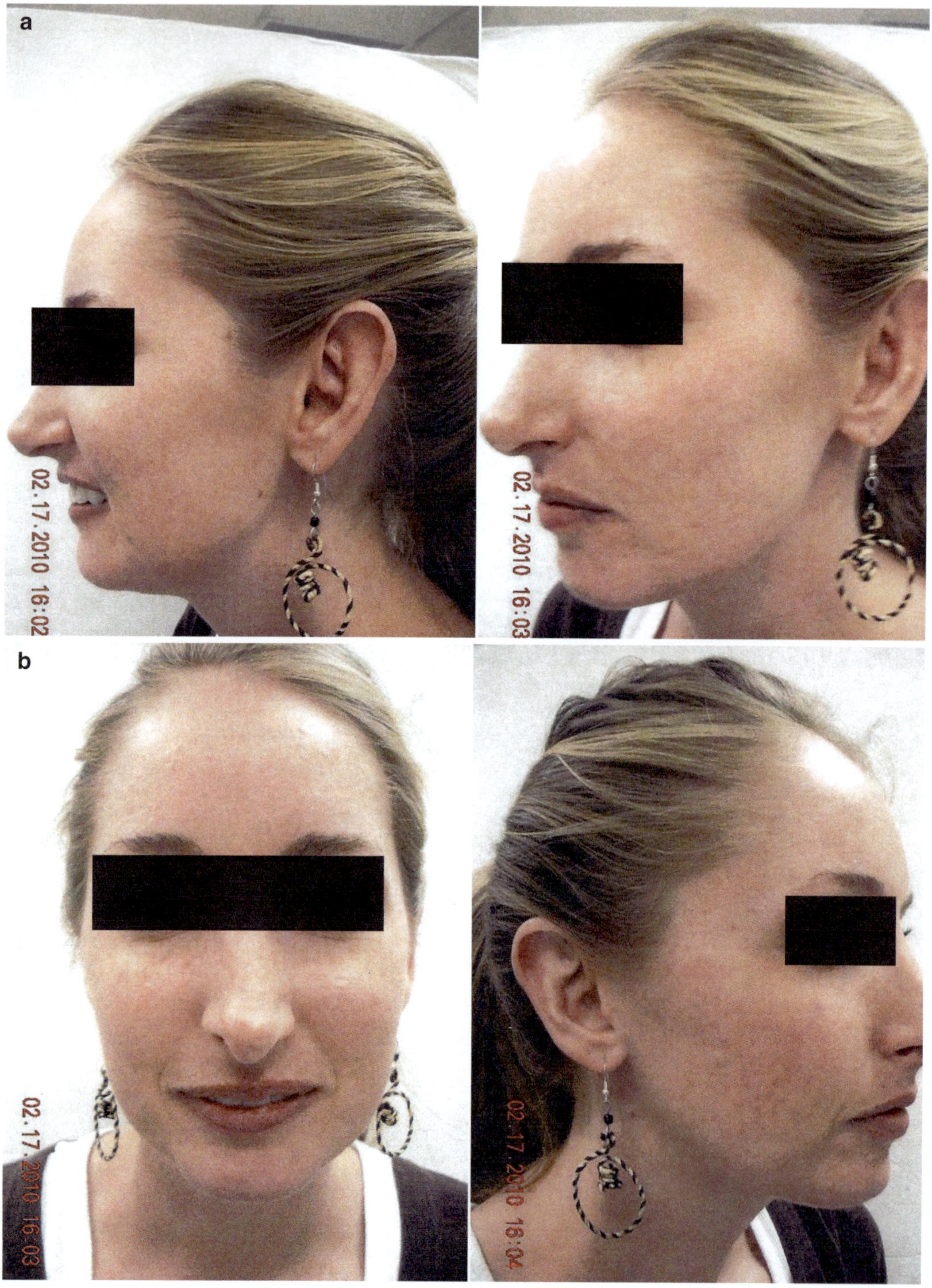

Fig. 40.4 (**a**, **b**) Postoperative patient after correction of prominent ears

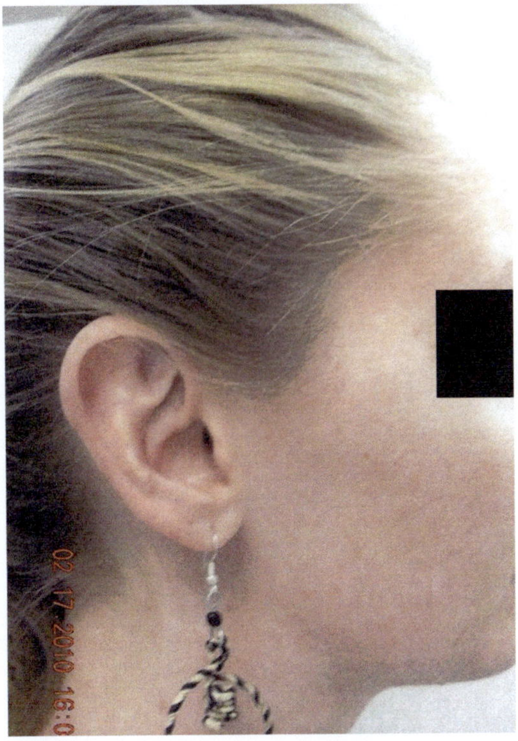

Fig. 40.5 Postoperative patient after correction of prominent ears

Paresthesia of the ear, especially to cold temperatures, may occur but typically improves over 4–6 months.

Suture extrusion and suture granuloma formation can occur, particularly in the retroauricular sulcus. This can be treated by simply removing the sutures and may be prevented by meticulous placement of the sutures by the surgeon. Keloids and hypertrophic scarring may occur, particularly in individuals with a prior history. The use of scar excision and serial intralesional steroid injections can be used for treatment of the condition [3].

Conclusions

Protuberant ears are a relatively common deformity. Successful surgical correction of this deformity in both the children and adults can produce high levels of patient satisfaction and can help treat psychological trauma produced from prominent ears. A thorough understanding by the surgeon of auricular anatomy and common causes of protruding ears, along with precise planning and technique for correction, can produce excellent cosmetic results.

References

1. Bisaccia E, Scarborough D. The Columbia manual of dermatologic cosmetic surgery. New York: McGraw-Hill; 2002.
2. Thorne CH. Otoplasty and ear reconstruction. In: Thorne CH, editor. Grabb and Smith's plastic surgery. 6th ed. Philadelphia: Wolters Kluwer; 2007. p. 297–311.
3. Wise JB, Shah AR, Constantinides M. Otoplasty. In: Lalwani AK, editor. Current diagnosis & treatment in otolaryngology-head & neck surgery. New York: McGraw Hill Medical; 2008. p. 940–8.
4. Dieffenbach JF. Die Operative Chirurgie. Leipzig: FA Brockhaus; 1845. Cited by Tanzer RC. Deformities of the auricle. In: Converse JM, editor. Plastic reconstructive surgery. 2nd ed. Philadelphia: Saunders; 1977. p. 1710.
5. Ely ET. An operation for prominence of auricles. Arch Otolaryngol. 1881;10:97–9.
6. Mustarde JC. The correction of prominent ears using simple mattress sutures: a ten-year survey. Plast Reconstr Surg. 1967;39(4):382–6.
7. Fritsch MH. Incisionless otoplasty. Laryngoscope. 1995;105(5 Pt 3 Suppl 70):1–11.
8. Converse JM, Nigro A, Wilson FA, Johnson N. A technique for surgical correction of the lop ear deformity. Plast Reconstr Surg. 1955;15(5):411–8.
9. Chongchet V. A method of antihelix reconstruction. Br J Plast Surg. 1963;16:268–72.
10. Stenstroem SJ. A natural technique for correction of congenitally prominent ears. Plast Reconstr Surg. 1963;32:283–93.
11. Bisaccia E, Scarborough DA. The surgical correction of the protuberant ear. Cosmet Dermatol. 1990;8:10–2.
12. Kurozumi N, Ono S, Ishida H. Non-surgical correction of a congenital lop ear deformity by splinting with Reston foam. Br J Plast Surg. 1982;35(2):181–2.
13. Matsuo K, Hayashi R, Kiyono M, Hirose T, Netsu Y. Nonsurgical correction of congenital auricular deformities. Clin Plast Surg. 1990;17(2):383–95.
14. Muraoka M, Nakai Y, Ohashi Y, Sasaki T, Maruoka K, Furukawa M. Tape attachment therapy for correction of congenital malformations of the auricle: clinical and experimental studies. Laryngoscope. 1985;95(2):167–76.
15. Hell B, Garbea D, Heissler E, Klein M, Gath H, Langford A. Otoplasty: a combined approach to different structures of the auricle. Int J Oral Maxillofac Surg. 1997;26(6):408–13.
16. Balogh B, Millesi H. Are growth alterations a consequence of surgery for prominent ears? Plast Reconstr Surg. 1992;90(2):192–9.
17. Warmuth IP, Bader R, Scarborough D, Bisaccia E. Otoplasty. Treatment of protuberant ears. Cosmet Dermatol. 1999;12(4):7–8.

18. Bradbury ET, Hewison J, Timmons MJ. Psychological and social outcome of prominent ear correction in children. Br J Plast Surg. 1992;45(2):97–100.
19. Elliott RA. Otoplasty. In: Regnault P, Daniel RK, editors. Esthetic plastic surgery. Boston: Little, Brown; 1984. p. 245–74.
20. Burres S. The anterior-posterior otoplasty. Arch Otolaryngol Head Neck Surg. 1998;124(2):181–5.
21. Becker OJ. Surgical correction of the abnormally protruding ear. Arch Otolaryngol. 1949;50(5):541–60.
22. Elliot RA. Otoplasty: a combined approach. Clin Plast Surg. 1990;17(2):373–81.
23. Davis J. Aesthetic and reconstructive otoplasty. New York: Springer; 1987. p. 37.
24. Spira M. Otoplasty: what I do now – a 30-year perspective. Plast Reconstr Surg. 1999;104(3):834–40.
25. Ducic Y, Hilger PA. Effective step-by-step technique for the surgical treatment of protruding ears. J Otolaryngol. 1999;28(2):59–64.
26. Lavy J, Stearns M. Otoplasty: techniques, results and complications – a review. Clin Otolaryngol Allied Sci. 1997;22(5):390–3.
27. Messner AH, Williams SC. Otoplasty: clinical protocol and long-term results. Arch Otolaryngol Head Neck Surg. 1996;122(7):773–7.
28. Calder JC, Naasan A. Morbidity of otoplasty: a review of 562 consecutive cases. Br J Plast Surg. 1994; 47(3):170–4.
29. Tan KH. Long-term study of prominent ear surgery: a comparison of two methods. Br J Plast Surg. 1986;39(2): 270–3.

Separating the Helix from the Antihelix: A New Concept in Prominent Ear Correction

41

Augusto Sette Câmara Valente

Introduction

The literature has published more than 200 techniques to correct protruding ears. This means that no isolated technique brings natural and permanent results in all kinds of folded antihelix deformities. Many different kinds of incisions, sutures, and cartilage-weakening procedures were created to correct a problem that affects 5 % of the Caucasian population. The stigma of protruding ears not only affects the socialization of the individual, but also leads to low self-esteem. The ears being on the face calls immediate attention to the problem, especially in men, since their haircuts do not allow them to hide the ear. Although the physiological consequences are negligible, the aesthetic and psychological effects on the patient can be substantial (Fig. 41.1).

The techniques described achieve satisfactory results, but few obtain what can be considered a perfect result, especially in ears with hard and thick cartilage. The separation of the helix and scaphoid fossa from the body of the ear (antihelix and concha), completely breaking the cartilage's inherent spring memory, allows the use of absorbable sutures to remodel it without any tension. This chapter is based on work published by the author in 2010 [1]. Modifications have been made to the original concept to improve the technique. A suture is introduced to align the helix with the new antihelix. In some ears whose deformity is in the middle and upper thirds of the ear, the originally described incision is used in part.

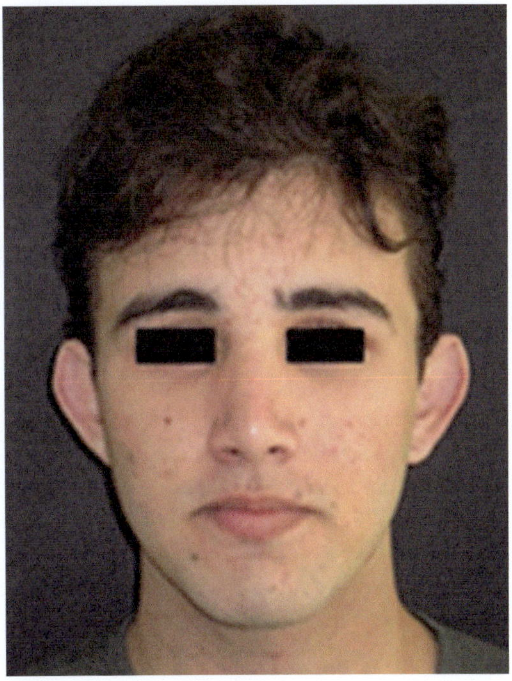

Fig. 41.1 The stigma of having protruding ears

History

In 1845, Dieffenbach [2] described the first treatment of protruding ear (posttraumatic) through the resection of the posterior skin and suturing of

A.S.C. Valente, M.D.
Rua Jose Negrao de lima 260,
Belvedere-Belo Horizonte, MG 30320280, Brazil
e-mail: augustoscvalente@gmail.com.br

M.A. Shiffman (ed.), *Advanced Cosmetic Otoplasty*,
DOI 10.1007/978-3-642-35431-1_41, © Springer-Verlag Berlin Heidelberg 2013

the auricular cartilage to the mastoid region. Ely [3] (1881) described his technique for correcting prominent ears by elective surgery: a postauricular skin excision, a conchomastoidal fixation, and conchal cartilage strip excision. Morestin [4] (1903) recognized the need for spring breakage to obtain definitive results. In 1910, Luckett [5] demonstrated that the deformity of protruding ears was chiefly the result of faulty folding of the antihelix. After this, several articles with various ideas for breaking the spring memory were published in the literature, especially involving complete or partial incisions of the cartilage in various forms and in various positions of the auricular pavilion.

Becker [6] introduced the concept of creating a tube of parallel incisions and use of sutures in 1952. This concept was redefined by Converse in 1953 and 1963 [7, 8]. In 1958, Gibson and Davis [9] published an article demonstrating the characteristic of the cartilage bending on the side opposite to its weakness. This concept was added to the technique of Mustardé [10], which used only mattress sutures to create the fold. Stenstrom [11] first abraded the cartilage and modeled the antihelix with sutures, decreasing the recurrence rate with this modification.

The concept of separating the antihelix from the helix was first described in 1963 by Chongchet [12]; later in 1964 came the ideas of Crikelair and Cosman [13], then Nordzell in 2000 [14] and Caouette-Laberge [15] in 2000. Their techniques exposed the anterior surface of the auricular pavilion and weakened the cartilage with striations made by partial incisions, drilling, and rasping. The incision placements broke the cartilage memory, but were not specific about the design of the antihelix, creating good but not perfect results. Furthermore, the helix was not firm, curving mainly on its medium third, which sometimes left a "dog ear" appearance as the end result.

Technique

Uncooperative patients and children receive general anesthesia. For other patients, only local anesthesia, possibly with the addition of intravenous sedation, is used. One percent lidocaine is used with epinephrine 1:200,000, asepsis is achieved with Betadine, and it is not necessary to cut the patient's hair. Local anesthesia is administered by regional, ring-like instillation of the anesthetic solution with subsequent infiltration of the entire posterior skin of the ear and the anterior region for designing the antihelix, facilitating making the mattress sutures (hydrodissection) [16].

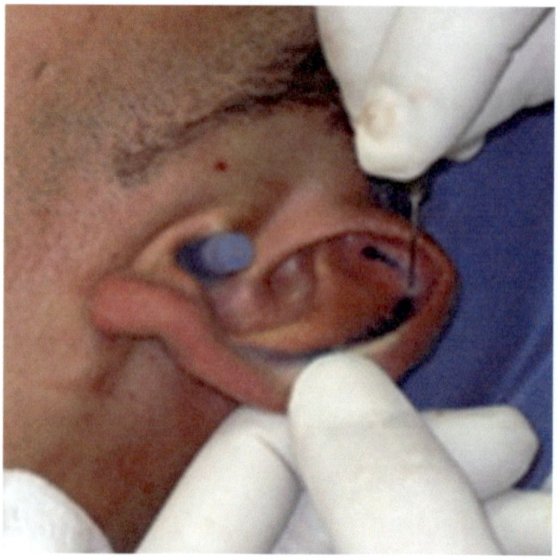

Fig. 41.2 Tattooing the cartilage with a needle on the superior and lateral border of the antihelix

The position of the antihelix is determined with the push-back finger maneuver. The cartilage is tattooed with methylene blue, and the needles are introduced through the full thickness of the ear in as many places as necessary in the superior and posterior border of the antihelix precisely from the beginning of the triangular fossa to the tail of the helix. These marks define the exact location of the posterior incision in the cartilage (Fig. 41.2).

A posterior skin incision is made in the form of a dumbbell, running almost the whole length of the ear, with two ellipses in the superior and inferior third and a narrow bridge in the middle third of the auricle. It is located in the projection of the antihelix's body that bends (Fig. 41.3). The placement of the incision is important for controlling the helix and the earlobe position. A narrow bridge incision in the middle third is necessary to avoid overcorrection of this seg-

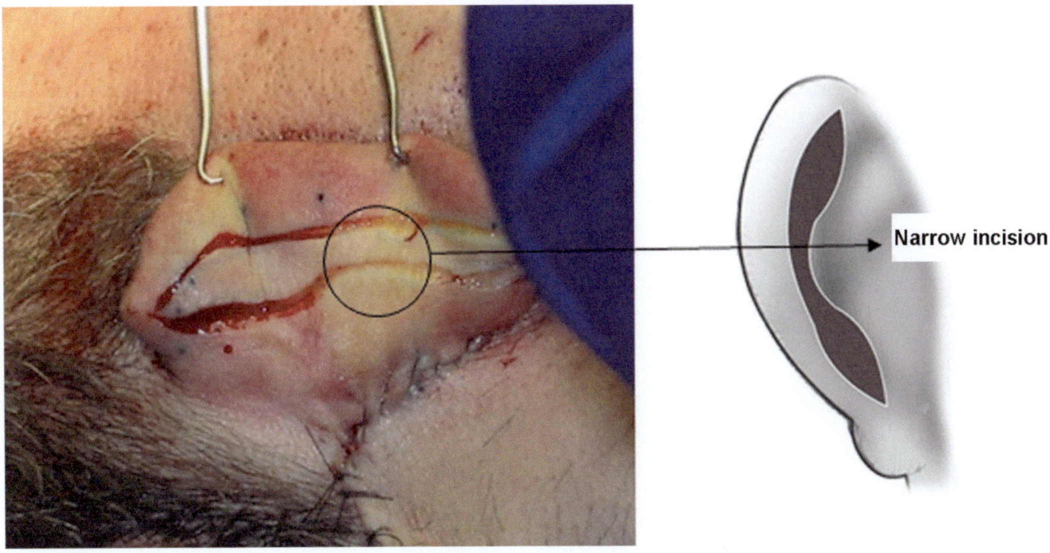

Fig. 41.3 Bielliptical posterior skin incision with a narrow bridge in the middle third of the ear. The narrow bridge is very important to avoid overcorrection. The sizes of the superior and inferior ellipses are determined based on the degree of ear prominence and are important for the correct helix and earlobe position

ment. The amount of posterior skin resection (size of the ellipses) defines the exact position of the helix and the earlobe.

The incised skin is removed, undermining the posterior surface of the cartilage. Hemostasis must be rigorous. After total exposition of the posterior side of the cartilage, the methylene blue marks are identified, and another mark is made on the cartilage line to be incised (Fig. 41.4). The complete incision in the cartilage includes the tail of the helix, going by the posterior border of the antihelix until the triangular fossa. At this point, the index finger is positioned at the anterior aspect of the ear, with the thumb holding the skin hooks to force the cartilage forward, facilitating the incision. When there is a normal positioning of the earlobe and the tail of a helix (the prominence involves only the middle and superior third), a partial incision is made as originally described, starting in the middle third of the antihelix and proceeding to the triangular fossa (Fig. 41.5). This modification allows shortening of the surgical time and reducing the trauma, but maintains the original idea and results.

Anteriorly, the antihelix's body is undermined with Stevens scissors to expose this structure completely. Three 4-0 polyglycolic acid mattress sutures are applied to reshape the new antihelix. It is not necessary to employ a nonabsorbable suture because the antihelix has lost its spring strength. The first suture is placed in the superior part of the antihelix, and this knot is tied with more slack than the second one, which is placed next to the first in the middle third of the antihelix. The third suture is placed more inferiorly in the region between the antitragus and the conchal

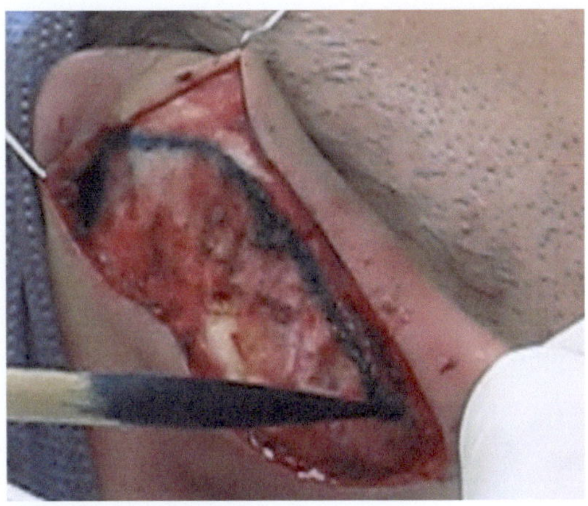

Fig. 41.4 Cartilage with marked tattooing points

cartilage to maintain the curve of the antihelix (Fig. 41.6). A fourth suture [17, 18] is applied to position the tail of the helix if there is an important lateral projection of this structure and the lobule. In cases in which the cartilage is very thick, it is necessary to make a parallel 10-mm incision to weaken the spring and facilitate the fold by suturing next to the antitragus region.

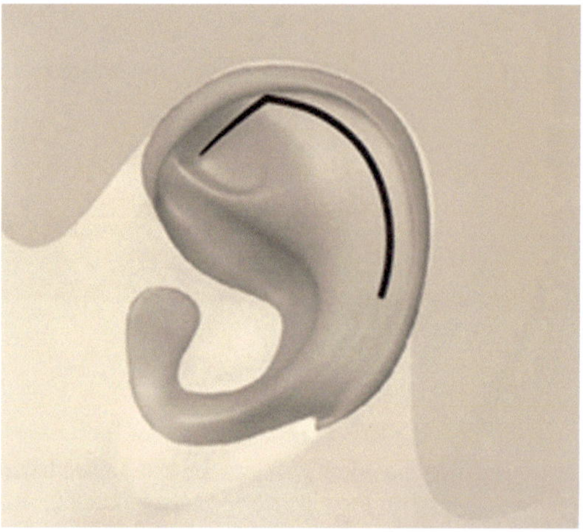

Fig. 41.5 Partial incision in the outer border of the antihelix, used in cases of superior and middle third prominence, as a modification of the original technique in these specific cases

The alignment point between the helix and the antihelix should be determined accurately to avoid distorting the anatomy of the ear (Fig. 41.7). Finally, as a refinement, a small strip of the cartilage is excised from the superior part of the lateral border of the newly shaped antihelical fold, close to the scaphoid fossa, to avoid any unexpected posterior projection of the cartilage at the back edge of the ear. This excision functions to simulate the natural shape of the antihelix, too (Fig. 41.8).

Great care should be taken in the reconstruction of the ear to obtain a perfect result with no recurrence.

The conchal cartilage should be operated upon only if a high degree of hypertrophy is present. In the author's view, the best way to do this is to set it back with a mastoid fixation [19] or an elliptical resection of the concha in the portion close to the cranium.

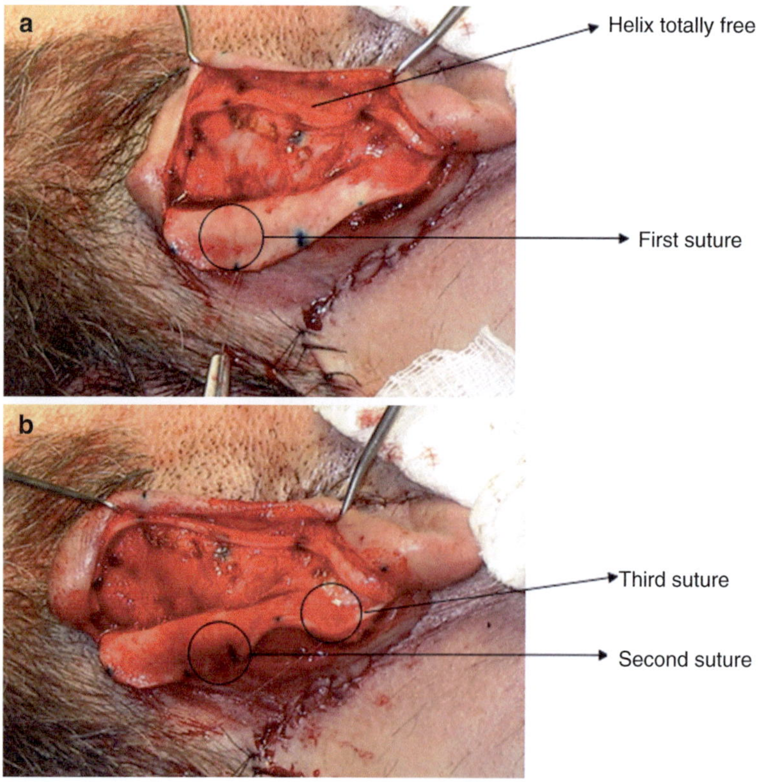

Fig. 41.6 (**a**, **b**) Three absorbable mattress sutures to reshape the new antihelix

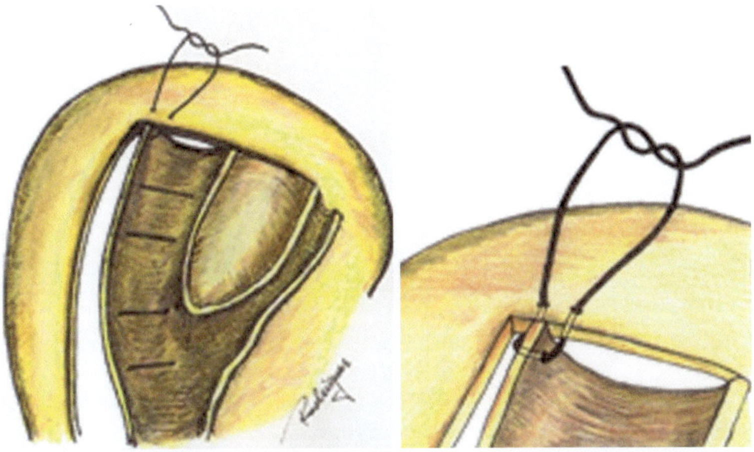

Fig. 41.7 The alignment point

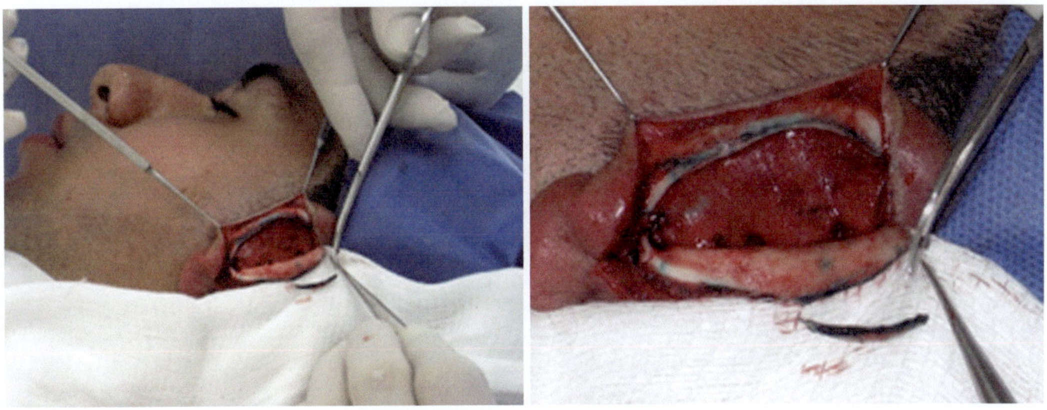

Fig. 41.8 A small strip of cartilage is cut off from the superior part of the lateral border of the antihelix to avoid posterior projection after surgery and simulates the natural shape of the antihelix

The ear dressing consists first of wet cotton soaked in 70 % alcohol, which is carefully molded into the concavities of the new ear's fold; a larger, dried portion of cotton is applied with a bandage placed around the head, which is kept in place for 4 days (Fig. 41.9). Because of the extensive undermining of the flaps, the dressing should never be tightened, thus preventing the occurrence of epidermolysis/necrosis.

Discussion

The strength and memory of the cartilage spring are the most difficult problems to solve in otoplasties, particularly when the cartilage is thick. Many authors have focused their efforts on weakening this region (the antihelix) and described a number of innovative ideas that have led to good, though not always perfect results. Moreover, the previously described procedures were time consuming, and some cases of irregularities in the antihelical fold were reported.

The general engineering of the ear spring results in a very strong and stable structure. The spring strength is determined by the complex strength of the fibers' distribution and continuity, which begins in the conchal region and is sustained in the helix. The helix acts as a framework, sustaining that structure to maintain the original position of the ear and the strength of the spring. If this distal continuity is broken, the spring loses strength because it has lost its support. A global view of the problem led the author

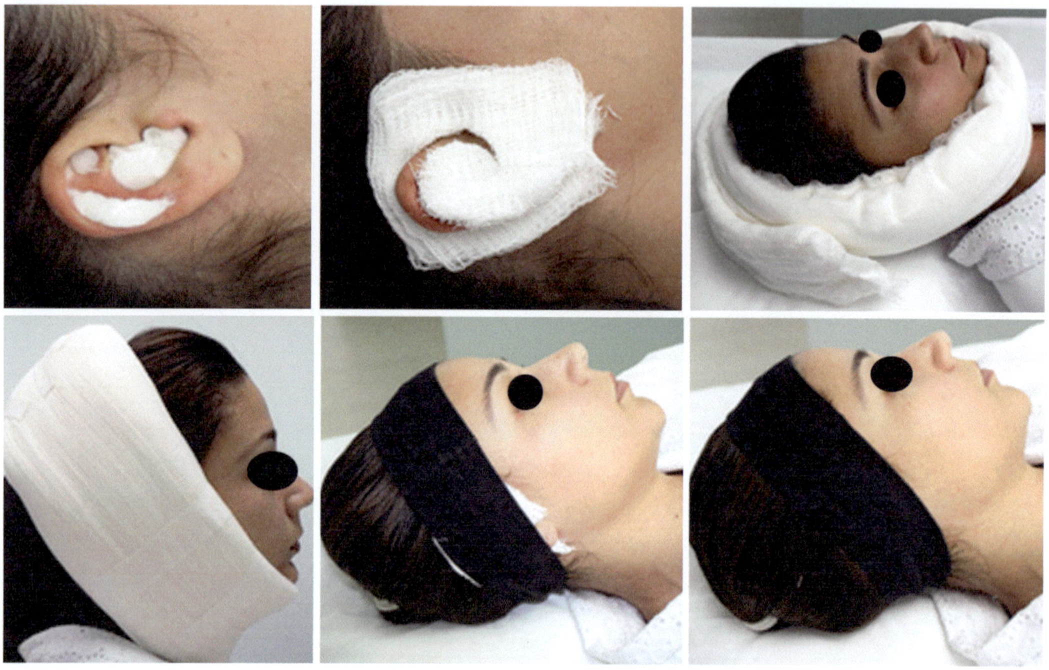

Fig. 41.9 Dressing. Cotton soaked in 70 % ethyl alcohol inside the ear's convolutions and a large dry cotton bandaged head to maintain the head's position at bedtime and to protect the new auricular pavilion

to conceive of another way to reshape this structure by deconstructing the ear, rebuilding it, and placing it in a new position to heal. This is the key point of this technique.

The separation of the helix/scaphoid fossa from the antihelix/concha breaks the spring force of the cartilage completely, facilitating the making of a new antihelix and the repositioning of the helix and the earlobe.

The precise location of the incision exactly according to the design of the antihelix creates two separate structures, the helix and the scaphoid fossa, from the antihelix and concha. The former is completely free for positioning in its proper position. The latter, now free from its distal support, tends, with its radial beams, to bend the antihelix. We use the cartilage spring strength in our favor (Fig. 41.10).

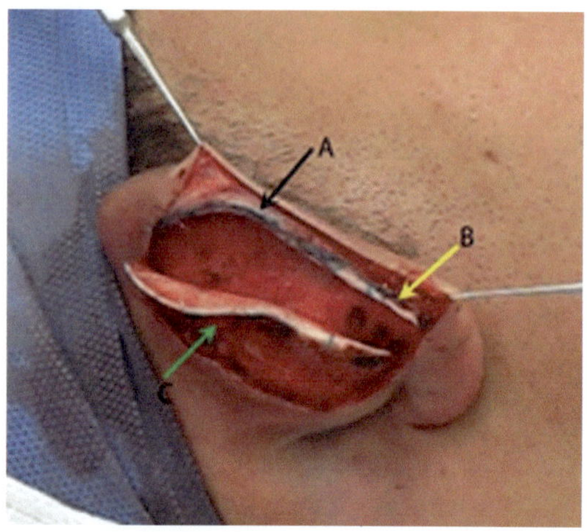

Fig. 41.10 Separating the helix from the antihelix. *Black arrow* (helix), *green arrow* (antihelix), and *yellow arrow* (tail of the helix). Notice how the posterior border of the antihelix is free to be folded

The techniques using sutures and weakening work well on fine cartilage, but the angle created at the outer edge of the antihelix is rounded and not 90°, as it would be a normal ear (Fig. 41.11). When bending to the antihelix, the helix also tends to bend, especially in its most cranial segment, because they are united. Thus, retaining part of the spring force predisposes to partial or total relapse.

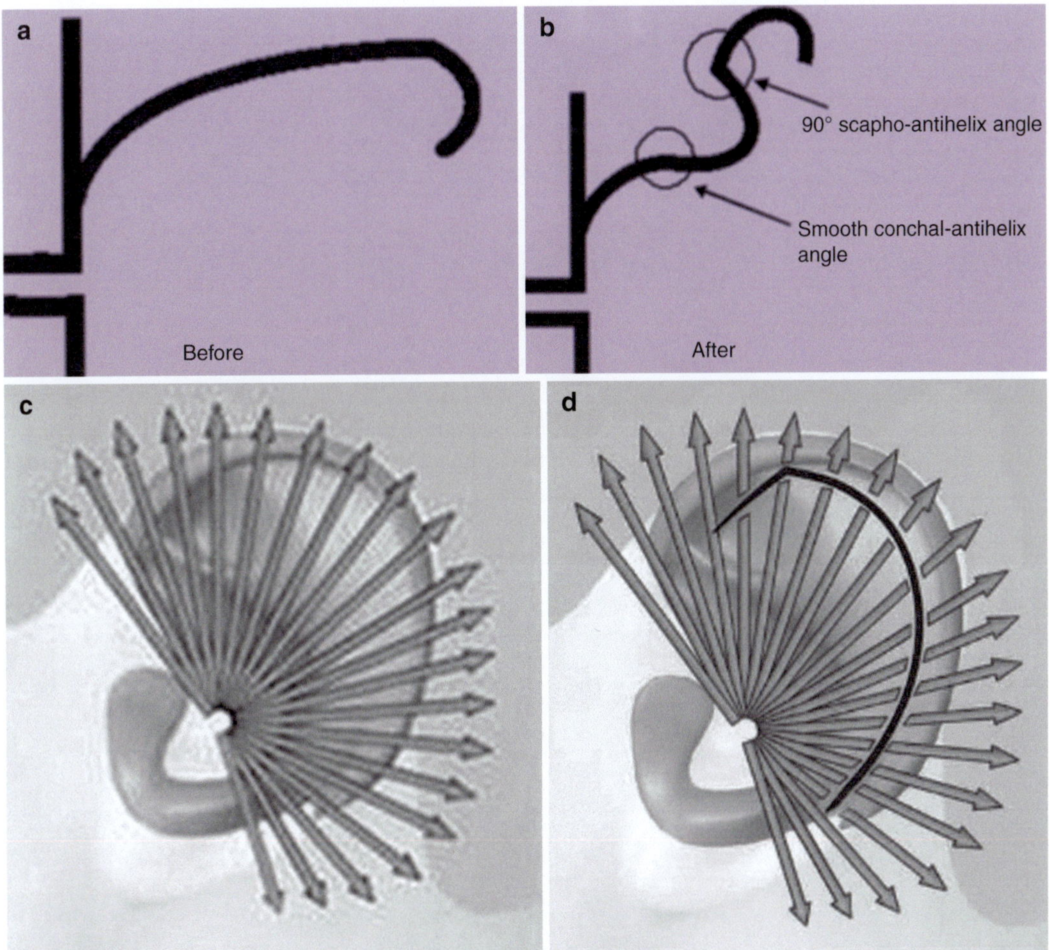

Fig. 41.11 (**a–d**) The leaf spring before and after applying the technique to create new and natural antihelix angles with the adjacent structures. The new angle is 90° with the scapha and helix smooth with the concha

The techniques that use complete incisions in the cartilage break the spring, but should be positioned exactly on the outer edge lateral and superior to the antihelix. The incision should be in exactly positioned to deconstruct the ear without leaving sharp edges at the postoperative site and maintaining the helix in a firm position for attachment to the scaphoid fossa.

The double incisions (parallel) in cartilage in techniques such as the Converse create short beams. The spring is extremely strong, and sometimes even a suture as thick as nylon 2–0 is unable to maintain the folding structure. This mainly occurs in thick cartilage. With another incision close to the concha, the opportunity is lost to use the leaf spring leaving the concha for our purposes. The advantage is to facilitate bending. The angle created by the incision in the region of the antihelix with the concha creates an angle that is not natural with sharp edges (Fig. 41.12).

All the techniques that use weakening of the cartilage – scoring, rasping, and especially partial incisions – are time consuming and can cause visible irregularities. With the incision described in this chapter, this becomes unnecessary. The modification added to the original technique proved fundamental when the

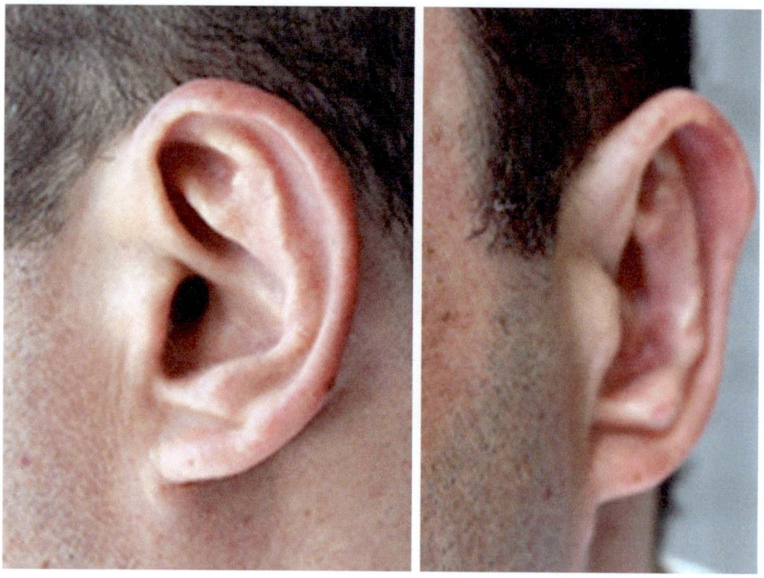

Fig. 41.12 Operated with the Converse technique. Note the unnatural angles created in the conchal-antihelix-scaphal region and the sharp edges. Also note the very short and strong leaf spring that lost its curvature, which was created with sutures with time

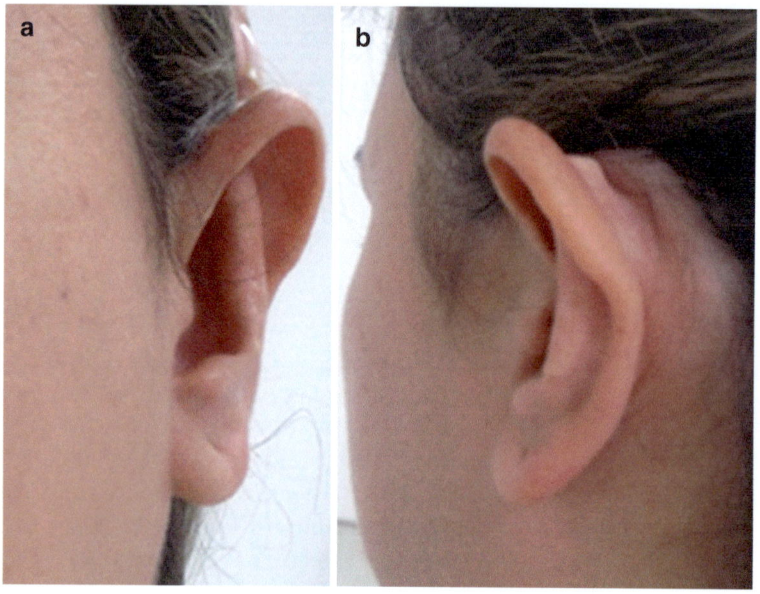

Fig. 41.13 (**a**, **b**) Complete recurrence of upper pole and a lack of alignment of the new antihelix in relation to the helix

author's cases no. 61 showed a misalignment of the two structures formed and an almost complete recurrence of the upper pole of the ear, the first time this has occurred (Fig. 41.13). It was clear that in certain patients resection of the upper skin ellipse was not enough for adequately positioning the helix and scapha. The alignment point was designed to solve this problem (Fig. 41.14).

In ears with prominence only in the region of the middle third and upper pole (Fig. 41.15), partial incision is extremely efficient (Fig. 41.16).

The postauricular incision associated with posterior undermining throughout obtained optimal results with an imperceptible scar.

The postoperative results followed the precepts of McDowel [20] and La Trenta [21] for aesthetic otoplasty (Fig. 41.17). The results are

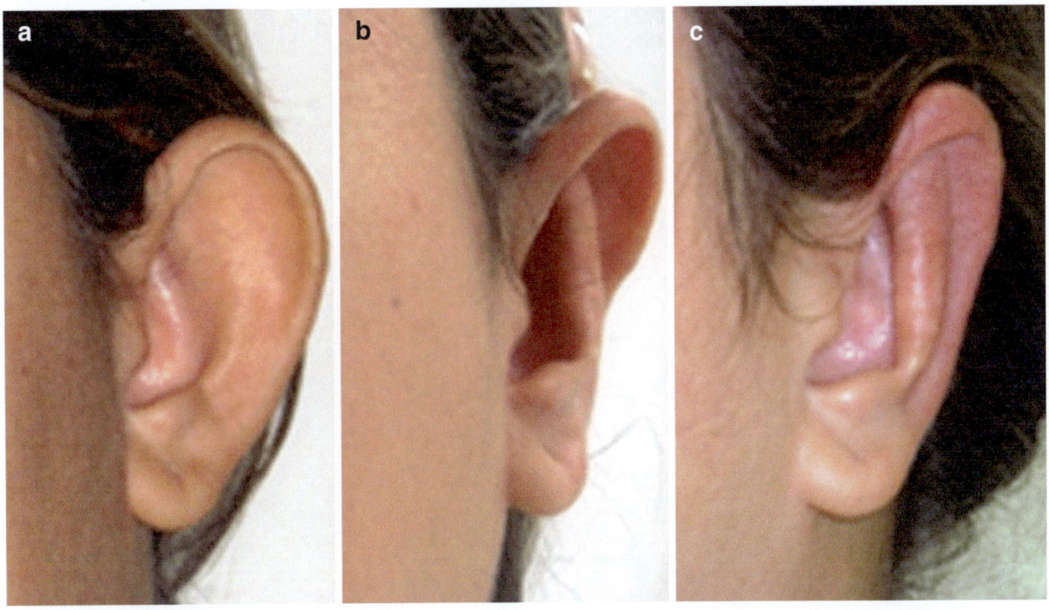

Fig. 41.14 (**a**) Preoperative 25-year-old. (**b**) Ten months postoperatively. (**c**) One month after reoperation

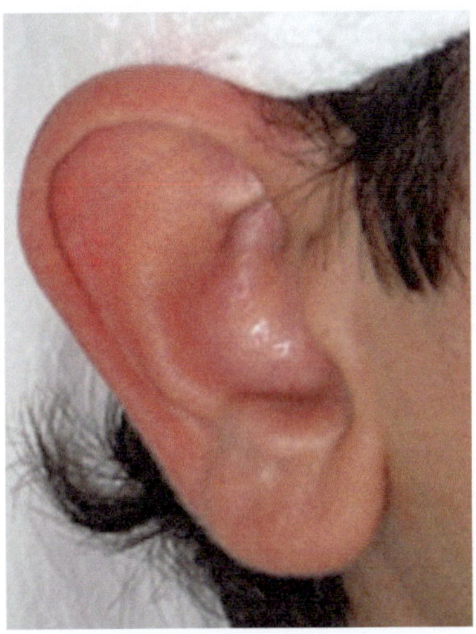

Fig. 41.15 Preoperative 14-year-old male. Note the prominence in the middle third and upper pole and the normal position of the inferior third and earlobe

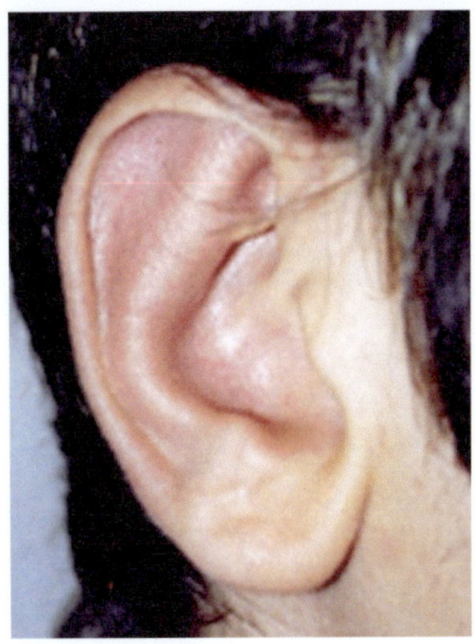

Fig. 41.16 One year after surgical correction. The result is very natural with partial incision

very natural looking, with the helix appearing straight and seeming to be beyond the antihelix from the frontal view. The antihelix contours appear smooth, round, and without irregularities, instead of being sharp, straight, or unnatural (Figs. 41.18, 41.19, 41.20, and 41.21).

Complications

Complications are the same as described in the literature – small hematomas, epidermolysis, retroauricular keloids, and late hypersensitivity – and the author has not experienced any cases of infection

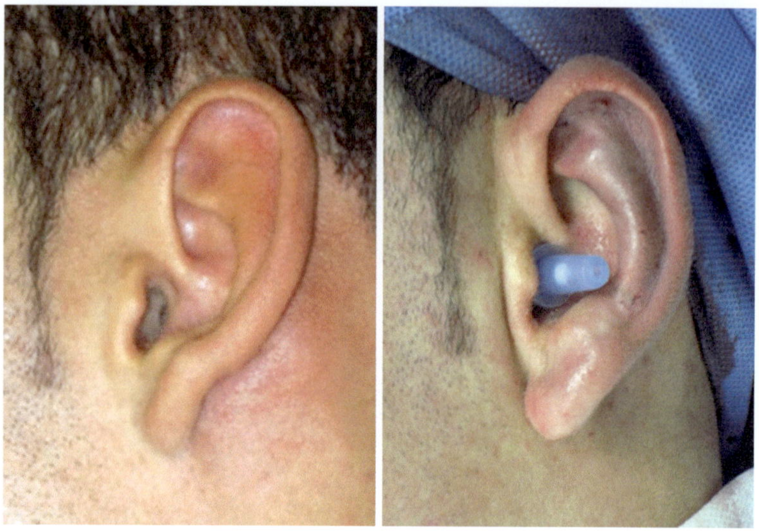

Fig. 41.17 (*Left*) Preoperative. (*Right*) Postoperative immediately after surgery

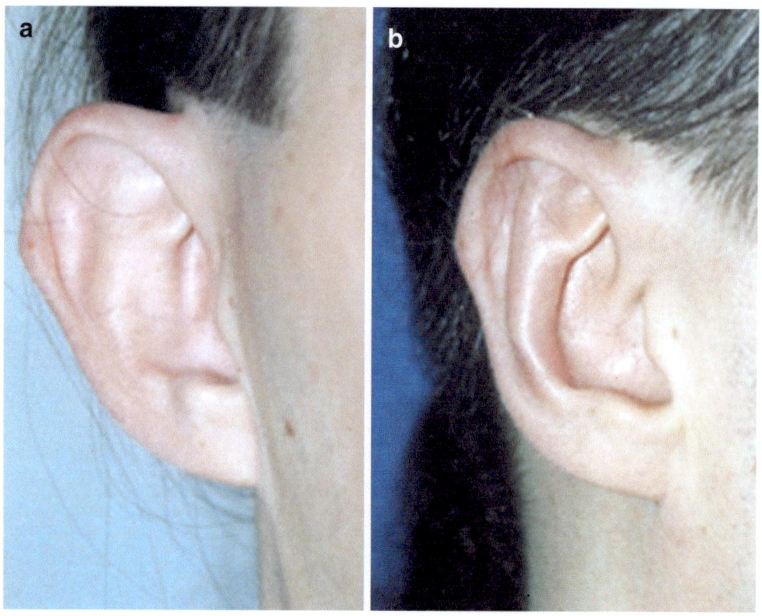

Fig. 41.18 (**a**) Preoperative 25-year-old male. (**b**) Eighteen months after correction of protruding ears

or dehiscence. All low rates are compatible with those reported in the literature [22]. Recurrences, which occurred mainly in the upper pole at the beginning of the series, have not occurred again so far in the last 26 patients since starting to use an alignment point. One patient presented with an unnatural, tube-like result (Fig. 41.22) caused by the sutures being very close to each other.

In a total of 86 patients, the satisfaction rate was 97.66 %. Very good results were achieved in 75 patients (87.22 %), good results in 9 patients (10.46 %), acceptable results in 1 patient (1.16 %), and a bad result in 1 (1.16 %) (Table 41.1).

Conclusions

Surgery for correction of prominent ears may at first seem to be a simple and easy procedure when we think that it only corrects the scaphocephalic angle to 30° in the preoperative and postoperative front view photos as a parameter of outcome. But if we think of the precepts of McDowell, La Trenta, and others, and the lateral and oblique views, the perfection of the structures becomes difficult to obtain because the ear is formed entirely of cartilage. This structure has a very powerful spring memory, and any incision or stitches made the

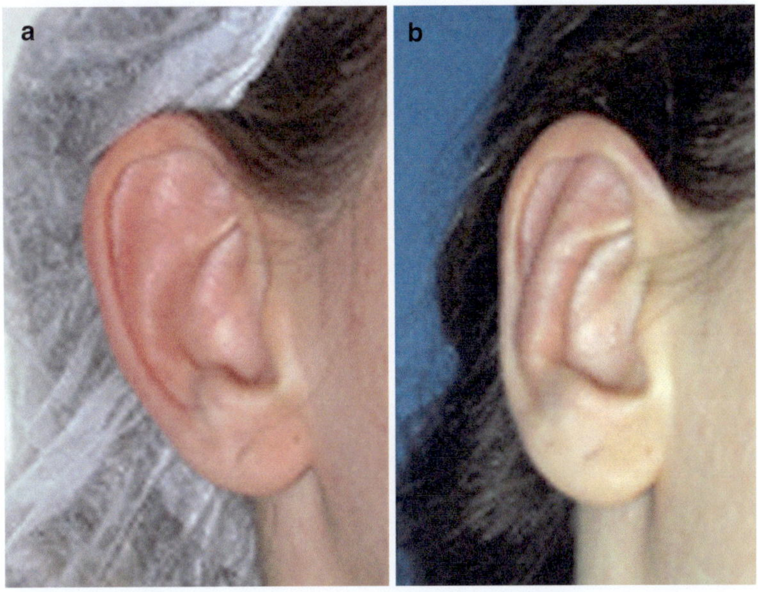

Fig. 41.19 (**a**) Preoperative 25-year-old female. (**b**) Three years after ear correction

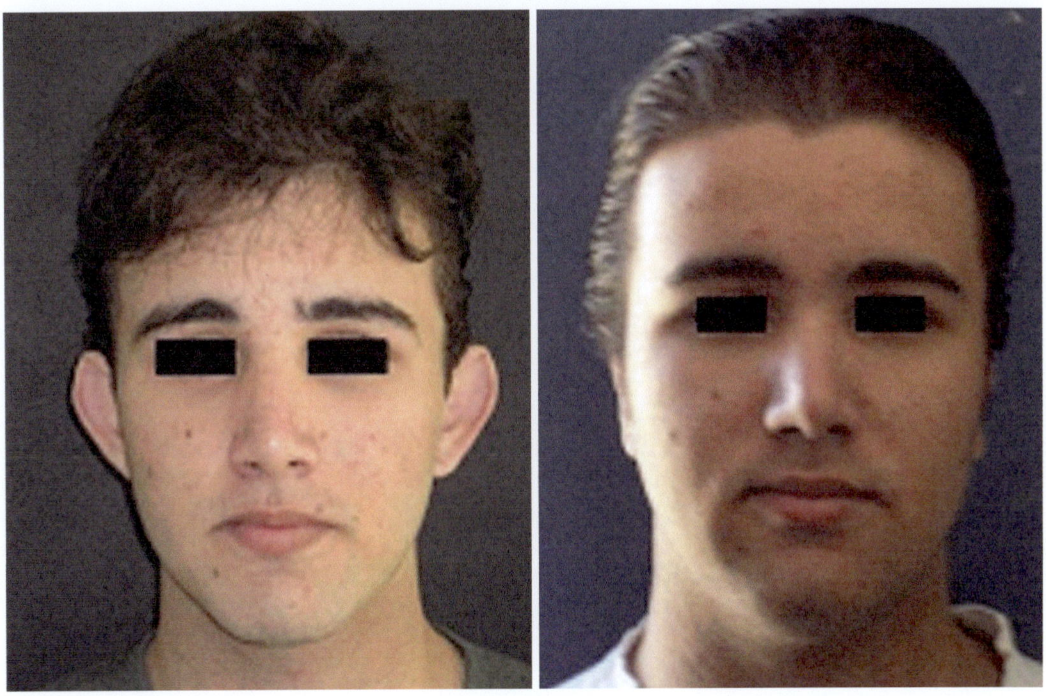

Fig. 41.20 (*Left*) Preoperative 15-year-old male. (*Right*) Five months after surgery

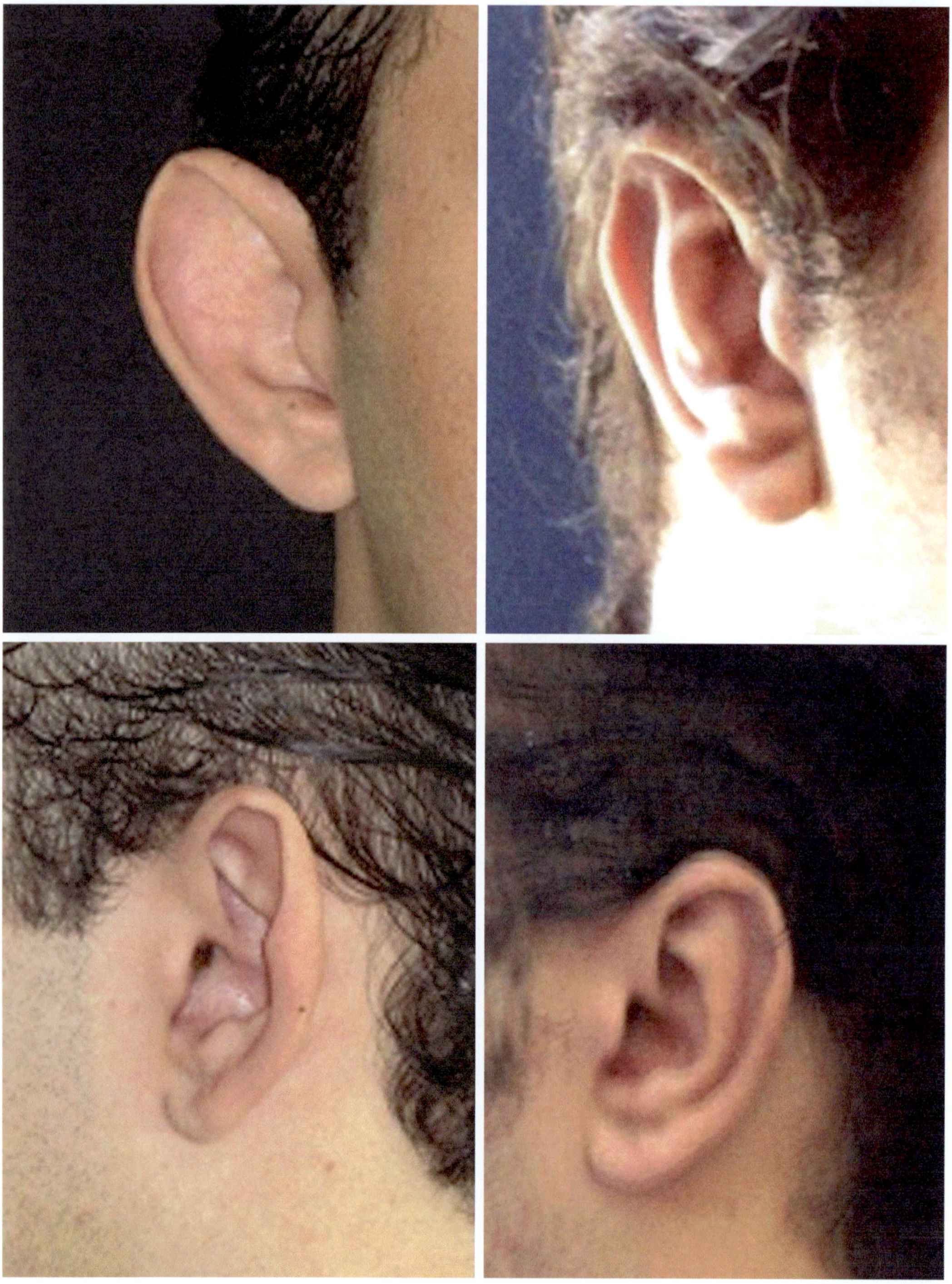

Fig. 41.20 (continued)

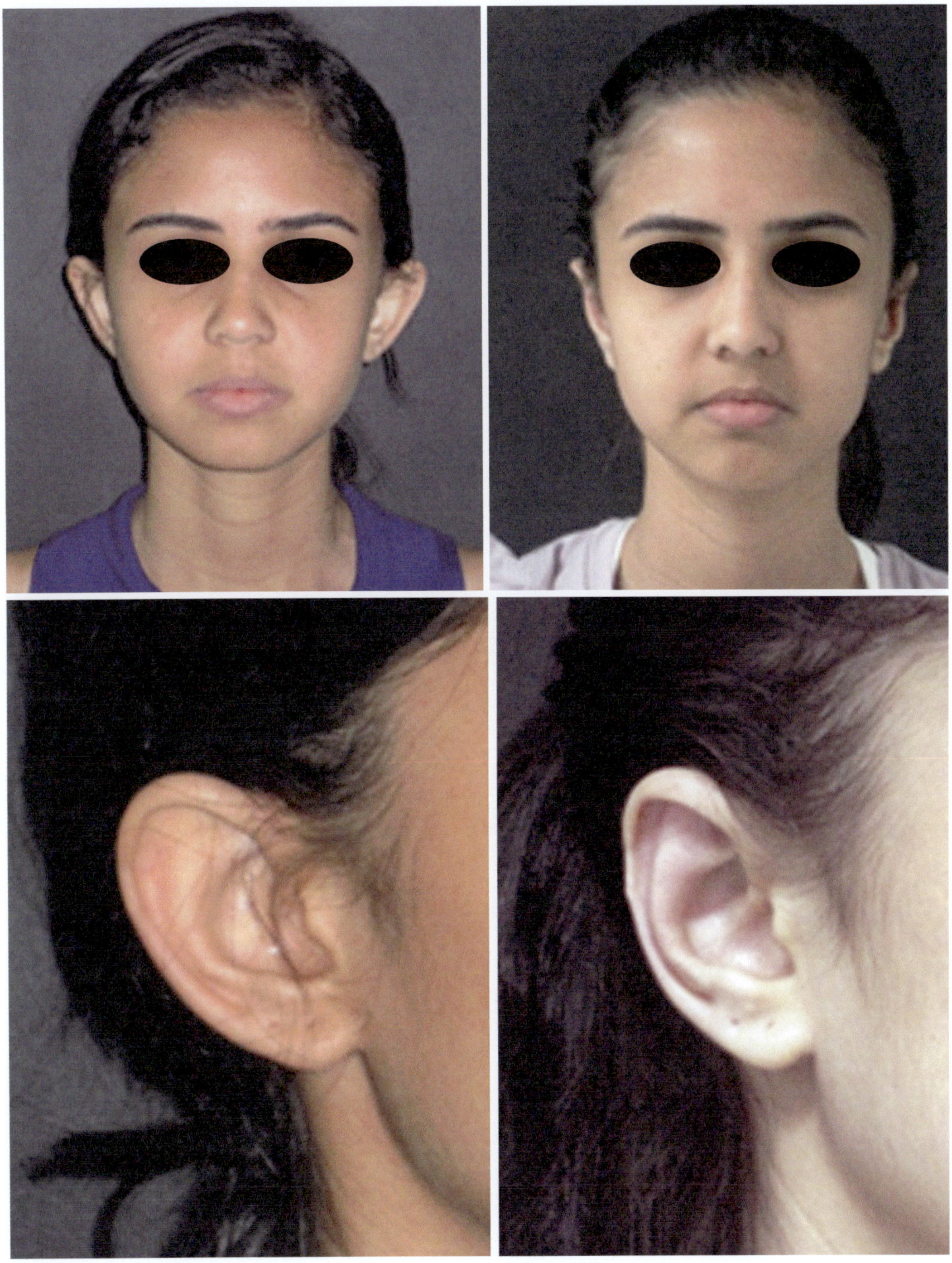

Fig. 41.21 (*Left*) Preoperative 18-year-old female. (*Right*) Postoperative

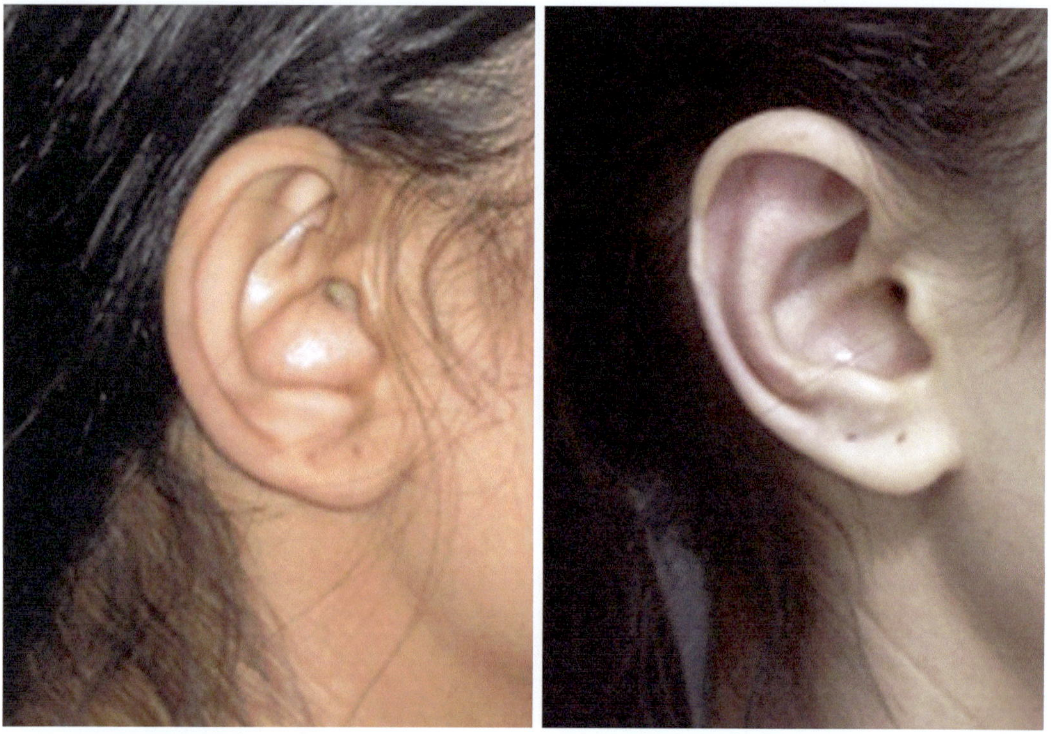

Fig. 41.21 (continued)

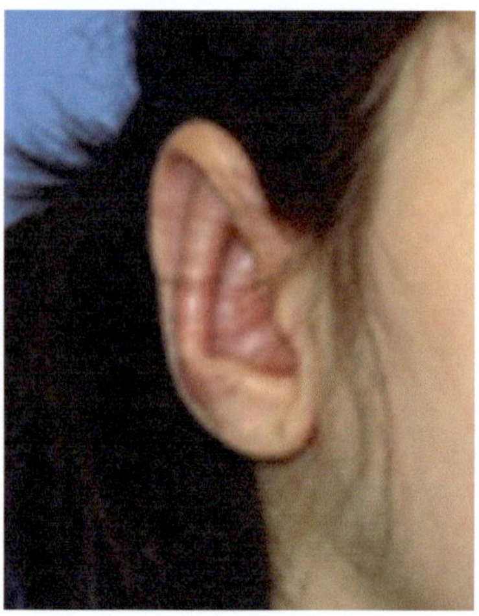

Fig. 41.22 Unnatural tube-like antihelix

wrong way can result in a deformity or change in the expected result.

The various techniques described currently use weakening (several types), sutures, and incisions of the cartilage. Based on what has been presented, complete incision of the cartilage breaks the spring memory, and this eliminates the need to weaken it. The placement of this incision should be specified in the design of the antihelix to create a new structure exactly as it should be, looking for that perfect result.

Only the use of sutures with or without weakening works well in thin cartilage, but it still does not define the correct angle created between the antihelix and helix/fossa scaphoid at 90°, which would be the most natural and furthermore may cause a fold in the cranial part of the helix since there is no physical separation between the two.

The cartilage incision in the region between the antihelix and concha creates an unnatural angle in this region and furthermore breaks the continuity of the beams' spring, which comes from the conchal region and ends at the free edge of the new antihelix, preventing the use of strength and the spring's memory in our favor.

The dressing should never be tight, because the detachments necessary to perform the technique leave the flaps sensitive and susceptible

Table 41.1 Satisfaction index

Satisfaction					
Very bad	Bad	Acceptable	Good	Very good	Total
0 (0 %)	1 (1.16 %)	1 (1.16 %)	6 (10.46 %)	75 (87.22 %)	86 (100 %)

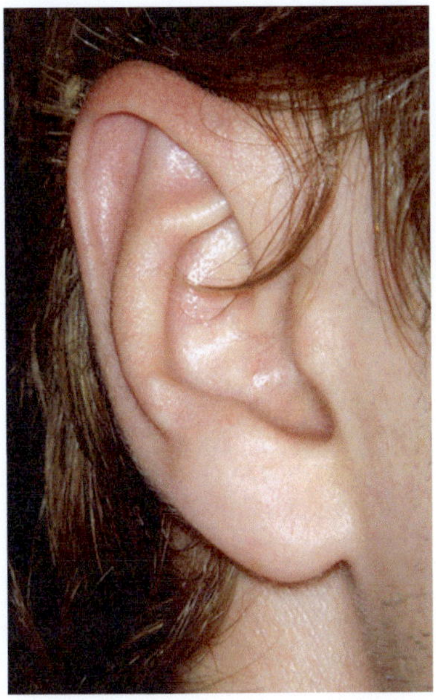

Fig. 41.23 The results are very natural looking, with the helix appearing straight and seeming to be beyond the antihelix on the frontal view. The antihelix contours appear smooth, round, and without irregularities

to compression. We believe that this technique is reproducible, and the results are natural-looking and have a very low rate of recurrence.

Every surgeon should handle the ear cartilage with care. Any incision made out of place may become visible and interfere with the results, which should not have signs of being an "operated" ear (Fig. 41.23).

References

1. Valente ASC. Separating the helix from the antihelix. A new concept in prominent ear correction. Aesthet Surg J. 2010;30(2):139–53.
2. Dieffenbach JE. Die operative Chirurgie. Leipzig: F. A. Brockhause; 1845.
3. Ely ET. An operation for prominent auricles. Arch Otolaryngol. 1881;10:97–9 (reprinted Rogers BO. Ely's 1881 operation for correction of protruding ears. A medical "first". Plast Reconstr Surg. 1968;42(6):582–6).
4. Morestin MH. De la reposition et du plissement cosmetiques du pavillon de l'oreille. Rev Orthop. 1903;4: 289–303.
5. Luckett WH. A new operation for prominent ears based on the anatomy of the deformity. Surg Gynecol Obstet. 1910;10:635–7.
6. Becker OJ. Correction of protruding deformed ear. Br J Plast Surg. 1952;5(3):187–96.
7. Converse JM, Nigro A, Wilson FA, Johnson NA. Technique for surgical correction of lop ears. Plast Reconstr Surg. 1955;15(5):411–8.
8. Converse JM, Wood-Smith D. Technical details in the surgical correction of the lop ear deformity. Plast Reconstr Surg. 1963;31:118–28.
9. Gibson T, Davis W. The distortion of autogenous cartilage grafts: its cause and prevention. Br J Plast Surg. 1958;10:257–74.
10. Mustardé JC. The correction of prominent ears using simple mattress sutures. Br J Plast Surg. 1963;16:170–8.
11. Stenstrom SJ. A "natural" technique for correction of congenitally prominent ears. Plast Reconstr Surg. 1963;32:509–18.
12. Chongchet V. A method of antihelix reconstruction. Br J Plast Surg. 1963;16:268–72.
13. Crikelair GF, Cosman B. Another solution for the problem of the prominent ear. Ann Surg. 1964;160: 314–24.
14. Nordzell B. Open otoplasty. Plast Reconstr Surg. 2000;106(7):1466–72.
15. Caouette-Laberge L, Guay N, Bortoluzzi P, Belleville C. Otoplasty: anterior scoring technique and results in 500 cases. Plast Reconstr Surg. 2000;105(2):504–15.
16. Brent B. Hydrodissection as key to a natural-appearing otoplasty. Plast Reconstr Surg. 2008;122(4):1055–8.
17. Webster GV. The tail of the helix as a key to otoplasty. Plast Reconstr Surg. 1969;44(5):455–61.
18. Beernink JH, Blocksma R, Moore D. The role of the helical tail in cosmetic otoplasty. Plast Reconstr Surg. 1979;64(1):115–7.
19. Furnas DW. Correction of prominent ears by conchamastoid sutures. Plast Reconstr Surg. 1968;42(3): 189–93.
20. McDowell AJ. Goals in otoplasty for protruding ears. Plast Reconstr Surg. 1968;41(1):17–23.
21. LaTrenta GS. Otoplasty. In: Rees TD, LaTrenta GS, editors. Aesthetic plastic surgery. 2nd ed. Philadelphia: Saunders; 1994. p. 891–921.
22. Janis JE, Rohrich RJ, Gutowski KA. Otoplasty. Plast Reconstr Surg. 2005;115(4):60e–72.

Balanced Otoplasty: Dividing the Ear into Vertical Thirds

42

Samuel M. Lam

Introduction

Otoplasty need not be as challenging an artistic endeavor as other facial cosmetic surgeries. A straightforward and systematic strategy as outlined in this chapter can help guide a surgeon to attain reproducible and aesthetically appealing outcomes. By dividing the ear into vertical thirds, a surgeon can identify the causative aesthetic problem and thereby correct it in a tailored and targeted manner. The upper third of the ear when prominent typically signifies the presence of a lop ear deformity in which the antihelical fold is diminished or altogether absent. Correction of this deformity involves Mustarde sutures to create a proper antihelical fold. The middle third of the ear, if prominent, usually reflects the overexuberant presence of the conchal cartilage, creating a cup ear deformity, which would mandate excision and reduction of the conchal bowl. Often neglected, the lower third of the ear can also manifest an enlarged, prominent, or protruding lobule that if ignored can lead to an unbalanced result with a nonaesthetically protruding lobule. Various strategies to reduce the lobule that will be discussed are a V–Y setback and cauda helicis fixation to the conchal bowl. This chapter will aim to describe the aesthetic principles, systematic planning, and surgical technique to create a balanced, natural, and aesthetic otoplasty result.

S.M. Lam, M.D.
Willow Bend Wellness Center, Lam Facial Plastic Surgery Center and Hair Restoration Institute, 6101 Chapel Hill Boulevard, Suite 101, Plano 75093, TX, USA
e-mail: drlam@lamfacialplastics.com

Principles and Strategy

All ears are not created equal. Besides the above considerations, ears can be asymmetrically protruding, differently shaped, and of different sizes. When trying to prioritize what would be the most important dimension to fix, the author tends to recall the time of performing reconstructive ear surgeries for skin cancer conditions. Whenever a cancer had to be removed, the ultimate goal would be focused on how the ears would look straight on from the frontal view, i.e., how much protrusion they would have off the head and to try to ensure that both ears would be protruding about the same degree. With bad technique, one ear could easily cup forward and protrude unnaturally. No other dimension was as important as how the ears appeared from the frontal view. Many times patients can become obsessed with the relative size differences of their ears or the fact that one ear shape is slightly or grossly different from the other ear. However, keeping in mind that the only time that both ears can be viewed at the same time is from the frontal view, it is not as important that the two ear shapes be of the same size and proportion because the viewer will never be able to see the two ears side by side to compare.

M.A. Shiffman (ed.), *Advanced Cosmetic Otoplasty*,
DOI 10.1007/978-3-642-35431-1_42, © Springer-Verlag Berlin Heidelberg 2013

After ensuring that the ears are protruding to the same degree, the second most important element to consider is how the shape of the ear itself looks from the side view. Because one size of the ear cannot be easily compared with the other size of the ear, size differences are not important. Instead, when looking at an ear from the side view, the ear should look like an ear, i.e., it should possess all the normal constituent elements of an ear like the helix and antihelix. So long as the protrusion from the frontal view is not compromised, the shape of the ear as viewed from the side takes secondary precedence.

An important element would be that the size of one ear should be similar to the size of the other ear. This size difference albeit difficult to appreciate can be deduced somewhat from the frontal view if grossly different in size and possibly with rapid turning of the head as the viewer sees one ear and then the other one. Despite this attribute ranking third in importance, it is actually almost impossible to fix without taking undue risk in violating the first two principles of normal protrusion and normal shape. As with cancer operations, tissue can be borrowed from the lobule and slid upward by making incisions along the inside of the helix, but this technique is more appropriate for skin cancer cases than for cosmetic reductive otoplasty.

How do these principles play out when working on real-case scenarios? Think of when one ear protrudes more than the contralateral side. When pulling the ear that is protruding out farther backward to match the other side, the antihelical fold sometimes can be deeper recessed due to the need for greater recession. This shape will obviously look different from the other side upon careful inspection, especially when the head is rotated to the side. Nevertheless, if we follow the principle that the ear should be as symmetrical as possible from the frontal view, i.e., the degree of protrusion should be as symmetrical as possible, then we are okay to ignore this slight difference. This limitation should be pointed out to a patient before surgery so that there is nothing unexpected afterward.

The term "telephone deformity" is well known and suggests that the ear is tucked too far backward to the cranium in the middle pole. An "antitelephone deformity" refers to pulling the upper pole too far back during a lop ear reduction. It is important that the ear not appear flat against the head no matter how much the patient is desirous of doing this, as it will appear unnatural. The ear should be resting 20°–30° naturally off of the mastoid. With experience, the surgeon need not measure the degree of protrusion on one side compared with the other but merely eyeballs the degree of setback and symmetry during the procedure.

For those just starting in the practice of otoplasty, more rigorous guidelines can be offered. Using Castroviejo calipers, the superior aspect of the helix should be approximately 10–12 mm from the cranium; the crural junction, at 16–18 mm; and the top of the external auditory canal, at 20–22 mm.

Another important concept that is overlooked is the relative position of the helix and the antihelix from the frontal view. When viewing an individual straight on, the helix should be ever so slightly lateral to the antihelix, i.e., the helix should not be hidden behind the antihelix. This problem can occur when the sutures are tied down too aggressively in a lop ear correction such that the antihelical fold dominates and covers the visibility of the helix from the frontal view. When tying down sutures during the procedure, the surgeon should always reference how the ear is shaping up from the frontal view as the first and foremost priority.

The sole exception when the antihelix can be tied down so that the helix is partially obscured is in an individual whose cartilage is very thick and would tend to rebound over time as the sutures relax and the ear begins to protrude slightly over time. The author believes that through-and-through cuts through the cartilage in the proposed region of the antihelical fold are verboten because it will frequently lead to the visibility of cut cartilage edges over time. Accordingly, a slightly overcorrection of the degree of setback of the ear is done when correcting a lop ear deformity because invariably there is some visible relaxation that can occur over time. This is especially true if the cartilage is stiff, rigid, and thick, as mentioned above. As always, it is important to explain this to a patient preoperatively so he or she does not perceive the surgery as a failure with some relaxation that is bound to occur.

Although through-and-through incisions through the proposed antihelix is unwise, partial scoring of the posterior aspect in the region of the antihelix truly can help reduce the tendency to relapse after a lop ear reduction. Technique will be explained in detail in the following section. When the cartilage is particularly rigid, it becomes imperative that the surgeon takes his time to score the posterior aspect of the cartilage in a deliberate and almost exhaustive manner to thin the cartilage down as much as possible.

Relaxation typically does not occur with cup ear reductions because I believe that some cartilage excision in the conchal bowl is critical to achieve the desired result. The precise technique will be described below. In the past, the author would not excise conchal cartilage but try to take the conchal bowl either back onto itself or onto the mastoid periosteum without predictable results. This is especially true when the conchal bowl cartilage is truly excessive in quantity, making a tack back to the mastoid virtually futile in the ability to achieve a durable result.

In general, even if there is some degree of conchal bowl excess but not a lot, the author will still prefer to excise a little bit of conchal bowl to break the recoil of the cartilage in an area that I deem safe, i.e., that should not create visible cut cartilage edges as would be visible by cutting along the region of the proposed antihelix. This is especially helpful when dealing with very thick, resilient cartilage in which the fear is that there would be total relaxation of the Mustarde sutures over time.

To determine how much lop ear deformity (absence of the antihelix), cup ear deformity (conchal excess), and lobular protrusion exist in a particular patient, the surgeon can stand in front of the individual and push back the top, middle, and bottom of the ear, respectively, to evaluate the relative contribution of each part of the ear to the observed deformity. Doing this is also very helpful in explaining to a patient what the precise mixture of aesthetic issues presents and how the surgery would be tailored accordingly. Also by doing this, sometimes the lobule that seemed to be okay becomes obviously protuberant when pushing back the upper two-thirds of the ear. In this case, a lobular reduction should be planned.

The two ways that are reliable methods to reduce the lobule include a V-to-Y setback and tacking the cauda helicis to the conchal bowl. Both methods can be combined as well when needed. When the lobule itself is too large and protrusive, the V-to-Y setback allows some reduction of the tissue from the posterior aspect of the lobule, permitting the ear to be reduced in size and somewhat retrodisplaced. When the ear lobule is just protruding out, securing a suture between the cauda helicis and the conchal bowl is a secure method of retrosetting the lobule and can be adjusted depending on how tight the suture is tied down. This is a more reliable method of lobule setback when the conchal cartilage is not resected as in a cup ear reduction. Sometimes both methods are helpful when used together to attain adequate lobular reduction.

In the past, the author would use 4-0 braided polyester fiber suture (Mersilene) for all otoplasties. However, there was a higher extrusion and infection rate noted with this braided suture. Further, when removing the suture in the office, it was quite painful for the patient and a more labor-intensive chore, pulling out a braided suture from the ear. Today, the author prefers 4-0 clear polypropylene (Prolene) suture as it is almost as easy to tack down as Mersilene with a much lower incidence of extrusion and infection, and when the suture extrudes, suture removal is almost entirely painless and easy to perform. The patient is always counseled that extrusion can occur but not to remove the sutures but to allow the author to do it, as needed. Typically the author does not like removing any sutures unless they are truly problematic prior to 6 months when I believe most of the scar tissue has become mature to hold the ear more durably in position.

Technique

Sedation, Preparation, and Anesthesia

When performing a reduction in the three vertical divisions of the ear, the author almost always proceeds with reducing the center (cup ear), then the top ear (lop ear), and then the lobule in that order. The technique will be described according to that sequence.

For children who would not tolerate intravenous sedation, then general anesthesia may be preferred. However, an increasing percentage of adults are now seeking reductive otoplasty later in life and can tolerate simple intravenous sedation with midazolam and fentanyl. Despite using sedation, the initial ring block can still be quite uncomfortable, so we make it a point to apply topical anesthetic cream for an hour circumferentially around the ear and directly on the ear (anteriorly and posteriorly) in order to minimize the potential discomfort.

The postauricular skin island planned for excision should be marked out before the patient is prepared and draped and after the anesthetic cream has been thoroughly removed. In a person with an obvious need for reductive otoplasty, a fusiform shape is removed running from 1 cm below the superior helix to 2 cm above the lobule, fanning from 5 mm superiorly to 1 cm at its greatest dimension (situated at the upper one-third of the planned excision) tapering downward to 2–5 mm inferiorly (Fig. 42.1). It is important to match the width on one side meticulously with the contralateral side using Castroviejo calipers. When performing nuanced, subtle otoplasty reductions, a proportionate degree of reduction in total amount of skin removed should be undertaken so that the ear is not inadvertently overpinned.

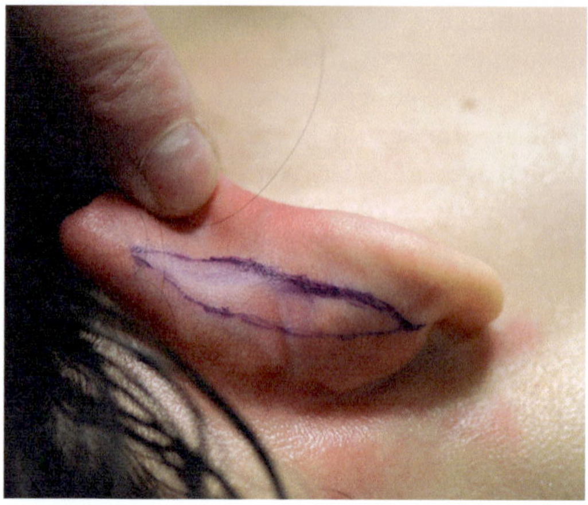

Fig. 42.1 The postauricular skin island planned for excision should be marked out before the patient is prepared and draped and after the anesthetic cream has been thoroughly removed. In a person with an obvious need for reductive otoplasty, I remove a fusiform shape running from 1 cm below the superior helix to 2 cm above the lobule, fanning from 5 mm superiorly to 1 cm at its greatest dimension (situated at the upper one-third of the planned excision) tapering downward to 2–5 mm inferiorly

The patient is then prepared with povidone-iodine solution to include both ears, the periauricular region, and the entire face. The reason for this extensive sterile preparation is that it is easy to touch the central face accidentally when performing bilateral otoplasty. The patient is draped with a sterile blue towel as a head wrap with both ears left exposed and remaining dressings applied circumferentially to maintain a sterile field. The patient has intravenous sedation administered. A 10-mL syringe containing a 50/50 mixture of 1 % lidocaine/l:100,000 epinephrine and 0.25 % bupivacaine is infiltrated as a ring block around each ear, i.e., 10 mL per each ear, taking care to be symmetrical in how the ring block is applied (Fig. 42.2). Additionally, 2–3 mL of 1 % lidocaine/l:100,000 epinephrine is infiltrated directly along the posterior aspect of the ear in the planned area of skin excision and the surrounding area (Fig. 42.3). Ten minutes is allowed to transpire for proper hemostasis and anesthesia to be established. It is critical not to infiltrate anesthesia along the anterior surface of the ear, which can lead to distortion and thereby inability to read what is going on during the procedure.

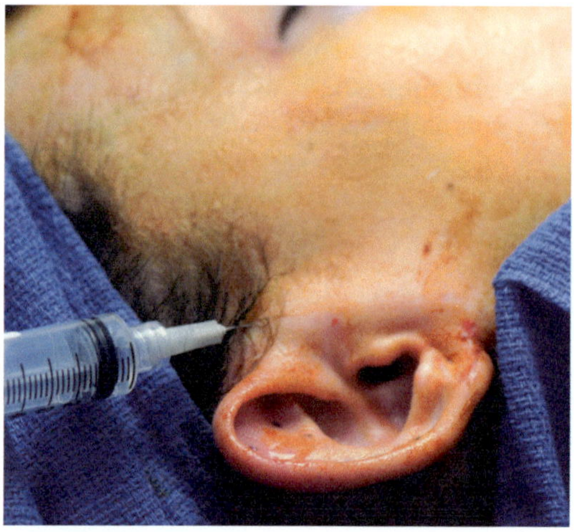

Fig. 42.2 A 10-mL syringe containing a 50/50 mixture of 1 % lidocaine/l:100,000 epinephrine and 0.25 % bupivacaine is infiltrated as a ring block around each ear, i.e., 10 mL per each ear, taking care to be symmetrical in how the ring block is applied

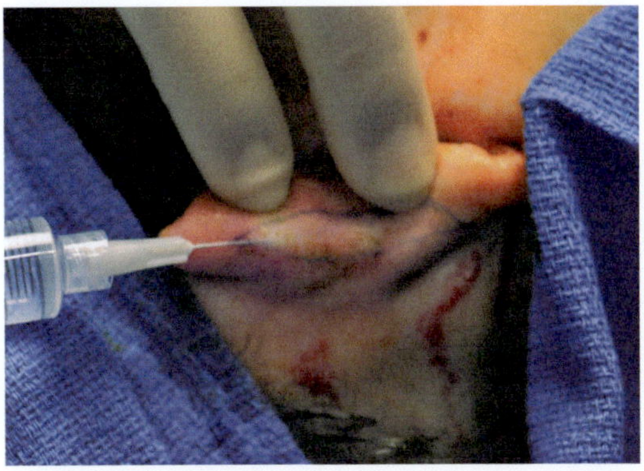

Fig. 42.3 Additionally, 2–3 mL of 1 % lidocaine/1:100,000 epinephrine is infiltrated directly along the posterior aspect of the ear in the planned area of skin excision and the surrounding area

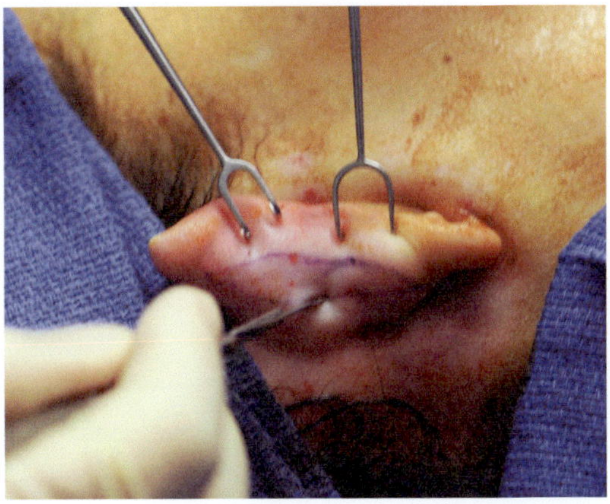

Fig. 42.4 The surgeon begins on one ear, incising the fusiform skin paddle with a Bard-Parker No.15 blade and discarding the removed skin

The surgeon begins on one ear, incising the fusiform skin paddle with a Bard-Parker No.15 blade and discarding the removed skin (Fig. 42.4). Hemostasis is achieved with bipolar cautery before proceeding. Medium-wide double-hooked retractors are enlisted to retract the ear, as the surgeon uses curved tenotomy scissors to spread and separate the skin from the underlying postauricular cartilage along the entire expanse of the postauricular surface (Fig. 42.5). Again hemostasis with bipolar cautery is attained as needed before proceeding.

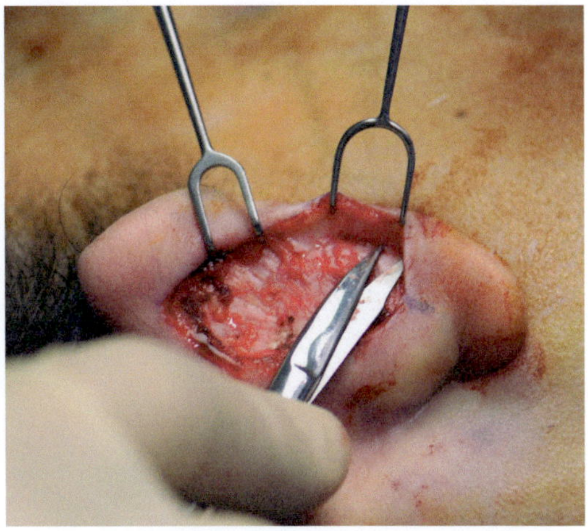

Fig. 42.5 Medium-wide double-hooked retractors are enlisted to retract the ear, as the surgeon uses curved tenotomy scissors to spread and separate the skin from the underlying postauricular cartilage along the entire expanse of the postauricular surface

Cup Ear Reduction

Twenty-five-gauge needles are used to penetrate the skin from the anterior to posterior side of the ear along the lateral curved edge of the conchal bowl to mark out the conchal bowl along the posterior aspect of the ear. Gentian violet can be used to connect the points along the posterior aspect to guide the first through-and-through incision through the conchal cartilage, taking care not to violate the anterior skin surface (Fig. 42.6). Approximately 2–4 mm of cartilage is then cut in a parallel arc medial to the previous incision and the ends joined to facilitate removal of this cartilage excess (Fig. 42.7). The curved tenotomy scissors are used to undermine under both cartilage edges approximately a centimeter on both sides so that the skin does not appear bunched up when the cartilage edges are closed together (Fig. 42.8). The cartilage is then closed with 2–3 interrupted 4-0 polypropylene sutures (Fig. 42.9).

Lop Ear Reduction

Multiple 25-gauge needles are placed through from the anterior to posterior side of the ear on both sides of the proposed antihelical fold to

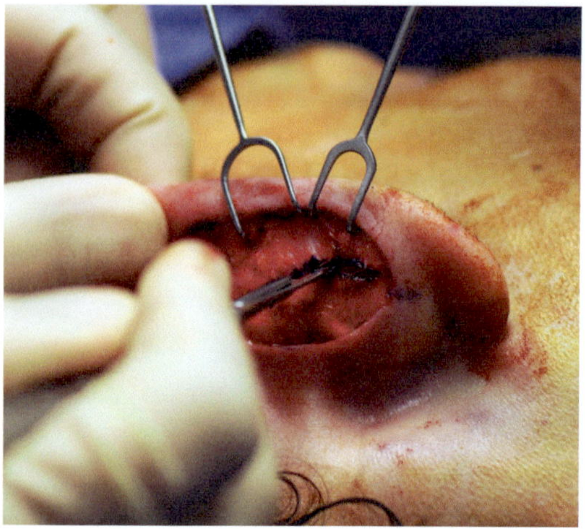

Fig. 42.6 Gentian violet can be used to connect the points along the posterior aspect to guide the first through-and-through incision through the conchal cartilage, taking care not to violate the anterior skin surface

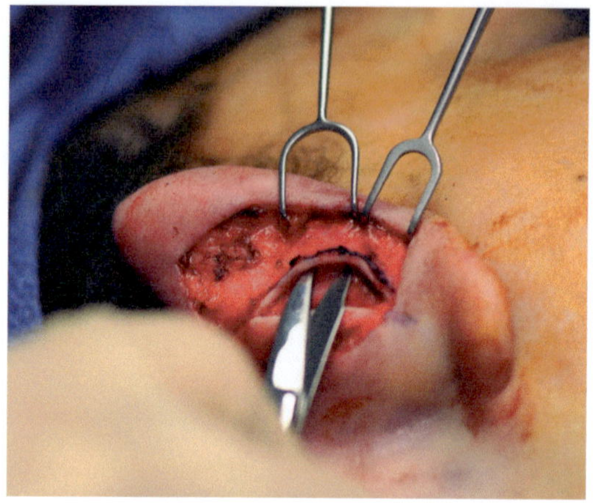

Fig. 42.8 The curved tenotomy scissors are used to undermine under both cartilage edges approximately a centimeter on both sides so that the skin does not appear bunched up when the cartilage edges are closed together

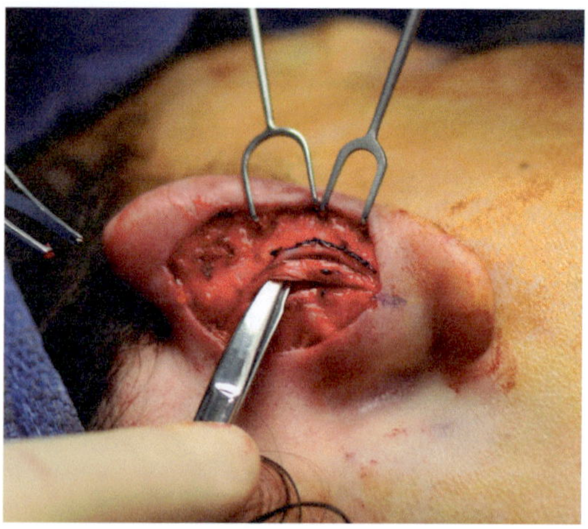

Fig. 42.7 Approximately 2–4 mm of cartilage is cut in a parallel arc medial to the previous incision and the ends joined to facilitate removal of this cartilage excess

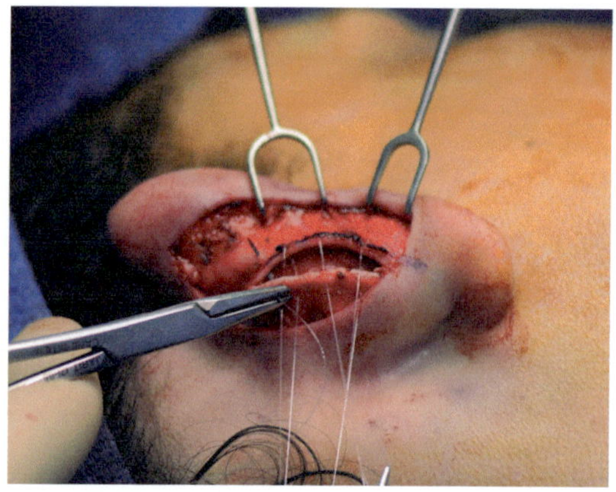

Fig. 42.9 The cartilage is closed with 2–3 interrupted 4-0 polypropylene sutures

correlate with where the mattress sutures will be placed. Typically 6–8 needles are placed to correspond with 3–4 sutures that will be used to recreate the antihelical fold with Mustarde sutures (Fig. 42.10). With the needles in place and the postauricular surface in view, the territory between the needles is scored in a partial thickness manner using a No.15 blade running vertically, horizontally, diagonally in one direction, diagonally in the opposing direction, and across until the cartilage is sufficiently weakened without fully penetrating with the knife to the other side (Fig. 42.11). In addition, the belly of the blade can be used to scrape the cartilage in the partially scored region of cartilage to further soften the cartilage to limit recoil. When the surgeon believes that the cartilage is sufficiently weakened, he can then progress with the suture placements.

Starting from the top, the 4-0 polypropylene suture is placed through the cartilage in a full-thickness manner ensuring that the needle penetrates all the way through the anterior perichondrium but not through the anterior skin.

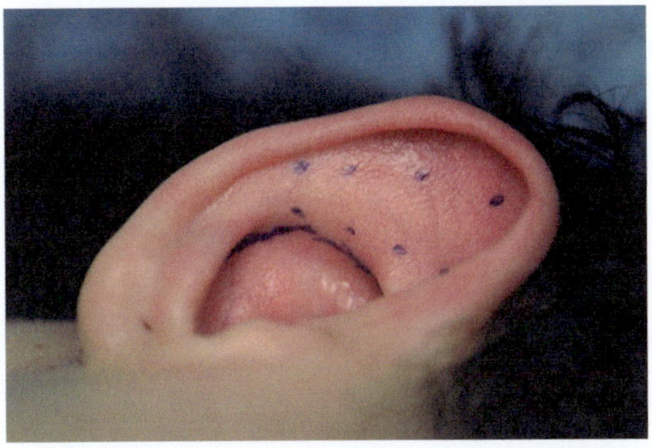

Fig. 42.10 Multiple 25-gauge needles are placed through from the anterior to posterior side of the ear on both sides of the proposed antihelical fold to correlate with where the mattress sutures will be placed. Typically 6–8 needles are placed to correspond with 3–4 sutures that will be used to recreate the antihelical fold with Mustarde sutures

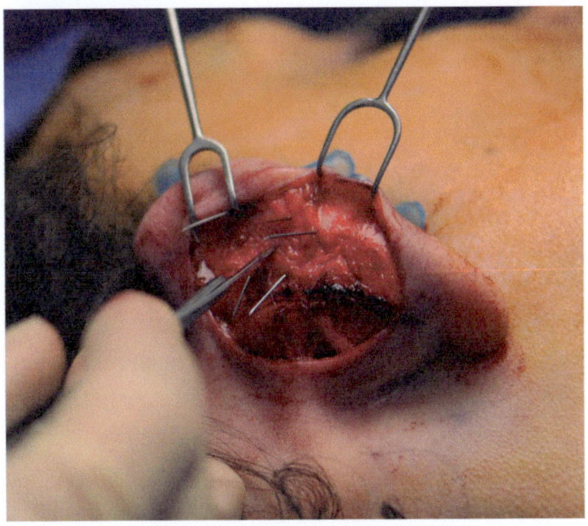

Fig. 42.11 With the needles in place and the postauricular surface in view, the territory between the needles is scored in a partial thickness manner using a No.15 blade running vertically, horizontally, diagonally in one direction, diagonally in the opposing direction, and across until the cartilage is sufficiently weakened without fully penetrating with the knife to the other side

The same needle is then passed through the corresponding 25-gauge needle point on the other side of the proposed antihelical fold in the same manner but backhanded to complete the mattress (Fig. 42.12). The suture is not tied down but tagged with curved or straight clamps. The two 25-gauge needles that were used as guides for the first suture are then removed. The same technique

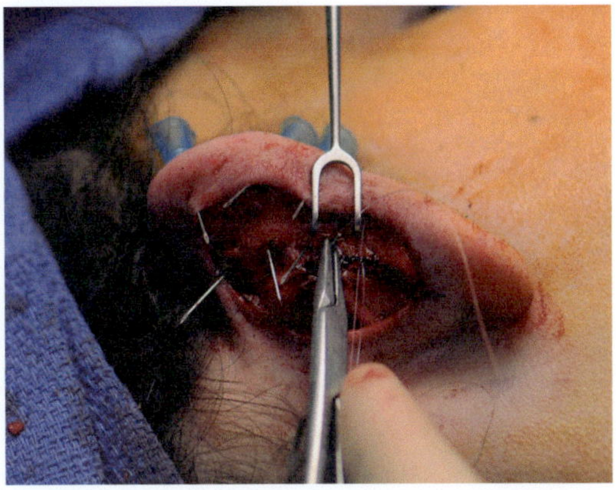

Fig. 42.12 Starting from the *top*, the 4-0 polypropylene suture is placed through the cartilage in a full-thickness manner ensuring that the needle penetrates all the way through the anterior perichondrium but not through the anterior skin. The same needle is then passed through the corresponding 25-gauge needle point on the other side of the proposed antihelical fold in the same manner but backhanded to complete the mattress

is continued along the entire length of the proposed antihelical fold, tagging but not tying down any of the sutures. The middle suture is then tied down with a surgeon's knot until the ear is positioned at about 80 % of the desired position and secured with remaining knots. The excess suture tails are then cut, saving the remaining needle and suture for use on the contralateral side if possible. Each additional mattress suture is tied down sequentially until the antihelical fold is fully formed, the ear is well positioned by inspecting the ear from a frontal view, and as mentioned before the helix is not entirely obscured by the antihelical fold from the frontal view.

Lobular Reduction

At this point, any lobular excess can be properly identified. If the lobular size is too large and protuberant, a V-to-Y closure can be done to draw the lobule backward and to reduce the size of the lobule somewhat. If the lobule is truly too large, a wedge excision may need to be undertaken, but this risks a visible incision from the frontal view that in most cases is not worth it. If the lobule is just somewhat protrusive relative to the reduced

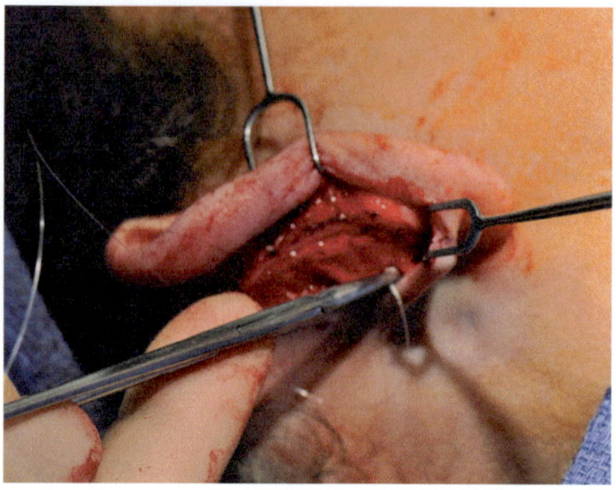

Fig. 42.13 If the lobule is just somewhat protrusive relative to the reduced upper two-thirds of the ear, then a 4-0 polypropylene suture can be passed through the cauda helicis and tacked back somewhere to the conchal bowl and tightness adjusted as the lobule begins to fall backward

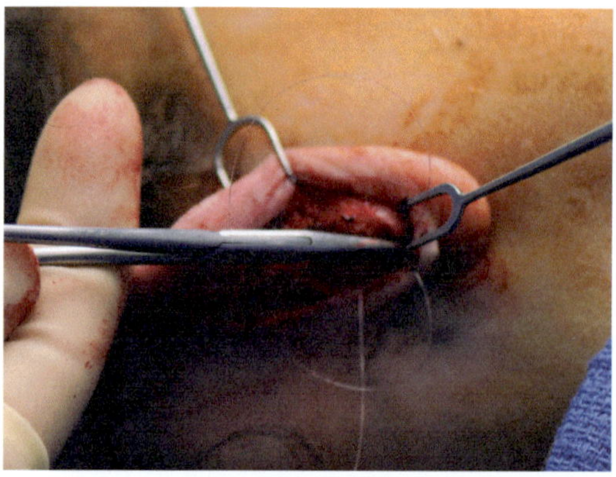

Fig. 42.14 This photograph shows the second pass of the lobule setback suture shown in Figure 42.13

upper two-thirds of the ear, then a 4-0 polypropylene suture can be passed through the cauda helicis (Fig. 42.13) and tacked back somewhere to the conchal bowl (Fig. 42.14) and tightness adjusted as the lobule begins to retrude backward. As a point of clarification, the cauda helicis is defined as the small appendage-like cartilage that signifies the very caudal border of the helical cartilage. It oftentimes needs to be dissected sharply with scissors to be readily identified, using palpation as a guide.

Skin Closure and Drain

When the ear looks good from a frontal position, i.e., the helix is not tucked too far back and the upper, middle, and lower poles look to be in alignment and in proportion, then the skin can be closed. A running 5–0 chromic suture is used to close the incision, leaving a small gap at the inferior aspect for a cut red rubber catheter tube that is left in place over night.

Contralateral Side

The contralateral side is approached in the exact same manner, taking care that when the head is turned to the other side, the recently operated-on ear is not bent and pinned unfavorably against the headrest/table. Some additional gauze padding can be secured to buttress the previously operated-on ear as it now presses more against the bed after the head is turned. When all of the Mustarde sutures have been tagged and are ready to be tied down, the surgeon should stand up and look down on the patient to evaluate the position of the ear relative to the other side when tying each knot down to ensure symmetry and similarity in curvature. In the past, the author would use calipers to measure the distance from ear to mastoid but has found that my eye is more accurate than these measurements can afford. It is imperative that the frontal view shows as symmetrical a result as possible. Sometimes that means bending one ear back more than the other ear to attain that frontal symmetry. However, it is also important to make sure that by bending one ear back farther than the other, the shape of the antihelix does not appear to be too distorted when pulled farther back than the other. A slight degree of greater curvature is accepted if it permits better frontal symmetry. Again, it is essential that the patient know that the ears may look different from a side or % view due to this fact in order to get a frontal view that looks more symmetrical. This limitation should be expressed in the preoperative encounter not ideally after the surgery has been completed. The difference between an education and an excuse is that an education is provided before the surgery and an excuse is offered afterward (Figs. 42.15 and 42.16).

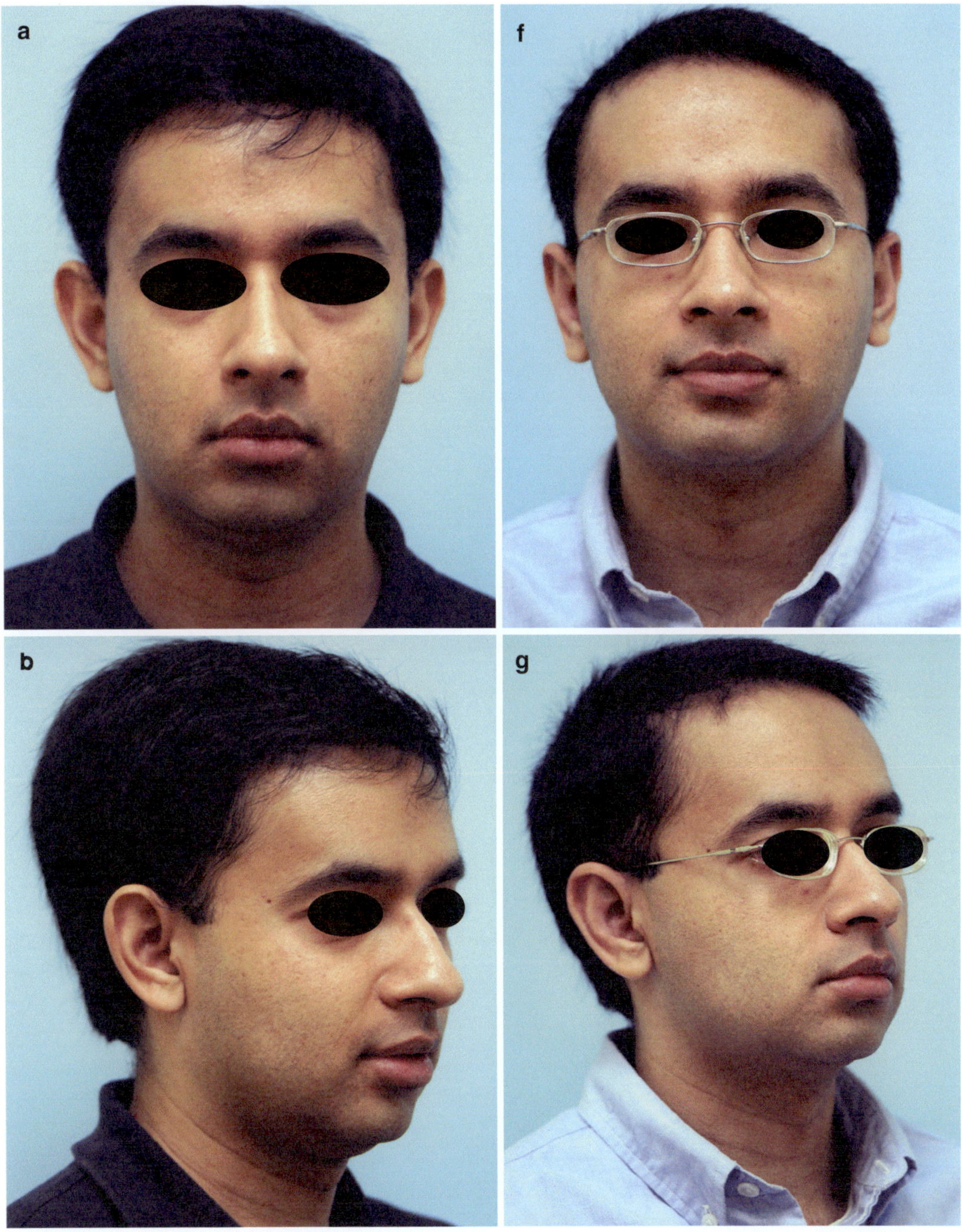

Fig. 42.15 (**a**) Preoperative 36-year-old gentleman. (**b**) One year after reductive otoplasty of a cup and lop ear deformity with good aesthetic improvement and improved symmetry in the result

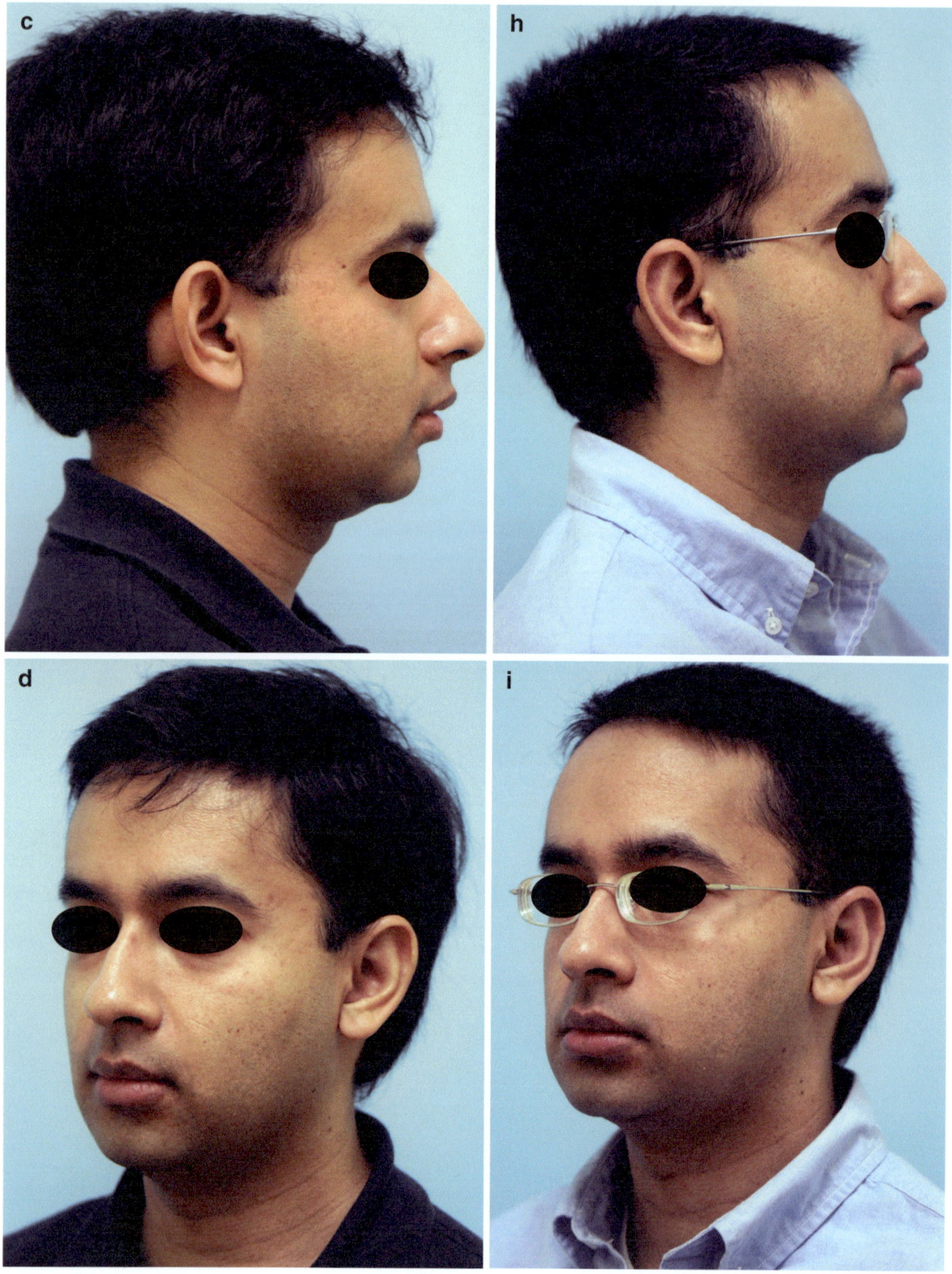

Fig. 42.15 (continued)

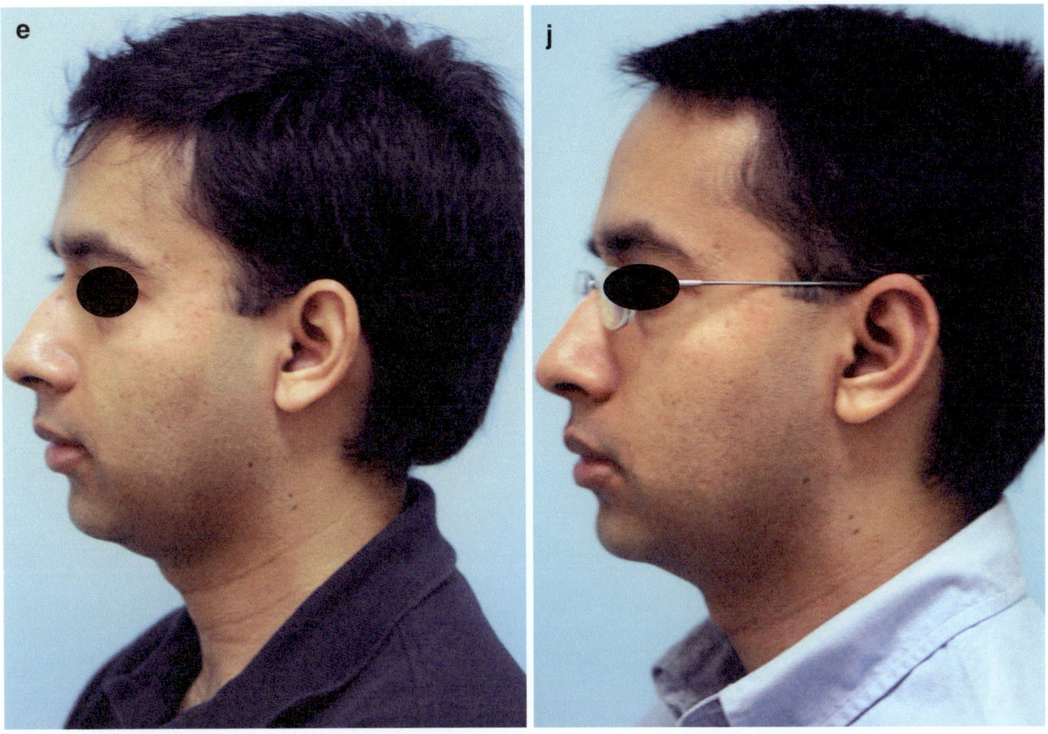

Fig. 42.15 (continued)

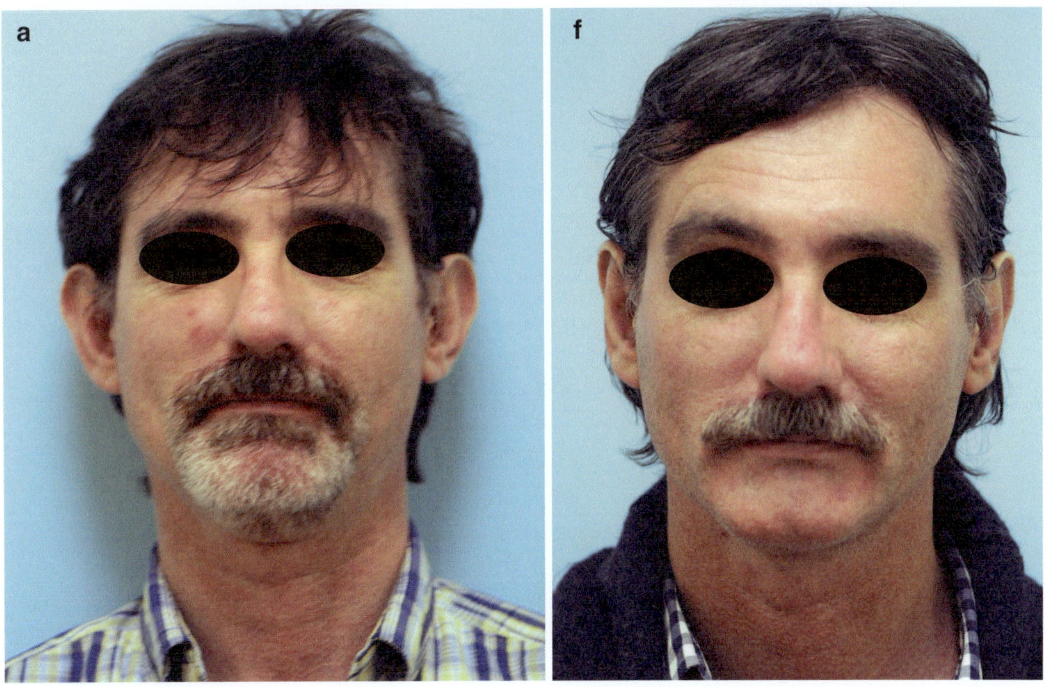

Fig. 42.16 (**a**) Preoperative 49-year-old gentleman. (**b**) One year after reductive otoplasty of a cup and lop ear deformity and lobule reduction with good aesthetic improvement and improved symmetry in the result

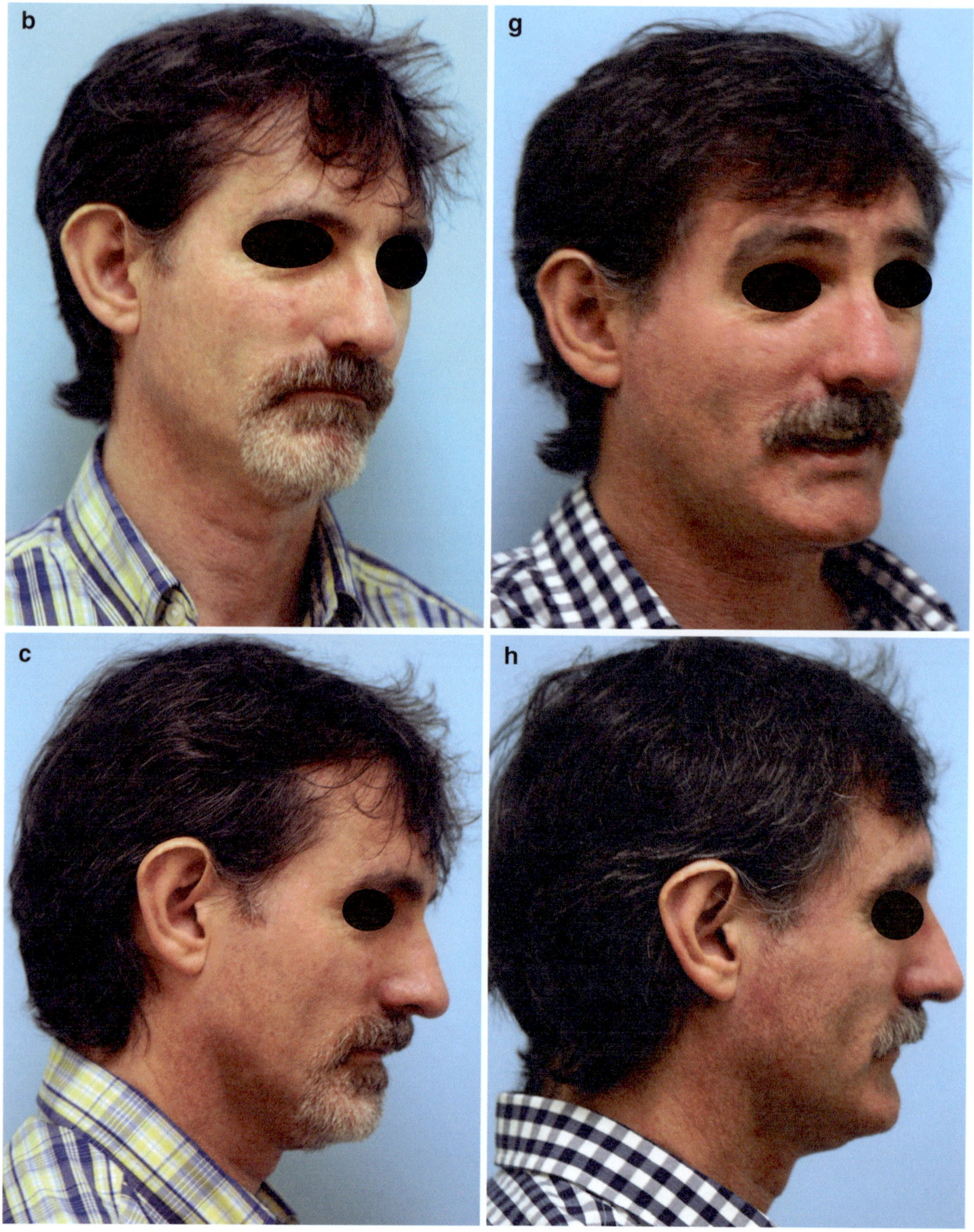

Fig. 42.16 (continued)

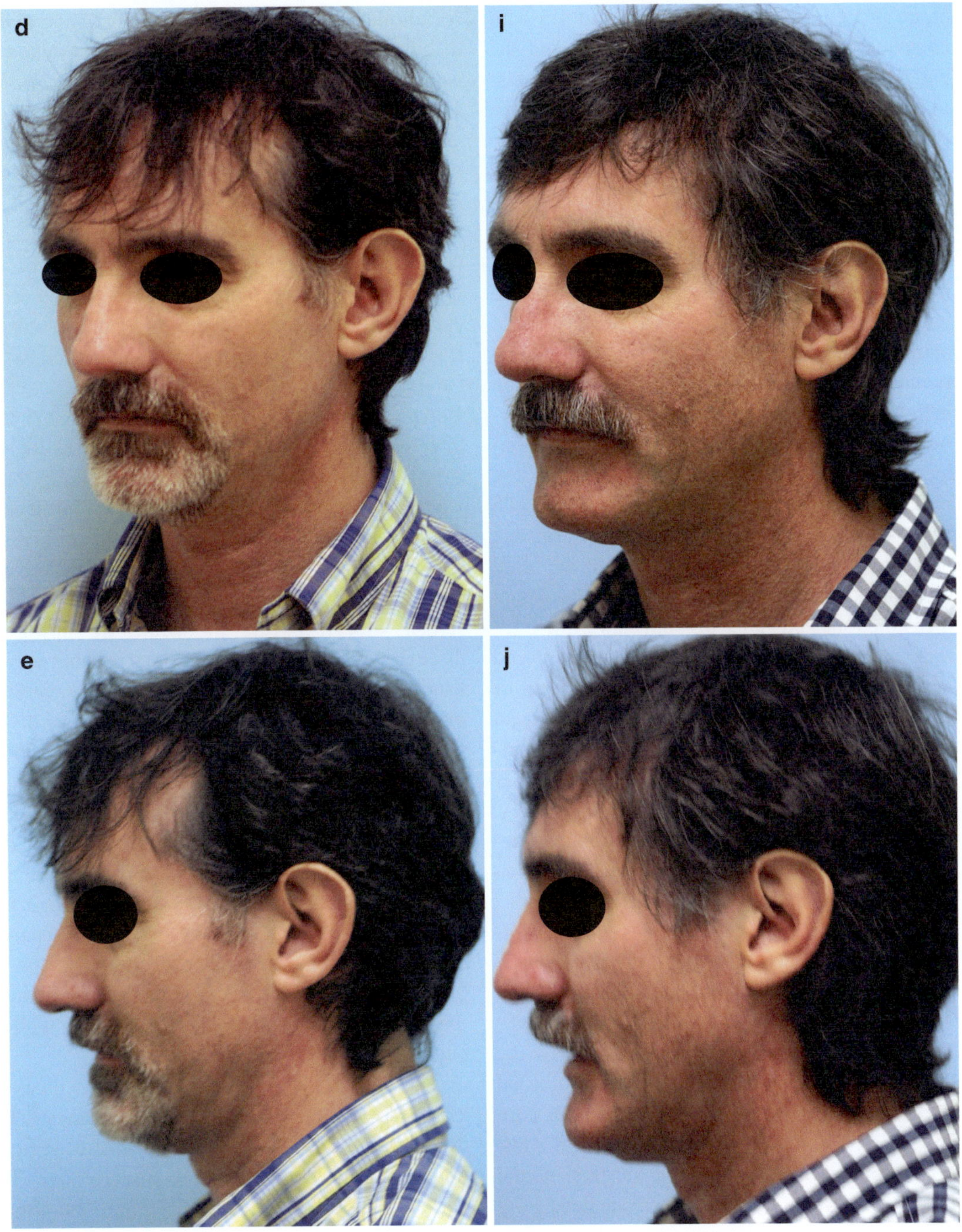

Fig. 42.16 (continued)

Bandage

At the completion of the case, all the povidone-iodine solution is gently but deliberately removed before dressing application. The patient is shown how the ears look at the end of the procedure if the surgery was performed under intravenous sedation rather than general anesthesia so that they do not fret that night of how their ears look and before greater edema sets in. Because the entire procedure takes between 1 and 1.5 h to complete, there is not a lot of edema and the patient can be shown the ears without much distortion. Clearly if there is significant edema, then the patient would not be shown the ears at the conclusion of the operative case.

On an adjacent Mayo stand, a metal basin is filled with non-sterile cotton balls impregnated thoroughly with mineral oil as well as conforming bandages. There is also a 5-mL syringe loaded with topical antibiotic ointment. Half a syringe of antibiotic ointment is injected along the postauricular incision on both sides. Then open cotton balls are fluffed and made sure that they are thoroughly soaked with mineral oil before conforming them carefully and attentively to the front and back sides of the ear on one side. A stacked pile of 4×4 gauze is placed on top, and the assistant holds that gauze in place on one ear as the same dressing is applied on the other ear. The assistant then holds stacked gauze on both ears while multiple layers of conforming bandage are placed around the head in two directions: from top of head to the neck and from the crown of the head to the neck. It is so important to place the bandage along these two vectors, or the bandage is liable to fall off the first night after the surgery, which can predispose toward hematoma formation and protracted edema. The bandage is then secured with multiple strips of clear plastic tape.

After Care and Recovery

The patient and family are advised that with the drains in place, they are intended to emit blood into the dressing and that the dressing can even be soaked up and soil the bed sheets. In addition, the first night following surgery as the bupivacaine wears off, the patient can have quite a bit of achiness and discomfort, and a prophylactic narcotic is advised to be given before retiring for the evening even if no pain has started. Typically, this discomfort is the most severe the night after surgery and greatly diminishes by the following day. When a conchal resection has been performed for cup ear reduction, the discomfort can linger somewhat longer for another day or two. For some patients, that discomfort can last up to a week but in my experience is typically much less after the first 1–3 days following surgery.

The next day the patient returns to the office with an athletic headband that has been previously purchased or that the office supplies. The dressing is carefully removed from the head by a combination of unwrapping it and cutting away the dressings. The drains are removed painlessly and the ears carefully inspected for edema and hematoma. If there is significant edema, the same operative bandage may be reapplied for another 2–3 days. However, this is only the situation in less than 5 % of cases in my experience. The postauricular incision is cleaned with hydrogen peroxide and the wound redressed with topical antibiotic ointment. The patient holds a mirror and the author stands behind the patient to show him how to apply the athletic headband. The fingers on both hands are spread widely, having the hands go upward through the headband on both sides pushing very firmly apart so that the headband is gently lowered over the head and the ears are not abraded or disturbed. The hands are slowly removed from the head one side at a time lowering the headband onto the ears in a gentle manner. At this point, the headband sometimes sits over the eyes, so that point is adjusted upward. Then if the headband is too tight (it should be snug but not overly tight), the author takes a pair of heavy scissors and a partial cut is made through the headband to alleviate the tension. This cut can be performed as many times as needed to relieve excessive tension without making the headband too slack.

The patient is advised to wear the headband 24 h a day for the first week and then thereafter only at night during sleep for a total of 6 weeks time. Chromic sutures tend to dissolve over a period of 2–3 weeks. If they are still present after the second week and they disturb the patient, then they can be removed as desired.

That patient is advised not to shower for 24 h after the procedure and then can resume normal showering thereafter. Bathtub bathing should be avoided especially considering that the presence of permanent sutures can become infected. This admonition should also apply to any other submersible activity like swimming for a period of at least 6 weeks. In fact, the author prefers no submersion for a minimum of 3 months if at all possible. Also, no contact sports for a minimum of 6 months would be advisable.

Patients are advised that at times the Mustarde sutures can become exposed and require removal. If this is the case, the patient should not attempt this by himself but come to the office for an easy removal. The author prefers to leave any exposed sutures for a minimum of 6 months so as to ensure that they do not compromise the tenacity of the position of the ear.

Patients are also warned that ears may relax somewhat during the recovery phase even for several months following the procedure especially with very thick cartilages that can recoil a bit over time. If patients are forewarned of this eventuality, they will not deem it a surgical error mandating a revision procedure. It is always emphasized that ultimate ear position can vary up to a year following a procedure.

Discussion

As with any cosmetic procedure, reproducibility of a result depends on the surgeon's experience and expertise with otoplasty. Learning from what works in one's hands is critical and only using the basis of what is written here as a guideline should be emphasized. The author constantly adapts small changes in the technique based on evaluating the results. This is a natural progression of any procedure, as mastery is only an asymptote in which one continues to improve but never attains it, especially for a mindful and diligent surgeon who cares about his results.

The author always undersells a patient on what is possible so that they are focused on improvement rather than perfection. When a patient insists on perfect symmetry, the author explains that is not possible based on the possibility of some relaxation in the ear position over time that can be somewhat variable. In addition, consent forms and also verbal reinforcement during the preoperative session "Should reiterate the two sides of the body are not the same and can never be made the same." One should remember the admonition that the difference between an education and an excuse is simply when it was told before or after surgery, respectively.

Complications

Despite rigorous preoperative counseling and meticulous surgical technique, complications can still arise. Any surgeon who has never experienced a complication simply has not operated on enough cases. That is the nature of the imperfect science of surgery.

The most common complication that I have seen with otoplasty is unfavorable relaxation of the Mustarde sutures. Since the author has incorporated more frequently the reduction of the conchal bowl, there has been a more reliable reduction in ear position with more stability in the results over time. Nevertheless, if the ears relax too much, a revision procedure is warranted, and this is the most common reason for a corrective procedure for me.

The second most common "complication" is extrusion of the Mustarde sutures over time that requires removal of them in the office setting. Before when 4-0 braided polyester (Mersilene) sutures were used, the removal process was gruesome and painful. Since converting to 4-0 clear polypropylene sutures, intermittent extrusion has not been encountered and removal of the suture is easy and painless. That is a big reason why polypropylene sutures are a preferred suture material.

At times some minor step-off deformities are seen at the conchal bowl from cup reduction that typically are very hard to notice unless closeup. Again, the author tries to explain the possibility of all "deformities" so that the patient will accept any minor flaws as normal rather than an unexpected deviation. To improve this situation, some filler material can be injected into the subcutaneous plane to soften any noticeable abrupt transitions.

The hardest thing to correct is an overcorrected ear. Once the scar tissue sets, an overcorrected ear possibly cannot be brought back to a less over-torqued position, at least in the author's hands. If the ear exhibits very resilient cartilage, the author tends to slightly overcorrect the ear with the knowledge that some relaxation will take place. Obviously, this maneuver should only be taken with experience that one's ears would relax. It is far easier to pull an ear farther back than to relax it when it is over pulled.

Conclusions

Otoplasty is a very rewarding cosmetic endeavor because it can almost be viewed as correcting a physical deformity that can be the source of teasing and low self-esteem for many individuals. Patients can be overwhelmingly satisfied with even the smallest degree of correction, and individuals are seeking this correction much more commonly later in life. In fact, the majority of my patients are adults rather than children who determine they would like some improvement in how they look later in life. This monograph is intended to guide a prospective surgeon through the trials, tribulations, and rewards of otoplasty through a single surgeon's experience with the procedure. Using a systematic approach to correct the ear and evaluating the ear as upper, middle, and lower deformities, the surgeon can achieve balanced results that are aesthetically pleasing without needing to be a supreme artist.

Reduction Otoplasty for Correction of the Large or Asymmetrical Ear

43

Christopher J. Coombs and Alex Yuen

Introduction

The pinna anatomically should sit within the boundaries of the middle 1/3 of the face (Fig. 43.1). It is usually only noticed in abnormality, which is particularly apparent with prominent ears. It has an extremely variable and intricate internal anatomy [15], but if the component subunits and proportions of the pinna have their appropriate anatomical relationships, then the external ear will be considered "normal."

A range of standard measurements for the external ear has been previously described [4]. The pinna, in appropriate proportion, is approximately 40–50 % longer than its width, with the length being 5.5–7 cm and the width 3–4.5 cm. [3, 4–6, 8–16]. Macrotia can be defined as a pinna that exceeds this normative data, but from an aesthetic point of view, macrotia can be said to exist when the pinna is larger than the boundaries of the middle 1/3 of the face (Fig. 43.1).

There are four main anatomical subunits of the pinna. These are the helix, the conchal bowl, the antihelix, and the lobe. It is the anatomical relationships of these that create the overall appearance of the pinna. In any aesthetic ear surgery, defining the anatomical difference will enable the surgeon to direct their surgery to return the subunit relationships to their appropriate proportions and relationships. In defining the anatomical issues in the large ear, it is useful to divide the ear into unequal 1/3s. The upper third is superior to the inferior crus, the middle third between the inferior crus and the incisura, and the lower third inferior to the incisura. Each of these "thirds" contributes approximately the following amounts to the overall length of the pinna: upper 1/3, 33 %; middle 1/3, 44 %; and 23 % for the lower third [16]. Knowing these proportions enables the surgeon to determine where the excess is in the large ear and also then create a surgical plan to address the excess.

Ear reduction is usually performed for one of two clinical presentations – either reduction of a truly large ear or to correct ear asymmetry, for example, with a unilateral lop ear deformity. In the situation of true macrotia, the excess is usually in the upper third with an increased scaphal height [7]. Also the earlobe can be increased in length (Fig. 43.2). In planning correction of the large ear, the surgeon may need to address both the scaphal and lobe excesses, in isolation or

C.J. Coombs, M.D., MBBS (Hons), FRACS (✉)
Department of Plastic and Maxillofacial Surgery, Microtia Service, Royal Children's Hospital, Flemington Rd, Parkville, VIC, Australia

The University of Melbourne, Grattan St, Parkville, VIC, Australia

Southern Plastic Surgery, 883 Hampton St, Brighton, VIC 3186, Australia
e-mail: chris@southernplasticsurgery.com.au

A. Yuen, MBBS, FRACS
Department of plastic Surgery
Royal Australasian College of Surgeons
Plastic Surgery Training Program,
16 Winfield Road, Balwyn North, VIC 3104, Australia
e-mail: ayuen7@hotmail.com

M.A. Shiffman (ed.), *Advanced Cosmetic Otoplasty*,
DOI 10.1007/978-3-642-35431-1_43,

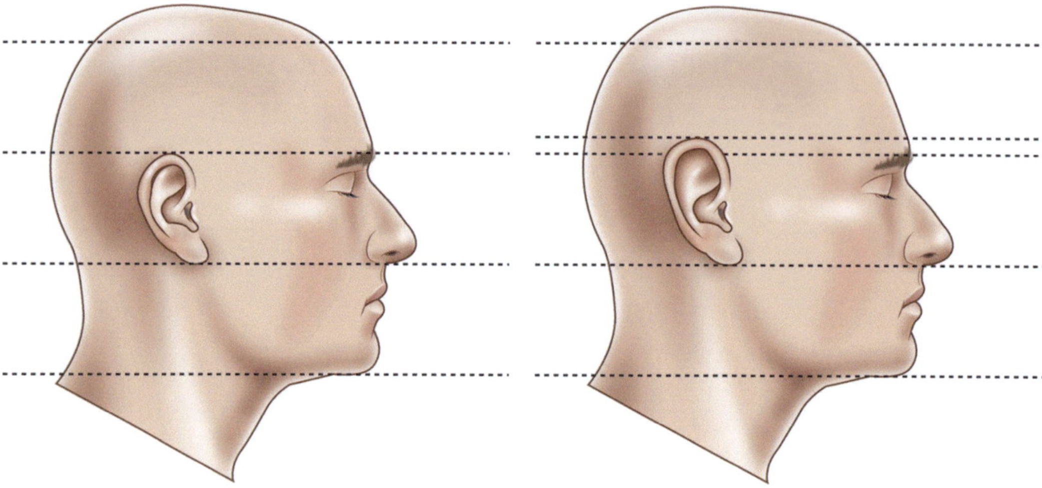

Fig. 43.1 The anatomical "correct" position of the pinna and when there is macrotia

simultaneously, with the aim being to recreate the appropriate internal proportions of the pinna and improved symmetry [18].

Historically, procedures have been described for ear reduction [2, 7, 17]. The first operations performed involved a full-thickness wedge resection of the ear's widest part with direct closure of the defect. Cupping of the ear and prominent scars resulted in poor aesthetic outcome. Later techniques described have placed the incisions at the edge of the helical subunit to improve the scars, using principles similar to the helical advancement flap described by Antia and Buch [1]. The key to a successful outcome for ear reduction surgery is appropriate preoperative assessment to determine where the excess is and strategic placement of incisions to hide the resultant scars at the junctions of the aesthetic subunits of the ear [18]. The placement of scars at the junctions of aesthetic subunits in the face leads to the least notable scars. Similarly, incisions on the anterior surface of the pinna at the junction of its anatomic subunits (the helical rim, the antihelix with the superior and inferior crura, the conchal bowl, and the lobe) will reliably produce scars that become virtually imperceptible.

The following procedure [18] follows these reconstructive and aesthetic principles. It can be used for correction of the scaphal height alone or for simultaneous correction of the scaphal height and the lobe length. It produces a consistent and predictable result, with excellent patient acceptance of the scars.

Operative Technique

Initially the length of the pinna is measured along its long axis. Analysis of the overall length is then done to determine the contribution of the upper, middle, and lower thirds to assess where the excess exists (Fig. 43.2). The required resection of the scapha, and amount of lobe lift, can then be determined to achieve the appropriate postoperative outcome in length reduction. The appropriate reduction in the scapha will result in a crescentic resection (Fig. 43.3) to reduce the upper third so that its postoperative height contribution is closer to 33 % of the overall height of

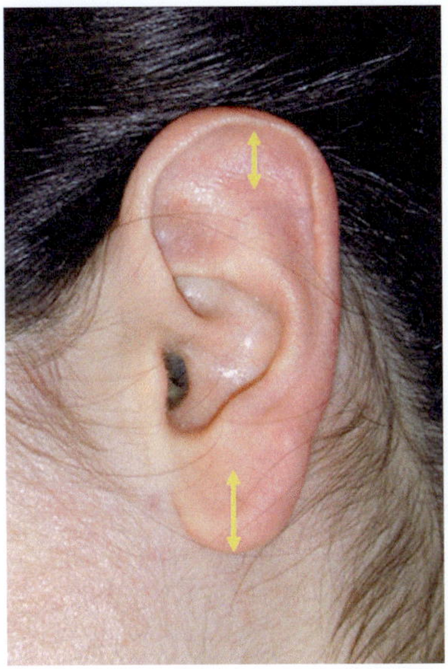

Fig. 43.2 Excess in both the *upper* and *lower* 1/3 of a macrotic ear

the pinna. The shape and position of the scaphal crescent will also determine the reduction in the upper third width, if this is required. The degree of lobe elevation also is estimated for recreation of its approximate 23 % contribution to the final overall height.

The procedure can be performed under local or general anesthesia. The incisions are marked, as is the amount of scaphal resection, which has been determined by careful preoperative assessment. The helical rim incision is taken inferiorly to the junction of the helical and earlobe subunits. This point is variable and needs to be determined for each patient by the surgeon. If there is excess length of the lobe and this requires elevation, then the helical incision is carried further inferoanteriorly in the groove the lobe creates with its junction with the antitragus and the inferior portion of the conchal bowl (Fig. 43.4).

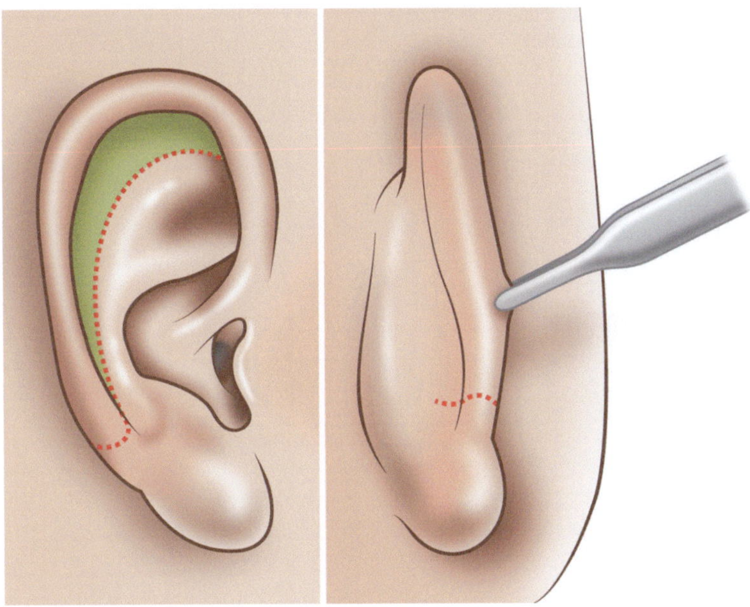

Fig. 43.3 Proposed incision and scaphal resection (in *green*)

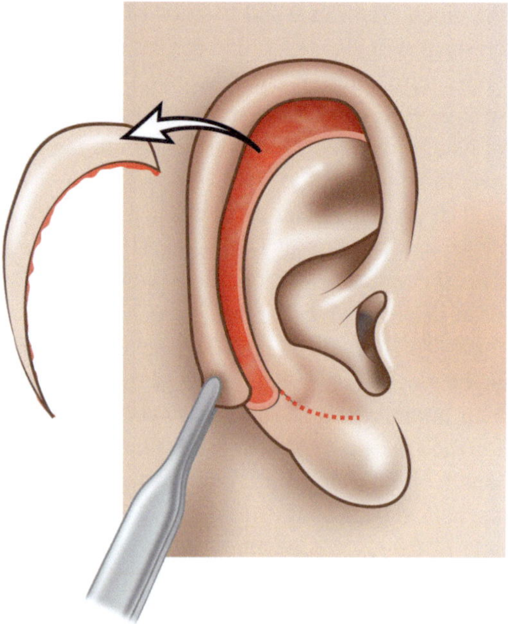

Fig. 43.4 *Dotted* representation of continued incision required for lobe elevation and chondrocutaneous scaphal resection, leaving postauricular skin intact

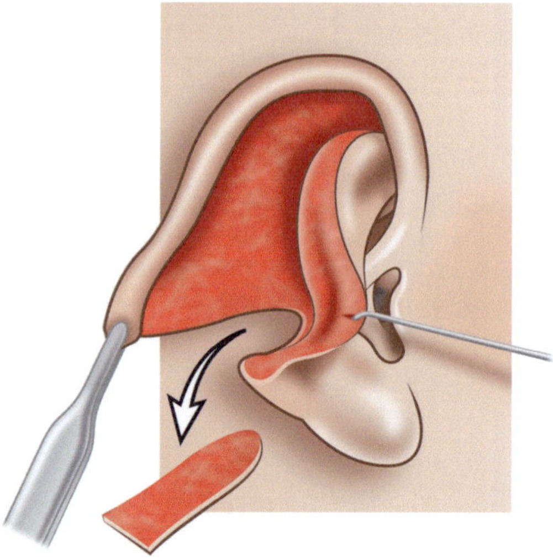

Fig. 43.5 Elevation of the superior postauricular skin flap with resection of the posterior "dog ear"

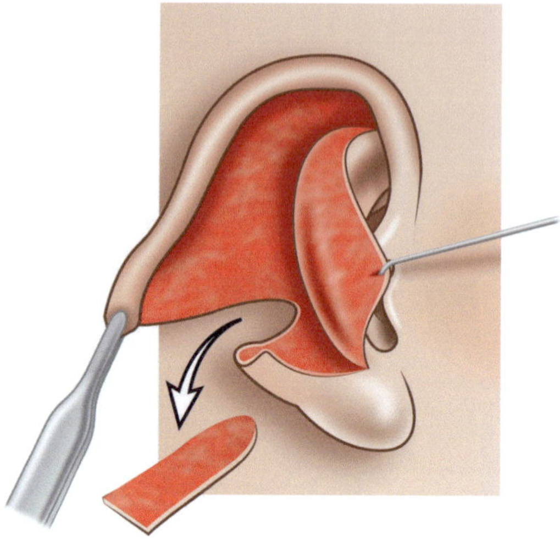

Fig. 43.6 Elevation of lobe if required on postauricular flap

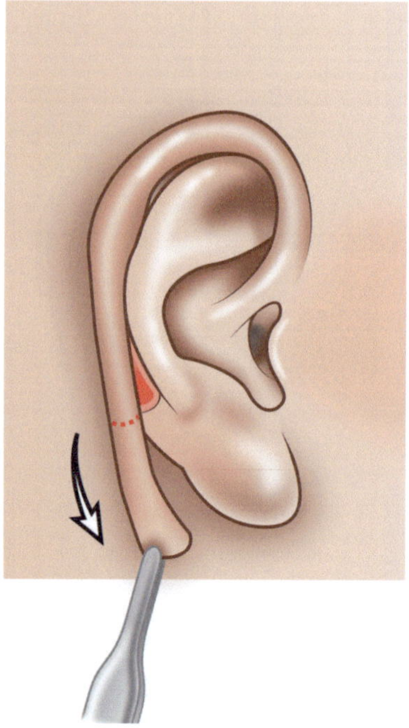

Fig. 43.7 Superior helical rim flap is advanced inferiorly to close the scaphal resection defect and rim resection amount determined

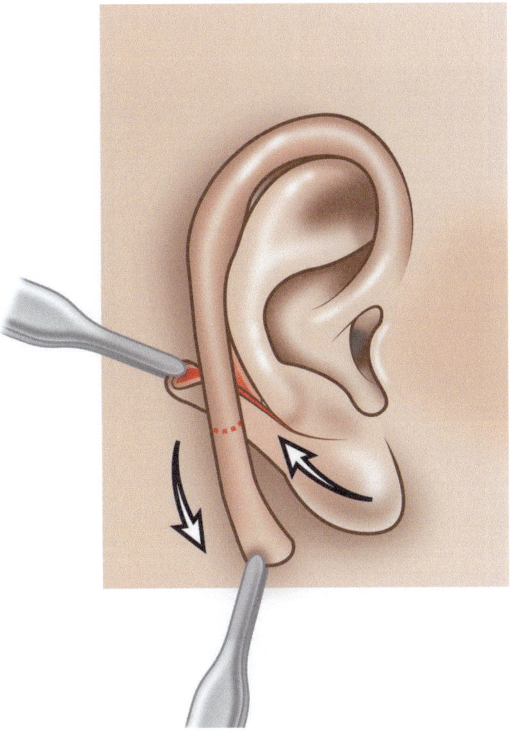

Fig. 43.8 Advancement and overlapping of both flaps when also elevating the earlobe to determine amount of resection

With the patient appropriately anesthetized and the incisions infiltrated with local anesthetic and epinephrine, the helical incision is initially made through the cartilage, leaving the postauricular skin intact. The predetermined scaphal crescent is then resected with the underlying cartilage (Fig. 43.4). The helical incision is continued inferiorly to the junction of the helical and earlobe subunits and then continued on to the posterior aspect of the pinna in a horizontal direction. The postauricular skin above the horizontal posterior incision is then raised from the posterior aspect of the ear cartilage just superficial to the perichondrium. This then creates a superior helical rim flap based on the postauricular skin to allow advancement of the rim in an inferior direction (Fig. 43.5).

If the lobe requires elevation to reduce its length, it is then also raised on the postauricular skin as a flap. The inferoanterior incision is continued in the groove between the earlobe and the antitragus and conchal bowl. The earlobe is then raised as a flap, similarly to the helical rim, based on the postauricular skin, which is dissected from the posterior aspect of the conchal bowl (Fig. 43.6). This dissection is carried as far as required to allow adequate elevation of the earlobe.

The helical rim on the flap of superior postauricular skin is then advanced inferiorly to close the scaphal defect, thus reducing the height of the upper 1/3 of the pinna. If the earlobe is not being altered, then following inferior advancement of the helical rim, the excess rim is marked and excised with the postauricular "dog ear" (Fig. 43.7). If the lobe is being elevated as well, then the ends of the superior helical rim and inferior earlobe are overlapped, and the appropriate excision of redundant tissue is performed (Fig. 43.8), again with the "dog ear" of the postauricular skin. Meticulous wound closure is then performed with particular attention given to approximation of the helical rim and lobe junction to avoid any "hour glassing" of the repair (Fig. 43.9).

Postoperatively the ears are dressed with a routine post-otoplasty dressing of gauze and head bandage for 5–7 days.

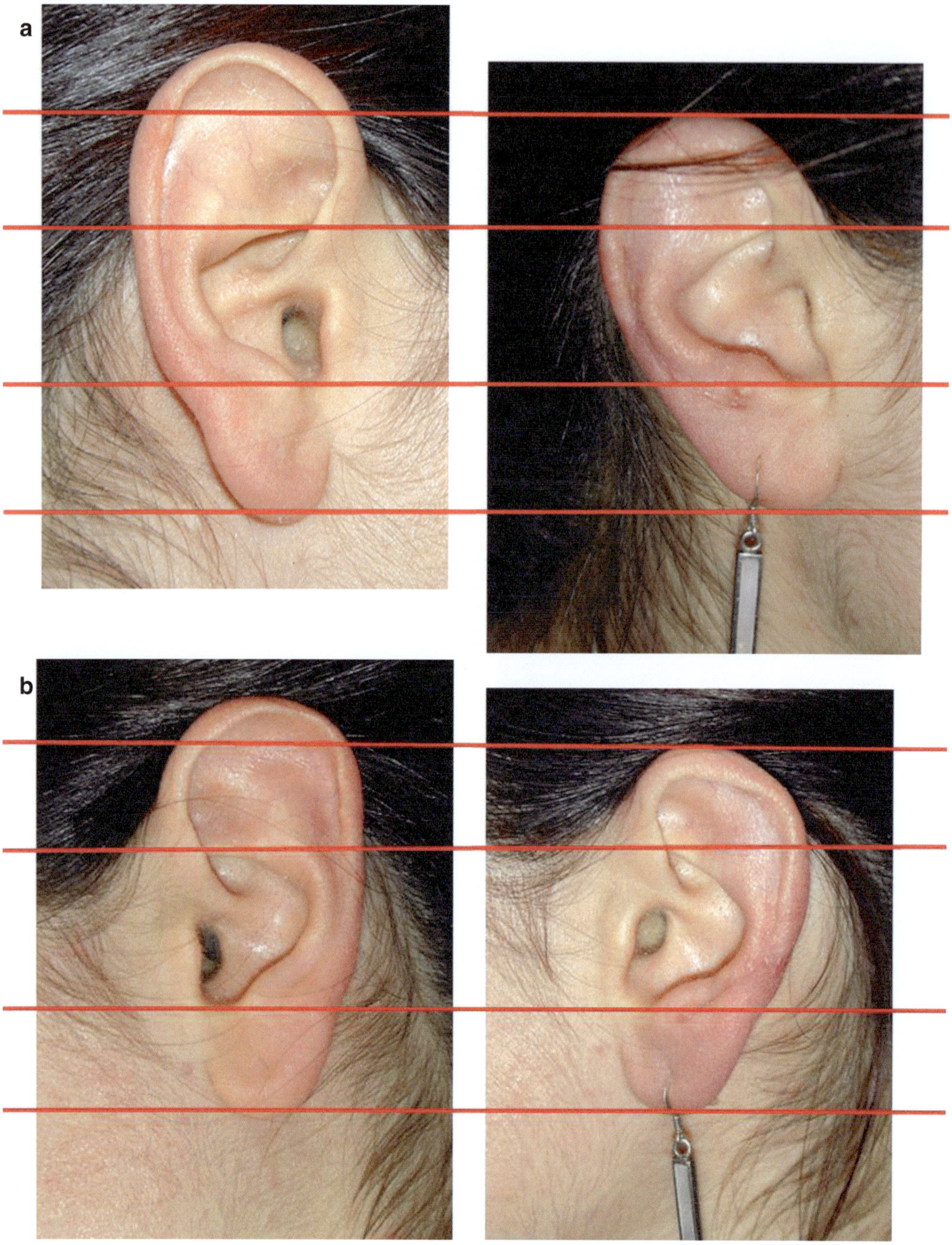

Fig. 43.9 Typical postoperative result showing reduction in *upper* 1/3 and elevation of *lower* 1/3. (**a**) Right ear. *Left* preoperative and *right* postoperative. (**b**) Left ear. *Left* preoperative and *right* postoperative

Conclusions

Reduction otoplasty can be a challenging procedure requiring accurate preoperative assessment and planning. The advantage of this technique is that it allows correction of the upper and lower third excesses simultaneously, thus restoring the appropriate internal proportions of the external ear while reducing the overall height of the pinna in a predictable and reproducible way. The resultant scars become imperceptible over time with their placement at the junctions of the pinna subunits.

References

1. Antia NH, Buch VI. Chondrocutaneous advancement flap for the marginal defect of the ear. Plast Reconstr Surg. 1967;39(5):472–7.
2. Argamaso RV. Ear reduction with or without setback otoplasty. Plast Reconstr Surg. 1989;83(6):967–75.
3. Broadbent TR, Mathews VL. Artistic relationships in the surface anatomy of the face: application to reconstructive surgery. Plast Reconstr Surg. 1957;20(1): 1–17.
4. Farkas LG. Anthropometry of normal and anomalous ears. Clin Plast Surg. 1978;5(3):401–12.
5. Farkas LG. Anthropometry of the normal and defective ear. Clin Plast Surg. 1990;17(2):213–21.
6. Farkas LG, Posnick JC, Hreczko TM. Anthropometric growth study of the ear. Cleft Palate Craniofac J. 1992;29(4):324–9.
7. Gault DT, Grippaudo FR, Tyler M. Ear reduction. Br J Plast Surg. 1995;48(1):30–4.
8. Hunt HI. War surgery of the face. Philadelphia: Lea and Febiger; 1926. p. 218.
9. Janis JE, Rohrich RJ, Gutowski KA. Otoplasty. Plast Reconstr Surg. 2005;115(4):60e–72.
10. Kotler HS, Robertson K, Tardy Jr ME. Pre- and postoperative management in otoplasty. Facial Plast Surg. 1994;10(3):244–54.
11. McDowell AJ. Goals in otoplasty for protruding ears. Plast Reconstr Surg. 1968;41(1):17–27.
12. Sheehan HL. General and plastic surgery with emphasis on war injuries. New York: Hoever; 1954. p. 331.
13. Skiles MS, Randall P. The aesthetics of ear placement: an experimental study. Plast Reconstr Surg. 1983; 72(2):133–40.
14. Smith HW. Calibrated otoplasty. Laryngoscope. 1979; 89(4):657–65.
15. Tolleth H. Artistic anatomy, dimensions, and proportions of the external ear. Clin Plast Surg. 1978;5(3): 337–45.
16. Tolleth H. A hierarchy of values in the design and construction of the ear. Clin Plast Surg. 1990;17(2): 193–207.
17. Yavuzer R, Sari A, Kandal S, Atabay K. A new ear reduction method without an anterior scar: posterior approach. Plast Reconstr Surg. 2003;112(2):701–2.
18. Yuen A, Coombs CJ. Reduction otoplasty: correction of the large or asymmetric ear. Aesthetic Plast Surg. 2006;30(6):675–8.

Correction of the Protruding Lobule 44

Cristina Isac and Aurelia Isac

Introduction

A key element to a successful otoplasty is the appropriate relationship between the lobule and the auricular cartilage architecture. If the lobule is not adequately managed, a telephone-ear or reverse telephone-ear deformity results.

The lobule is the lower non-cartilaginous third of the auricle. It should rest in a straight line with the helical cartilage when viewed from the front. Lobule prominence is thought to be determined by either excess skin or fibrofatty tissue behind the lobule or the protrusion or excessive length of the tail of the helix which pulls the lobule laterally (Fig. 44.1).

Failure to correct lobular protrusion during otoplasty will cause this deformity to appear even more conspicuous [1]. Actually, in most of the cases, after setting back the auricle and recreation of the antihelical fold, the lobule will almost always appear protruding. That is why lobule protrusion correction may be necessary in every case.

C. Isac, M.D., Ph.D. (✉)
Department of Plastic Surgery,
University of Medicine and Pharmacy "Carol Davila",
Bucharest, Romania

Department of Plastic Surgery,
University Hospital for Plastic Surgery and Burns,
Calea Grivitei 218, Sector 1, Bucharest, Romania
e-mail: ina@drisac.ro; inaisaac@yahoo.com

A. Isac, M.D., Ph.D.
Department of Plastic Surgery,
University Hospital for Plastic Surgery and Burns,
Calea Grivitei 218, Bucharest, Romania
e-mail: ireliflorin@yahoo.com

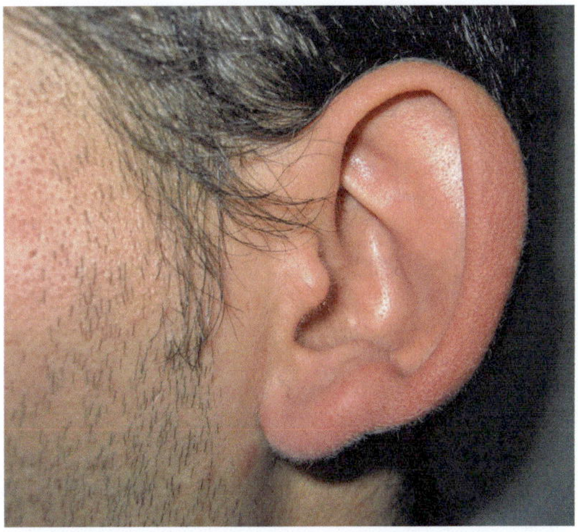

Fig. 44.1 Protruding lobule determined by laterally situated helical tail

Techniques to Correct the Protruding Lobule

Lobule setback is a difficult part in otoplasty. Few techniques have been described to resolve this deformity. In some cases, recreation of the antihelical fold may control the lobule position, since the lobule is attached to the helical framework [1, 2].

In case of a mild protrusion, retrolobular skin excision may achieve correction. Different skin excision patterns of the lobule have been described: fishtail, dumbbell, tennis racket shape, swallowtail, and rhomboid (Fig. 44.2). Many surgeons prefer elongating the postauricular skin excision inferiorly on the posterior aspect of the lobule in a widened shape-open book [1] or diamond shape [3]. Other approaches have included skin wedge

M.A. Shiffman (ed.), *Advanced Cosmetic Otoplasty*,
DOI 10.1007/978-3-642-35431-1_44, © Springer-Verlag Berlin Heidelberg 2013

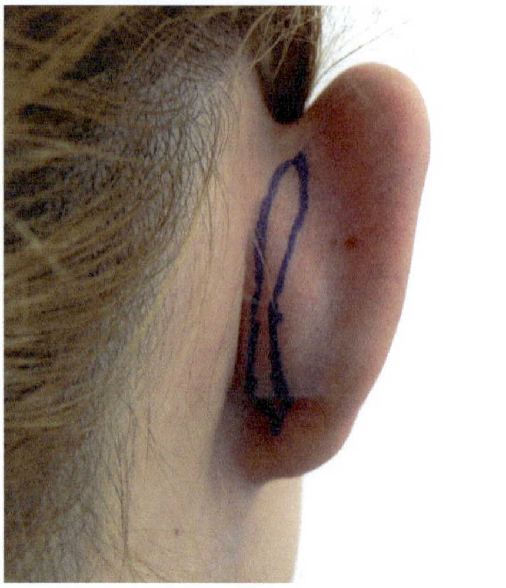

Fig. 44.2 Rhomboid excision from the posterior part of the lobule

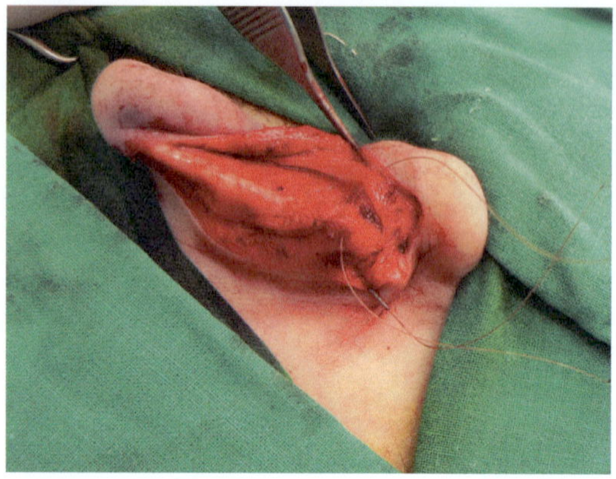

Fig. 44.3 The authors' preferred method: full-thickness incision and separation of the helical tail from the newly formed antihelix with 180° cartilage folded back and sutured; the helical tail is set back by a single horizontal mattress suture to the most inferior part of the concha

excisions on the medial aspect of the lobule [4–6] or curvilinear excisions along the inferior aspect of the lobule, anterior to the lobule-cheek junction [4]. However, skin excision should not encroach the retrolobular sulcus in order not to blunt it. In addition to the fishtail or elliptical skin excision, Karagoz et al. [7] excise one or more extra triangle-shaped skin islands at the lateral and inferior aspects of the elliptical excision to improve surgical results, stating that with regard to the lobule, two resections yield better results than a single excess resection.

Most authors agree that the lobule resting position is mainly determined by the relative position of the helical caudal end to the conchal bowl. This means that controlling the helical tail would effectively control the position of the lobule. Goulian and Conway [8] described the helix and concha as two separate units and advocated dissection of the plane between them to restore their relative orientation. Separating the helical tail from the concha allows repositioning of the cauda helicis [9], which, in turn, being attached to the cephalic portion of the lobule allows lobular position changing. The helical tail can then be approximated to the concha with different suture techniques.

Webster [10] identifies the tail of the helix as the key to otoplasty and recommends suturing the tail of the helix to the posterior side of the concha with one or two permanent horizontal mattress sutures. This is our preferred technique, also (Fig. 44.3). A full thickness that separates the helical tail from the newly formed antihelix is needed to allow the cartilage to be folded 180°. The lobule, which is attached to the helical tail, can then be set back by a single horizontal mattress suture which approximates the cauda helicis to the concha (Fig. 44.4).

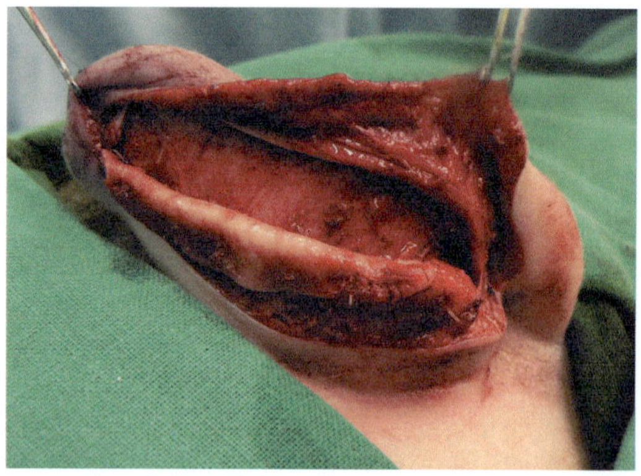

Fig. 44.4 Authors' technique of cartilage folding and the helical tail-concha suture in place to set back the lobule

Bauer et al. [11], by contrary, believes that the main cause of prominent lobule is not the helical tail, but the conchal shape. He advises against freeing the helical tail (which is a duplication of the inferior part of the helix) from the anterior skin because this maneuver will diminish the effectiveness of correction of the lobule prominence.

The conchal excision which he believes is a key point in prominent ear correction softens the cartilage spring in the helical tail, allowing the lobule to be more easily recessed. He addresses lobule prominence only by varying the closure of the posterior diamond-shaped inferior portion of the excised skin to different positions until the lobule setback is the desired one.

Siegert [12] uses one or multiple sutures from the dermis to the most inferior portion of the concha for lobule setback. The anchorage to the dermis should be strong enough but not too superficial so as to produce tethering of the skin or suture visibility. The path of each arc of mattress suture should be wide enough to allow strong anchorage of the intervening fibrofatty tissue of the lobule [1, 12]. A small anterior stab incision may be performed in the lobule to facilitate passage of the suture via an anterior or posterior approach [1]. Spira [13] uses a single similar dermal-mastoid 5-0 PDS suture placed in the primary incision line.

Gosain uses a dermal-mastoid periosteum suture to fix the lobule [4]. The point of suture placement is determined as the closest point on the medial surface of the lobule to the retrolobular sulcus which controls the lobule position and minimally alters the sulcus. Gosain uses a laterally extended small incision through the point of control and passes a single 3-0 PDS suture from the point of control to the mastoid fascia and the medial aspect of the postauricular skin incision. The main advantage of this technique is, as its author states, the stable result in time with no recurrence.

Thorne [14] excises a triangle of skin from the medial surface of the lobule. When the defect is closed, the suture incorporates the posterior surface of the concha.

Some authors advocate weakening the cartilage by scoring the helix of the tail or incising along its scaphal attachment prior to suturing [1], while others prefer its excision [15]. Adamson and Litner [1] states that by excising the tail of the helix, we only forfeit suture control of the lobule. Many authors also underlined the importance of leaving the tail of the helix and its attachment to the anterior skin intact as it is this attachment that allows lobule reposition [4, 5, 16, 17].

Helical tail fixation to the concha by means of sutures may be combined with posterior lobular skin excision.

If the lobule is not adequately managed, a telephone-ear or reverse telephone-ear deformity results. On the other hand, excess resection of the earlobule yields an either flat or stretched lobule.

In addition to being prominent after the setback of the ear, the lobule may also appear too long compared to the new shape of the auricle. Rodriguez-Camps shortens the lobule in almost every case with the use of a specific design [18].

Conclusions

Compared to the luxurious number of techniques which address the antihelical fold recreation and conchal setback published over the years, surprisingly very few procedures have been described for lobular protrusion. This is even more astonishing as inadequate lobule positioning may alter the result of an otherwise perfectly performed otoplasty.

References

1. Adamson P, Litner J. Adjunctive procedures: management of the helix, scapha and lobule. In: Adamson P, editor. Aesthetic otoplasty (Thomas procedures in facial plastic surgery). Shelton: People's Medical Publishing House USA Ltd; 2011. p. 45–53.
2. Beernink JH, Blocksma R, Moore WD. The role of the helical tail in cosmetic otoplasty. Plast Reconstr Surg. 1979;64(1):115–7.
3. Bauer B. Evolution and refinements in otoplasty techniques. In: Nahai F, editor. The art of aesthetic surgery- principles and techniques. St. Louis: Quality Medical Publishing; 2005. p. 1463–95.
4. Gosain AK, Recinos RF. A novel approach to correction of the prominent lobule during otoplasty. Plast Reconstr Surg. 2003;112(2):575–83.
5. Mustarde JC. The correction of prominent ears using simple mattress sutures. Br J Plast Surg. 1963;16: 170–8.
6. Furnas DW. Correction of prominent ears by conchomastoid sutures. Plast Reconstr Surg. 1968;42: 189–93.
7. Karagoz H, Eren F, Ulkur E. A new skin excision pattern to correct protruding earlobe deformity in prominent ears. Aesthetic Plast Surg. 2012;36(1):215–7.
8. Goulian D, Conway H. Prevention of persistent deformity of the tragus and lobule by modification of the

Luckett technique of otoplasty. Plast Reconstr Surg. 1960;26:399–404.

9. Caouette-Laberge L, Guay N, Bortoluzzi P, Belleville C. Otoplasty: anterior scoring technique and results in 500 cases (review). Plast Reconstr Surg. 2000;105(2): 504–15.
10. Webster G. The tail of the helix as a key to otoplasty. Plast Reconstr Surg. 1969;44(5):455–61.
11. Bauer B, Margulis A, Song DH. The importance of conchal resection in correcting the prominent ear. Aesthet Surg J. 2005;25(1):72–9.
12. Siegert R. Correction of the lobule. Facial Plast Surg. 2004;20(4):293–8.
13. Spira M. Otoplasty: what I do now-a 30-year perspective. Plast Reconstr Surg. 1999;104(3): 834–42.
14. Thorne C. Otoplasty. Plast Reconstr Surg. 2008;122(1): 291–2.
15. Nachlas NE, Duncan D, Trail M. Otoplasty. Arch Otolaryngol. 1970;91(1):44–9.
16. Elliot Jr RA. Otoplasty: a combined approach. Clin Plast Surg. 1990;17(2):373–81.
17. McDowell AJ. Goals in otoplasty for protruding ears. Plast Reconstr Surg. 1968;41(1):17–27.
18. Rodriguez-Camps S. Our procedure for integral aesthetic otoplasty. Aesthetic Plast Surg. 1997;21(5):332–8.

Repair of Split Earlobe with Free Conchal Cartilage Sandwich Graft

45

Rajiv Agarwal

Introduction

The ear is one of the most visible facial feature in a profile view, and hence its cosmetic concerns are frequently requested for correction. A torn earlobe is by far the commonest cosmetic problem of the ear requiring surgery. Torn earlobes result from various forms of trauma, including babies pulling on earrings, entanglement in telephone cords [1], hairbrushes and clothing, spousal abuse, and last but not the least by use of heavy earrings over a period of time [2]. In many Asian countries, especially India, ear piercing is practiced as a ritual and is customary for all girls to have their ears pierced at the age of 1 year. This practice makes the human earlobe the most used and albeit abused part of the body by metal ornamentations.

Many techniques have been published for the repair of earlobe tears [3–10]. These techniques consist of simple suturing of the tear, use of flap for preservation of earhole besides description of many different types of flaps to provide strength to the earlobe below the repaired earhole. All these surgical methods inadvertently tend to add to further scarring and weakening of the earlobe tissues, thus predisposing the earlobe to recurrent tears.

The earlobe anatomically consists of skin layer and subcutaneous tissue only with no internal architectural support of cartilage, muscle, or fascial tissue. The soft structure of the earlobe is hence not strong enough to withstand the continuous trauma associated with long-term earring use with its attendant problems of superadded incidental trauma due to inadvertent pulling of earring or even surgical scarring which is unwittingly contributed by repeated repairs of split earlobe.

A new technique has been developed which strengthens the earlobe with locally available conchal cartilage and provides the necessary reinforcement of earlobe tissues, preventing further recurrence following surgery. This technique also allows simultaneous creation of a centrally located earhole, thus eliminating the waiting period between earhole repair and reperforation. A new classification scheme and anatomy of acquired cleft earlobes is also described [11, 12].

Technique

Anesthesia

The operation is performed under local anesthesia as an outpatient procedure. The center of the earlobe is marked and tattooed. The edges of the split earlobe are first infiltrated with 2 % xylocaine mixed with adrenaline solution. Thereafter,

R. Agarwal, M.D.
Department of Plastic Surgery,
K.G Medical University,
Lucknow, India
e-mail: drrajivagarwal@gmail.com

M.A. Shiffman (ed.), *Advanced Cosmetic Otoplasty*,
DOI 10.1007/978-3-642-35431-1_45, © Springer-Verlag Berlin Heidelberg 2013

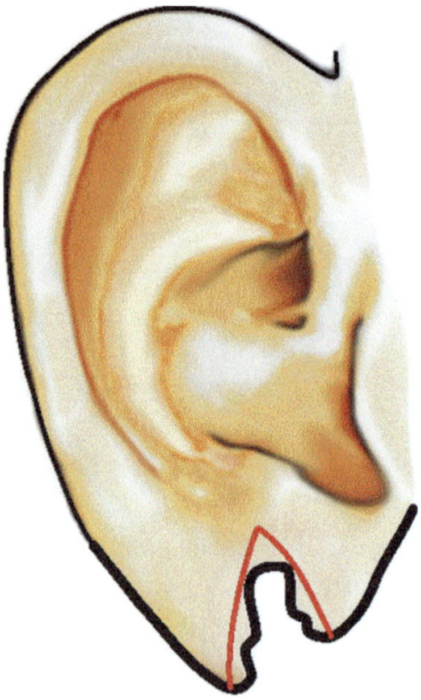

Fig. 45.1 Marking (in *red color*) for paring the edges in a case of right-sided total split of the earlobe with fibrosis and retraction of the earlobe halves

the same solution is infiltrated along a line located between the auriculocephalic sulcus and the helical border on the posterior surface of the ear. The plane of injection is between the skin and the conchal cartilage. Ten-minute time is allowed after injection to take advantage of the vasoconstrictor effect of the adrenaline and also for the swelling of local anesthetic to subside.

Paring the Edges

A stay suture at the apex of the earlobe is used to stabilize the lobe. Two stay sutures may be used on each side if there is total cleft of the earlobe. The cleft edges are pared using a #11 blade and the intervening inrolled skin tissue is discarded (Fig. 45.1). The same blade is used to create a pocket in both the split halves of the earlobe. The depth of the pocket should be two third of the diameter of the respective split half of the earlobe. Care is exercised so as not to unduly thin any of the split halves, thus maintaining adequate thickness of the tissue on all sides of the pocket. Hemostasis is maintained.

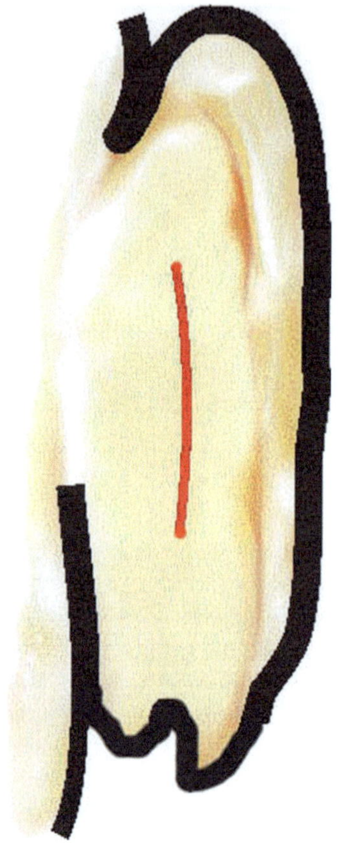

Fig. 45.2 Curvilinear incision located on a line between the auriculocephalic sulcus and the helical margin. Length of incision is usually 3–4 cm

Harvesting the Cartilage Graft

A curvilinear incision is made along a line midway between the auriculocephalic sulcus and the helical margin (Fig. 45.2). Skin flaps are reflected on both sides to expose the conchal cartilage. A disc of conchal cartilage of size commensurate with the created pocket is marked out and dissected out. The diameter of the conchal cartilage graft should be two thirds of the diameter of the repaired earlobe and usually measures 1.5 cm. for one side (Fig. 45.3). For bilateral cases, cartilage grafts may be taken from both the sides. Adequate care should be taken to not damage the skin of the anterior aspect of the concha. The donor site is closed after ensuring hemostasis. The harvested conchal graft should be inspected for

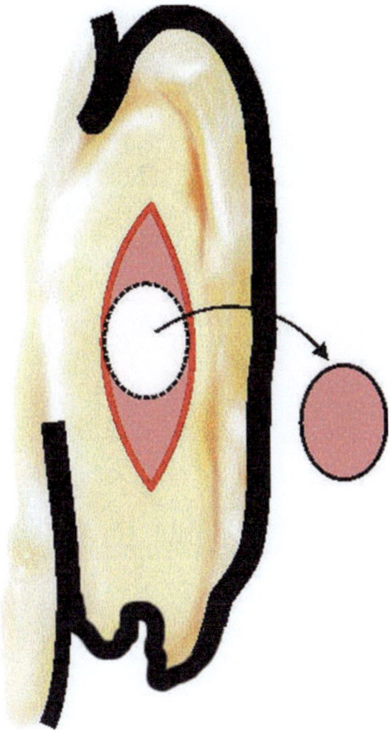

Fig. 45.3 Harvested conchal cartilage disc measuring approximately 1.5 cm in diameter

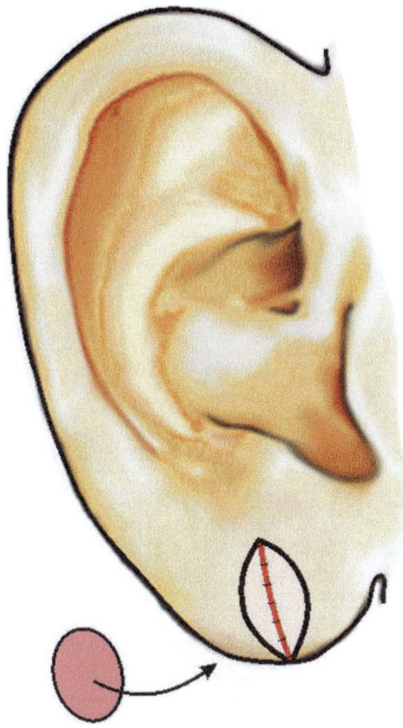

Fig. 45.4 Repaired posterior layer of the split earlobe in preparation for making a "bed" for the conchal cartilage graft

any thickenings, and if present, they should be shaved off using a # 11 blade.

Placement of the Graft in the Earlobe

The posterior layer of the split earlobe is closed first using 5/0 PDS so as to create the bed for the graft (Fig. 45.4). Next the harvested graft is placed in the earlobe pocket with the concavity facing anteriorly (Fig. 45.5). Care should be exercised so that any significant contour curvatures of the graft disc be corrected by scoring the graft on the opposite side. The anterior layer of the earlobe is then repaired in single layer using 6/0 PDS, taking care to maintain the shape of the earlobe (Fig. 45.6).

Simultaneous Creation of New Central Earhole

A new earhole is created at a central location on the repaired split earlobe at the marked site.

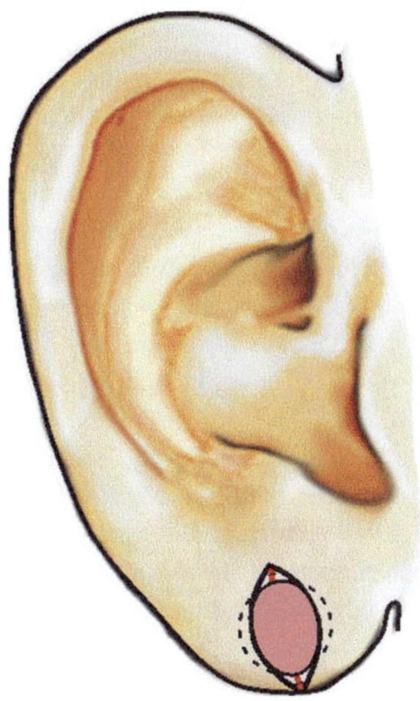

Fig. 45.5 Placement of the conchal cartilage graft over the repaired posterior layer. The graft is placed snugly in the pocket that is created in the earlobe on both the sides of the cleft

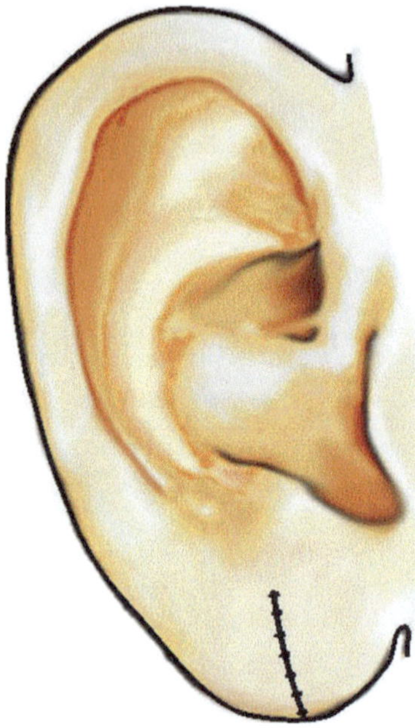

Fig. 45.6 The appearance after final closure of the anterior layer over the previously placed conchal cartilage graft

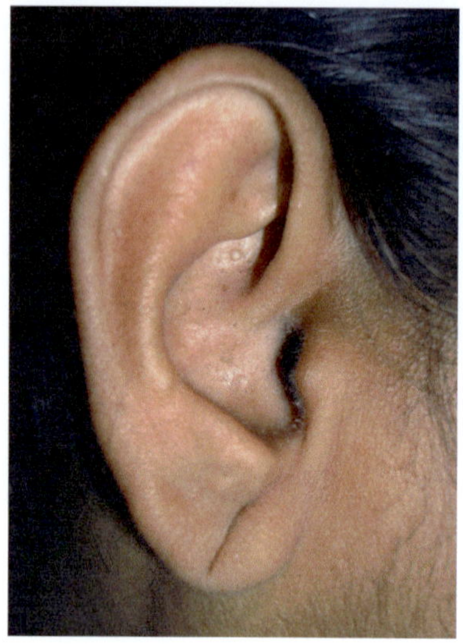

Fig. 45.7 Split right earlobe in a 42-year-old female showing the unique axis of splitting of the earlobe. The axis of splitting was 29° from the craniocaudal axis of the ear

A # 16 needle is taken and pierced from posterior to anterior direction at the proposed site of earlobe. The needle tip goes through posterior earlobe skin, new conchal graft, and the anterior earlobe skin. A stud type of gold ear jewelry presterilized in Lysol solution is taken and is simply inserted into the needle tip hole. The needle along with the stud is now withdrawn toward the posterior side and needle is taken out. The stud is now capped easily, completing the procedure. Alternatively, an intravenous cannula of 18 G is taken and passed through the proposed site of earhole. The stilette is removed and a ~5-mm length of distal sheath is cut and left behind in the new hole. The sheath can be even used for wearing artificial jewelry in those patients with positive history of metal allergy. Subsequently, as the tract epithelializes, the sheath is removed and the earhole can then be used for wearing appropriate metal jewelry.

Postoperative Care

Postoperatively, the ear cavity is packed with gauze soaked in antibiotic solution, and retroauricular support dressing is also given for 48 h to prevent auricular hematoma. An antibiotic ointment is freely applied over the earlobe reperforation site, and free rotation of the stud bar is checked. The patient is instructed to keep the stitch line clean with dilute hydrogen peroxide solution and Q tip along with twice daily application of antibiotic ointment. Twice daily circular motion of the stud is also recommended after application of lubricating ointment.

Patients are instructed to continue wearing light jewelry for at least 2 months after surgery.

Anatomy of the Split Earlobe

The pathological anatomy of the split of the earlobe is unique and interesting. It has been observed that the axis of the splitting of the earlobe does not correspond to the anatomical craniocaudal axis of the ear but is directed in a down and out position starting from the original centrally located earhole. This particular axis of tear was found to be present in both incomplete and complete splitting of the earlobes caused due to constant pulling by the earrings (Fig. 45.7).

On analysis using clinical goniometry and CAD measurements of these cases, the axis of splitting is a function of the relative position in which that individual holds the head while awake and performing various tasks. The vertical axis of the ear in normal head-holding position is inclined at an angle of approximately 25°±5°, and this fact determines the axis of the splitting of the ear. It is clear that gravity combined with weight of the earring contributes to the oblique axis of the split [12].

Table 45.1 Classification of acquired split earlobe deformity [11]

Type	Description
Type I	Stretched out hole of earlobe more than twice the original diameter[a]
Type II	Near total split of earlobe. A thin rim of soft tissue remaining
Type III	Total split of earlobe with preservation of soft tissue
Type IV	Total split of earlobe with fibrosis and retraction of earlobe halves
Type V	Single/multiple tears of earlobe with fibrosis and loss of soft tissue

[a]A normal earhole would be defined as one that is located in a central aesthetic location on the earlobe, is horizontally oriented, and allows snug fitting of a regular earring

A New Classification for Split Earlobe Deformity

The split earlobe deformity can present in a variety of combinations and degrees of split ranging from an elongation of the earhole to total split of the earlobe. Moreover, there are other variables that also need to be taken into consideration while planning repair for split earlobe, especially the condition and volume of the soft tissues and also multiplicity of the tears.

No formal classification for acquired split earlobe exists currently in the literature. Boo-Chai (1961) [3] described two types of acquired clefts: complete and incomplete. This classification however does not give enough details of the split earlobe.

A new classification system for grading the split earlobe based on its severity and also condition of the soft tissues is described. This classification system is helpful for planning the type of surgical treatment (Table 45.1). All the acquired split earlobes have been classified into five types with type I having minimal and type V having maximum deformity (Figs. 45.8, 45.9, 45.10, 45.11, and 45.12) [11]. The type of surgical repair for these grades of split ear should

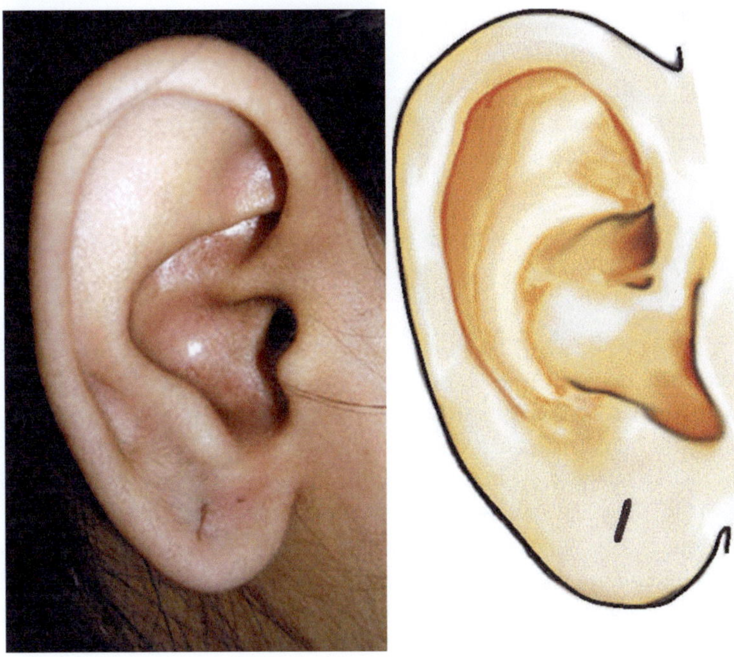

Fig. 45.8 Clinical photograph of right ear of a 21-year-old woman with type I classification of acquired split earlobe deformity

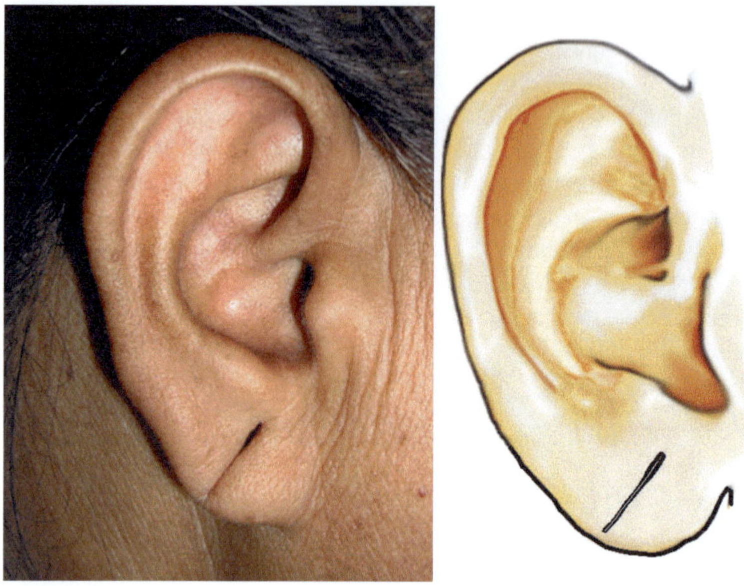

Fig. 45.9 Clinical photograph of right ear of a 45-year-old woman with type II classification of acquired split earlobe deformity

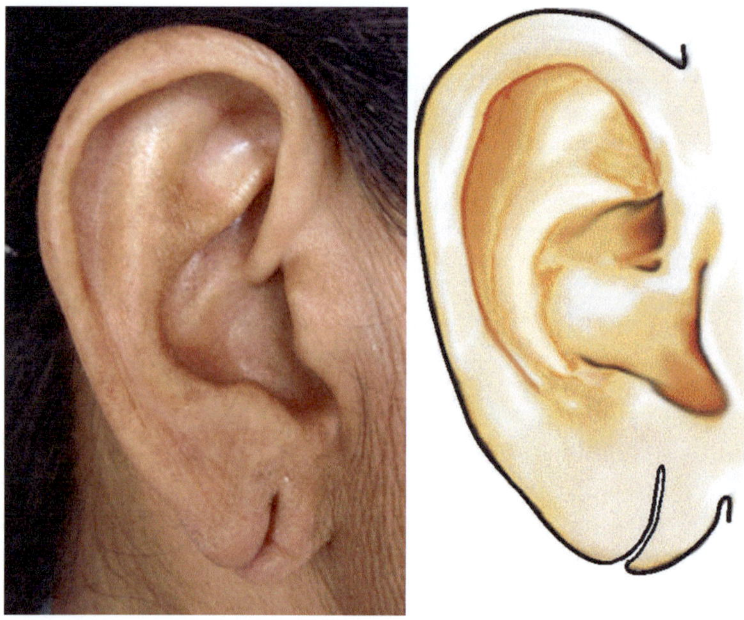

Fig. 45.10 Right ear of a 42-year-old woman with type III classification of acquired split earlobe deformity

take into account the various local factors including the quality of soft tissues, number of times the repair has been done previously, and the extent of split. Traditional repairs may be used for the treatment of types I to III, but we recommend the conchal cartilage graft sandwich technique for all the types of split earlobe except type I, where any of the traditional techniques may be used.

Discussion

The split earlobe deformity occurs primarily in women as they are akin to wearing heavy jewelry for a long duration. The splitting may be observed in age group ranging from 18 to 62 years; the average age of involvement is usually 35 years. Both the sides of the ear may be involved by the splitting forces. Majority of the women have had

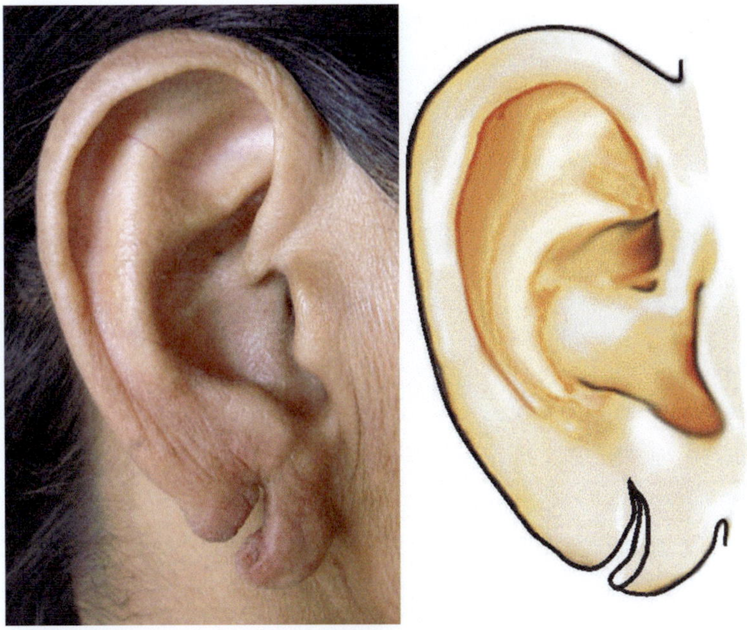

Fig. 45.11 Right ear of a 40-year-old woman with type IV classification of acquired split earlobe deformity

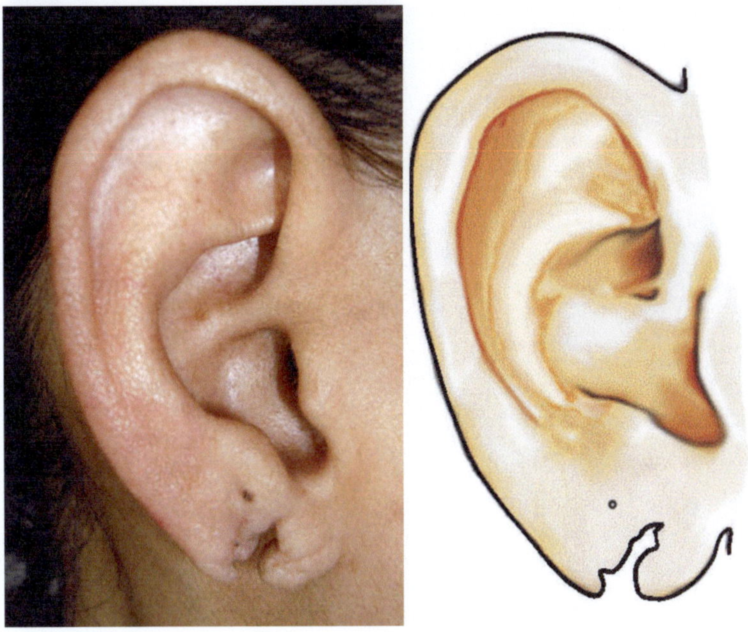

Fig. 45.12 Right ear of a 42-year-old woman with type V classification of acquired split earlobe deformity

three constant predetermining factors for the torn earlobe. Firstly, they have been using heavy jewelry for extended period of time. A positive history of acute pull on the earring was present in all the cases at some point. A positive history of metal allergy in the form of metal dermatitis of the earlobe may also be present.

The results of the repair of split earlobe using the conchal cartilage graft have been shown in a representative patient in Fig. 45.13. No recurrence of split was reported in the current series. The diameter of the earhole has remained constant over a follow-up period ranging from 1 to 3 years. The patients have been instructed to wear

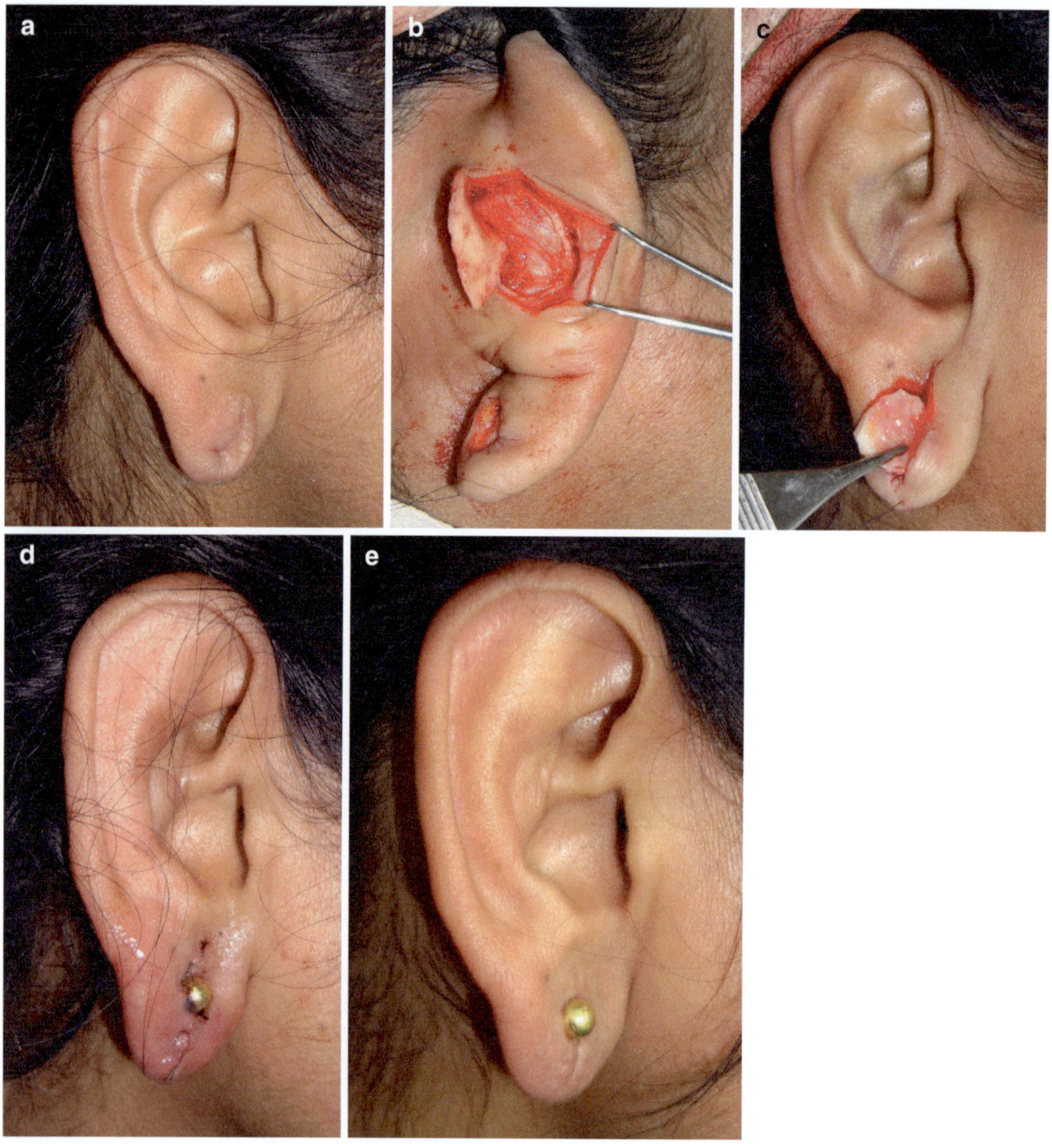

Fig. 45.13 (**a**) Right ear of a 45-year-old woman with type II classification of acquired split earlobe deformity before surgery. The tissues are torn and loose. (**b**) Intraoperative showing harvesting of conchal cartilage. (**c**) Intraoperative showing insertion of conchal cartilage disc into the earlobe. (**d**) Early postoperative showing suture line with simultaneous reperforation in a central location. (**e**) Follow-up showing well-healed suture line with the new earhole. The earlobe looks rejuvenated due to volume restoration, shape, and strength afforded by the conchal graft

light jewelry routinely, but occasional usage of heavy jewelry is also permissible with this technique.

The cartilage graft has settled well in this group of patients. The earlobe feels stiff for few weeks after surgery but gradually softens over a period of time. There has been no report of cartilage exposure or extrusion in this series. The conchal graft donor site has also healed well in this series. The scars have matured well and there has been no residual deformity of ear following removal of conchal graft. A granuloma was reported in one patient that healed completely after local curettage.

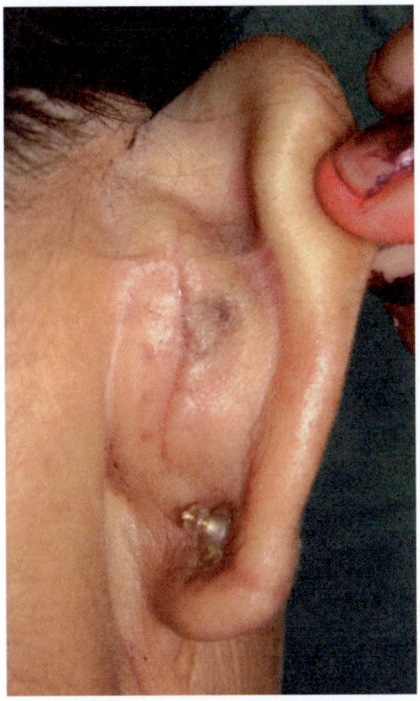

Fig. 45.14 Clinical photograph of a patient after conchal cartilage graft procedure showing minimal donor site deformity and scarring

The patients have been followed up for a period ranging from 6 months to 3 years. Six patients complained of residual swelling and hardness of the earlobe during the first 2 weeks after surgery. One patient developed a small granuloma at the site of the new earhole. This however responded with change in the earrings. No other problems have been reported by the patients in this series. The donor site has healed well in all the patients without any problem or deformity (Fig. 45.14).

The ears command a position of prominence and contribute to key aesthetic beauty of the face. The earlobe is one of the most visible parts of the face and is also the commonest site of the body which is used for metal ornamentations. Women and men alike enjoy wearing ear jewelry to enhance their appearance and to fulfill socioreligious obligations. Rings, posts, studs and many other trendy designs of earrings have adorned ears since ancient times.

In India, earlobes are universally pierced as a ritual before the age of 1 year among females of all races and also in specific castes of males too in adolescent age. The earlobes consequently are made to bear the brunt of metal ornaments very early on in life. The initial ear ornament is commonly either a stud or a small ring, but later on in adolescence and later years, there is a gradual shift to "danglers" and often heavy earring use. These types of earrings especially in young mothers are prone to being yanked by children, or they may suffer similar kind of acute severe pull or entanglement due to other reasons [1]. This acute event initiates a "tear" of the earhole which becomes the starting point for a split earlobe.

The split earlobe is a troublesome problem to the plastic surgeon because of high incidence of recurrence after repair. Many different techniques have been described in the literature for repair. These techniques range from excision of skin of the cleft edges and resuturing to fashioning different designs of flaps of skin on the anterior and/or posterior aspects of the earlobe. These techniques may or may not be combined with preservation of the original earhole repair [4]. There are several disadvantages with these techniques. Repair of split earlobe by either a straight line or any form of Z-plasty closure [5–10] introduces a scar right across the central "aesthetic" axis of the earlobe which constitutes an area of weakness in the earlobe. When a reperforation is being done, it has to be done on any one side of the scar, thus making the new hole in a paracentric position on the earlobe. These repairs subject the patient to a 3–4-weeklong waiting period between the repair and reperforation. The Z-plasty design often leads to lengthening of the earlobe, thus causing distortion of the shape of the lobe making the earlobe pointed in shape. There is also a possibility of an oblique retear as the upper limb of the repaired Z lies directly below the hole which slants downward. All in all, these Z-plasty techniques aim at introducing tongue of tissue below the repaired earhole for support, but given the compromised, scarred, and ischemic conditions of the soft tissues of the earlobe, these repairs eventually give way leading to enlarged earholes over time especially if the patient goes back to wearing heavy earrings.

It is interesting to study the likely cause(s) of elongation and splitting of the earlobe. Two important reasons have emerged as the inciting causes of split earlobe. The usual inciting factor is the acute tugging of the pendant earring by small children. This event leads to a skin breach in the lower part of the earhole which becomes a path for subsequent tear of the lobe. Dibbell [13] has also reported acute lacerations of the earlobes from forcible traction causing their clefts, and these findings have also been reported by Boo-Chai [3].

Raveendran and Amarasinghe [14] have reported a new theory of splitting of the earlobe as due to the allergy of metals used in the earring. We have also observed that earrings made of artificial metals lead to increased incidence of infection, granuloma formation, or even keloid formation at the local site. These factors found in 11 cases of this series lead to complete blockage of the earlobe necessitating a later redo piercing and leaving behind a potential weakness in the soft tissues which is prone to subsequent splitting of the earlobe. We have henceforth advised all of our patients to bring gold ear studs only for the procedure of simultaneous repiercing at the time of repair. Cornetta and Reiter [15] have devised a novel technique for those having metal hypersensitivity. They have described the use of the distal shaft of an intravenous catheter as an earring post sheath that allows hypersensitive individuals to wear earrings in pierced ears on a limited basis. McDonagh et al. [16] in a large study of 612 consecutive patients undergoing routine patch tests for suspected allergic contact dermatitis found that many women who have had their ears pierced gave a history of cutaneous reactions to metallic jewelry and almost one third were sensitive to nickel. They were of the opinion that ear piercing seems to induce nickel allergy which may result in lifelong morbidity and difficulty in employment. Jewelry suppliers should be encouraged to provide nickel-free earrings to reduce the frequency of this apparently avoidable problem. In the current series, all the women were preoperatively assessed for history of metal allergy, and those with suggestive symptomatology were pierced using intravenous catheter. Once the fistula was well formed, these women resumed earrings.

The human earlobe is composed of skin and subcutaneous tissue which is predominantly fat. There are no tough supporting tissues present in the earlobe and it is devoid of any inherent structural support. It is clear that an acquired traumatic split in the earlobe causes scarring, ischemia, and weakening of the earlobe. Repeated attempts at surgical repair further weaken and cause cicatricial volume atrophy of the earlobe and predispose to recurrent tears. Given such circumstances, we have devised a new technique whereby a healthy disc of conchal cartilage is harvested and placed in the earlobe at the time of repair. This cartilage disc has been found to provide many advantages and overcomes the disadvantages found with the traditional techniques.

The cartilage provides a buttress support to the ear and prevents retear as the new hole is done through the center of this disc. It restores the soft tissue volume of the ear, thereby improving earlobe aesthetics. Thirdly, it allows the creation of a central aesthetic earhole. Fourthly, it allows simultaneous reperforation at the time of repair and cuts down the waiting period completely, leading to high degrees of patient satisfaction and acceptability to this procedure. The conchal cartilage is an ideal support tissue for split earlobe repair as it is a standard donor source of cartilage and is located in the same surgical field.

There has been no recurrence or enlargement of the earhole following introduction of the conchal cartilage graft. Concha of one side is adequate to provide enough tissue for repair of both the earlobes, leaving behind the other concha for future requirements. In the event of theoretical possibility of enlargement of the earhole, a second hole can be conveniently made through the conchal graft at a nearby location, after repair of the previous hole.

The use of a conchal cartilage "sandwich" graft for repair of split earlobe seems justifiable as earlobe tears are limited to the area of the earlobe and perforations of the cartilaginous part of the ear by metal ornamentations is seldom seen. This is attributable to the fact that the metal ornament derives strong support of the cartilage that it pierces. A further similarity is also found in case of nose perforations which seldom tear. These perforations too are transcending the alar cartilage which provides enough structural support to resist tears.

Recently Mischkowski et al. [17] have also recommended conchal grafts as ideal cartilage graft material for reconstructive procedures. They believe that no other biological or alloplastic material approaches the qualities of fresh autogenous cartilage in terms of safety, durability, and versatility.

The only disadvantage with this technique has been a residual stiffness of the earlobe consequent to the use of the cartilage graft. However, only one patient complained about this and the stiffness resolved with time. Secondly, this is usually not a problem in majority of the cases as the earlobes are already covered by the metal ornaments and are hence inaccessible to the palpating finger of the patient.

There have been no reports of recurrence of splitting of earlobe following introduction of conchal cartilage discs at the time of repair. The earhole size also did not change over the follow-up period of 3 years. Additionally, there have been no reports of perichondritis in the earlobe in the operated patients, and all of them have tolerated these cartilage grafts well under cover of systemic perioperative antibiotics.

Conclusions

The conchal cartilage graft sandwich procedure allows immediate reperforation of the repaired earlobe at the time of repair in a central aesthetic location along with providing necessary strength to the earlobe, thus preventing recurrence in primary and recurrent split earlobe.

References

1. Niamtu J. Eleven pearls for cosmetic earlobe repair. Dermatol Surg. 2002;28(2):180–5.
2. Altchek E. Tearing of an earlobe by weight of a telephone earpiece on an earring. Plast Reconstr Surg. 1977;59(4):564.
3. Boo-Chai K. The cleft earlobe. Plast Reconstr Surg Trans Bull. 1961;28:681–8.
4. Pardue AM. Repair of torn earlobe with preservation of the perforation for an earring. Plast Reconstr Surg. 1973;51(4):472–3.
5. Hamilton R, LaRossa D. Method for repair of cleft earlobes. Plast Reconstr Surg. 1975;55(1):99–101.
6. Abenavoli FM. Split earlobe: repair using a half Z-plasty technique. Plast Reconstr Surg. 1996;98(2):372–3.
7. Agarwal R. Repair of cleft earlobe using double opposing Z-plasty. Plast Reconstr Surg. 1998;102(5):1759–60.
8. Gajiwala K. Repair of the split earlobe using a half Z-plasty. Plast Reconstr Surg. 1998;101(3):855–6.
9. Fatah MF. L-plasty technique in the repair of split ear lobe. Br J Plast Surg. 1985;38(3):410–4.
10. Staiano JJ, Niranjan NS. Split earlobe repair using a double-flap technique. Ann Plast Surg. 2001;47(1):89–91.
11. Agarwal R, Chandra R. A new technique for repair of acquired split-ear-lobe deformity: the free conchal cartilage sandwich graft. J Plast Reconstr Aesthet Surg. 2010;63(3):499–505.
12. Agarwal R, Chandra R. The anatomy of split ear lobe. J Plast Reconstr Aesthet Surg. 2008;61 Suppl 1:S114.
13. Dibbell DG. Split earlobe deformities. Plast Reconstr Surg. 1970;45(1):77.
14. Raveendran SS, Amarasinghe L. The mystery of the split earlobe. Plast Reconstr Surg. 2004;114(7):1903–9.
15. Cornetta AJ, Reiter D. Ear piercing for individuals with metal hypersensitivity. Otolaryngol Head Neck Surg. 2001;125(1):93–5.
16. McDonagh AJ, Wright AL, Cork MJ, Gawkrodger DJ. Nickel sensitivity: the influence of ear piercing and atopy. Br J Dermatol. 1992;126(1):16–8.
17. Mischkowski RA, Domingos-Hadamitzky C, Siessegger M, Zinser MJ, Zoller JE. Donor-site morbidity of ear cartilage autografts. Plast Reconstr Surg. 2008;121(1):79–87.

46 Prominent Lobule Correction in Otoplasty: With Step-by-Step Description of the "Y to V Setback" Technique

Yigit Ozer Tiftikcioglu and Ufuk Bilkay

Introduction

Otoplasty for correction of prominent ear deformity is well established despite the variety of techniques. It is possible to obtain successful results with alternate techniques based on surgeon preference or specific needs of the patient [1–16]. Maybe one of the most common long-term complications of the operation is an unnatural "operated" look of the ear. Intermingled recesses and folds constitute the complex anatomy of the auricle as we know it. This seemingly chaotic arrangement is in harmony and the human eye is very quick to detect any alterations to it [17]. Although most patients are satisfied as long as their ears are less visible than before, an unnatural looking ear will attract more attention than before, leading to annoying inquiries. Our current aim in otoplasty must be further refinement of the surgical technique in order to address finer details such as Stahl's ear, prominent Darwin's tubercle, and lobule prominence.

Disharmony of the lobule with corrected cartilage framework of the auricle is one of the common reasons of an "operated" look. The lateral surface of the lobule may be facing anteriorly as part of a cup ear deformity, or the rest of the ear may be normal as an isolated lobule deformity. Careful assessment of the lobule position during preoperative examination of an otoplasty patient is essential. However, normal lobules may also become relatively prominent after medialization of the helix and related structures, leaving the lobule in place. Therefore one should carefully reassess the alignment of the lobule with rest of the auricle after completion of the major steps of any otoplasty technique. The above-mentioned condition may result in a secondary lobule deformity if left untouched.

Misalignment of the lobule may result in "telephone ear" or "reverse telephone ear" deformities. If the lobule is readily movable together with the cartilage framework, it is possible to correct it together with no further intervention. However, such medial movement as a whole is often inadequate and further correction of lobule position is required.

Although earlobes are significant anatomic structures with regard to normal facial appearance, there are not many articles addressing this issue [7–10]. Review of the literature shows that some surgeons prefer skin excisions and others suggest correction of cartilage framework for correction of the lobule deformity [2].

Gosain prefers suturing of the tail of the helix to the conchal rim to correct lobule position [2, 13]. However, it is sometimes impossible to move the

Y.O. Tiftikcioglu, M.D. (✉) • U. Bilkay, M.D.
Department of Plastic, Reconstructive and Aesthetic Surgery, Ege University Medical School, Bornova-Izmir TR-35100, Turkey
e-mail: drtiftikcioglu@yahoo.com; ubilkay@hotmail.com

Electronic supplementary material
The online version of this chapter (doi:10.1007/978-3-642-35431-1_46) contains supplementary material, which is available to authorized users.

M.A. Shiffman (ed.), *Advanced Cosmetic Otoplasty*,
DOI 10.1007/978-3-642-35431-1_46, © Springer-Verlag Berlin Heidelberg 2013

lobule by manipulating the cartilage framework. On the other hand, buckling of the cartilage framework may cause unwanted irregularities elsewhere.

Advocates of skin excision believe that the prominence of the lobule is caused by skin excess [2]. Postauricular skin excision may be extended inferiorly to provide lobule setback, or a separate wedge excision from the posterior surface of the lobule may be performed [2, 3]. Although it may sound simple, these excisions are tricky and over-excision may cause iatrogenic lobule deformities. It is usually difficult to plan the amount of skin excision beforehand.

Spira used a single dermomastoid suture to medialize the lobule [2]. This is a very useful trick but necessitates dissection of the mastoid area that is prone to bleeding and hematoma formation.

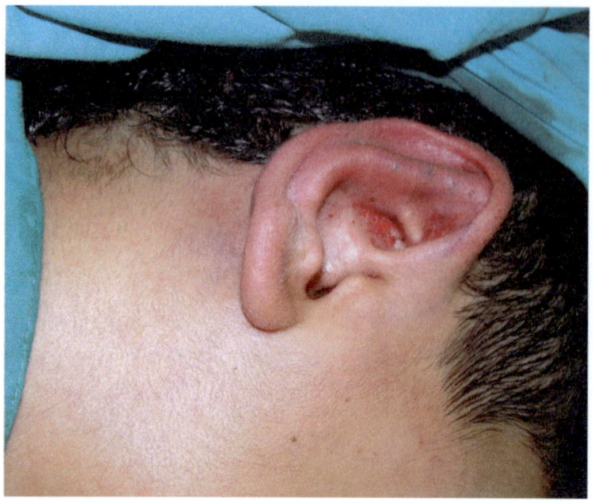

Fig. 46.1 A routine otoplasty was first performed with Mustarde conchoscaphal sutures and Furnas conchomastoid sutures. After the completion of otoplasty, the lobule is still very prominent despite proper medialization of cartilage framework

Authors' Preferred Technique

The preferred technique is Y to V setback of the lobule. It may be used as the last step of a routine otoplasty operation or for correction of isolated or secondary prominent lobule deformities. This technique is simple and easy to learn. The technique enables manipulation of the lobule independent from the cartilage framework. It enables sensitive calibration of the amount of setback and skin excision. Deep dissection that may lead to hematoma is unnecessary. Step-by-step illustration of the technique is as follows:

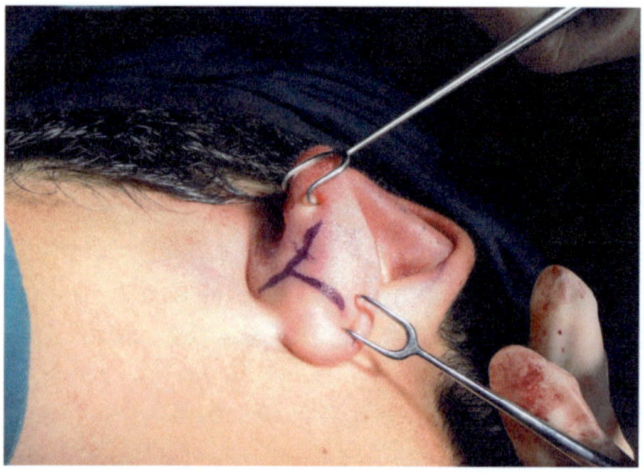

Fig. 46.2 A horizontal "Y" shape is marked on the posterior surface of the lobule so that the arms of the "Y" point the lateral edge of the lobule and the foot points the planned direction of medialization

Step 1

In this case a routine otoplasty was first performed with Mustarde conchoscaphal sutures and Furnas conchomastoid sutures. After the completion of otoplasty, the lobule is still very prominent despite proper medialization of cartilage framework (Fig. 46.1).

Step 2

A horizontal "Y" shape is marked on the posterior surface of the lobule so that the arms of the "Y" point the lateral edge of the lobule and the foot points the planned direction of medialization (Fig. 46.2).

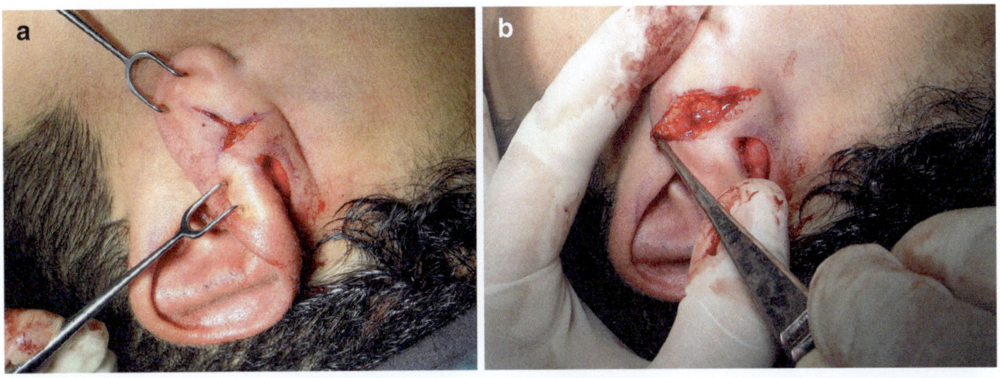

Fig. 46.3 (**a**) The "Y"-shaped incision is made. (**b**) A triangular skin flap is elevated from the area between the arms of the "Y"

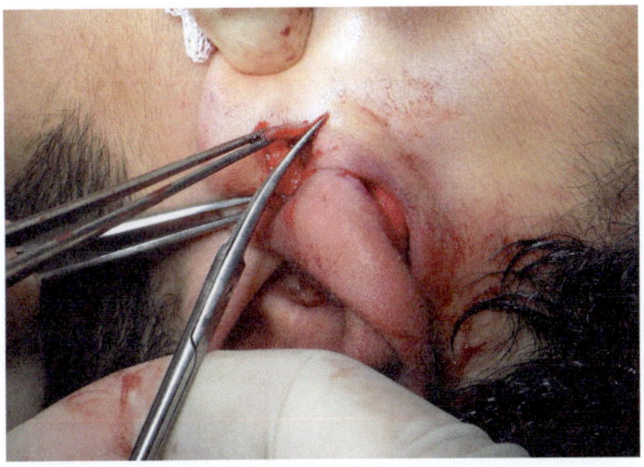

Fig. 46.4 The triangular flap is advanced medially toward the mastoid to be anchored to the tip of the foot of the "Y"-shaped incision. At this stage the new position of the lobule is checked, and the incision may be elongated medially if further medialization is necessary

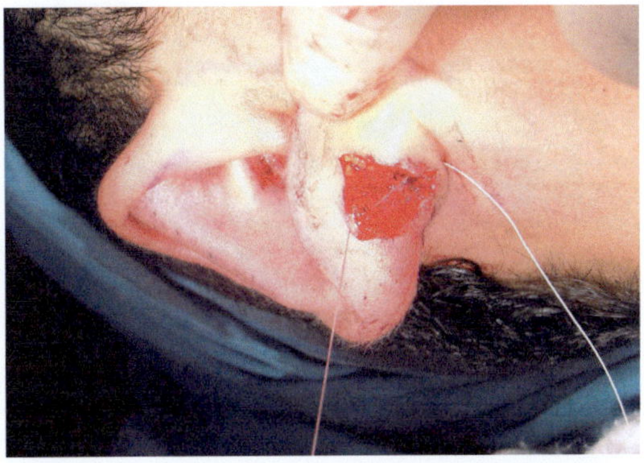

Fig. 46.5 The base of the flap is fixed with 3/0 polypropylene to the mastoid fascia. Excess skin at the sides of foot of the "Y" may be excised

Step 3

The "Y"-shaped incision is made. A triangular skin flap is elevated from the area between the arms of the "Y" (Fig. 46.3).

Step 4

The triangular flap is advanced medially toward the mastoid to be anchored to the tip of the foot of the "Y"-shaped incision. At this stage the new position of the lobule is checked, and the incision may be elongated medially if further medialization is necessary (Fig. 46.4).

Step 5

The base of the flap is fixed with 3/0 polypropylene to the mastoid fascia. Excess skin at the sides of foot of the y may be excised (Fig. 46.5).

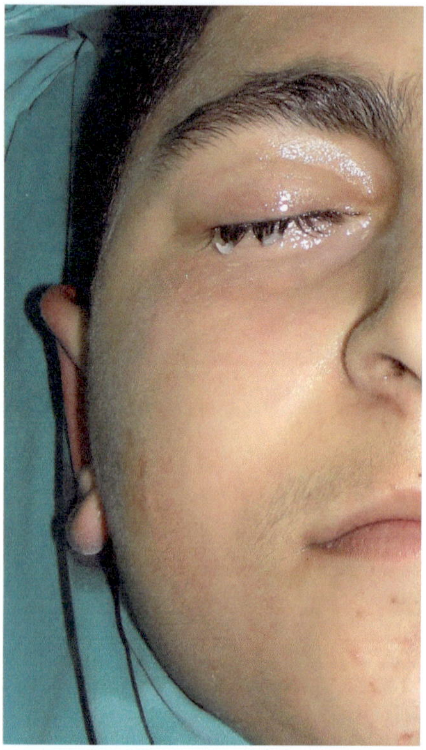

Fig. 46.6 The final result after the remaining skin incisions are sutured with 4/0 polypropylene

Step 6

Remaining skin incisions are sutured with 4/0 polypropylene and the procedure is finished (Fig. 46.6).

Conclusions

The procedure is easy to learn and the results are excellent (Fig. 46.7).

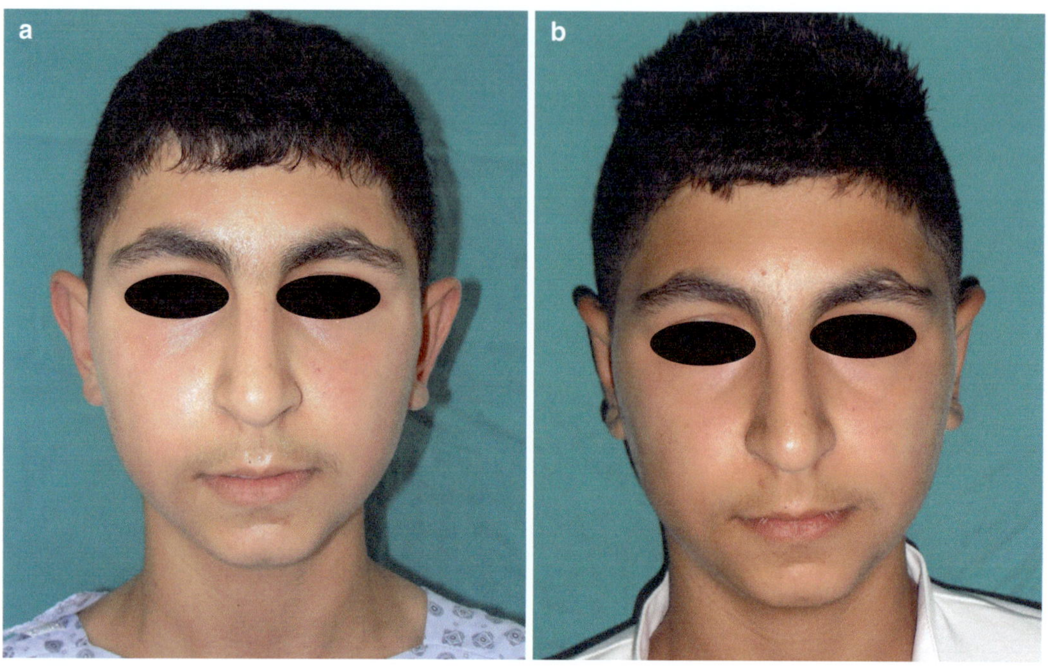

Fig. 46.7 (**a**) Preoperative. (**b**) Postoperative

References

1. Siegert R. Correction of the lobule. Facial Plast Surg. 2004;20(4):293–8.
2. Gosain AK, Recinos RF. A novel approach to correction of the prominent lobule during otoplasty. Plast Reconstr Surg. 2003;112(2):575–83.
3. Ellis DA, Keohane JD. A simplified approach to otoplasty. J Otolaryngol. 1992;21(1):66–9.
4. Schwentner I, Schmutzhard J, Deibl M, Sprinzl GM. Health-related quality of life outcome of adult patients after otoplasty. J Craniofac Surg. 2006; 17(4):629–35.
5. Becker DG, Lai SS, Wise JB, Steiger JD. Analysis in otoplasty. Facial Plast Surg Clin North Am. 2006; 14(2):63–71.
6. Nuara MJ, Mobley SR. Nuances of otoplasty: a comprehensive review of the past 20 years. Facial Plast Surg Clin North Am. 2006;14(2):89–102.
7. Yuen A, Coombs CJ. Reduction otoplasty: correction of the large or asymmetric ear. Aesthetic Plast Surg. 2006;30(6):675–8.
8. Mattheis S, Siegert R. Techniques in otoplasty. HNO. 2006;54(8):643–52.
9. Bajaj Y, Rokade A, De PR. Otoplasty: experience with a modification using a drill, and literature review. J Laryngol Otol. 2007;121(1):61–4.
10. Emery BE. Otoplasty. Facial Plast Surg Clin North Am. 2001;9(1):147–57.
11. Sevin K, Sevin A. Otoplasty with Mustarde suture, cartilage rasping, and scratching. Aesthetic Plast Surg. 2006;30(4):437–41.
12. Gosain AK, Recinos RF. Otoplasty in children less than four years of age: surgical technique. J Craniofac Surg. 2002;13(4):505–9.
13. Gomulinski L, Mauduy M, Saterre J. Our experience of otoplasty based on the study of the cartilaginous frame, especially the tail of the helix (about 244 cases and 22 anatomical dissections). Ann Chir Plast Esthet. 2005;50(3):206–15.
14. Adamson PA, Litner JA. Otoplasty technique. Facial Plast Surg Clin North Am. 2006;14(2):79–87.
15. Elliott Jr RA. Otoplasty: a combined approach. Clin Plast Surg. 1990;17(2):373–81.
16. Furnas DW. Correction of prominent ears with multiple sutures. Clin Plast Surg. 1978;5(3):491–5.
17. Bilkay U, Tiftikcioglu YO, Kapi E, Ozek C. Y-to-V setback for prominent lobule correction in otoplasty. Ann Plast Surg. 2011;66(6):623–6.

Compression Treatment of Ear Keloids by a Modified Oyster Splint Technique

47

Jessica C. Hassel, Alexander Kreuter, and Alexander J. Hassel

Introduction

Keloids can develop after injuries, surgical interventions, or skin piercings at certain predilection sites, such as neck, shoulders, breast, and ears. Keloids are benign fibrous proliferations, histologically characterized by excessive deposition of dermal collagen in a frequently mucinous matrix, due to increased collagen synthesis in fibroblasts and decreased collagen degradation [1]. Pathophysiologically keloid formation is still not fully understood. Mitogens like the insulin-like growth factor (IGF), the vascular endothelial growth factor (VEGF), and the transforming growth factor beta (TGF-beta) seem to play a distinct role in this process [2–4]. Foreign-body reactions, frequently observed after ear piercing, wound infections, as well as continuous tension on wounds after surgery or by heavy earrings, also promote keloid formation. Besides, there seems to be a genetic disposition for keloid formation in persons with black skin, certain HLA-types, and blood group A. Keloids may develop at any age, but young persons are most frequently affected [5]. Interestingly, after ear piercing, keloids seem to occur mainly in patients who were 12 or older when the piercing was done [6].

Although keloids are benign, they mean a substantial cosmetic disfigurement to the patients, especially if they occur on the ears, leading to a reduction of patients' quality of life. In addition, they can be itchy and painful. Treatment of ear keloids is still a major challenge. Because of the high recurrence rates of up to 80 %, surgical removal should be performed only in combination with other therapies [7]. Various postoperative treatments, such as topical silicone gels, intralesional corticosteroids with or without cryotherapy, radiotherapy, or compression therapy, may be used [5]. Although there is little evidence from controlled clinical studies, the most promising proceeding seems to be a combination of therapies [8].

Topical application of silicone gel sheets is intended to soften hypertrophic scars and reduce pruritus by skin hyperhydration [9]. For most of keloid formations, however, this therapy alone is usually insufficient. Injection of corticosteroids intralesionally is another common keloid therapy. Corticosteroids reduce collagen synthesis and increase collagenase activity [10]. However, in case of large keloids, particularly those developing on ears, this therapy is often unsuccessful,

J.C. Hassel, M.D. (✉)
Department of Dermatology, National Center for Tumor Diseases, University Hospital Heidelberg, Im Neuenheimer Feld 460, Heidelberg 69120, Germany
e-mail: jessica.hassel@med.uni-heidelberg.de

A. Kreuter
Zahntechnik Alexander Kreuter (Dental Laboratory), Reuenthaler Straße 7, Weilbach 63937, Germany
e-mail: alexander.kreuter@gmx.de

A.J. Hassel, M.D.
Department of Prosthodontics, Heidelberg University Hospital, Im Neuenheimer Feld 400, Heidelberg 69120, Germany
e-mail: ahassel@gmx.net

M.A. Shiffman (ed.), *Advanced Cosmetic Otoplasty*,
DOI 10.1007/978-3-642-35431-1_47, © Springer-Verlag Berlin Heidelberg 2013

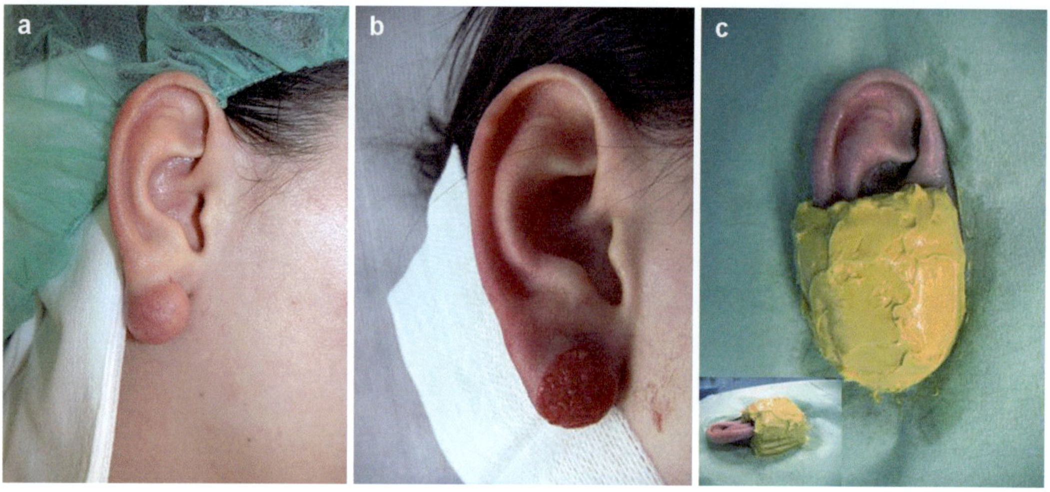

Fig. 47.1 Operation and silicone impression. (**a**) A 16-year-old girl with ear keloid upon presentation. (**b**) Clinical finding at 3 days postoperatively. (**c**) Silicone impression on ear after creation

even if combined with cryotherapy [11, 12]. Repeated cryosurgery alone may be an effective therapy of small keloids but often causes hypopigmentation [5]. Immediate postoperative irradiation of ear keloids can be successful [13], probably by destruction of the fibroblasts. But since there have been isolated reports of skin tumor development after keloid irradiation [14, 15], this option should be chosen only after careful consideration and failure of other therapies, especially in children [16].

Pressure therapy can be a good postoperative option [17]. The pressure applied should exceed the capillary pressure to generate local hypoxia which can be seen by blanching of the skin [18]. This will reduce tissue metabolism and inhibit fibroblast proliferation. Compression has also been shown to increase collagenase activity and stabilize mast cells, which leads to a reduction of pruritus. To treat earlobe keloids, a large variety of compression splints, made of metal or acrylic or equipped with magnets, have been developed [17, 19, 20]. However, the auricle is difficult to treat by compression because of the pressure sensitivity of the auricular cartilage. Here, mainly techniques that are common in dentistry and dental engineering are used [21–23]. The authors combined a modified "oyster splint" technique with intraoperative corticosteroid injection and topical application of a silicone gel sheet.

Technique

Keloid Excision

To minimize trauma and prevent tension on the wound, we prefer the shave excision of the keloid if possible (Fig. 47.1). Aim of the excision should be to restore the shape of the ear, not to excise the keloid completely [24]. Shave excision has another advantage, namely, to avoid sutures which could promote keloid formation by a foreign-body reaction. To optimize the aesthetic outcome, depending on the location of the keloid, excision and wound adaptation with sutures may be needed, however. After excision we inject triamcinolone acetonide intralesionally and place a hydrogel bandage on the wound to promote secondary healing by moist wound conditions [25].

Taking the Impression

Within the first week after surgery, the wound is protected by an adhesive film dressing (e.g., Hydrofilm®, Hartmann), and the ear is isolated with Vaseline. To protect the ear canal, a foam pellet is inserted. The impression is then taken with a two-phase, addition-cured silicone (e.g., Epiform®, Institut Schilling GmbH). Use of silicones guarantees a detailed impression and they are easy to remove from the skin. First, a thin, mobile silicone phase is used to

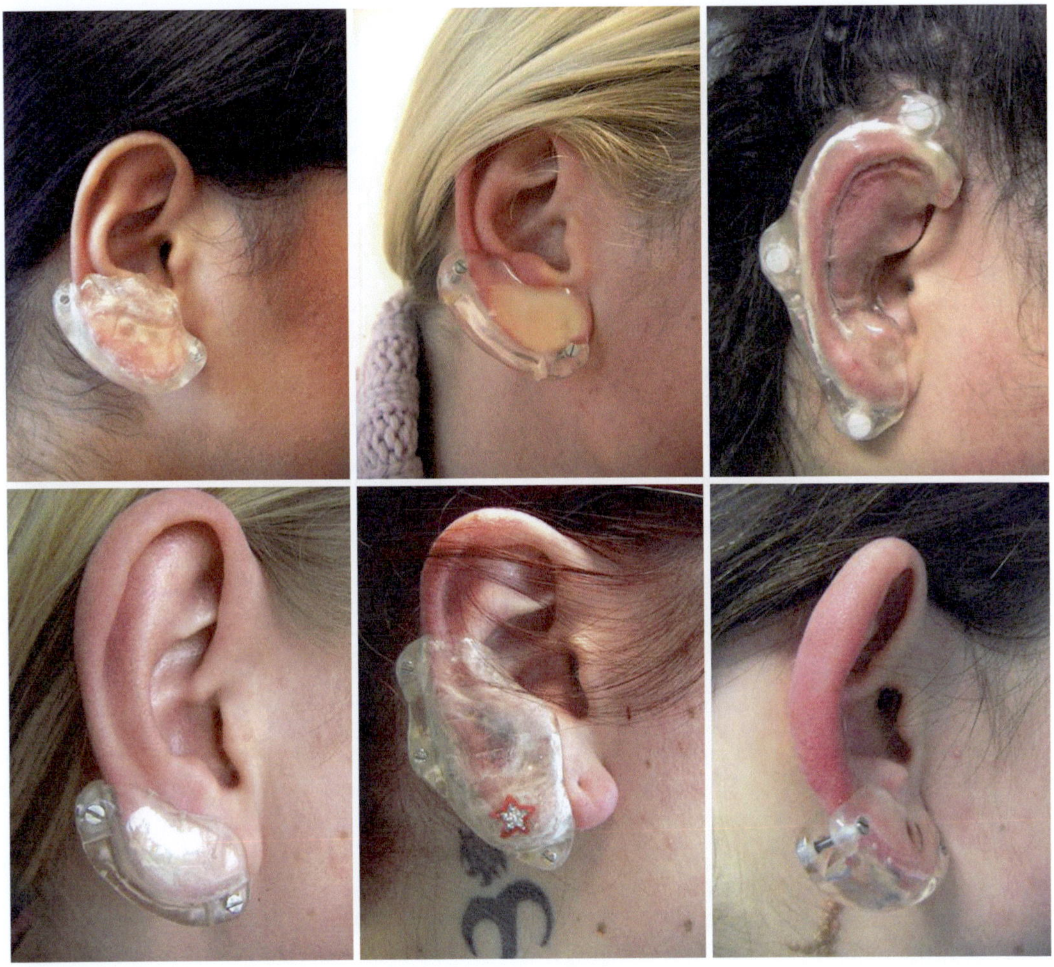

Fig. 47.2 Individual splints depending on ear shape and keloid location

obtain a detailed impression, without deformation of the ear, and covering approximately 1 cm of adjacent skin. A more viscous, yet still mobile, component is then used to complete the impression. The layer should be of sufficient thickness for stability (Fig. 47.1). While taking the impression, it is important to avoid air bubbles, to obtain an exact negative model of the ear. After setting of the silicone, it can be easily removed from the ear. The wound is covered with a silicone gel sheet (e.g., Cica-Care®, Smith and Nephew) and fixed with a bandage [25].

Fabrication of the Oyster Splint

The silicone impression is given to a dental laboratory to fabricate an accurate, true-to-scale stone model. On this model the "oyster splint," an acrylic resin splint consisting of two shells, is made. The splint is provided with nylon or metal screws to be able to adjust the pressure exerted on the patient's ear. A detailed description of the splint fabrication technique has been published [26]. To obtain a good functional compressive device, it is important to communicate with the dental laboratory and give an exact drawing on the parts of the ear which have to be covered. The oyster shells cover the part of the ear which was previously affected by the keloid, avoiding the ear opening. Use of transparent acrylate enables close observation of the underlying skin. If desired, decorative features can be incorporated [25]. With this technique very individual splints are made (Fig. 47.2).

Table 47.1 Patient follow-up (FU)

ID	Location of ear keloid	Duration of therapy (months)	Compliance	Recurrence	FU/time of recurrence (months)
1	Back of right ear	24	+	No	72
	Top of left ear	12	+	No	26 (Fig. 47.3)
2	Right lobulus	0	–	Yes	5
3	Right helix (3 in row)	22	–	Yes	24
4	Both lobuli	11	+	No	49
5	Right lobulus	0	–	Yes	8
6	Right lobulus	12	+	No	37
7	Right lobulus	24	–	Yes	25
8	Left lobulus	24	–	Yes	26
9	Left lobulus	24	–	Yes	25
10	Right lobules	3	–	Yes	3 (Fig. 47.4)
11	Right lobulus	12	+	No	31 (Fig. 47.3)
12	Right lobulus	>15	+	No	15
13	Right lobulus	>6	+	No	6
14	Left lobulus	>7	+	No	7
15	Left lobulus	2	–	Yes	4
16	Left lobulus	>13	–	Partially	13
17	Right lobulus	>7	+	No	7

Adjustment of the Oyster Splint

The pressure generated by the oyster splint is adjusted in such a way that the underlying skin turns pale, i.e., anemic, but the splint is not painful to wear. The method proposed by Mercer and Studd [22] was modified in so far as a silicone gel sheet is applied between the wound and the splint, to protect the fresh wound or hydrate the fresh scar and increase patient comfort. The splint should be worn 23 h a day. It is recommended to remove the splint for 1 h a day to enable care of the skin and cleaning of the device. During the first week, the patient's ear should be examined for pressure lesions. If necessary, the respective splint areas are abraded. If pressure seems to be too low (loosening of the splint, no blanching of the underlying skin), acrylic material can be added to the region of the splint corresponding to the keloid.

The duration of compressive therapy should at least be 6–12 months. If patients are wearing the splint regularly, no additional therapy is needed. However, a wearing time of less than 20 h a day – caused by incompliance or problems getting the splint on – is not enough to prevent keloid formation [27]. Then additional steroid injections into the developing keloid can be given to have time to solve the problem. Treatment cannot be stopped until there is no longer any activity in the scar.

Follow-Up of Patients

A group of 23 patients with a follow-up of at least 6 months have been treated with this technique by the authors from 2007 to 2012. The first important step to be successful with this treatment is to take time for detailed information about treatment options, the elaborateness of this method, and the importance of absolute compliance to make sure that only very motivated patients decide to take this treatment. Otherwise compliance and success will be poor. Despite this proceeding, six of the patients decided not to wear the splint after fabrication and did not return for recall visits. The median age of the 17 remaining patients was 18 years at operation (age range – 14–37 years); 82.4 % of them were female (Table 47.1). Two patients were not able to fix the splint properly to the ear and therapy had therefore to be stopped; both of them got a recurrence (Table 47.1). Thus, 15 patients were treated with this pressure device. However, of those, only half were compliant in wearing the splints for the supposed times; the other half stopped therapy too early or wore the splint in a kind of "on and off strategy," only applying the splint when they felt the keloid started to develop again. This explains times of 2 years followed by a recurrence; the scar never had time to settle down. Importantly, the incompliance of patients was never based on pain during wearing [27] but on the elaborateness of the method being always reminded of their keloid. Of six patients with recurrences, four decided not to do any treatment at that time. Two patients were referred to radiation oncologists because they had multiple local treatments already before the pressure device was made and felt not to be able to achieve compliance. They received 20 Gy (6-MeV electrons, 5×4 Gy) to the keloid area immediately after reexcision of the keloid. However, even with this treatment, the keloid recurred a few months after irradiation.

Some of the patients had additional corticosteroid injections into the developing keloid. But, according to our experience, this should be limited to give the patient a second chance for compliance when he realizes that the keloid will definitely recur. Otherwise it just prolongs time for definite recurrence. Our experience shows that success of this treatment depends strongly on compliance. By patient questionnaires we found out that to prevent the keloid formation, the splint has to be worn every day for at least 20 h for between 6 and 12 months [27]. Prolongation of therapy was always based on initial incompliance or problems to get the splint on. However, patients who managed to wear the splint appropriately were very happy about the cosmetic outcome (Fig. 47.3) [28]; most of them had several unsuccessful treatments before.

Discussion

Ear keloids continue to be a therapeutic challenge. The compression treatment by this modified oyster splint technique can be a very successful method to prevent the recurrence of ear keloids after surgical removal. However, it has to be taken into account that the duration of this therapy is long and its success largely depends on the daily wearing time of the splint, i.e., on patient compliance. Of course patients in addition have to have a certain manual dexterity in handling the splint screws. Putting the splint together with magnets might be easier but would not assure pressure adjustment. Figure 47.4 shows how the pressure is responsible for keloid prevention. This 16-year-old girl had a recurrence of the keloid just in an area where the splint did not cover the scar sufficiently. Regular follow-up examinations, allowing the clinician to check, among other factors, whether or not the patient properly applies the splint, are indispensable to this treatment. However, only one of ten patients considered the effort involved in this therapy unjustifiable [27].

As compliance is so important, it appears sensible to carefully select the patients for this therapy and inform them about the effort involved, in order to prevent a course of treatment that would be frustrating for both patient and clinician. High patient motivation is the basic prerequisite for a successful treatment and for satisfaction with both the method and the result. This technique can easily be combined not only with the use of silicone gel sheets but also with other therapy options, such as intralesional injection of steroids. This combination, however, was necessary mainly in those patients who did not wear their splints for more than 20 h/day [27]. If compliance did not improve, it was not able to prevent keloid formation.

Most of the patients had already undergone several other therapies, including surgery, intralesional corticosteroid injection, and/or cryotherapy. None of these therapies had prevented their ear keloids from recurring, which suggests that these ear keloid treatments may not be successful without any compression therapy. Postoperative irradiation is described to be successful with a relapse rate of 16 % after 5 years [13]. The two patients referred for radiation therapy suffered a recurrence. However, they received fractionized radiotherapy with doses of five times 4 Gy instead of a single 10-Gy dose 24 h after excision. But, in our opinion radiation therapy should only be the

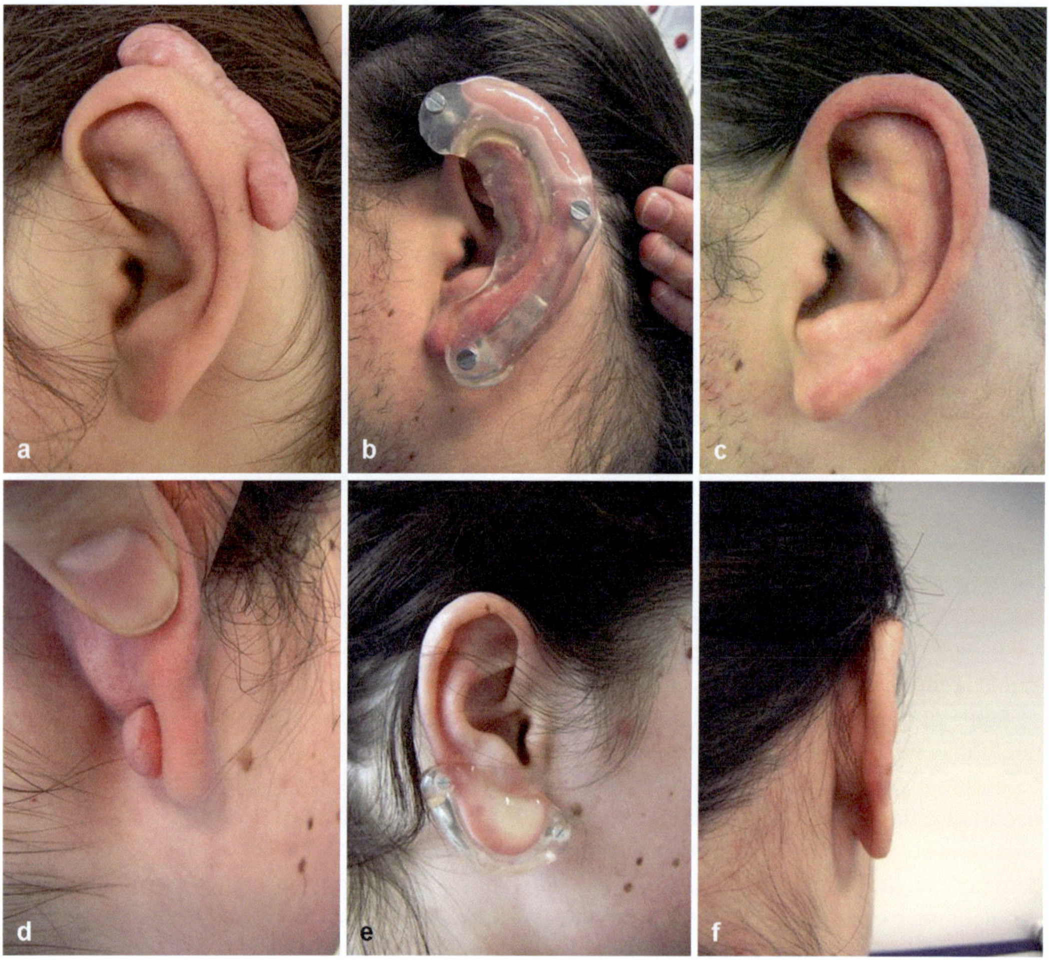

Fig. 47.3 Outcome of patients: (*top*) An 18-year-old man at presentation (**a**), wearing the splint (**b**), and 2 years after operation (**c**). (*Bottom*) A 22-year-old woman at presentation (**d**), wearing the splint (**e**), and 2 years after operation (**f**)

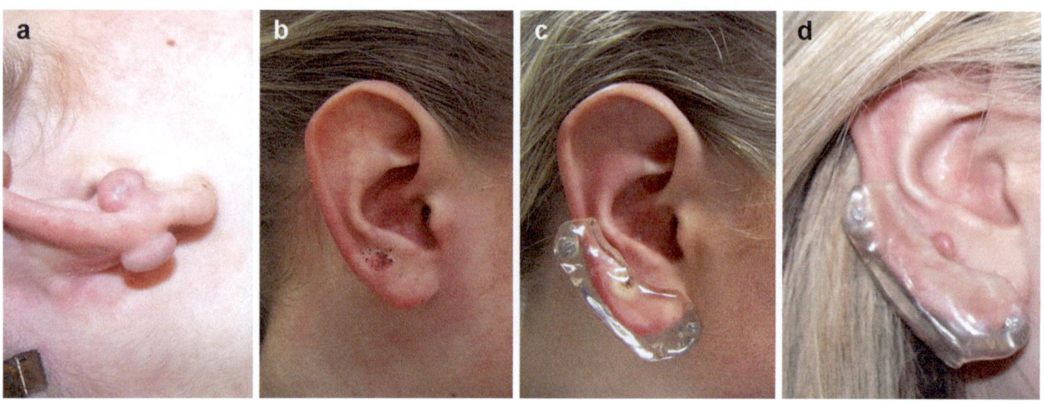

Fig. 47.4 Case of recurrence: (**a**) A 16-year-old girl at presentation. (**b**) Three days after operation. (**c**) Wearing the splint. (**d**) Three months later with a recurrence where the splint did not cover sufficiently. This case demonstrates how important sufficient pressure is to prevent a recurrence

last resort when treating ear keloid patients, who are usually very young, because it may involve the risk of causing skin cancer [14, 15].

Conclusions

Although it requires considerable time and effort, the modified oyster splint technique seems to be a promising keloid therapy with only minimal side effects. However, it is not suitable for any patient. The keloids have to be limited to the ears, i.e., a region on which pressure can be exerted by the compression splint, and the patients have to be highly compliant and show a certain manual dexterity in applying the splint.

References

1. Abergel RP, Pizurro D, Meeker CA, Lask G, Matsuoka LY, Minor RR, et al. Biochemical composition of the connective tissue in keloids and analysis of collagen metabolism in keloid fibroblast cultures. J Invest Dermatol. 1985;84(5):384–90.
2. Phan TT, Lim IJ, Bay BH, Qi R, Longaker MT, Lee ST, et al. Role of IGF system of mitogens in the induction of fibroblast proliferation by keloid-derived keratinocytes in vitro. Am J Physiol Cell Physiol. 2003;284(4):C860–9.
3. Le AD, Zhang Q, Wu Y, Messadi DV, Akhondzadeh A, Nguyen AL, et al. Elevated vascular endothelial growth factor in keloids: relevance to tissue fibrosis. Cells Tissues Organs. 2004;176(1–3):87–94.
4. Liu W, Wang DR, Cao YL. TGF-beta: a fibrotic factor in wound scarring and a potential target for anti-scarring gene therapy. Curr Gene Ther. 2004;4(1):123–36.
5. Olabanji JK, Onayemi O, Olasode OA, Lawal OA. Keloids: an old problem still searching for a solution. Surg Pract. 2005;9:2–7.
6. Mall JW, Pollmann C, Müller JM, Büttemeyer R. Keloidbildung des Ohrläppchens nach Ohrlochstechen. Chirurg. 2002;73(5):514–6.
7. Berman B, Bieley HC. Adjunct therapies to surgical management of keloids. Dermatol Surg. 1996;22(2):126–30.
8. Hackert I, Aschoff R, Sebastian G. The treatment of keloids. Hautarzt. 2003;54(10):1003–15.
9. Gold MH, Foster TD, Adair MA, Burlison K, Lewis T. Prevention of hypertrophic scars and keloids by the prophylactic use of topical silicone gel sheets following a surgical procedure in an office setting. Dermatol Surg. 2001;27(7):641–4.
10. Diegelmann RF, Bryant CP, Cohen IK. Tissue alpha globulins in keloid formation. Plast Reconstr Surg. 1977;59(3):418–23.
11. Griffith B, Monroe CW, McKinney P. A follow-up study on the treatment of keloids with triamcinolone acetonide. Plast Reconstr Surg. 1970;46(2):145–50.
12. Sclafani AP, Gordon L, Chadha M, Romo 3rd T. Prevention of earlobe keloid recurrence with postoperative corticosteroid injections versus radiation therapy: a randomized, prospective study and review of the literature. Dermatol Surg. 1996;22(6):569–74.
13. Ragoowansi R, Cornes PG, Glees JP, Powell BW, Moss AL. Ear-lobe keloids: treatment by a protocol of surgical excision and immediate postoperative adjuvant radiotherapy. Br J Plast Surg. 2001;54(6):505–7.
14. Botwood N, Lewanski C, Lowdell C. The risks of treating keloids with radiotherapy. Br J Radiol. 1999;72(864):1222–4.
15. Epstein R, Hanham I, Dale R. Radiotherapy induced second cancers: are we doing enough to protect young patients? Eur J Cancer. 1997;33(4):526–30.
16. Saladi RN, Persoud AN. The causes of skin cancer: a comprehensive review. Drugs Today (Barc). 2005;41(1):37–53.
17. Brent B. The role of pressure therapy in management of earlobe keloids: preliminary report of a controlled study. Ann Plast Surg. 1978;1(6):579–81.
18. Rockwell WB, Cohen EK, Ehrlich HP. Keloids and hypertrophic scars: a comprehensive review. Plast Reconstr Surg. 1989;84(5):827–37.
19. Chang CH, Song JY, Park JH, Seo SW. The efficacy of magnetic disks for the treatment of earlobe hypertrophic scar. Ann Plast Surg. 2005;54(5):566–9.
20. Snyder GB. Button compression for keloids of the lobule. Br J Plast Surg. 1974;27(2):186–7.
21. Sela M, Taicher S. Prosthetic treatment of earlobe keloids. J Prosthet Dent. 1984;52(3):417–8.
22. Mercer DM, Studd DM. "Oyster splint": a new compression device for the treatment of keloid scars of the ear. Br J Plast Surg. 1983;36(1):75–8.
23. Bahmer FA, Scheicher S, Zilz W. Treatment of earlobe keloids by the "oyster-splint technique" according to Mercer and Studd. Akt Dermatol. 1993;19:64–6.
24. Cosman B, Wolff M. Correlation of keloid recurrence with completeness of local excision. Plast Reconstr Surg. 1972;50(2):163–6.
25. Hassel JC, Löser C, Voigtländer V, Rammelsberg P, Hassel AJ. Treatment of ear keloids by the oyster splint technique. Cosmet Med. 2007;6:269–73. No additional issue number.
26. Kreuter A, Hassel JC, Voigtländer V, Rammelsberg P, Hassel AJ. Interdisziplinäre Behandlung von Ohrkeloiden – die "Austernschalentechnik". Quintessenz Zahntech. 2006;32(4):394–8.
27. Hassel JC, Löser C, Koenen W, Kreuter A, Hassel AJ. Promising results from a pilot study on compression treatment of ear keloids. J Cutan Med Surg. 2011;15(3):130–6.
28. Hassel JC, Roberg B, Kreuter A, Voigtländer V, Rammelsberg P, Hassel AJ. Treatment of ear keloids by compression, using a modified oyster splint technique – a case report. Dermatol Surg. 2007;33(2):208–12.

Part IV

Postoperative

A New Postoperative Otoplasty Dressing Technique Using Cyanoacrylate Tissue Adhesives

48

Volker Wedler, Miriam Vetter, and Matthias Foehn

Introduction

Otoplasty is a commonly performed operation in plastic surgery. The obvious goal of cosmetic surgery of prominent ears is to normalize the shape and position of both ears with maximal symmetry [1]. Usually both ears have to undergo a surgical procedure, but sometimes, a unilateral procedure is performed. In general, otoplasty surgery patients are children; however, in the authors' department, most patients are adults. It is technically difficult to apply a postoperative dressing because of its tendency to slip. The dressings for adults are different than those for children. An attractive appearance in public and for the possibility of returning to work is important. The aim of the dressing is to maintain the desired shape and position postoperatively. Another goal is to prevent hematoma or loosening of the dressing. Classic otoplasty dressings have been described as variants on a cotton wool pad placed over either a dry dressing or a Vaseline gauze securing each ear in position. Usually an elastic bandage is bonded around the head. Problems and complications of postoperative ear dressings are loosening, especially during the night; postoperative discomfort; and even skin necrosis because of the wrapping being too tight [2–6].

Technique

After the surgical procedure, the authors use the cyanoacrylate tissue adhesives for closing the skin. It is necessary to clean the wound thoroughly and then apply the bonding in thin layers with a light, brushing stroke while holding the edges of the wound together. After that, we fixate the concha at the mastoid also using the bonding (Fig. 48.1). It is

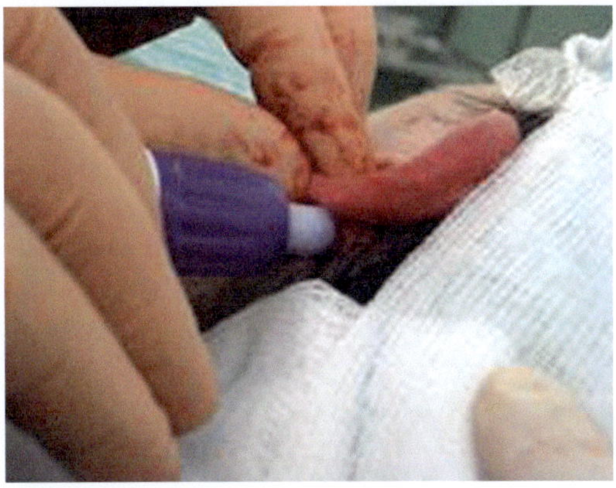

Fig. 48.1 Fixing the concha with adhesive at the mastoid

V. Wedler, M.D. (✉)
Department of Plastic, Reconstructive and Aesthetic Surgery, Kantonsspital Frauenfeld/Münsterlingen, Waldeckstrasse, Frauenfeld CH-8500, Switzerland
e-mail: volker.wedler@stgag.ch, info@wedler.ch

M. Vetter, M.D.
Department of Plastic, Reconstructive and Aesthetic Surgery, Kantonsspital Frauenfeld, Pfaffenholzstrasse 4, Frauenfeld 8501, Switzerland
e-mail: dr.miriam.vetter@web.de

M. Foehn, M.D.
Department of Plastic and Hand Surgery, University Hospital Centre Freiburg, Hugstetter Strasse 55, Freiburg im. Breisgau D-79106, Germany
e-mail: matthias.foehn@uniklinik-freiburg.de

M.A. Shiffman (ed.), *Advanced Cosmetic Otoplasty*,
DOI 10.1007/978-3-642-35431-1_48, © Springer-Verlag Berlin Heidelberg 2013

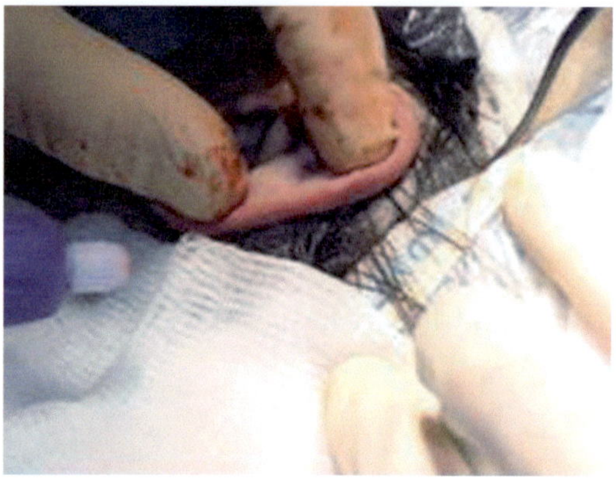

Fig. 48.2 Pressing the concha to the head area until the liquid adhesive is dried

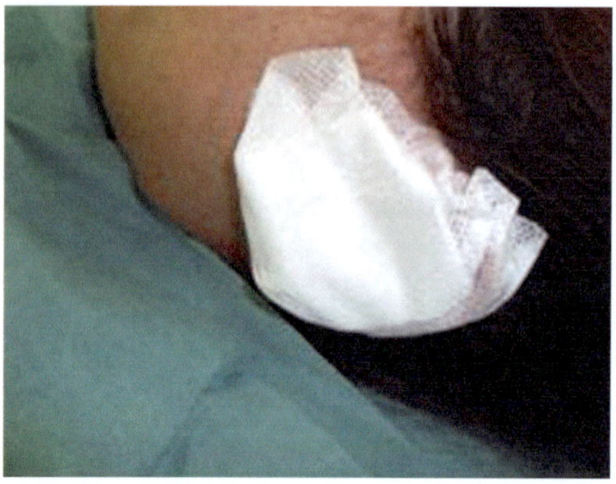

Fig. 48.3 Plaster in the required size is placed over the ear

essential to press the concha to the head area until the liquid adhesive is dried (Fig. 48.2). Then a flat piece of cotton wool pad and a piece of adhesive tape or plaster in the required size is placed over the ear. This causes compression to avoid postoperative hematomas. No huge dressing is needed, and no around the head taping is necessary (Fig. 48.3). Four to 6 days after the surgical procedure, we remove the plaster or cotton wool pad. The bonding scab usually is removed after 10–14 days, sometimes earlier.

Discussion

This otoplasty dressing technique is simple, economical, and very convenient and comfortable for the patients. There are no further costs because of the use of the cyanoacrylate tissue adhesive that is used for skin closure in the same surgical procedure. The cyanoacrylate tissue adhesive is a liquid bonding agent that holds many cuts, wounds, and incisions together as effectively as sutures [7, 8]. It is especially desirable for the sensitive skin of the face [9]. It is waterproof, so patients can shower immediately after removing the plaster [9]. We have not noticed any allergic reaction after using the bonding. In case of emergency or if examination is required, it can be easily removed. It is rare to not be possible to apply the tissue adhesive, even in very hairy patients with deep hairlines.

References

1. Aygit AC. Molding the ears after anterior scoring and concha repositioning: a combined approach for protruding ear correction. Aesthetic Plast Surg. 2003;27(1):77–81.
2. Bartley J. How long should ears be bandaged after otoplasty? J Laryngol Otol. 1998;112(6):531–2.
3. Bhatti AF, Chapman TW, Orlando A. Practical tips for otoplasty. Plast Reconstr Surg. 2006;117(1):329–30.
4. Krupp S, Asse N'Dri H. Otoplasty without a conformer dressing. Ann Plast Surg. 1991;26(4):407–12.
5. McIntire MR, Morgan RF, Kenney JG, Edgerton MT. Postoperative protection for the external ear. Ann Plast Surg. 1983;11(3):261–2.
6. Simo R, Jones NS. Head bandaging following otoplasty—how we do it. J Laryngol Otol. 1994;108(5):410–2.
7. Shapiro AJ, Dinsmore RC, North Jr JH. Tensile strength of wound closure with cyanoacrylate glue. Am Surg. 2001;67(11):1113–5.
8. Toriumi DM, O'Grady K, Desai D, Bagal A. Use of octy-2-cyanoacrylate for skin closure in facial plastic surgery. Plast Reconstr Surg. 1998;102(6):2209–19.
9. Maw JL, Quinn JV, Wells GA, Ducic Y, Odell PF, Lamothe A, et al. A prospective comparison of octylcyanoacrylate tissue adhesive and suture for the closure of head and neck incisions. J Otolaryngol. 1997;26(1):26–30.

Head Bandage After Otoplasty

49

Ahmad A. Orabi

Background and Rationale

Whatever the otoplasty technique followed, surgeons usually advocate or even necessitate applying a well-molded padded head bandage following otoplasty [1, 2]. However, the purpose of postoperative head bandage is controversial, and many have persuasively argued against their use. Suggested benefits [3–8] included hematoma prevention and absorption of blood trickling, splinting, and protection:

1. Prevention of hematoma, reduction of postoperative bleeding, and absorption of blood trickling [1, 6, 9]. Hematoma is one of the most feared sequelae in the early phase of postoperative period [10]. The usual culprits leading to this complication are insufficient intraoperative hemostasis or other errors in surgical technique. Less commonly, rebound vasodilatation from local anesthetics, hypertension, preexisting coagulopathy, and postoperative trauma can be involved [10, 11]. There is no evidence to support the view that the head dressing has a hemostatic role [12], and some feel that a head bandage could not be tied so tight as to prevent hematoma without causing a pressure sore to the forehead or pinna [13].

   Previous studies suggested no increase in the incidence of hematoma when head dressings were not used [1, 6, 13, 14].

   Postoperative bleeding is a warning sign for possible hematoma. Indeed, both share the same etiology. Again, it has to be also noted as a general surgical principle that early postoperative bleeding is prevented by meticulous intraoperative hemostasis and not by dressings [6]. Bleeding is classified as such significant, if it necessitates a bandage change [10] or return to the hospital for advice [1]. Studies in which head bandages were not used did not report comparatively higher incidence of significant postoperative bleeding [1, 6, 13, 14]. Powell [1] stated that the padded bandage absorbs any trickle of blood and the patient might inconveniently return to hospital with a minor bleeding. However, the majority of his patients managed to mop this satisfactorily with a tissue, and if the parents and patients are warned and reassured at the time of discharge, this problem would not be serious.
2. Splinting and help to mold the newly shaped ear [7, 9, 15]. Interestingly, it was Stenstrom [3] himself who alluded to the fact that no special care needs to be taken to consolidate or preserve the shape and position of the ears. In Powell study [1] as well as recent studies [6, 13, 14], there were no reported increase in early recurrence of ear prominence where no head bandage was used and regardless of the technique used, i.e., suture or cartilage sculpting techniques. The follow-up in most of these studies was too short to comment

A.A. Orabi, M.D., MSc, FRCSEd (Oto), FRCSEd (ORL-HNS)
Director, Otolaryngology-Head and Neck Surgery, Anas Consultancy Ltd for Specialized Medical Services, 2 Thistle close, NR5 9HR, Norwich, United Kingdom
e-mail: aaorabi@doctors.org.uk

M.A. Shiffman (ed.), *Advanced Cosmetic Otoplasty*,
DOI 10.1007/978-3-642-35431-1_49, © Springer-Verlag Berlin Heidelberg 2013

on late recurrences or long-term satisfaction. However, in one quasi-randomized controlled study [13], there was no difference in long-term satisfaction scores (median: 38 months). Therefore, some doubt is casted on the suggestion that a head bandage promotes the contouring of the re-draped skin, and it is stated if the result achieved at surgery is good, it will remain so. Furthermore, wound strength is still minimal after a week, and healing takes at least 6 weeks before scarring has matured enough. If the bandage does act as a splint, then it should be kept on for up to 6 weeks [16].

3. Protection of the ear from potential injury in the immediate postoperative period, thereby preventing early recurrence [1, 12]. However, using a removable elastic sports headband or crepe bandage especially at night for 3–8 weeks to prevent inadvertent folding of the ear was suggested [1, 12, 14, 17–20]. Shokrollahi and Tanner [21] described how the ears do not require extra protection during the initial postoperative period, thus negating the need to have the traditional head bandage. In at least 3 of the – no head bandage – studies [6, 13, 14], none of their patients was reported to suffer postoperative injury to the pinna. The ears are usually sensitive and uncomfortable postoperatively if manipulated and therefore likely to provide sufficient disincentive to patients tempted to touch them or allow siblings pulling at them [6, 14]. It does appear that using a head bandage for the protection of the ear has been overestimated.

Types of Head Dressings/Bandages (Fig. 49.1)

The type of head bandage used depends on surgeon's choice. It may be fluff gauze supportive dressing with a circumferential gauze [22] or crepe bandage, a silicone foam ear dressing with a protector [23], a custom-made ear guard constructed with Orthoplast sheet and leather straps [24], a wrestling head gear [2], or kraft paper [3]. The presence of different types of head dressings indicates that no single type has been found universally ideal. Some are considerably more complicated and difficult to apply or difficult to remove and reapply if needs be, and some are uncomfortable to wear at night especially in hot weather. On the other hand, some can slip off easily and may allow the ear to be folded in an unfavorable position during sleep [2].

Duration of Head Bandage Application

Stenstrom [3] stated that early removal of dressing did not endanger the surgical outcome. Reported duration of head bandage application varies from a few hours to 10 days [1, 11, 18, 19, 25, 26] and even 2 weeks [20] following surgery followed by a further period of night protection for a variable length of time up to 6 months [12]. The duration for which they are applied depends on the set protocol in an institution or the personal preference of the surgeon [12]. Bartley [16] suggested the use of a head bandage for no more than 24 h. Ramkumar et al. [12] study, limited to 2 months follow-up, showed no benefit from the application of a formal head bandage for any longer than 1 day.

Possible Problems and Complications

Use of head bandage itself can lead to many complications:

1. Slippage and frequent need to re-bandaging [17]. This is the most frequently encountered problem [16, 17, 23, 27, 28] (ranging from 40 to 67 % within a week of the operation), and in many cases, it would appear to migrate placing unexpected tensions on the ear [16]. This can be troublesome leading to recurrent visits to hospital, inconvenience, and distress. Furthermore, in one audit [28], bandage redressing was found to correlate heavily to a higher complication rate although it was difficult to ascertain the unidirectionality of such correlation. Various modifications to the technique and type of head bandaging and some tips have been suggested to reduce such slippage particularly at night [29, 30], but none has been substantiated.

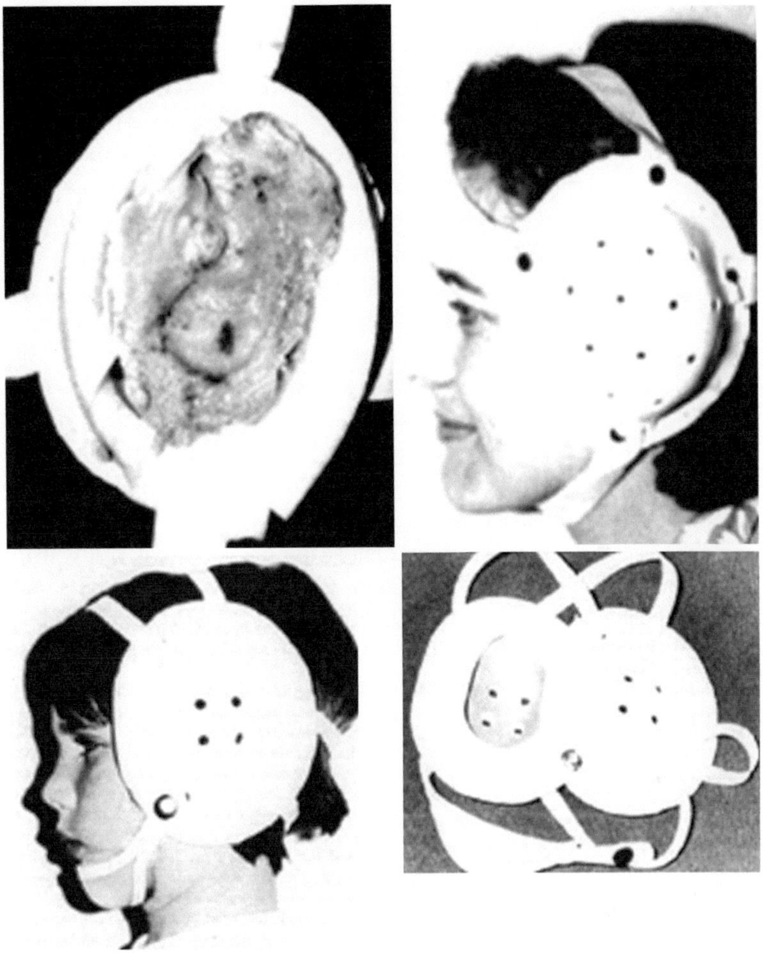

Fig. 49.1 Examples of Head dressings: *Top*: Silicone foam mould secured in the ear protector (*left*) and the ear protector (*right*) [23]. *Bottom*: Westling head gear device showing the cup-shaped protective aluminum supports [2]

2. Pressure necrosis of the anterior skin and cartilage of the pinna and skin of forehead [1, 10, 14]. It is the result of obstruction of the venous circulation in the subdermal plexus caused by excessive pressure from inappropriately tight dressings [10]. Necrosis can also occur secondary to an expanding hematoma or infection as well as technical errors such as excess diathermy. Anterior cartilage scoring techniques pose a particular danger as anterior dissection can cause anterior hematoma, which in turn may lead to anterior skin necrosis followed by chondritis and eventually resulting in permanent cartilage irregularities. Further factors include the potential development of a sharp antihelical fold as well as excessive diathermy on the undersurface of the anterior skin resulting in a compromise of what is already thin fragile skin [10, 15].
3. Potential for obscuring early recognition of complications such as infection and hematoma.
4. Conductive deafness due to packing of the ear with proflavin or cotton wool blocking the external auditory meatus [6, 12].
5. Postoperative nausea and vomiting from packing of the concha [6, 12, 14, 31] by stimulating a branch of the vagus supplying the concha and the posterior wall of the external auditory meatus (Arnold's nerve).
6. Smell of coagulated blood in the hair [16].
7. Discomfort and itching due to sweating provoking an attempt to scratch the ear under the dressings [6, 12].
8. Health economic-related issues such as increase theater time, reduced cost-effectiveness for both hospital and parents/patients that is associated with unscheduled related visits, as well as

increased return time to normal activity [16, 17, 28]. Patients are more willing to return to work or school if they do not have embarrassing head dressings on [6].

Some of these problems are considered trivial and are usually not mentioned in the patient record. However, they can cause significant problems and embarrassment to patients [1, 16]. Practical disadvantages might therefore outweigh the theoretical advantages of head bandage.

Alternatives to Head Dressings and Bandages

Alternative methods have been introduced to avoid the use of the head bandage such as use of tulle gras [1], Steri-Strips [6], and 2-octyl-cyanoacrylate (Dermabond®, Ethicon, Inc., Somerville, NJ) skin adhesive [9, 14, 21]. The advantages of the latter besides comfort and acceptability include the ability to form a sealed, flexible membrane with antimicrobial properties over the incision and strong adherence to skin edges providing additional support [14]. It can be used for skin closure [9, 14, 21, 32] and as a glue dressing to hold back the posterior pinna against the postauricular mastoid area [9, 21, 32]. There were no complications attributable to such use of current tissue glues with longer chain molecule [15].

Level of Evidence

Advocates for using head bandages following otoplasty claim theoretical benefits that have never been substantiated. The level of evidence in studies arguing against its use is not high either. Powell [1] using the anterior scoring technique in his prospective study suggested that a postoperative padded head dressing is not required in a well-motivated patient. However, he considered all his patients as homogenous non-head bandage group despite using a head protective bandage in 33 out of 40 patients for a varying duration ranging from the period of recovery from general anesthesia to the next postoperative day. Furthermore, he followed up his patients for 30 days only. Orabi et al. [13] in their quasi-randomized controlled study concluded that patients' satisfaction and complications following otoplasty were not influenced by omitting head bandage use, particularly when cartilage plication technique was used. Wong and Sylaidis [6] in a prospective study using posterior cartilage scoring and/or posterior suture conchoplasty found no increased risk of hematoma or of early recurrence in their patients where they used a single Steri-Strip only to dress the wound. They have used, however, historical controls from other studies. Bovill et al. [14] retrospective comparative study using modified Mustarde technique has the same conclusion. However, their Dermabond group still used a headband for 24 h a day for the first week and then at night for the subsequent week; therefore, it was not purely a non-head bandage group. The follow-up for these studies was variable and ranged from 1 to 38 months.

Recommendations for Future Studies

Therefore, there remains a need for large prospective single-blinded randomized controlled structured trials with large comparative sample size where a head bandage is not used. Study designs with self-controls are particularly relevant here. The outcome measures should include the long-term satisfaction and objective cosmetic measurements (e.g., using McDowell's basic goals of otoplasty [33]), complications (including delayed), as well as unscheduled visits. The trials should ideally include stratification for different operative techniques as well as degree and type of deformity. Limandjaja et al. [10] also recommended, when calculating complication incidence, a minimum follow-up period of 2 years, considering each operated ear as an independent variable and only including bilateral primary procedures.

References

1. Powell BW. The value of head dressings in the postoperative management of the prominent ear. Br J Plast Surg. 1989;42(6):692–4.
2. McIntire MR. Postoperative protection for the external ear. Ann Plast Surg. 1983;11(3):261–2.
3. Stenstrom SJ, McIntire MR, Morgan RF, Kenney JG, Edgerton MT. A simple operation for prominent ears. Acta Otolaryngol. 1967;63(S224):393–402.
4. Mustarde JC. The correction of prominent ears using simple mattress sutures. Br J Plast Surg. 1963;16:170–8.
5. Stark RB. Otoplasty. Aesthetic plastic surgery. 1st ed. Boston: Little and Brown; 1980. p. 345–61.
6. Wong MC, Sylaidis P. Head dressings for pinnaplasty: a tradition not supported by evidence. Br J Plast Surg. 2001;54(1):81–2.
7. Georgiade GS, Riefkohl R, Georgiade NG. Prominent ears and their correction: a forty-year experience. Aesthetic Plast Surg. 1995;19(5):439–43.
8. Spira M. Otoplasty: what I do now- a 30-year perspective. Plast Reconstr Surg. 1999;104(3):834–40.
9. Vetter M, Foehn M, Wedler V. A new postoperative otoplasty dressing technique using cyanoacrylate tissue adhesives. Aesthetic Plast Surg. 2010;34(2): 212–3.
10. Limandjaja GC, Breugem CC, Mink van der Molen AB, Kon M. Complications of otoplasty: a literature review. J Plast Reconstr Aesthet Surg. 2009;62(1):19–27.
11. Adamson PA, McGraw BL, Tropper GJ. Otoplasty: critical review of clinical results. Laryngoscope. 1991;101(8):883–8.
12. Ramkumar S, Narayanan V, Laing JH. Twenty-four hours or 10 days? A prospective randomised controlled trial in children comparing head bandages following pinnaplasty. J Plast Reconstr Aesthet Surg. 2006;59(9):969–74.
13. Orabi AA, Chintamani BH, Timms MS. Is a head bandage useful after otoplasty? A quasi-randomized controlled study of complications and patient satisfaction. Ear Nose Throat J. 2009;88(10):E17–22.
14. Bovill ES, Boulton R, Wharton S. Use of Dermabond as a dressing for prominent ear correction: a sound alternative to head dressing. J Plast Reconstr Aesthet Surg. 2010;63(6):1065–6.
15. Patel AJ, Price RD. The use of tissue glue in prominent ear correction surgery. Aesthetic Plast Surg. 2011;35(2):245–7.
16. Bartley J. How long the ears should be bandaged after otoplasty? J Laryngol Otol. 1998;112(6):531–3.
17. Bradbury ET, Hewison J, Timmons MJ. Psychological and social outcome of prominent ear correction in children. Br J Plast Surg. 1992;45(2):97–100.
18. Nachlas N. Otoplasty. In: Papel I, Larrabee GW, Holt SP, Sykes J, editors. Textbook of facial plastic and reconstructive surgery. 3rd ed. New York: Thieme; 2009. p. 429.
19. Horn CE. Treatment of congenital auricular deformities. In: Thomas JR, editor. Advanced therapy in facial plastic and reconstructive surgery. Shelton: Peoples Medical Publishing House-USA; 2010. p. 519.
20. Weerda H. Abnormalities. In: Weerda H, editor. Surgery of the auricle: tumours-trauma-defects-abnormalities. New York: Thieme; 2007. p. 130.
21. Shokrollahi K, Tanner B. "Glue ear": beginning of the end for head bandages after prominent ear correction? J Plast Reconstr Aesthet Surg. 2008;61(9):1077.
22. Converse JM, Wood-Smith D. Technical details in the surgical correction of lop ear deformity. Plast Reconstr Surg. 1963;31:118.
23. Tegtmeier RE. A silicone foam ear dressing. Plast Reconstr Surg. 1977;60(1):131–2.
24. Tanzer RC, Chaisson R. A protective guard for use during reconstruction of the auricle. Plast Reconstr Surg. 1974;53(2):236–8.
25. Bull TR. Otoplasty: Mustarde technique. Facial Plast Surg. 1994;10(3):267–76.
26. Beasley NJ, Jones NS. Otoplasty- the problem of the deep conchal bowl. J Laryngol Otol. 1996;110(9): 864–88.
27. Jeffery SL. Complications following correction of prominent ears: an audit review of 122 cases. Br J Plast Surg. 1999;52(7):588–90.
28. Self AC, Madani H, Senior N, Howes S, Dheansa BS. Ear dressings post pinnaplasty. J Plast Reconstr Aesthet Surg. 2010;63(6):555.
29. Simo R, Jones NS. Head bandaging following otoplasty- how we do it. J Laryngol Otol. 1994;108(5): 410–2.
30. Nassab R, Soueid A, Ahmad F, Dhital S, Juma A. A clinical tip for prominent-ear-correction dressings: a simple advice for prevention of slippage. J Plast Reconstr Aesthet Surg. 2009;62(5):668.
31. Ridings P, Gault D, Khan L. Reduction in postoperative vomiting after surgical correction of prominent ears. Br J Anaesth. 1994;72(5):592–3.
32. Davis M, Lidder S, Nakhdjevani A, Pereira J. Ideal pinnaplasty dressing-glue versus bandage. Presented at the British Association of Plastic, Reconstructive and Aesthetic Surgeons Winter Scientific Meeting, London, Dec 2008.
33. McDowell AJ. Goals in otoplasty for protruding ears. Plast Reconstr Surg. 1968;41(1):17–27.

50 Postoperative Care Using a Silicone-Based Occlusive Dressing

Jonathan K. Frankel and Diana C. Ponsky

Introduction

As our understanding of the healing process evolves, we continue to search for the optimal dressing to apply in the immediate postoperative setting. The recent utilization of occlusive dressings has improved results of some facial plastic surgery procedures such as facial laser resurfacing [1]. Dermatologists have found a significant reduction in pain, erythema, and edema with the use of silicone occlusive dressings [2]. The curves and contours of the ear, however, present a unique obstacle and preclude application of most occlusive dressings. A malleable silicone-based occlusive dressing has many properties that make it a superior postoperative dressing in otoplasty, as will be discussed in this chapter.

There are several requirements that must be considered in choosing an appropriate otoplasty dressing. In any surgical procedure, the dressing must keep the wound clean, as protection from bacteria decreases the risk of infection and promotes healing. Secondly, surgical dressings that maintain a moist environment increase the rate of epithelialization by preventing wound desiccation and subsequent necrosis [3, 4]. Furthermore, it is important that the dressing provides protection from physical trauma. A physical barrier will help prevent alteration of the cosmetic results achieved by the surgeon's meticulous work. Without adequate protection, the surgical site risks distortion from a postsurgical hematoma, increased scarring from trauma-induced inflammation, disruption of the suture line, or necrosis caused by trauma to the auricular vascular supply.

The traditional non-occlusive dressing, consisting of a plastic hard cup with a padded base (Glasscock, Otomed, Lake Havasu City, AZ), provides protection from trauma but does not adequately meet the aforementioned requirements of an effective otoplasty dressing. The nonremovable, customized occlusive dressing is a superior protective barrier as compared to the Glasscock and also enhances healing by maintaining a moist, virtually bacteria-free environment.

A silicone-based occlusive dressing (Diamond Seal, Snowden-Pencer, Genzyme Biosurgery, Cambridge, MA) has proven to be an excellent option for otoplasty with no documented dressing-related complications [5]. It is composed of nontoxic semitransparent silicone, which solidifies when mixed with the enzymatic catalyst. This easily moldable dressing takes approximately 5–10 min to solidify after the catalyst is introduced. The silicone dressing presents several benefits to the patient and surgeon and should be

J.K. Frankel, M.D.
Department of Otolaryngology, University Hospitals, Case Western Medical Center, Cleveland, OH 44106, USA
e-mail: jkfrankel@gmail.com

D.C. Ponsky, M.D. (✉)
Department of Otolaryngology-Facial Plastic and Reconstructive Surgery, University Hospitals, Case Medical Center, 11100 Euclid Avenue, Mailstop LK5045, Cleveland, OH 44106, USA
e-mail: dianaponsky@yahoo.com

M.A. Shiffman (ed.), *Advanced Cosmetic Otoplasty*,
DOI 10.1007/978-3-642-35431-1_50, © Springer-Verlag Berlin Heidelberg 2013

considered in every otoplasty case. The benefits are as follows:

1. Quick and easy—takes an average of about 10–15 min to apply and does not significantly lengthen the operative time. This benefits both the patient, as anesthesia time is minimized, and the surgeon, as efficiency is maximized.
2. Precise—enables the surgeon to create a mold customized to the patient's unique auricular anatomy.
3. Discrete—minimal bulk as compared to the Glasscock dressing. It does not require a head wrap and can be covered with a hat or wrap if the patient so desires. This diminishes any sense of embarrassment that patients may otherwise experience.
4. Semitransparent—allows for monitoring of the wound for infection and assurance of proper healing.
5. Secure—is not easily moved from the initial placement, which is especially advantageous in pediatric patients. The traditional non-occlusive dressing can become dislodged easily and create pressure points. Pressure points decrease vascular supply, thus increasing the risk of infection and necrosis of the surgical site.
6. Safe—nontoxic, does not pose a risk to hearing, and has not been associated with any postsurgical complications in the authors' experience.

Procedure

The auricle and surrounding area is prepared for surgery using a sterile technique. A water-based surgical lubricant is combed into the postauricular hair in an anterior to posterior direction, preventing the hair from interfering with the procedure and dressing application. It is important to ensure any hair contacted by the silicone is cleaned thoroughly before the dressing solidifies.

Following the otoplasty procedure, a piece of cotton is dampened with saline solution and placed into the external ear canal. This prevents silicone from entering the external ear canal and contacting the tympanic membrane. A tail is left on the dampened cotton, which, when later removed, serves as a window within the solidified silicone to the ear canal. A bolster of moist-squeezed-dry cotton is subsequently placed in the conchal bowl. The obliteration of dead space by the bolster minimizes the necessary amount of silicone and ensures that the sensitive conchal tissue is not incidentally probed during later removal of the dressing. The bolster is then secured with an absorbable suture, usually 5.0 fast-absorbing plain gut. The use of the silicone dressing obviates the need to bolster the ear with dental roll and suture.

After preparing the ear for the dressing, a medical-grade silicone and catalyst are mixed in the Diamond Seal dual plunger syringe. The mixture is injected onto the auricle and spread evenly from the concha to the posterior aspect of the helix. After conforming the silicone mixture to the auricular contours, the surgeon smoothes the surface using Surgilube water-based surgical lubricant to prevent the dressing from adhering to the surgical gloves. When the surgeon is satisfied with the dressing, it is left for about 5 min or until fully solidified. Finally, the damp piece of cotton is removed, leaving an auditory window. It should be noted that newly produced silicone tends to solidify more slowly, but this should not affect the effectiveness of the dressing. The surgeon should expect to become efficient and skilled at molding the dressing within just a few trials.

The patient is seen 5 days postoperatively, and the dressing is removed. By this point, the surgeon can expect reepithelialization of the suture line and near-to-complete resorption of 5-0 or 6-0 fast-absorbing plain gut sutures. The sebaceous secretions produced by the skin provide natural lubrication and allow for easy and painless removal of the dressing. If there are adherent portions of the dressing, they can be gently undermined with a lacrimal probe or comparable instrument.

The use of silicone-based occlusive dressing is not only better tolerated by patients than the traditional non-occlusive dressing, but it also improves cosmetic results. It is a technique that can be used for nearly any otoplasty case, and it is foreseeable that these dressings will soon become the standard of care. Although particularly useful for otoplasty (Figs. 50.1, 50.2, and 50.3), silicone-based occlusive dressings offer many benefits to the patient and surgeon and show promise in many other areas of facial plastics.

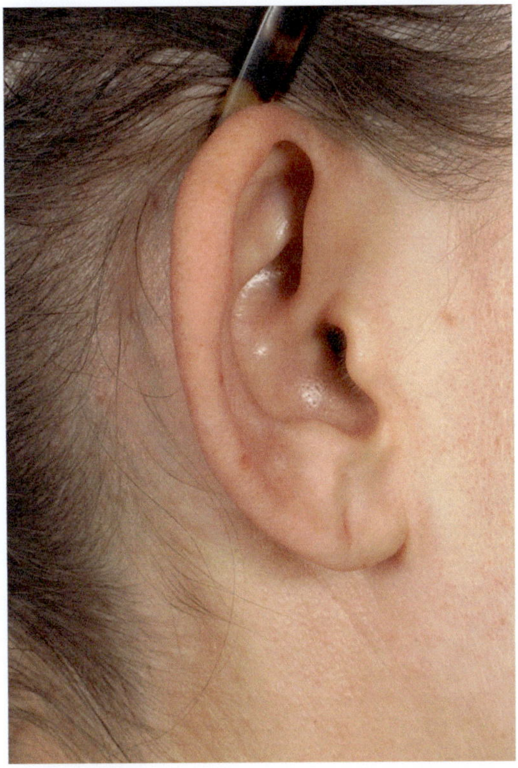

Fig. 50.1 Preoperative photo of a patient presenting for otoplasty

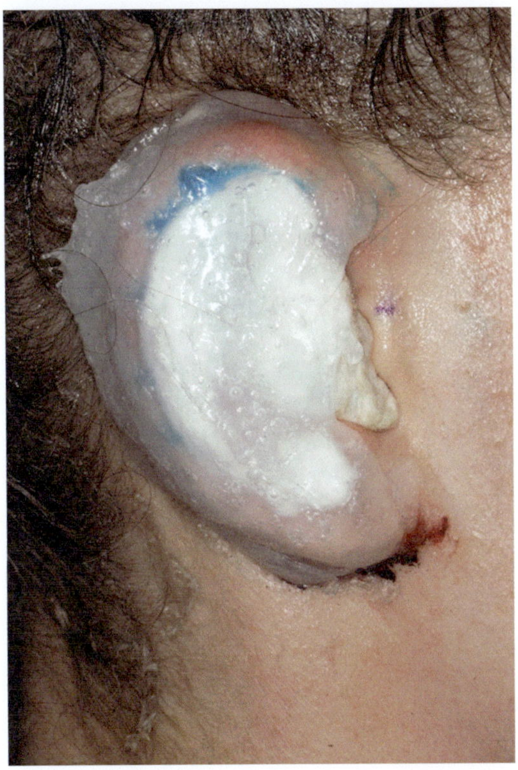

Fig. 50.2 Silicone-based occlusive dressing following otoplasty

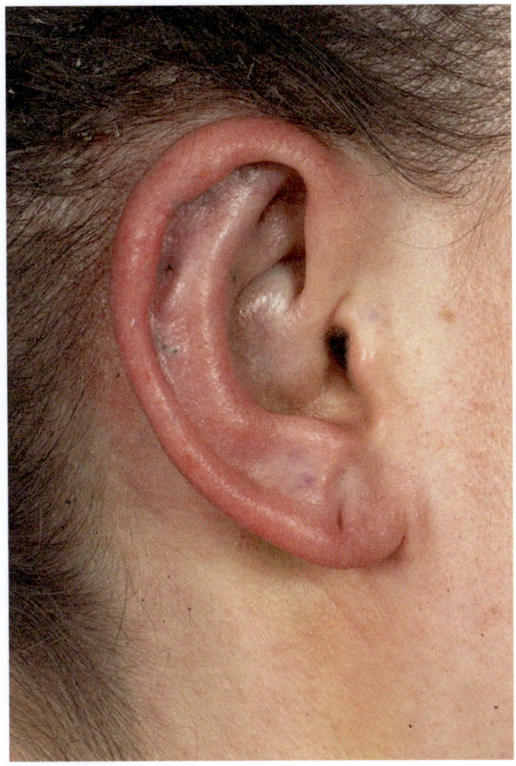

Fig. 50.3 Five days postoperative

References

1. Michelow BJ, Varghai A, Movassaghi K, Guyuron B. A new dressing for laser-treated areas. Plast Reconstr Surg. 2002;110(4):1150–7.
2. Suarez M, Fulton Jr JE. A novel occlusive dressing for skin resurfacing. Dermatol Surg. 1998;24(5):567–70.
3. Kannon GA, Gerrett AB. Moist wound healing with occlusive dressings. A clinical review. Dermatol Surg. 1995;21(7):583–90.
4. Vogt PM, Andree C, Brueing K, Liu PY, Slama J, Helo G, et al. Dry, moist, and wet skin wound repair. Ann Plast Surg. 1995;34(5):493–9.
5. Tang CJ, Ponsky DC. Seal it and reveal it: postoperative otoplasty care using a silicone-based occlusive dressing. Otolaryngol Head Neck Surg. 2010;142(4):621–3.

Part V

Complications of Otoplasty

Otoplasty Complications

51

Melvin A. Shiffman

Introduction

Cosmetic otoplasty is a frequently performed procedure. For the prominent ear, there are many different approaches to correct the various problems, and this may lead to a variety of complications. There are other cosmetic problems that may be treated including scars, especially keloid scars, traumatic injuries, and resection of tumors. Complications can arise from cosmetic otoplasty, most of which are well known. The surgeon performing otoplasty should be aware of the possible complications, their cause, and their treatment.

Complications

Angulation of Incision

Farrior (2000) [1] reported angulation of the partial incisions on the anterior surface resulting from the incision having been carried too deep.

Asymmetry [2]

Asymmetry may exist before otoplasty is performed. If asymmetry occurs postoperatively, correction may be avoided if the asymmetry is minor. Surgical correction would depend on the cause of the asymmetry (i.e., too tight or too loose a suture on one side, too much or too little skin excision on one side).

Bleeding and Hematoma [1, 3, 4]

The cause of bleeding after otoplasty can be from inadequate hemostasis, hypertension, rebound vasodilatation from local anesthetics, postoperative trauma, or preexisting coagulopathy. Surgical intervention is necessary to control bleeding vessels and evacuate blood clots. Failure to remove an expanding hematoma in a timely fashion may result in tissue necrosis or chondritis.

Cartilage Irregularities [5, 6]

Palpable and visible cartilage edges or irregularities of the cartilage can be caused by full-thickness cartilage incisions (cartilage splitting) or some sculpting techniques that weaken the cartilage.

Cartilage Necrosis [2]

This may occur from not draining a hematoma early enough and the hematoma causing excessive pressure on the cartilage. The necrotic area should be excised. There will probably be a deformity that will need filling.

M.A. Shiffman, M.D., J.D.
Section of Surgery, Newport Specialty Hospital,
17501 Chatham Drive, Tustin, CA 92780-2302, USA
e-mail: medicinepluslaw@yahoo.com,
shiffmanmdjd@gmail.com

M.A. Shiffman (ed.), *Advanced Cosmetic Otoplasty*,
DOI 10.1007/978-3-642-35431-1_51, © Springer-Verlag Berlin Heidelberg 2013

Chondritis and Perichondritis [6]

Typically, clinical signs of infection (i.e., pain increasingly resistant to analgesics, swollen erythematous ear) begin 3–5 days after surgery. Chondritis may require drainage and debridement of infected cartilage. Appropriate perioperative antibiotics and drainage of any collection of serum or blood can prevent chondritis.

Granulomas [4]

Braided nonabsorbable sutures are more likely to cause granulomas than monofilament nonabsorbable sutures. Removal of the suture and granuloma would be necessary. Monofilament nonabsorbable sutures, nylon or polypropylene, may erode through skin causing fistulas or granuloma.

Grisel's Syndrome [7–12]

Grisel's syndrome is a non-traumatic subluxation of the atlanto-axial joint caused by inflammation of the adjacent tissues found primarily in children. This may occur in association with any condition that results in hyperemia and pathological relaxation of the transverse ligament of the atlanto-axial joint. Several common otolaryngeal conditions have been associated with the syndrome: pharyngitis, adenotonsillitis, tonsillar abscess, cervical abscess, and otitis media. Moreover, the syndrome has been observed after numerous otolaryngologic procedures such as tonsillectomy, adenoidectomy, and mastoidectomy. Non-traumatic subluxation of the atlanto-axial joint should be suspected in cases of persistent neck pain and stiffness

Early management, consisting of cervical immobilization and medical treatment, is considered the key factor for a satisfactory outcome.

Hypersensitivity [2]

Postoperative hypersensitivity is the result of nerve endings being irritated or cutaneous nerves growing back. This will usually subside with avoidance of pressure on the ear and mild pain medication such as Tylenol.

Infection [2, 4, 13, 14]

Infection is usually diagnosed because of excessive pain, erythema, fever, or purulent drainage. The wound has to be opened, cultured, and thoroughly cleansed with antibiotic solution and oral antibiotics then used for at least 7 days. Culture and sensitivity (C&S) of the pus may take a few days to be reported, and the antibiotics may have to be changed depending on the results. Failure to treat the infection early and adequately may result in perichondritis, chondritis, and cartilage necrosis [2, 14].

Overcorrection

The flattened appearance of the ear after otoplasty and the helix no longer visible from the frontal view is due to overmedialization of the entire ear leaving the auriculomastoid angle less than 30° [3]. Overcorrection of the middle third of the ear results in prominent inferior pole and contributes to the "telephone deformity" [2, 14].

Overcorrection of the superior and inferior poles results in the "reverse telephone ear" deformity [2, 3].

Obliteration of the External Ear Canal [3, 4, 15, 16]

Surgical deformity from anterior displacement of the concha produces obliteration of the ear canal. The origin is from setback of an extensively hypertrophic concha with conchomastoid sutures alone.

This can be prevented by careful preoperative planning and sticking to the plan in excising the concha. Treatment requires excision of the undercorrected concha and lateral based conchal flap [15].

Pain

Excessive postoperative pain may be a warning sign of a developing hematoma. The dressing should be removed and the wound examined for swelling and fluctuant mass indicating a hematoma. Treatment requires exploring the wound to find the source of bleeding for electrocoagulation and evacuation of the hematoma. A drain may be used for 24–48 h to detect further fresh bleeding and to drain any residual blood.

Recurrent Deformity [3, 4, 14]

Recurrence of the initial ear deformity may be caused by trauma, patient manipulation, insufficient cartilage weakening, suture failure, or suture insufficiency. This may be the result of relying on skin excision to retain correction.

Reverse Telephone Deformity [3, 4, 16]

This is produced by unequal setback of the auricle where the concha is relatively prominent with respect to the superior pole and inferior poles. The deformity is caused by failure to address the prominent concha while focusing on the deformity of the antihelical fold. The conchal setback is done too excessively, and the concha rolls in the sagittal plane, pushing the tragus laterally and narrowing the outer segment of the external auditory canal.

Prevention requires conchal resection, if indicated, and proper placement of the conchomastoid suture. Treatment involves surgical replacement of the conchomastoid suture.

Scarring [4]

Baker and Converse (1979) [17] reported hypertrophic and keloid scars in 11 % of African American ears and 2.1 % in Caucasian ears. Hypertrophic or keloid scars occur in about 15 % of blacks, Hispanics, and Asians [18, 19].

The opening for earrings may be a source of keloid scarring. Excess tension on the closure may result in a widened scar. Careful and conservative skin resection can help limit excessive scar formation [6].

About 80 % of hypertrophic scars will resolve without treatment, but 80 % of keloid scars will recur, although many times with some improvement, with treatment. Treatment may include intralesional steroid (triamcinolone) alone or in combination with 5-fluorouracil or bleomycin, excision with or without irradiation, cryotherapy with or without intralesional steroid, and compression therapy.

Skin Necrosis

Necrosis of the skin is usually the result of postoperative compression dressings being too tight or by excessive electrocoagulation under the skin. This may result in wound dehiscence.

Suture Extrusion [1, 2, 4, 14]

Extrusion of sutures may result from permanent sutures being placed too close to the skin and excessive tension of the cartilage. Infection can cause sutures being extruded. If suture extrusion is a late complication, probably no surgery will need to be performed as long as the ear retains its corrected shape.

Telephone Ear Deformity [3–5, 16]

This deformity is created by unequal setback of the auricle where the superior and inferior poles of the ear are still protuberant in relationship to the middle third of the ear.

The cause is attributed to inadequate correction of the superior pole; uncorrected prominent helical root; excessive tightening of the conchomastoid sutures; excessive tightening of the concho-scaphoid sutures (especially in the middle third); excessive removal of skin, soft tissue, or cartilage in the middle third of the ear; and uncorrected lobule.

Prevention includes tightening the middle suture last to avoid potential overcorrection, avoiding excess removal of cartilage, and determining if the lobule and helical tail have to be corrected once the conchal and antihelix are treated. Treatment requires replacement of the Mustardé sutures and the Furnas conchomastoid sutures to obtain the antihelical fold and conchal position. If the lobule, helical root, or superior pole has not been initially improved, then these have to be corrected.

Undercorrection

Farrior (2000) [1] described a patient who required opening of the superior third of the incision for placement of a horizontal mattress suture near the superior crus because of the failure to place a suture above the level of the junction of the crus that is usually done to create a more normal contour.

Undercorrection of the superior helix and lobule results in a relatively prominent superior third of the ear called the "telephone deformity" [2, 14]. Undercorrection of an overdeveloped conchal bowl can result in a "reverse telephone ear" [2, 3].

Unrealistic Expectations of Patient

Unrealistic expectations of the patient should be detected by the surgeon before operating on the ears. This requires listening to what the patients have to say about what they want done and the results they expect. A careful discussion of the surgical procedure and the limitation of results from any complications should be held.

Wound Dehiscence

Dehiscence may occur from loss of skin sutures from trauma, too loosely tied sutures, skin necrosis, or wound infection.

References

1. Farrior RT. A facial plastic surgeon's perspective. In: Romo III T, Millman AL, editors. Aesthetic facial plastic surgery: a multidisciplinary approach. New York: Thieme; 2000. p. 427–43.
2. Nachlas NE. Otoplasty. In: Papel ID, editor. Facial plastic and reconstructive surgery. New York: Thieme; 2002. p. 309–21.
3. Adamson PA, Strecker HD. Otoplasty techniques. Facial Plast Surg. 1995;11(4):284–300.
4. Owsley TG, Biggerstaff TG. Otoplasty complications. Oral Maxillofac Surg Clin North Am. 2009;21(1):105–18.
5. Walter C, Nolst-Trenite GJ. Revision otoplasty and special problems. Facial Plast Surg. 1994;10(3):298–308.
6. Sclafani AP. Otoplasty. 2011. http:emedicine.co/article839886-treatment#a17. Accessed 26 Sept 2011.
7. Samuel D, Thomas DM, Tierney PA, Patel KS. Atlanto-axial subluxation (Grisel's syndrome) following otolaryngological diseases and procedures. J Laryngol Otol. 1995;109(10):1005–9.
8. Gourin CG, Kaper B, Abdu WA, Donegan JO. Nontraumatic atlanto-axial subluxation after retropharyngeal cellulitis: Grisel's syndrome. Am J Otolaryngol. 2002;23(1):60–5.
9. Bocciolini C, Dall'Olio D, Cunsolo E, Cavazzuti PP, Laudadio P. Grisel's syndrome: a rare complication following adenoidectomy. Acta Otorhinolaryngol Ital. 2005;25(4):245–9.
10. Rinaldo A, Mondin V, Suárez C, Genden EM, Ferlito A. Grisel's syndrome in head and neck practice. Oral Oncol. 2005;41(10):966–70.
11. Deichmueller CM, Welkoborsky HJ. Grisel's syndrome–a rare complication following "small" operations and infections in the ENT region. Eur Arch Otorhinolaryngol. 2010;267(9):1467–73.
12. Durst F, Staudenmaier R, Pilge H, Lauen J, Prodinger P, Holzapfel K, et al. Grisel's syndrome after otoplasty. HNO (Hals-, Nasen-, Ohren-Heilkunde). 2012; 60(2):135–40.
13. Elliott Jr RA. Complications in the treatment of prominent ears. Clin Plast Surg. 1978;5(3):479–90.
14. Campbell AC. Otoplasty. Facial Plast Surg. 2005;21(4):310–6.
15. Spira M, Stal S. The conchal flap as an adjunct in otoplasty. Ann Plast Surg. 1983;11(4):291–8.
16. Hoehn JG, Ashruf S. Otoplasty: sequencing the operation for improved results. Plast Reconstr Surg. 2005;15(1):5–16.
17. Baker DC, Converse M. Correction of protruding ears: a 20-year retrospective. Aesthetic Plast Surg. 1979;3(1):29–39.
18. Shiffman MA. Causes of and treatment for hypertrophic and keloid scars with a new method of treating steroid fat atrophy. Int J Cosmet Surg Aesthet Dermatol. 2002;4(1):9–14.
19. Shiffman MA. Uncovering scars. Healthy Aging. 2007;3(2):23–6.

Understanding and Correcting the Unfavorable Results After Otoplasty

52

Ashley K. Lentz and Bruce S. Bauer

Introduction

It has been well documented in the literature that ear deformities can result in significant psychological and emotional distress [1, 2]. Children who have prominent ears are perceived as "normal" with a "minor cosmetic defect" yet are ridiculed far more often than children with more significant craniofacial defects. This finding is attributed to the belief that major craniofacial anomalies evoke a sense of pity, and therefore, teasing is not acceptable [3]. Therefore, patients that undergo otoplasty have motivations for the procedure which include improved cosmetic outcome while seeking to stop all social stigmata of their original defect. As such, a less than perfect outcome is not tolerated. Any perceived postoperative deformity or asymmetry can render patients angry and distrustful. When faced with revision otoplasty, the surgeon should go to great lengths to carefully analyze the post otoplasty deformity and develop a well-organized plan for the correction. Without a corrective strategy, one is likely to encounter further complications and unwanted outcomes.

A.K. Lentz, M.D. (✉)
Division of Plastic and Reconstructive Surgery, Department of Surgery, University of Florida College of Medicine, PO Box 100138, Gainesville, FL 32610, USA
e-mail: lentz@surgery.ufl.edu

B.S. Bauer, M.D.
Section of Pediatric Plastic Surgery, Division of Plastic and Reconstructive Surgery, NorthShore University Health System, University of Chicago Medical School, Chicago, IL, USA

Department of Surgery, University of Chicago, Pritzker School of Medicine, 501 Skokie Blvd, Northbrook, IL 60062, USA
e-mail: bbauer@northshore.org

Anatomy and Etiology of the Prominent Ear

Anthropometric studies have been performed to better define the anatomy of a normal ear [4]. These measurements do not function as an absolute guide but rather set guidelines for defining the ideal ear. Attempts for a clear definition of prominent ears using comparative anatomy have revealed that perception of prominence is multifaceted and subjective [5]. Therefore, actual measurements to define prominent ear are not absolutely necessary, as recognition of prominence is typically innate.

Two etiologies are commonly described for prominent ear. The first is effacement of the antihelical fold, with an obtuse scaphoconchal angle [6]. This causes the upper third of the ear to project outward (Fig. 52.1). The second, conchal hypertrophy, causes total displacement of the entire ear from the head (Fig. 52.2) [7]. Additional etiologies include the presence of an abnormal skull shape due to plagiocephaly (Fig. 52.3) or a heart-shaped face with a broad intertemporal distance tapering toward a narrow face and mandible (Fig. 52.4). In each of the later two cases, the ear

M.A. Shiffman (ed.), *Advanced Cosmetic Otoplasty*,
DOI 10.1007/978-3-642-35431-1_52, © Springer-Verlag Berlin Heidelberg 2013

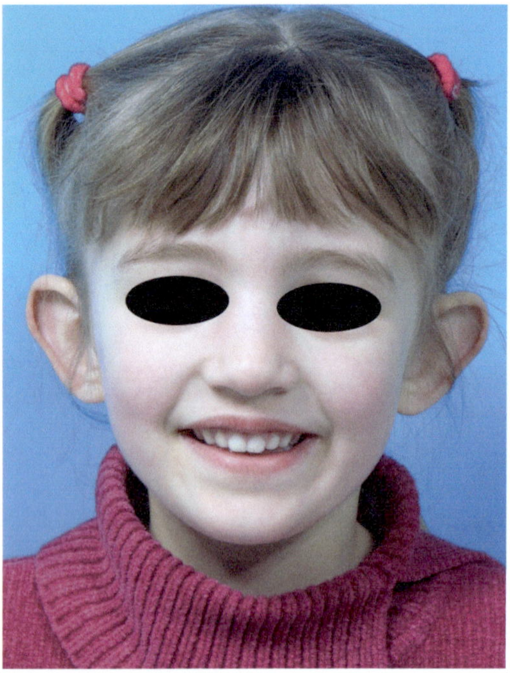

Fig. 52.1 Effacement of the antihelical fold, with an obtuse scaphoconchal angle causing the upper third of the ear to project outward

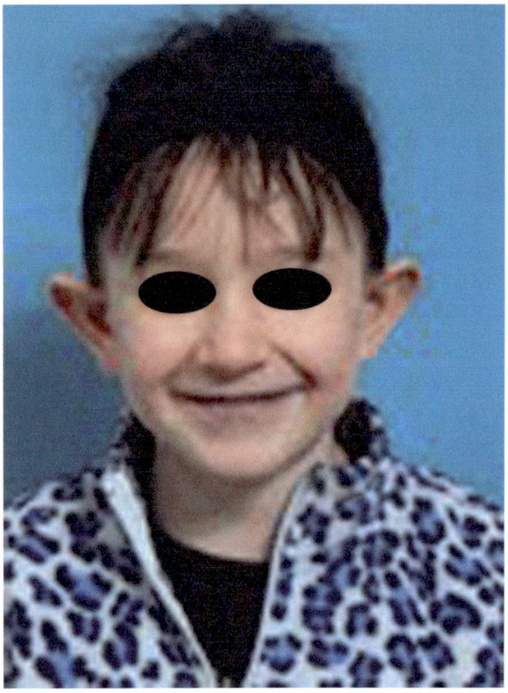

Fig. 52.2 Conchal hypertrophy causing total displacement of the entire ear from the head

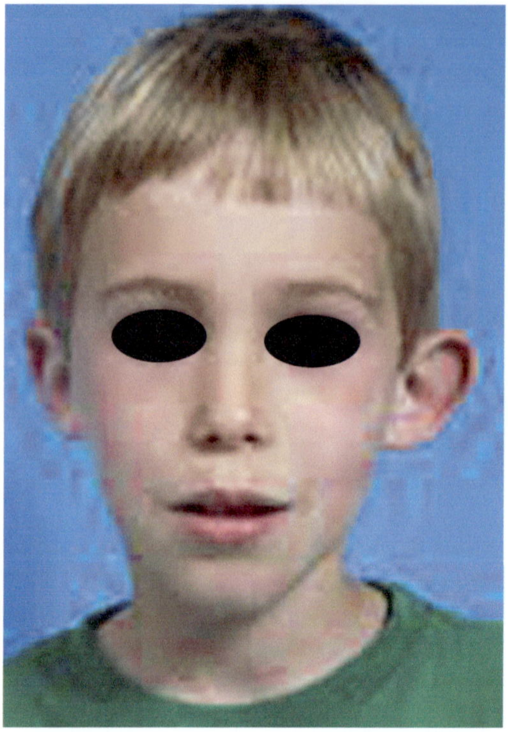

Fig. 52.3 Presence of an abnormal skull shape due to plagiocephaly

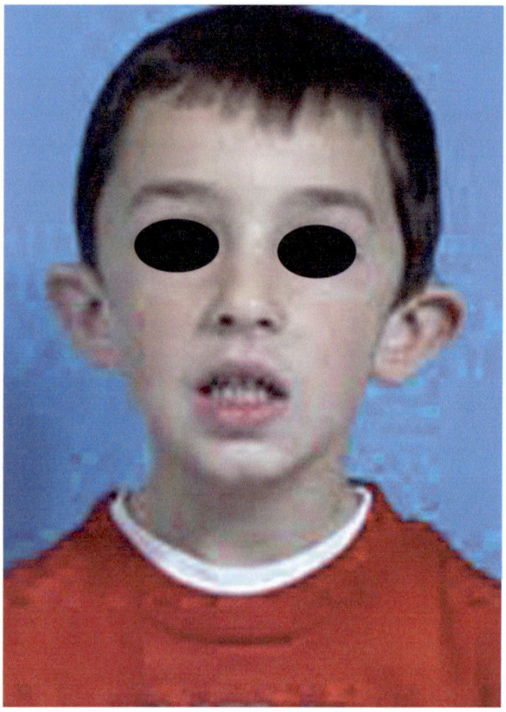

Fig. 52.4 Heart-shaped face with a broad intertemporal distance tapering toward a narrow face and mandible

sits on a sharply inclined cranial base, creating a unilateral prominence in the former and bilateral in the later.

Goals for Otoplasty

In 1968, McDowell [8] described six basic goals for otoplasty. These include (1) complete correction of the upper third of the ear; (2) preservation of the visualization of bilateral helices from the front view; (3) smoothing and regularity of the helical line; (4) avoidance of postauricular sulcus distortion; (5) no creation of a plastering appearance of the ear to the skull, meaning preservation of the normal values of distance between the mastoid and the helix; and (6) the position of each ear should remain symmetrical within 3 mm at any given point. Achievement of these goals is not possible without a critical evaluation of the ear anomaly and a well-thought-out plan for surgical correction.

Dieffenbach [9] originally described the excision of postauricular skin and placement of conchomastoid sutures. Since that time, numerous otoplasty techniques have been described to address the effacement of the scaphoconchal angle, the lack of an antihelical fold, the conchal hypertrophy, and the lobular deformity. The chosen surgical technique should address the underlying pathology in order to achieve the desired outcome.

Etiology of Post Otoplasty Deformities

Post otoplasty deformities most typically present as errors of overcorrection or undercorrection. Most often, the deformity is of mixed origin. Undercorrection is rather straightforward while overcorrection can present one of the most challenging problems in surgery of the external ear.

Undercorrection often occurs when absorbable sutures are used for correction of ear position and cartilage tension is no longer restrained once the sutures absorb. Permanent sutures should be used with full-thickness bites through the cartilage including both surfaces of perichondrium so as to avoid sutures cutting through with secondary loss of correction. Undercorrection also occurs when cranial and skeletal asymmetry goes unrecognized, and the repair fails to address the need for asymmetrical correction of each ear. If conchal hypertrophy is ignored and surgery aims to correct only the antihelix and scaphoconchal effacement, then prominence will remain with anatomic distortion. Finally, the lobule must always be included in the preoperative analysis. If there is lobular hypertrophy or inadequate positioning of the lobule, it requires correction at the time of otoplasty. Release or resection of the cartilage at the antitragus-conchal junction is often necessary in order to prevent the outward thrust on the lower third of the ear. Skin resection alone cannot reposition the lobule properly.

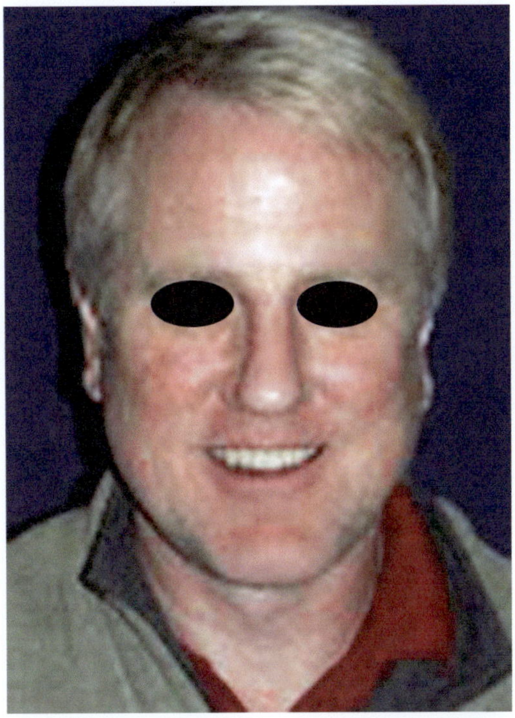

Fig. 52.5 Over-resection of skin and cartilage damage at varying degrees lead to overcorrection with a "pinned back" appearance, as there is loss of the visibility of the helix from the frontal view

Over-resection of skin and cartilage damage at varying degrees lead to overcorrection. Patients will complain of a "pinned back" appearance, as they lose the visibility of the helix from the front view (Fig. 52.5). Most often, this tends to occur when conchal hypertrophy is not addressed.

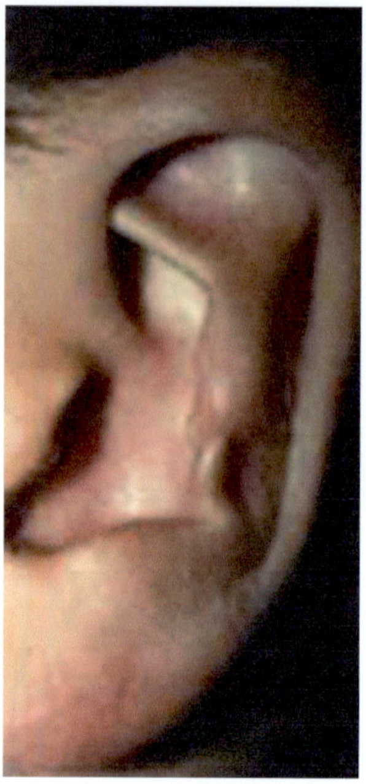

Fig. 52.6 A sharp, unnatural antihelical edge with disruption of the smooth cartilage results from fracturing of the cartilage and loss of smooth cartilage contour

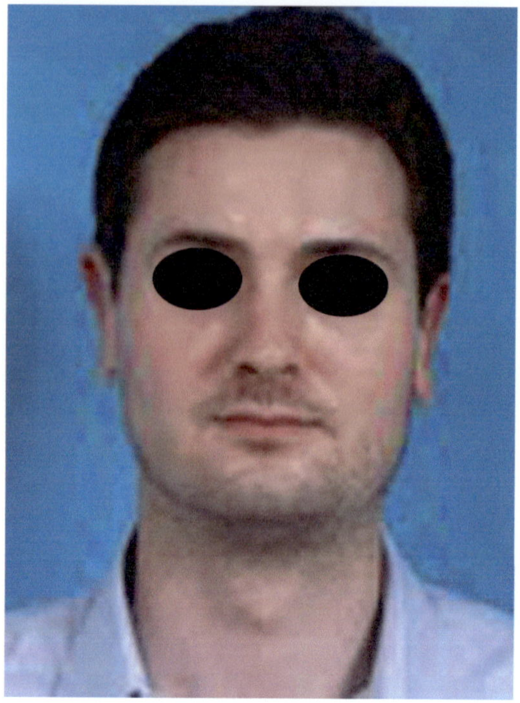

Fig. 52.7 The telephone deformity

Balance and shape of the ear must be maintained, and aggressive scoring of the cartilage to overcompensate for conchal hypertrophy will cause irregularities along the antihelix and crura. A sharp, unnatural antihelical edge with disruption of the smooth cartilage results from fracturing of the cartilage, and loss of smooth cartilage contour is perhaps the greatest challenge in repairing overcorrection (Fig. 52.6). The authors' current otoplasty technique arose out of an understanding of how this secondary deformity could be avoided with a chondrocutaneous-conchal resection as the means of helping to "break the spring" of the antihelix and allow the antihelix to be reshaped without any disruption of either surface. This technique of conchal resection allows for final reshaping with the use of suture placement alone.

The telephone deformity is the prime example of post otoplasty complication of mixed origin (Fig. 52.7). In these cases, there is overcorrection of the middle third of the ear due to over-resection of the skin. The skin resection should be carefully tapered in this region to smoothly follow the line of the upper-third correction. If lobular hypertrophy goes unrecognized and untreated, it creates a prominent lower third of the ear as compared to the middle third.

Algorithm-Based Approach to Revision Otoplasty

Revision otoplasty requires attention and understanding of not only the original etiology of prominent ear but also the state of the post otoplasty deformity. A logical and well-thought-out surgical plan should be implemented in order to achieve proper correction. First, the surgeon must have a thorough discussion with the patient

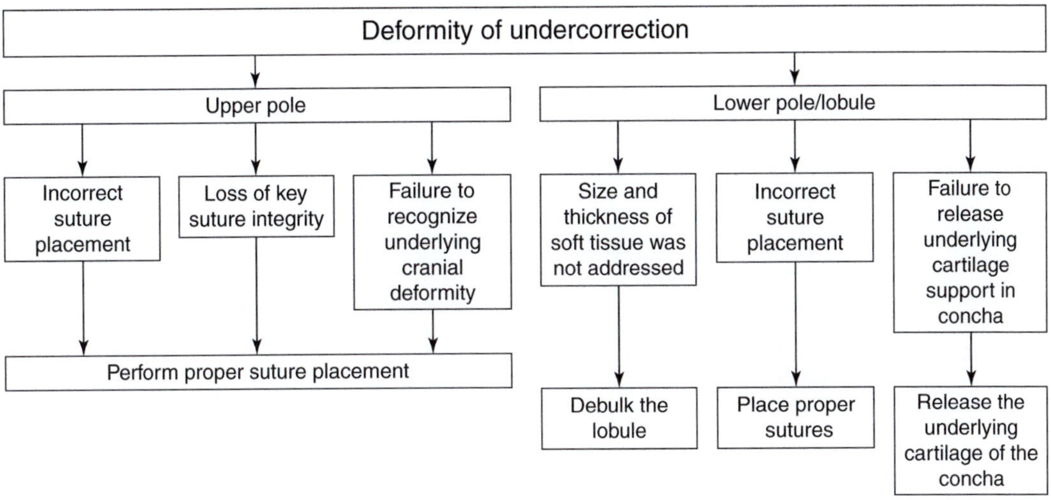

Fig. 52.8 Deformity of undercorrection

to determine expectations and willingness to achieve optimal outcomes. Patients must have realistic goals, as correction can be difficult in the case of overcorrection, and some cases may require multiple revisions in order to achieve the optimal outcome. The anatomy of the previously operated antihelix and concha will dictate the number of steps needed for correction of the deformity. In simpler cases, placement or release of sutures is all that is required to repair the deformity. In contrast, cartilage grafting may be required in more complex post otoplasty deformities [10].

Undercorrection is straightforward, and reoperation includes resection of residual conchal hypertrophy, replacement of cartilage-shaping sutures, resection of excess skin, and correction of lobular excess (Fig. 52.8). In the case of conchal hypertrophy, we recommend an anterior approach for resection as this allows the ear to fall or "spring back" into the correct position. A minimal amount of skin is removed during conchal harvest. The concha and skin should be sutured prior to proceeding to the next stage of repair. Conchal excess exerts a posterior force on the antihelix and creates a prominent sharpened edge. For this reason, the conchal hypertrophy should be addressed prior to cartilage reshaping.

Overcorrection requires greater thought and technical expertise. The operative plan typically requires a strategy to correct cartilage and skin defects. Careful analysis will dictate your need for cartilage grafting and need for skin grafts or flaps in order to modify shape and skin deficiency (Fig. 52.9).

Skin shortage is classically seen in the middle third of the ear, and this defect requires skin replacement. While in early approaches to correction of this deformity, we released scar and adhesions holding the cartilage in its overcorrected position, followed by placement of a full-thickness skin graft to the defect, the extent of cartilage release was limited by needing to maintain a vascular bed for the graft. With additional experience it became clear that a postauricular transposition flap could be used to avoid this potential limitation of the correction and also allow placement of stenting cartilage grafts when needed. The flap may be designed from an area of relative skin excess above or below and

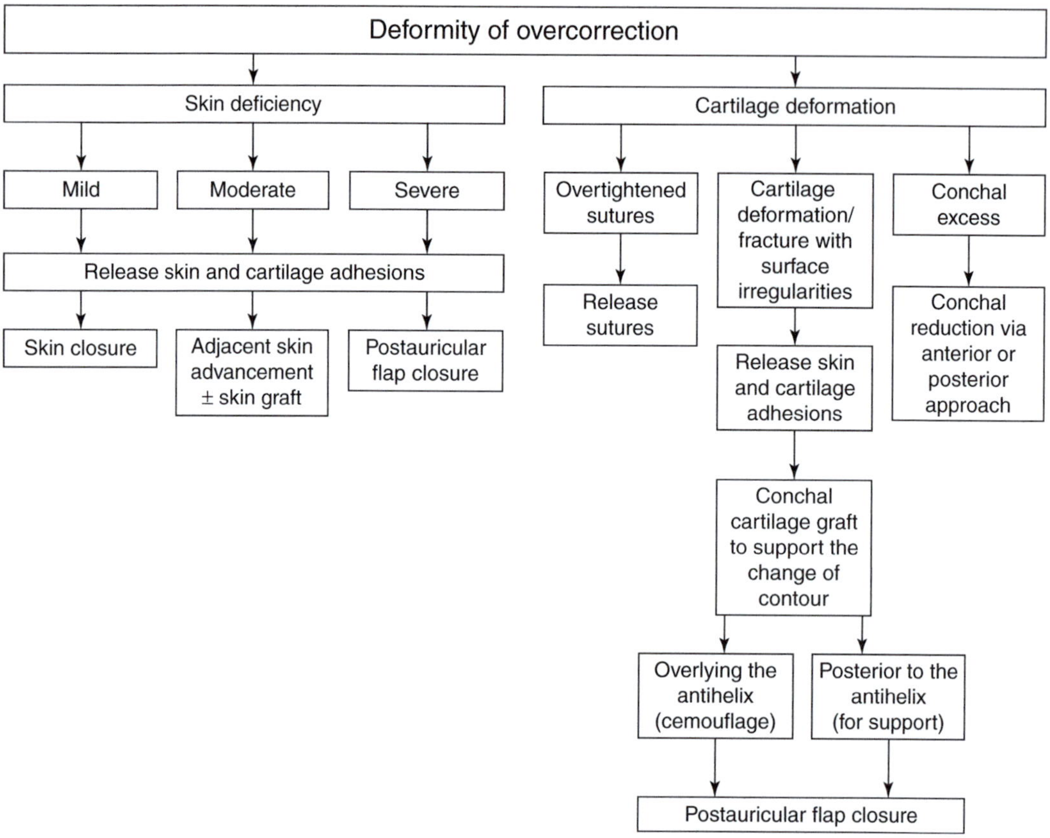

Fig. 52.9 Deformity of overcorrection

rotated 180° in the deficient middle third (Fig. 52.10). It is important to maintain the underlying fascia in these flaps in order to preserve the vascularity.

The sharp, unnatural appearance of an overcorrected antihelix is the most difficult deformity to correct. The goal is to achieve a smooth surface of the antihelix. Very few reports exist to describe the correction of antihelical deformities [11]. A posterior approach is designed to allow wide access to release the sutures and fibrous cartilage adhesions deforming the cartilage. Meticulous dissection in the loose plane above the perichondrium by aligning the scissors with the surface of the cartilage and the use of cut/spread motions is necessary to expose the cartilage (Fig. 52.11). This technique prevents further damage of the remaining cartilage. The cartilage should be carefully unfolded and inspected for quality. At this point, harvested cartilage grafts are added posteriorly to reinforce the fracture sites and to stent open the collapsed antihelical fold (Fig. 52.12). Clear nylon sutures are used to secure the grafts in multiple planes to avoid shifting of the grafts. On occasion, the posterior cartilage grafts do not provide enough correction, and an anteriorly placed graft is required to camouflage severe distortion. The skin in this area is densely adherent to the scared cartilage, and special care must be given to avoid disruption of the skin envelope. Costal cartilage may be needed in cases of conchal cartilage shortage.

In severe cases, attempts for correction of the skin deficiency and cartilage disruption may be better tackled in a multistaged approach. First, provide additional skin with either a graft or a transposition flap. A second stage is used to perform cartilage grafts and suture reshaping.

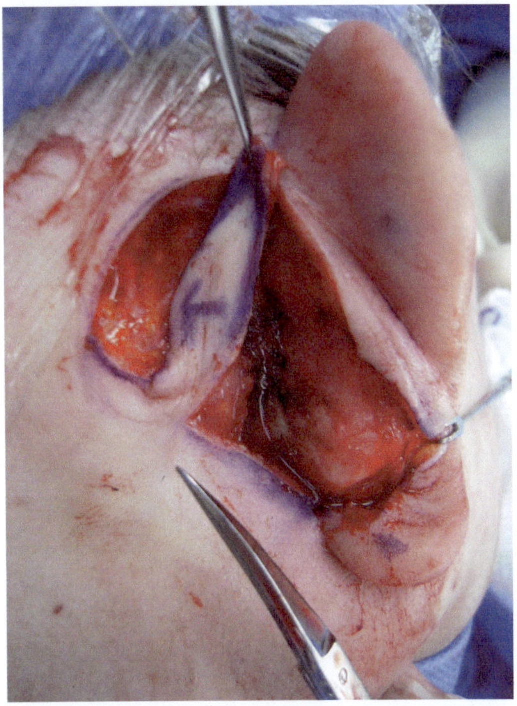

Fig. 52.10 The flap may be designed from an area of relative skin excess *above or below* and rotated 180° in the deficient middle third

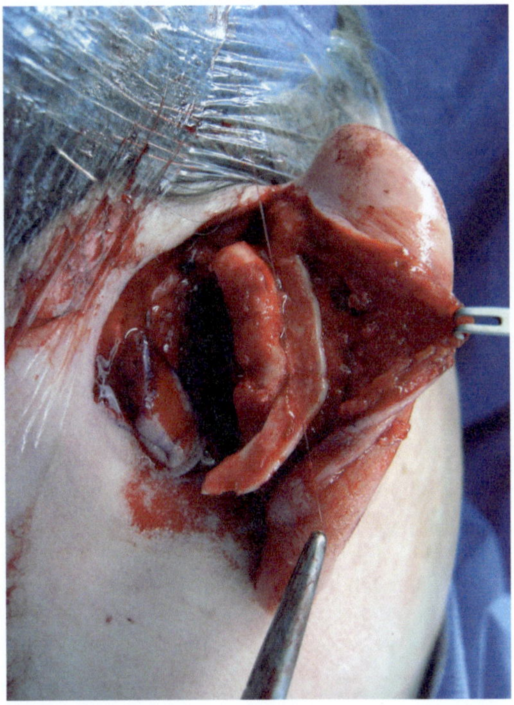

Fig. 52.12 Harvested cartilage grafts are added posteriorly to reinforce the fracture sites and to stent open the collapsed antihelical fold

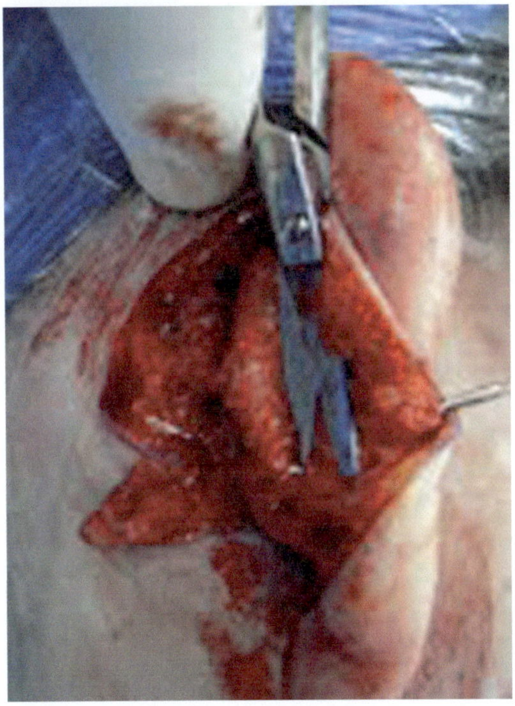

Fig. 52.11 Dissection in the loose plane above the perichondrium by aligning the scissors with the surface of the cartilage and the use of cut/spread motions is necessary to expose the cartilage

Conclusions

Patients seek otoplasty for cosmetic and emotional reasons. When there is a less than perfect outcome, patients express dissatisfaction and reconstruction. If the baseline ear anatomy goes unrecognized and the treatment plan for repair incorrect, then post otoplasty deformities will arise. Adequate analysis of the ear will help determine the cause of the deformity.

The common post otoplasty deformities include the following: (1) loss of the postauricular sulcus, (2) loss of the helical rim visibility, (3) irregular antihelical surface, (4) sharp antihelical fold, (5) residual prominence, (6) telephone ear deformity, and (7) asymmetry. The loss of the postauricular sulcus is due to aggressive skin resection, thereby obliterating the space between the posterior auricle and the mastoid. Overtightened sutures cause loss of helical rim visibility. Cartilage disruption and fracture create an irregular antihelical surface or, worse, a sharp, unnatural appearance. Inadequate conchal reduction also causes a sharp unnatural antihelix. Undercorrection of the superior one-third of the ear results in residual prominence. Mixed errors of over- and undercorrection lead to a telephone ear deformity and asymmetry. A telephone ear deformity may have excess middle-third ear skin excision or a hypertrophied lobule, whereas asymmetry can occur with overcorrection due to overtightened sutures, or undercorrection may be present due to an unrecognized skull base deformity.

An algorithm-based approach is helpful when determining the best solution for reconstruction. Careful attention to the underlying pathology and a detailed approach to repair are necessary. Patients must have a realistic understanding of the limitations for revision and the possibility for multiple stages. Thorough preoperative discussion will empower the patient to understand the complexities of repair and ultimately result in an acceptable outcome.

References

1. Bradbury ET, Hewison J, Timmons MJ. Psychological and social outcome of prominent ear correction in children. Br J Plast Surg. 1992;45(2):97–100.
2. Cooper-Hobson G, Jaffe W. The benefits of otoplasty for children: further evidence to satisfy the modern NHS. J Plast Reconstr Aesthet Surg. 2009;62(2):190–4.
3. MacGregor FC. Ear deformities: social and psychological implications. Clin Plast Surg. 1978;5(3):347–50.
4. Farkas LG. Anthropometry of normal and anomalous ears. Clin Plast Surg. 1978;5(3):401–12.
5. Driessen JP, Borgstein JA, Vuyk HD. Defining the protruding ear. J Craniofac Surg. 2011;22(6):2102–8.
6. da Silva Freitas R, Sanchez ME, Manzotti MS, Baras F, Ono MC, de Oliveira e Cruz GA. Comparing cephaloauricular and scaphaconchal angles in prominent ears and control subjects. Aesthetic Plast Surg. 2008;32(4):620–3.
7. Bauer BS, Song DH, Aitken ME. Combined otoplasty technique: chondrocutaneous conchal resection as the cornerstone to correction of the prominent ear. Plast Reconstr Surg. 2002;110(4):1033–40; discussion 1041.
8. McDowell AJ. Goals in otoplasty for protruding ears. Plast Reconstr Surg. 1968;41(1):17–27.
9. Dieffenbach JF. Die operative Chirurgie. Leipzig: F. A. Brockhause; 1845.
10. Lentz AK, Plikaitis CM, Bauer BS. Understanding the unfavorable result after otoplasty: an integrated approach to correction. Plast Reconstr Surg. 2011;128(2):536–44.
11. Widgerow AD. Revision otoplasty: the contracted antihelical fold. Plast Reconstr Surg. 2002;110(3):827–30.

Solving Sharp Edges of the Antihelix After Otoplasty

53

Renato da Silva Freitas, Maria Cecilia Closs Ono, and Nivaldo Alonso

Introduction

Prominent ear deformity is the most common ear malformation. The incidence in Caucasian population is 5 % with 8 % of those having a positive family history [1]. When correcting the deformity, the surgeon must have a thorough knowledge of the normal anatomy to achieve an acceptable result [2]. The most common auricular deformities are poorly developed antihelical fold and the formation of excessive conchal cartilage. Such deformities eliminate the distinction between the conchal cavity and scapha, resulting in the lateral projection of the ear [3]. Various surgical techniques (more than 200) have been proposed for the treatment of this deformity [3]. Some studies have presented techniques using a total cartilage incision to treat the prominent ear and avoid its recurrence [4, 5]. Pitanguy described a technique in which an island of cartilage is created on the anterior surface of the ear that is pushed forward to resemble a smooth antihelical fold by suturing of edges of the wound after resection of a generous ellipse of skin from the posterior surface [6]. Other surgeons have published studies presenting their successful experience with this technique [7]. The authors, however, have seen several cases of secondary deformities utilizing this technique, presenting with a good antihelical fold, but with excessive sharpness evident, providing a deformed antihelix due the cartilage island. A novel solution for correction of this deformity is described by the authors.

Technique

A posterior incision along the previous scar was performed until the cartilaginous surface, and then undermine over the perichondrium. After a complete releasing of the posterior skin, the anterior surface was carefully undermined, with care taken to avoid skin laceration. The cartilage island was identified and kept untouched on the surface. A diamond drill with pineapple shape point was utilized to trim the sharp borders (Fig. 53.1). After careful hemostasia, the skin envelope was draped over the cartilage and sutured. A compressive dressing associated to four sutures crossing all the layers are used to redrape the skin and avoid hematoma. Follow-up of these patients demonstrated great improvement of the ear contours (Figs. 53.2 and 53.3).

R.da Silva Freitas, M.D. (✉)
Department of Plastic Surgery, Federal University of Parana, Rua General Carneiro 181 9o. Andar, Curitiba, PR 80000-000, Brazil

Universidade Federal do Paraná
Livre-Docente pela USP, Curitiba, PR, Brazil
e-mail: dr.renato.freitas@gmail.com

M.C.C. Ono, M.D.
Rua Rosa Kaint Nadolny, 190, ap 701, Campo Comprido, Curitiba, PR CEP 81200-525, Brazil
e-mail: mccono@gmail.com

N. Alonso, M.D.
Av Pavao 130, apto 162, Moema, São Paulo, SP 04516-010, Brazil
e-mail: nivalonso@gmail.com

M.A. Shiffman (ed.), *Advanced Cosmetic Otoplasty*,
DOI 10.1007/978-3-642-35431-1_53, © Springer-Verlag Berlin Heidelberg 2013

Discussion

Among the surgical goals in the otoplasty is to produce a smooth, rounded, and adequate prominent antihelical fold. The majority of the patients presenting for otoplasty are happy with decreased projection of the helix. But some patients do not wish stigmata of the procedure. Many techniques have been published, using sutures, transection, or scoring for antihelical fold reconstruction. When a complete incision is performed on the ear cartilage, it is possible to achieve sharp borders of the antihelix, a potentially undesirable result [5].

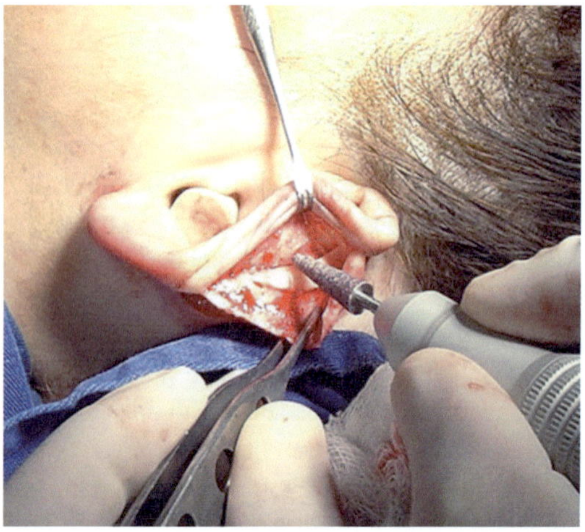

Fig. 53.1 Utilizing the drill to trim the borders of cartilage

Luckett was the first to describe the cartilage incision [4]. He described a crescent-shaped segment of skin and cartilage and sutured the edges to create a new antihelical fold. Pitanguy [6] presented his technique using an island of cartilage that is pushed forward to create the new antihelix. Balogh and Millesi [5] have used a sutured 2-mm strip of cartilage behind the cartilage edge to avoid sharpness of the new antihelix. However, they presented the same complication presented in this chapter in 9 cases out of a total 77 cases operated. Recently, a new study was published using this island technique in 278 patients, but the authors did not mention the occurrence of sharping edges of the new antihelical fold [7].

Antihelical fold deformity can follow various techniques. The severity of the deformity guides the treatment. The procedure we have described can repair this complication after ear cartilage incision, especially when the main problem is the acute and unnatural borders of the antihelical fold. However, there are more severe cases in

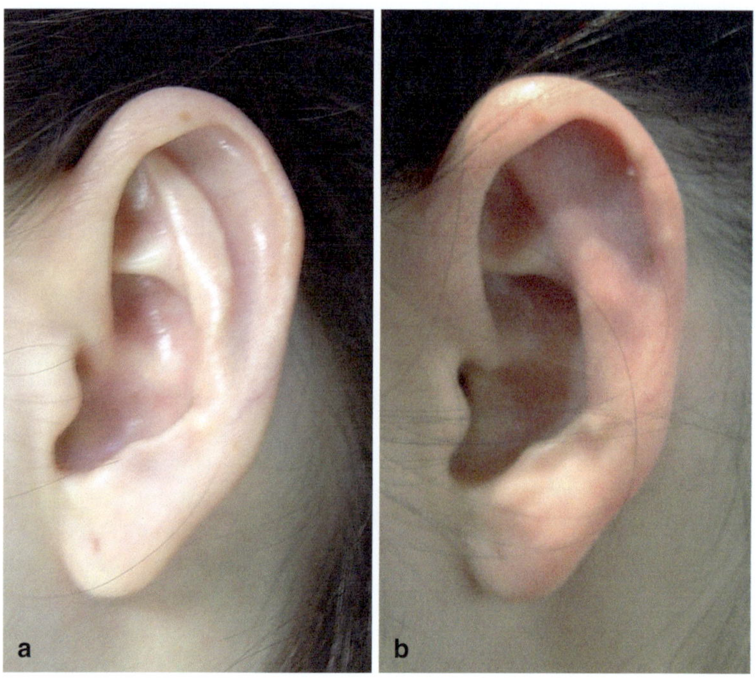

Fig. 53.2 (**a**) Preoperative patient who had otoplasty 2 years before and now complains about the appearance of her ears. (**b**) Six months postoperative

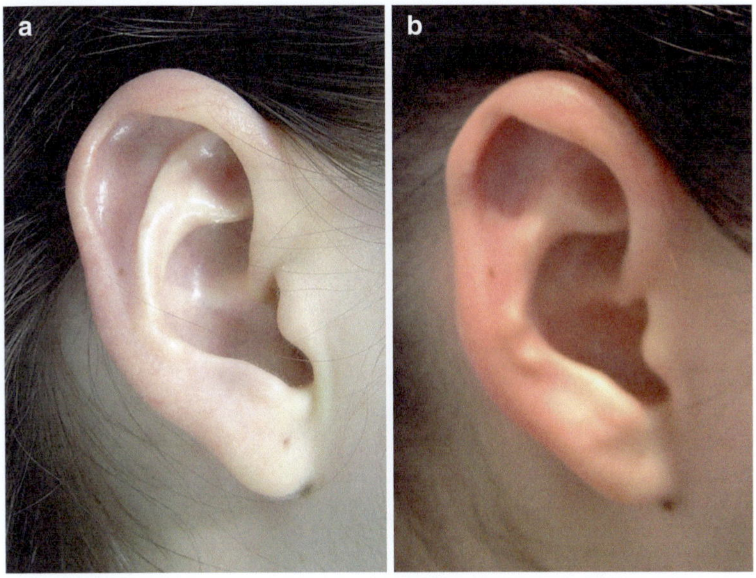

Fig. 53.3 (**a**) Preoperative patient. (**b**) Postoperative following Pitanguy technique otoplasty

which it is necessary to consider the use of a conchal or costal cartilage frame to substitute the antihelical fold deformity [2].

The authors believe that the surgeon should avoid complete cartilage incision, primarily on the antihelix, to prevent the occurrence of an unnatural and unpleasant result.

References

1. Kelley P, Hollier L, Stal S. Otoplasty: evaluation, technique, and review. J Craniofac Surg. 2003;14(5):643–53.
2. Firmin F, Sanger C, O'Toole G. Ear reconstruction following severe complications of otoplasty. J Plast Reconstr Aesthet Surg. 2008;61 Suppl 1:S13–20.
3. Panettiere P, Marchetti L, Accorsi D, Del Gaudio GA. Otoplasty: a comparison of techniques for antihelical defects treatment. Aesthetic Plast Surg. 2004;27(6):462–5.
4. Rogers BO. The classic reprint. A new operation for prominent ears based on the anatomy of the deformity by William H. Luckett, M.D. (Reprinted from Surg Gynec & Obst, 10:635–7, 1910). Plast Reconstr Surg. 1969;43(1):83–6.
5. Balogh B, Millesi H. Are growth alterations a consequence of surgery for prominent ears? Plast Reconstr Surg. 1992;90(2):192–9.
6. Pitanguy I, Müller P, Piccolo N, Ramalho E, Solinas R. The treatment of prominent ears: a 25-year survey of the island technique. Aesthetic Plast Surg. 1987;11(2):87–93.
7. Werdin F, Wolters M, Lampe H. Pitanguy's otoplasty: report of 551 operations. Scand J Plast Reconstr Surg Hand Surg. 2007;41(6):283–7.

Prophylactic Z-Plasty to Prevent the Notch Deformity of the Helical Rim Following the Wedge Excision of the Ear

54

Peter Kim

Introduction

Wedge excision is a popular and a well-documented surgical procedure of removing a wide range of skin lesions and cancers of the ear. It is a simple and an effective treatment. But not too infrequently, notch deformity of the helical rim is noted postoperatively (Fig. 54.1). Such deformity is well accepted in majority of cases and can be hidden behind the longer hair, but in some cases, it leads to patient dissatisfaction. Application of Z-plasty [1] in these instances can effectively prevent helical rim notch deformity, and this chapter will illustrate this technique.

Technique

Basal cell carcinoma (BCC) of the ear was excised using Mohs surgery to enable maximum amount of soft tissue for the ear reconstruction (Fig. 54.2). The ear was wedge excised, and when the surgical margins of the wedged ear were approximated, the "notch" deformity of the helical rim was noted. If the ear was to be approximated in its current state, a postoperative ear with a notch deformity can be predicted. In order to prevent this complication, Z-plasty was fashioned prophylactically. A 60° Z-plasty incision was made; the two triangular flaps were elevated and transposed and then sutured. Sutures were removed after 1 week, and a 3-month postoperative outcome was satisfactory with no notch deformity.

Discussion

The ear is an important aspect of facial aesthetics. One of the cosmetically pleasing aspects of a natural ear is an ear with a smooth and uninterrupted helical contour. Disturbances in this contour, such as the notch deformity following a wedge excision, can produce cosmetic concerns and patient dissatisfaction. A major cause of notch deformity of the helical rim appears to be related to excess closure tension on the rim [2]. This produces tissue ischemia in short term (dehiscence) which can manifest as a contour defects both immediately at the time of surgery as well as gradually over the longer term as the result of distensae striae.

Z-plasty was initially described by Fricke in 1829 and William Horner in 1837 [3], and Z-plasty is one of the oldest and most recognized form of skin flap surgery. In Z-plasty, Z-shaped skin incision is made to allow the two triangular flaps to be elevated and interdigitated (transposed) as to produce a change in the direction of the central limb (Fig. 54.3). When this principle is applied in the skin surgery of the

P. Kim, M.D., MBBS
Simply Beautiful Cosmetic Surgery & Laser Clinic,
4 Farnell Street, West Ryde, Sidney,
NSW 2114, Australia
e-mail: dr.peterkim@yahoo.com.au

M.A. Shiffman (ed.), *Advanced Cosmetic Otoplasty*,
DOI 10.1007/978-3-642-35431-1_54, © Springer-Verlag Berlin Heidelberg 2013

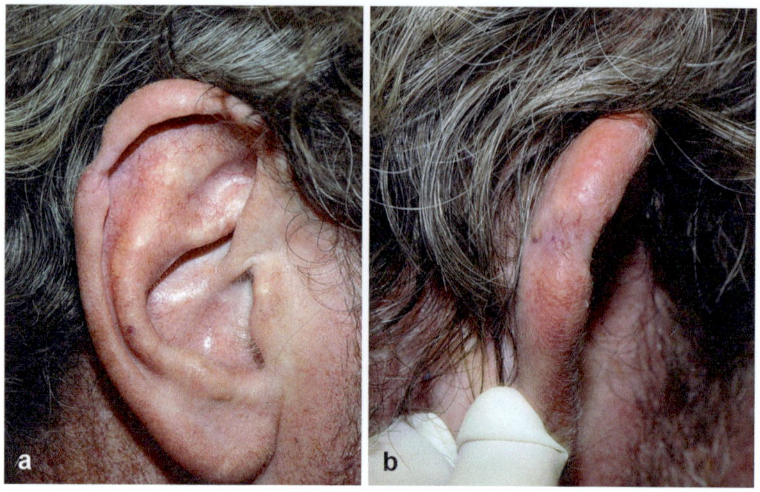

Fig. 54.1 **a**) Notch deformity of the helical rim. **b**) Following a wedge excision

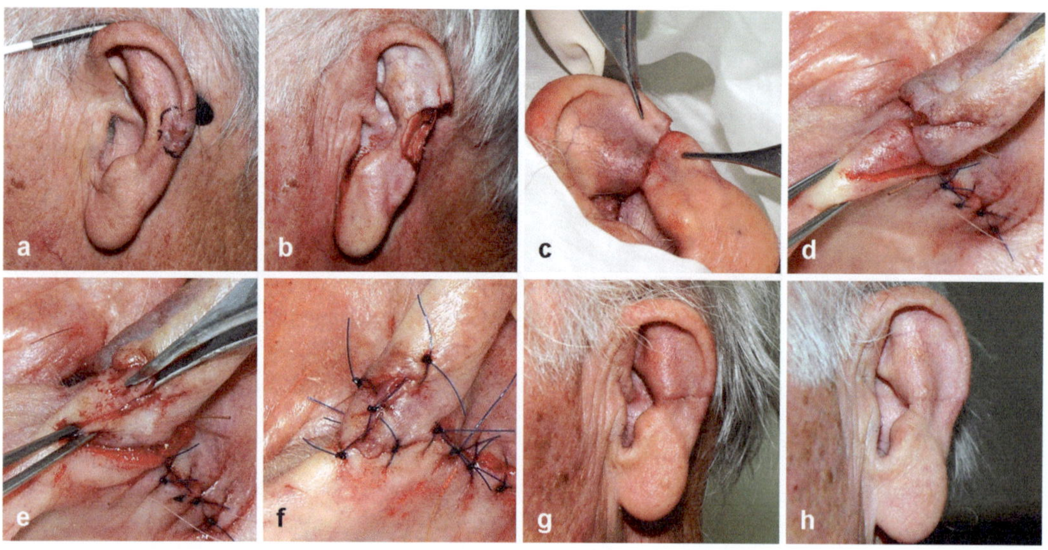

Fig. 54.2 Application of Z-plasty prophylactically to prevent notch deformity of the helical rim. (**a**) Basal cell carcinoma (BCC) of the ear. (**b**) BCC excised using Mohs surgery to enable maximum amount of soft tissue for the ear reconstruction. The ear was wedge excised. (**c**) When the surgical margins of the wedged ear were approximated, the "notch" deformity of the helical rim was noted. (**d**) Z-plasty was fashioned prophylactically. Z-plasty incision, 60°, was made. (**e**) Two triangular flaps were elevated and transposed. (**f**) Sutured. (**g**) Sutures removed after 1 week. (**h**) Three months' postoperative outcome was satisfactory with no notch deformity

ear, an effective correction of the scars and helical rim contour deformities can be achieved by changing the direction of scar (from transverse to parallel Z-plasty). This is one of the oldest and most recognized forms of skin flap surgery.

1. Tissue lengthening along the rim
2. Interrupting scar linearity (zigzag scars are less perceptible)
3. Producing a smooth and continuous helical rim curvature

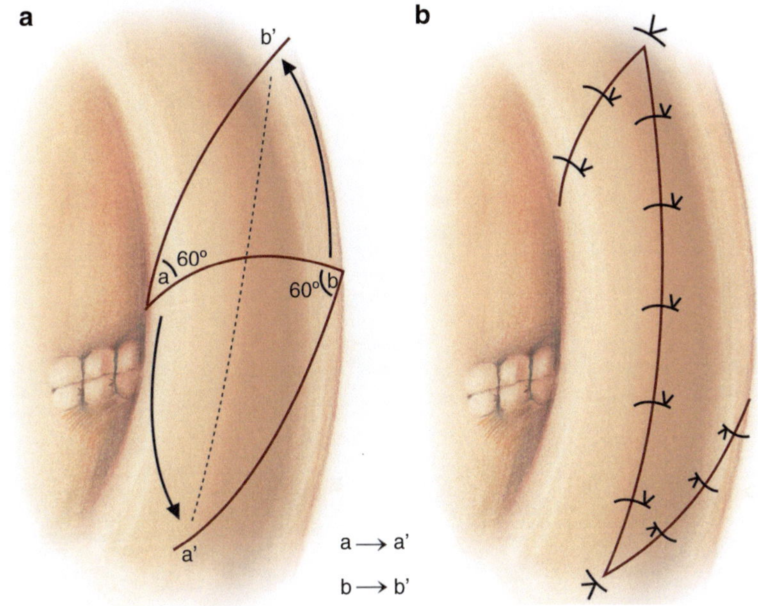

Fig. 54.3 (**a**, **b**) Standard 60° Z-plasty when applied in ear

In the ear, Z-plasty is commonly used to treat the postoperative depressed scar or a preexisting dermatological deformity [4]. However, where the postoperative notch deformity can be intraoperatively predicted, such as in this case following a wedge excision, prophylactic Z-plasty can prevent such deformity and in turn produce a more cosmetically satisfying outcome, without significantly increasing the morbidity.

Conclusions

Prophylactic Z-plasty following a wedge excision of the ear lesion offers a surgeon a simple and an effective one-stage procedure that can prevent the unsightly notch deformity of the helical rim.

References

1. Kim P. Prophylactic Z-plasty – correcting helical rim deformity from wedge excision. Aust Fam Physician. 2010;39(9):649–50.
2. Holzmann RD, Guldbakke KK, Schanbacher CF. Bilateral advancement flaps with helical rim Z-plasty. Modification for management of ear defects. Dermatol Surg. 2008;34(3):374–7.
3. Hodges A. Z-plasty.A-Z of plastic surgery. Oxford: Oxford University Press; 2009.
4. Lee PK, Ju HS, Rhie JW, Ahn ST. Two flaps and Z-plasty technique for correction of longitudinal ear lobe cleft. Br J Plast Surg. 2005;58(4):573–6.

Otoplasty Revision

55

Philip A. Young

Introduction

Perhaps the most important point to emphasize when discussing the topic of revisional surgery for otoplasty is prevention. It is much more complicated to revise an unwanted result than getting it right the first time around. Of course, that principle can likely be applied to all aspects of surgery. But, this chapter would be amiss if it did not mention some important points about prevention. Importantly, the goal in otoplasty is to pin back the ears to the degree that the patient desires. This could be variable based on for whom you are performing the otoplasty. So a generous discussion with your patient is paramount in deciding just how much setback they are wanting. If you do not talk to your patients, it does not matter how well you do the otoplasty; you might still be wrong if you do not achieve what they want. So our discussion again goes back to prevention. Find out what your patient wants and document it. You will then have a better chance of making them happy. There are ideals in the literature, however. This is likely going to be covered in other chapters. But based on the author's theory on aesthetics [1], the ears should protrude about one iris width from the side of the head. One and a half iris widths of ear protrusion is probably the upper extreme of normal; anything more than that would be interpreted by the viewer as excessive. Most people like their ears protruding about an iris width without them knowing how the author's theory applies to ear aesthetics. In addition, if there is any way that you would choose to skew whether the upper, middle, or lower third is more protruding, it is always better to allow the upper third to protrude the most then middle and then lower in that order (Fig. 55.1).

This chapter is based strongly on the author's experience but is undoubtedly influenced by a gestalt created by extensive background reading. In the video case a specific case will be illustrated that carries with it some of the more extreme techniques that are needed in an otoplasty revisional case.

P.A. Young, M.D.
1810 116th Ave NE #102,
Bellevue, WA 98004, USA
e-mail: dryoung@drphilipyoung.com,
payoung88@gmail.com

General Prevention and Personal Thoughts on Otoplasty and the Revisional Approach

The upper third of the ear is the area that is most likely to recur following an otoplasty. It has been found that the relapse of this area is most likely due to loosening of the sutures. There may not be something that can be done about recurrence in this area, but these are some points that can be suggested. A 4-0 Mersilene is likely the most common suture to be used in Mustarde-type sutures (Fig. 55.2) [2, 3] for reconstruction of the superior crus of the antihelix. The benefit of this suture is the braided,

M.A. Shiffman (ed.), *Advanced Cosmetic Otoplasty*,
DOI 10.1007/978-3-642-35431-1_55, © Springer-Verlag Berlin Heidelberg 2013

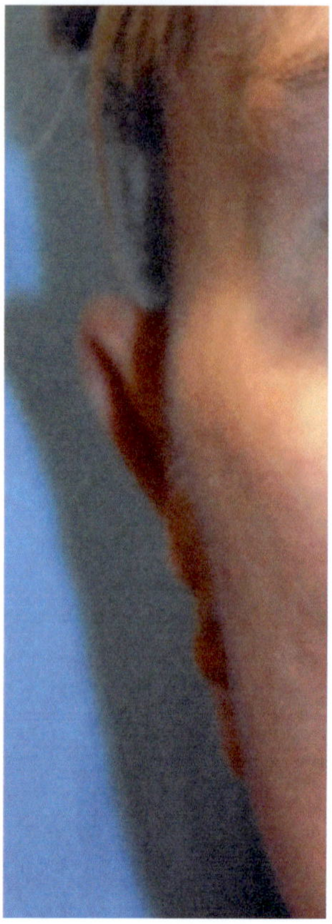

Fig. 55.1 Overcorrected ear. The ear is barely visible. In the middle and lower thirds, only 2–4 mm of ear is showing lateral to the side of the face. The superior third is showing approximately 8–9 mm. From the frontal view, you should be able to see the helix, and the antihelix should be more medial than the helix

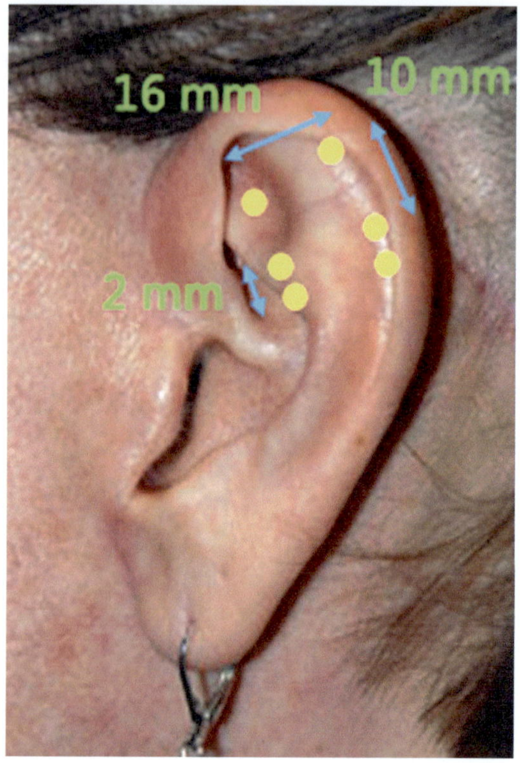

Fig. 55.2 The Mustarde sutures. The markings for the Mustarde sutures are 16 mm apart across the width of the superior crus of the antihelix. They are 10 mm apart lengthwise. The next horizontal mattress sutures are set 2 mm from the previous one. These numbers can vary depending on the person and the shape that you want to achieve

nonabsorbable qualities that prevent pull-through and absorption of the suture. This suture has a long history of success among surgeons who perform otoplasty. Because braided sutures are more likely to get infected, 4-0 clear nylon is used as do many surgeons currently. Although this suture is more likely to pull through, the author concentrates on getting full-thickness bites including the perichondrium when performing Mustarde sutures. With 4-0 Mersilene, the closer you are to the skin surface, the greater is the possibility of issues such as infection, suture abscesses, and rejection of the suture. An erroneous approach to the upper third is to depend on the Mustarde sutures to do most of the pinning back of the ears. The fault here is that when Mustarde sutures are relied on more than other techniques, one often tends to set back the helical rim so that the antihelix covers the helix on frontal view. This situation does not represent the ideal. This can be a telltale sign of a poor and unthoughtful otoplasty. It is much better to rely more on the conchal setback (Fig. 55.3) [4] to mostly pin back the ears and more of a subtle bend and creation of the antihelix that can give a more natural look. With that approach, the recreated antihelix has less pressure placed on it by the sutures and is thus less likely to be affected by pull-through of the sutures and recurrence of the prominent upper third. Also you are more likely to have a better result where the helix is positioned more laterally than the antihelix.

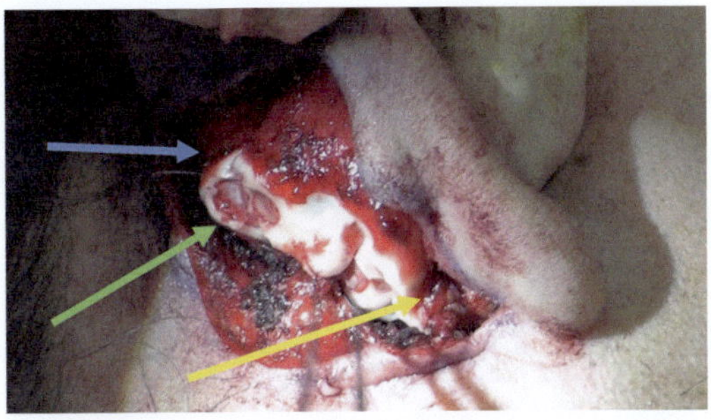

Fig. 55.3 Conchal setback. The 15 blade can be directed at the concha and specifically address each quadrant of the ear. This is done incrementally and reassessed to assure the most perfect amount of setback. The *green arrow* indicates the area that has been shaved. The *blue arrow* shows the direction and exposure that you must approach and achieve to medialize the superior third. The *yellow arrow* indicates the exposure you need to achieve to treat the inferior strut of the conchal bowl to medialize this area

Conchal Setback and Mustarde Sutures Specifics

Start out the otoplasty with the conchal setback [4], then shave the back of the concha with the 15 blade to weaken the concha. This is done from upper third to lower third. Most of the setback is achieved when the 15 blade is concentrated over the struts that actually protrude the ear. Wide exposure is key to allow you to weaken the upper and lower third, not just the middle third. In Fig. 55.3, the blue and yellow areas indicate the areas that require more exposure to approach the upper and lower third supporting struts of the concha that need to be weakened to medialize these quadrants. This is done in a gradual manner to achieve just the right amount of total ear setback with the goal being the patient's desired amount of setback. In Fig. 55.3, the green arrow shows the area that has been shaved. In actuality, the shaving of the concha need not be so extensive that the other soft tissue is exposed on the other side of the cartilage. This figure is meant to illustrate this point. Doing this may weaken the concha to such a degree that you have bunching in the conchal bowl which is undesirable. It is much better to gradually thin the concha carefully so that a large expanse of cartilage is thinned evenly and sufficiently to medialize the ear without much pressure placed when assessing the ear intraoperatively. If you do encounter areas of bunching, tacking sutures can be done with 5-0 fast gut to allow these areas of soft tissue to adhere to the adjacent underlying postauricular areas. Another reason for recurrence is an overdependence on the conchal mastoid sutures and less on the conchal shaving. I believe conchal shaving is essential in getting more long results with medialization. If there is little antihelical bend, I might be conservative in the conchal setback superiorly in order to allow the Mustarde sutures to medialize the upper third and create the antihelix bend to the desired amount. But I always have in mind that the less dependence on the Mustarde sutures, the better it is for more long-term results. After each round of shaving, the frontal view is checked to make sure that the concha is not over weakened and to get just the right amount of setback. This is perhaps the key to the best results. The concha is set back with 4-0 clear nylon placed sequentially and incrementally in number. The antihelical bend is created with the Mustarde sutures. The Mustarde sutures are placed through stab incisions from the anterior side with an 11 blade. This makes it easier to judge the amount of bend that would be created. This approach puts both less strain on the Mustarde sutures and allows me to get more accurate and aesthetic results. It also allows less strain on the conchal mastoid sutures and the possibility of weakening the cartilage that is used for these sutures when you put the sutures from behind.

In Fig. 55.2, the yellow dots show where the Mustarde sutures will be placed. Sixteen millimeters is the distance across the width of the antihelix. The sutures are placed 10 mm apart in the vertical dimension, lengthwise along the antihelix, as shown. The next horizontal mattress suture is 2 mm apart. These measurements are more the classical approach. In reality, you can determine where you want the antihelical bend by bending the helix and mapping the light reflex that you see. The bend will usually also create a highlight, and the edge of the highlight is where you can make the sutures enter. The classical measurements are just a guideline, and they can be quite variable depending on the person. As you move more inferiorly, the width of the horizontal mattress sutures also gets closer than

16 mm. Instead of 16 mm, the author often finds that 14 and 13 mm are for the first Mustarde horizontal suture and 12 and 10–9 mm are for the second Mustarde sutures. At times, the author finds, however, that only the first suture and second one are needed for support.

Undercorrection: General Thoughts

Undercorrection of the otoplasty is a much easier situation in an otoplasty revision [5] case than the overcorrected ear from otoplasty. Undercorrection is revised most of the time by redoing the procedures [6, 7] that were done in the original surgery. Some general personal thoughts on undercorrection in the revision setting and the use of Mustarde sutures and conchal setback will be presented here. Most of the time, undercorrection can be corrected by further conchal setback and conchal weakening in the particular section of the ear where the undercorrection is located. You can reference the above pointers on how to achieve that. Removal of more mastoid fascia can also be done in the superior, middle, or lower third to further medialize the ear in each of these areas prior to the conchal setback. This is not necessary in most situations and that the conchal setback with shaving is more than effective. There are many instances when after the conchal setback and the Mustarde sutures are done, the superior and anterior attachment of the helix can assume an odd appearance in that portion of the ear. A bowed and protruding helix is sometimes the result near the anterior attachment of the helix. Tacking of the superior and anterior helix to the deep temporal fascia can be done with a 4-0 nylon to address this issue (Fig. 55.4). Locating where to place the nylon sutures is paramount. You have to test different areas in this location to achieve the desired results. The more anteriorly the suture is placed, the more tension is created, and you can actually get some lateralization to the helix. Whereas a more posterior and superior suture will more medialize the ear at the superior third. Also carrying out the Mustarde sutures again and tying these sutures more aggressively can further medialize the upper third if this is the cause. You can determine if you need Mustarde sutures when you have no significant antihelical fold and the concha appears to be set back enough already. Again, the details on the Mustarde sutures and the conchal setback were explained earlier and in other chapters.

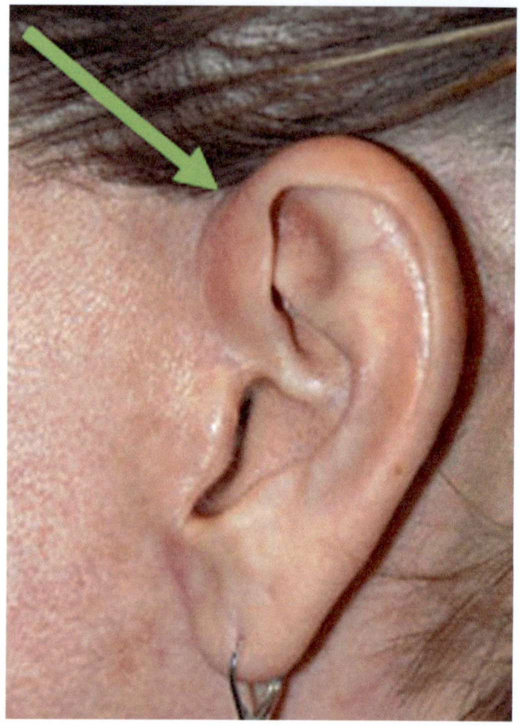

Fig. 55.4 Tacking the superior anterior attachment of the helix (*Green arrow*). This is a common area to create an odd bowing effect after Mustarde sutures and conchal setback. Tacking this down will get an even better result for your patient

Undercorrected Upper Third

Further setback of the upper third can be accomplished by more aggressive Mustarde sutures being careful not to hide the upper helical rim behind the antihelix on frontal view. Also, as mentioned earlier the anterior and superior attachment of the helix can be set back through a separate incision or an extension of the original incision (Fig. 55.4). The goal here is to tack the helix in this area to the temporal fascia. If you want to avoid suture failure this time and would like to support your revised Mustarde suture, one

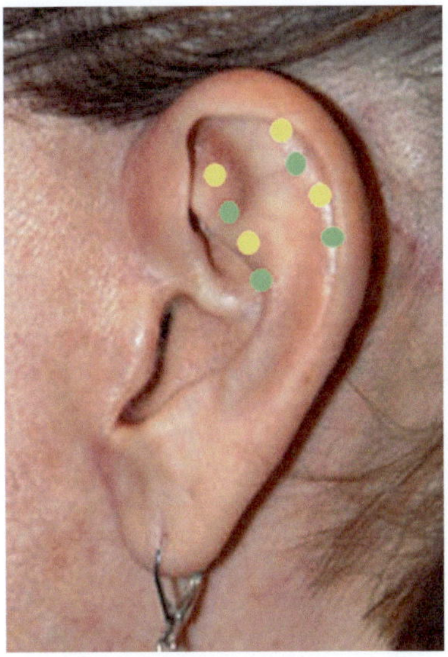

Fig. 55.5 If you want to avoid suture failure this time and would like to support your revised Mustarde suture, one option is to stagger the Mustarde suture and have them overlap with each set of horizontal mattress sutures separated by 5 mm. The *yellow dots* represent the first Mustarde suture, and the *green dots* represent the second set

option is to stagger the Mustarde suture and have them overlap with each set of horizontal mattress sutures separated by 5 mm (Fig. 55.5).

If the undercorrection of the upper third is not due to the lack of the antihelical bend, treatment of the conchal bowl may be what will be needed. As discussed earlier, most conchal setbacks are concentrated on the projection of the middle third. The lack of exposure and treatment of the upper third strut within the conchal bowl during the original procedure could be the cause of the excessive lateral position that persists in the otoplasty revision. So one needs to prudently decide if it is the Mustarde sutures or the conchal setback or both that are needed. The key to this decision is whether there is present an adequate bend in the antihelix. If there is a deficiency, you will need to determine if Mustarde sutures will be enough to medialize the upper third to the ideal degree without hiding the helix behind the antihelix. If this is not enough, it may still require conchal bowl shaping. Further conchal setback, when required, necessitates aggressive exposure of the upper thirds conchal strut and further incremental shaving and conchal mastoid sutures to create the ideal position of this section.

Undercorrected Middle Third

The undercorrected middle third will require more conchal shaving, setback, and possible removal of soft tissue beneath the conchal bowl. Thoughtful and incremental changes will achieve the best results based on preoperative patient counseling. Conchal shaving and setback should be more than enough to medialize any section of the ear, and the removal of soft tissue is not really necessary. It is important to make sure that it is truly an undercorrected middle third and not an overcorrected upper and lower third. In this situation, further medialization of the middle third will lead to an overcorrected ear as a whole. This would be the worst situation and the most difficult to reverse depending on the maneuvers that were used to achieve this state.

Undercorrected Lower Third

For the undercorrected lower third, further conchal setback requires aggressive exposure of the conchal bowl inferiorly. Further shaving of the inferior strut of the concha with mastoid conchal sutures will be the most effective move to medialize the lower third. In addition to more aggressive conchal setback, removing the cauda helicis can help medialize the lower third. Although this is often suggested in reality, the removal of the cauda helicis has less effect on lower third than concentrating on the inferior strut of the concha for more medialization. More aggressive skin removal is another adjunct to medialize the lower third but less accurate and reliable. There are many variations in drawing the skin resection to help medialize the lower third. The dumbbell excision of skin is often done in the original otoplasty to help medialize the upper and lower third. This can be done again during the revision in a more aggressive manner. Another consideration is to tack the earlobe in a more medial position by extending the incision inferiorly and tacking the earlobe to the deep soft tissue in this area. Aesthetic judgment will determine where and how the incision is extended to achieve the results you want. The inferior incision starts at the inferior end of the original postauricular incision but is located just under the lobule. You have to determine where you want the earlobe to be more medialized, and this will guide you on how you place your incision. However, all of these other options are inferior to the thoughtful treatment of the inferior conchal strut with shaving and sutures. These adjunctive maneuvers can optimize the conchal setback revision of the lower third but are not necessary in my opinion.

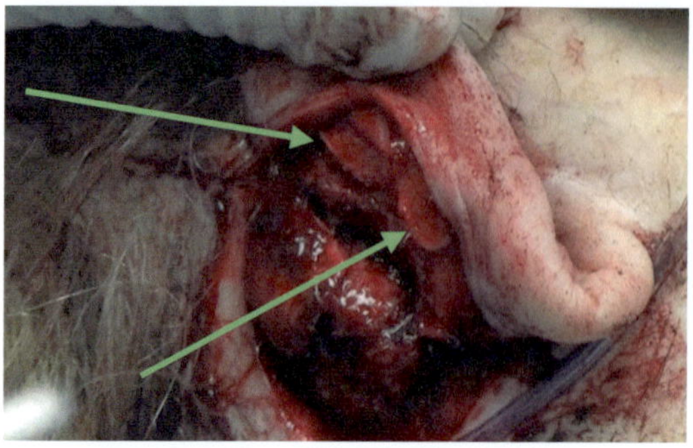

Fig. 55.6 Antihelix with grafts in place. Dissection is required with scissors to spread and cut through scar tissue holding the overly aggressive antihelical bend. Cartilage grafts are in place (as indicated by the *green arrows*) to maintain the correction for the long term

Overcorrection of the Upper Third

Reversing the Mustarde Sutures

Overcorrection after otoplasty is the much more complicated situation. In the upper third, it can entail over tightening of the Mustarde sutures. In this situation it may be that the helix is not visible on frontal view or contributing to the overmedialized state. The approach entails loosening the bend of the antihelix by cutting through sutures and scar tissue. Through the postauricular incision, the iris scissors is used to incrementally incise and spread through the scar tissue just under the antihelix. A cartilage bar that is straight or bent less than the current bend in the antihelix is an important consideration in supporting the reversal of the overly aggressive Mustarde sutures. Strong sutures to hold these grafts in place are necessary to resist recontracture of this area (Fig. 55.6). Through-and-through sutures to tack these support grafts are also a consideration to strengthen the position of these grafts with 4-0 fast gut. Reverse Mustarde sutures are also an option or can be done in conjunction with these other maneuvers with the goal of bending the antihelix in the opposite way. These sutures can be done in an analogous way that lateral crural horizontal mattress sutures are done to support the lateral crural from a convex to straight shape. One could choose to place these support sutures for additional support even with cartilage grafting and the other methods mentioned.

Reversing the Conchal Setback in the Upper Third

Less commonly, an overcorrected upper third is due to an aggressive setback of the concha in this area. Because the conchal setback is mostly directed towards the middle third, I often find that this is not the reason that the upper third is overcorrected. As I will explain in more detail below in the overcorrection of the middle third, release of adhesions of the conchal bowl will precede the use of cartilage batten-type grafts to the concha. The goal is grafting cartilage to support the strut that usually holds the upper third in a more lateral position within the concha. To support this, more grafting in the middle third can be used to support the upper third cartilage strut grafts. This is done in much the same way as in Fig. 55.6. The difference is that these grafts are placed where the struts were originally and some overlap is helpful for support. Other options exist when cartilage is scarce. Rotating mastoid and postauricular tissue based anteriorly can be done to lateralize the upper third. If this tissue is not enough, you can rotate a superficial temporal fascial flap based on the superficial temporal artery. Medpor or rib cartilage can also be carved to lateralize the upper third but are second choices and should be discussed with your patients in greater details.

Cartilage Grafts

The lack of cartilage may become an issue in this situation. Obvious possible sources include nasal septum, rib, or the other ear. You can also consider the ipsilateral or contralateral tragal cartilage, caudal helicis cartilage, or conchal bowl that is not contributing to the ultimate shape of the ear. In regard to the tragal cartilage, preserving the portion of this cartilage that immediately protrudes laterally to the external auditory canal is prudent to maintain the shape of the tragus. For conchal bowl cartilage sources, taking the parts of the cartilage that are not part of the struts that are protruding the ear is important to maintain the amount of protrusion that you would like to maintain. This usually limits conchal cartilage that is at the base of the bowl.

Skin Component

One of the biggest issues with overcorrection in any section of the ear is the loss of skin. Without the outer lining, all other attempts to revise the overcorrected ear will not be effective. The extremely strong pressures from the contracture will ultimately destroy any scar release, cartilage grafting, and other measures that are done. There are many possibilities for correction. A V-Y advancement is a possible way to recruit skin to the postauricular area directed to the area of the ear that needs the most skin. This can be designed from behind the ear to recruit skin from the postauricular area (Fig. 55.7). The width of the V should approximate the area that is in need of lateralizing the most. If at all possible, it is desirable to have the Y limb close along the hairline. Another option is the use of two separate fusiform shapes that can be recruited from different sections of the ear (upper, middle, lower third) based on a subcutaneous pedicle to augment the skin where it is needed. Figure 55.7 shows these flaps that were used to augment the middle third

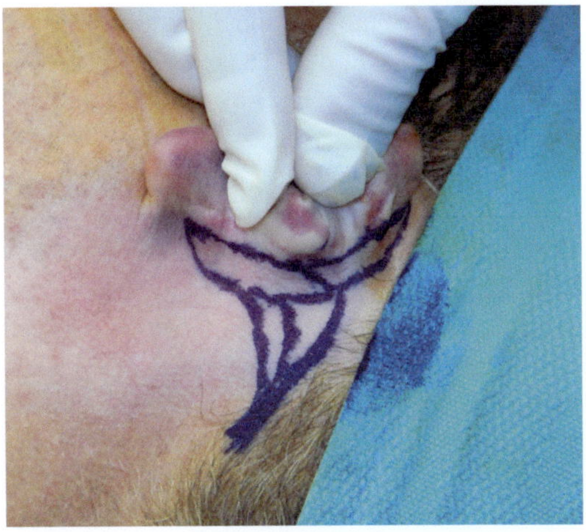

Fig. 55.7 Options for skin replacement. This is an example of skin flaps that can help augment the middle third. The fusiform shapes denote options for subcutaneous pedicled flaps that can be advanced into the middle third. Additional skin can also be recruited through a V-Y advancement with the superior limb oriented along the postauricular hairline as shown. Variations of this can be tailored for the upper and lower third of the ear

in this particular patient. A variation of this can be done for the upper and lower third as well. You must plan the flaps so that when they are advanced, the widest portion is at the most medialized location that you are trying to correct and the advancement and the width of the flaps will also support the parts of the ear that also need to be lateralized. A posterior hairline incision can be used to advance a rotational flap of skin to this area as well. The length of the hairline incision will depend on the amount of skin that will need to be recruited. A transposition flap from the preauricular area can be considered if the patient is agreeable to an incision in this area. Full-thickness skin grafts from the opposite ear or other areas are other possibilities if regional skin flaps are not enough. With full-thickness skin grafts, the revision otoplasty could be approached in a staged fashion. The full-thickness skin graft is done a few weeks to months in advance before cartilage grafting, and other maneuvers are done to revise the otoplasty. If done in one stage, rotating mastoid fascia or superficial temporal fascia based on the superficial temporal artery should be considered to support the skin graft. Others have suggested recruiting skin from one of the other sections of the ear (upper, middle, or lower third) to supply skin from an area that is overcorrected to the area of deficiency [5] through transposition flaps.

Overcorrection of the Middle Third

With the middle third an overcorrection can lead to a telephone ear deformity where the middle third is brought in more relative to the upper and lower thirds of the ear. The main cause of this is too much of a conchal setback in the middle third area or not enough conchal setback in the upper and lower thirds. For the upper third, overly aggressive Mustarde sutures are also a consideration. Thinking about these points is an important determination before deciding to revise any otoplasty. An adequate discussion with your patient is paramount to find out what they would like. Computer imaging is helpful to find an agreement of a shape that you are both trying to achieve and that improvement and not perfection is the goal. If the overcorrection is due to an over aggressive conchal setback, augmentation is necessary.

Reversal of the Conchal Setback and Element of the Conchal Bowl

Knowledge of how each section of the ear is affected by the conchal bowl is important in understanding how to revise the overcorrected or undercorrected state. The superior third supporting strut is rather straight and perpendicular to the surface of the head compared to the middle strut. The middle third is more curved to the bowl's base, while the inferior third can be in between the two. Variations exist. Most of the time there will be remnant cartilage in the concha that when supported by stronger cartilage grafts will allow the concha to resume a shape more like the conchal's original shape. Release of scar tissue causing the concha to adhere to deeper tissues is a necessary first step. The new grafts that are supporting the struts should have adjacent grafts in the location of the other struts for support or collapse is a likely possibility. Depending on which

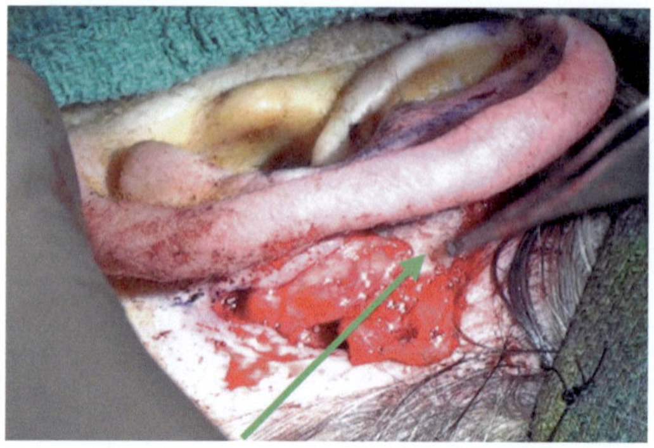

Fig. 55.8 Medpor in place to help lateralize the ear. The *green arrow* and Adson forceps are pointing to the Medpor in the postauricular space to help lateralize the ear. Mastoid fascia anteriorly based and flipped to cover the Medpor implant is shown just below. There is another rotated flap based on an inferior pedicle that is also being rotated upwards to the Medpor

section of the ear is overcorrected, the grafts will need to be done in the upper, middle, or lower third. The overcorrected ear and how it is related to the conchal setback procedure in the section of the middle ear is most often overcorrected by the conchal setback. Supporting soft tissue around the grafts that will fill in possible dead space and also support the cartilage grafts holding the ear laterally can be helpful to add additional support. If the struts are not able to recreate the strength of the original struts holding the ear in a more lateral position, a rib cartilage graft carved to fit may be necessary using Burt Brent's microtia approach. An alternative is the rotation of mastoid fascia to lateralize the ear in the right amount or rotating superficial temporal fascia with the same intent as mentioned previously. Medpor blocks are another option that can be carved to emulate the original conchal shape also through incorporating Burt Brent's microtia approach (Fig. 55.8). A vascular bed is necessary when contemplating Medpor or complications could arise. With any of these approaches, a prerequisite is sufficient outer lining. Many times, it is the lack of skin from overly aggressive skin resection that has caused the ear to become too medialized. Hence, replacing the skin component is likely the first objective to getting a sufficient result as discussed previously. If this is not accomplished, it is my experience that other procedural steps like cartilage grafting, release of scar tissue, reversing sutures, and all other maneuvers will be done in vain.

Telephone Ear Deformity

Again, when considering the overcorrection of the middle third, you need to determine if the middle third is actually ideally set back and the upper and lower thirds are more protruding or if the middle third is really overcorrected. If the middle third is ideal and the upper and lower thirds are protruding more than ideal (telephone ear deformity), then you may need to set back the upper and lower third. This is done by getting wide exposure of the upper and lower thirds to further weaken the concha bowl and the struts that are holding these areas in a more protruding manner (Fig. 55.3). Most of the time, the conchal weakening was concentrated on the middle third in the original procedure because surgeons are less likely to get the wider exposure to approach these superior and inferior areas to set back the upper and lower thirds. So in the revision, you must adequately expose the struts that are holding the upper and lower thirds more laterally than the middle third. Following this, further weakening and mastoid conchal sutures will allow you to set back the upper and lower third into a more ideal position. If the middle third is the section that is overcorrected, augmentation and reversal of the conchal setback is required as explained above.

Overcorrection of the Lower Third

For the lower third, the discussion will repeat some of the same issues discussed above. In regard to the specifics of the lower third, it is more natural that the lower third is more medial than the middle and upper third. The upper third can tolerate the most lateral position. This subconsciously emulates the desired shape of the face, with the width of the face at the level of eyes being more attractive when it is wider than the lower third of the face. If you are in a position where the upper and lower thirds are medialized more than the middle third, it is a better option to concentrate on lateralizing the upper third before the lower third for this reason. A medialized lower third is much more easily tolerated from an aesthetic standpoint than a medialized upper third.

Reversing the Conchal Setback in the Lower Third

For an overcorrected lower third, cartilage grafting the inferior struts of the conchal bowl is one option. A single strut is likely to bend one way or the other. One should support the strut with another strut, most likely in the area of the middle third to support the strut holding the lower third in a more lateral position. If these struts are not strong enough to hold the ear laterally, a total graft with a strut carved out for the inferior and middle third may be needed. This can be done with a rib graft or Medpor block carved to emulate the conchal bowl in these areas. As mentioned before, rotating a mastoid fascial graft based anteriorly can be an option. The superficial temporal parietal fascia is complicated because this rotated flap will likely also lateralize the superior and middle third and you will have to determine if this is what you want to achieve. Also this flap has a longer distance to reach for the inferior third and is a second choice after the mastoid flap and other options.

Reversing Overcorrection of the Lower Third Created by Overly Aggressive Skin Resection

Support for the skin lining is essential as described in the other sections. Over-resection of skin in the lower third is more a common situation than in the upper and lower third because resection of skin has been taught to be one of the main ways to medialize the lower third. In addition to the V-Y advancement, full-thickness skin graft, and posterior hairline incision and rotation, a preauricular rotation flap could be considered (at the expense of an incision in the preauricular area) as a source of skin. A preauricular skin flap is perhaps best used to replace skin in the lower third as compared to the middle and upper

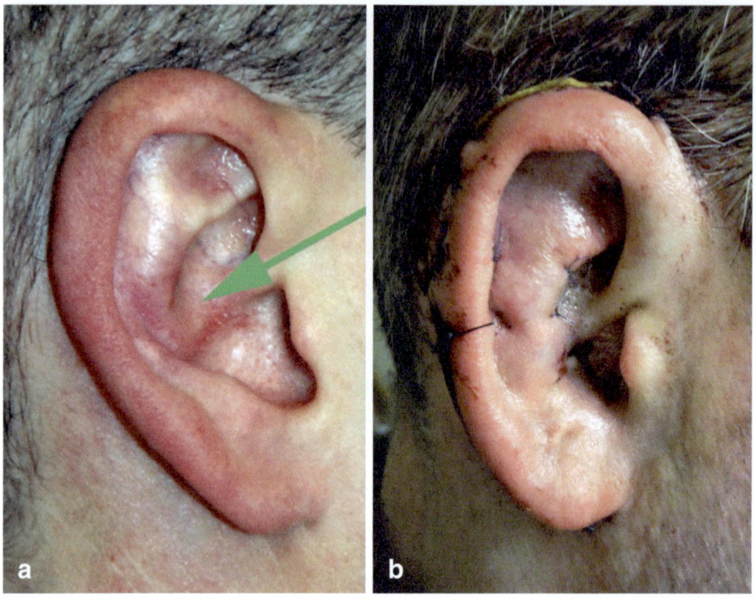

Fig. 55.9 Antihelix irregularity. (**a**) The area of depression was excised and the two halves connected. With a mastoid facial graft, minced cartilage was used to further shape this area (*Green arrow*). (**b**) Immediately postoperative after correction of antihelix irregularity. The irregularity was corrected by excising the depression reconnecting the antihelix and then shaped further with a mastoid fascia and minced cartilage underneath

third. Another option is a tissue expander prior to the otoplasty revision. This option, in my experience, is the most unpopular of all the options. In the situation where the upper or middle third has a surplus of skin, a rotation flap from this location can be swung inferiorly to allow the lower third to become more lateralized. But as stated earlier, cartilage grafting is essential in holding any section of the ear in a more lateral position, whether it is upper, middle, or lower third of the ear, for the long term.

Sharp Edges and Irregularities

The Mustarde sutures and conchal setback when done right should have the least risk of having these issues. Many other techniques require incisions through the antihelix and helix that can lead to sharp edges and irregularities that people often seek remedy. Also rasping, burring, and other forms of abrasion to weaken the front portion of the ear to allow bending can lead to irregularities. Prevention is also a key here as well, and the author uses Mustarde sutures, conchal setback, and the suture at the anterior superior helix attachment for most all otoplasty prominent ear situations. Figure 55.9 shows an antihelix irregularity that the patient said looked "broken." This was repaired by excising the depressed area and connecting the two edges. To further soften the ear, a mastoid fascial graft was incorporated over the repaired area and minced cartilage added to add structure and shape to the antihelix. This case illustrates how you can approach sharp edges and irregularities. Most sharp edges can be excised and shaped to blend in with the surrounding cartilage. The use of scissors, rasps, and power burs can aid in achieving this. If augmentation is necessary, cartilage grafts can be used to help shape different portions of the ear. Morselizing the edges of the grafts can help them blend in with the native cartilage. Minced cartilage can give you some ability to mold the shape that you want. Because the skin in this area is so thin, a fascial graft is a necessity to help your corrections and grafts blend in. The fascial graft can also allow you to contain minced cartilage in the location you want and help you mold them into the shape you want as well.

References

1. Young PA, Sinha U, Rice D, Stucker F. Circles of prominence: a new theory on facial aesthetics. Arch Facial Plast Surg. 2006;8(4):263–7.
2. Mustarde JC. The correction of prominent ears using simple mattress sutures. Br J Plast Surg. 1963;16:170–8.

3. Pearl CB, Wallace RD. New technique for marking the location of Mustardé horizontal mattress sutures. Plast Reconstr Surg. 2009;123(5):1468–70.
4. Furnas DW. Correction of prominent ears by conchamastoid sutures. Plast Reconstr Surg. 1968;42(3):189–93.
5. Lentz AK, Plikaitis CM, Bauer BS. Understanding the unfavorable result after otoplasty: an integrated approach to correction. Plast Reconstr Surg. 2011; 128(2):536–44.
6. Janz BA, Cole P, Hollier LH, Stal S. Treatment of prominent and constricted ear anomalies. Plast Reconstr Surg. 2009;124(1 Suppl):27e–37.
7. Thorne CH. Otoplasty. Plast Reconstr Surg. 2008; 122(1):291–2.

Part VI

Outcomes

Sensibility of the Ear After Otoplasty

56

Pedro Soler Coltro and Marcus Castro Ferreira

Introduction

Prominent ear is a common congenital deformity of the ear, an incidence of about 5 % in Caucasian population. There is inadequate formation of the antihelix fold as well as conchal hypertrophy, scaphoconchal angle greater than 90°, and forward lobule. Prominent ears may cause psychological disorder, emotional stress, behavioral disturbance, and restriction of social interaction in children, adolescents, and adults. The treatment of prominent ears involves reshaping of the antihelical fold, correction of the conchal defect, and lobule repositioning, the primary responsibilities for the anatomical defects [1, 2]. Usually a combination of techniques is used based on each particular case and each degree of ear deformity [3, 4].

Tactile sensibility of the ear skin is from branches of the cervical plexus and branches of V, VII, IX, and X cranial nerves [1, 2]. The posterior surface of the ear receives sensory innervation from the cervical plexus: the greater auricular nerve (branches of C2 and C3) and the minor occipital nerve (branch of C2). The anterior surface (helix, antihelix, tragus, and lobule) is innervated by the greater auricular and auriculotemporal nerve (branch of mandibular division of trigeminal nerve). Concha and external auditory canal receive sensory innervation from the posterior auricular nerve (branch of the facial nerve), the Arnold's nerve (auricular branch of the vagus nerve), and the Jacobson's nerve (branch tympanic of the glossopharyngeal nerve) (Fig. 56.1).

Assessment of cutaneous tactile sensibility may be carried out by some neurosensory tests, based on the knowledge of skin innervation [5]. The group A-beta nerve fibers are responsible for conducting touch stimuli including both those from slow- and fast-adaptative sensory receptors. The slow-adaptative fibers conduct pressure perception, constant touch, and texture and their skin receptors are the Merkel and Ruffini cells. The fast-adaptative fibers provide motion and vibration perception and their cutaneous receptors are the Meissner and Pacini cells [6]. The best approach for measurement of cutaneous tactile sensibility should include both static pressure sensation (slow-adaptative fibers) and motion sensation thresholds (fast-adaptative fibers), allowing monitoring before and after surgical treatment [7, 8].

The Semmes-Weinstein monofilaments are known as a test to evaluate touch sensibility of the skin. It examines only the slow-adaptative sensory fibers and their peripheral receptors. The fast-adaptative fibers can be evaluated by another

P.S. Coltro, M.D. (✉)
Division of Plastic Surgery, Faculty of Medicine, University of São Paulo, Alameda Jauaperi 943 apto 172, Indianópolis, São Paulo, SP 04523-014, Brazil
e-mail: pscoltro@hotmail.com

M.C. Ferreira, M.D., Ph.D.
Division of Plastic Surgery, University of São Paulo, Avenida Doutor Arnaldo 455, Cerqueira César, São Paulo, SP 01246-903, Brazil
e-mail: mcastroferreira@uol.com.br

M.A. Shiffman (ed.), *Advanced Cosmetic Otoplasty*,
DOI 10.1007/978-3-642-35431-1_56, © Springer-Verlag Berlin Heidelberg 2013

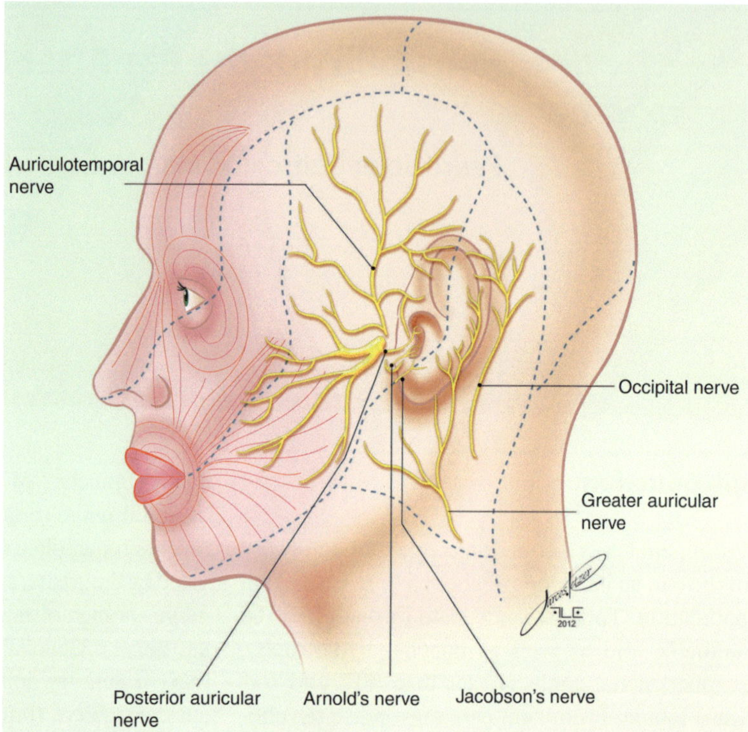

Fig. 56.1 Innervation of the skin of the external ear

test using vibration producing instruments, as diapasons [6]. In 1989, Dellon et al. [9, 10] introduced a new test using the Pressure Specified Sensory Device™, PSSD, a device that quantifies the level of pressure from 0 to 100 g/mm² applied by metal prongs to the skin. The thresholds of pressure necessary for the patient to feel the stimulus, both statically and in moving, assess both the slow- and fast-adaptative fibers.

Plastic surgeons from the University of São Paulo, Brazil, have employed this device in order to better study changes in sensibility that occur in the postoperative period of a number of conditions treated by plastic surgery, including trauma, aesthetic procedures, but mostly importantly, diabetic neuropathy [11–15].

Temporary or permanent changes on skin sensibility may occur in the postoperative period after plastic surgery procedures, especially when there is extensive skin and subcutaneous tissue dissection. The surgery of prominent ear involves dissection of its cutaneous posterior surface and we supposed that otoplasty might cause some impairment in the ear sensibility of the skin.

The authors could not find studies that objectively compare the sensibility of the skin of the ear before and after surgery for prominent ears and, therefore, studied the tactile sensibility on the skin of the ear before and after otoplasty for prominent ears measuring the cutaneous pressure thresholds with the Pressure Specified Sensory Device™ (PSSD). Furthermore, vibration and hot/cold sensibility were also evaluated [16].

Study of Sensibility of the Ear's Skin

A prospective study was conducted with 15 patients presenting bilateral prominent ears [16]. They were submitted to bilateral otoplasty by the same surgeon and in all of them the following anatomical deformities were observed: conchal hypertrophy, scaphoconchal angle greater than 90°, absence of the antihelical fold, and forward lobe. Exclusion criteria included previous ear and other surgery on the periauricular region and systemic comorbidities that could alter the sensibility, such as diabetes or neurological disorders.

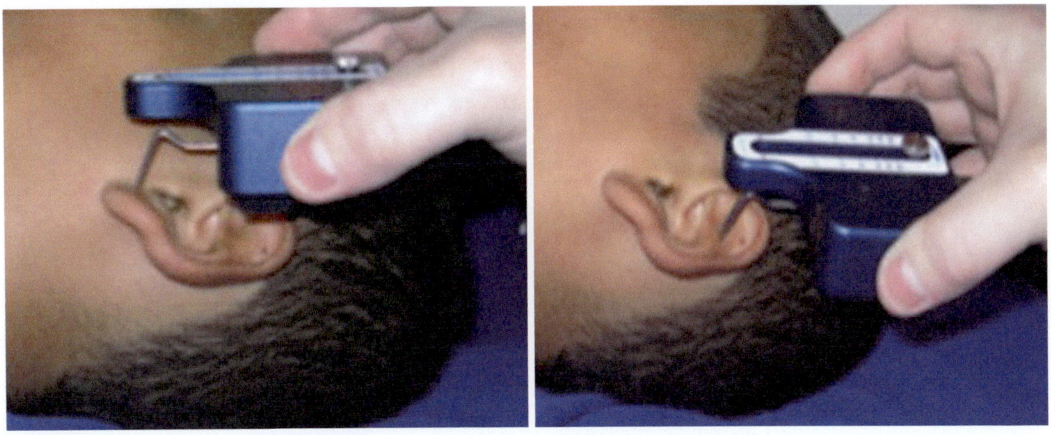

Fig. 56.2 Performing the test: a metal rod transducer of PSSD touching the ear

Local anesthesia was used, blocking the main nerve branches of the ear, the mastoid region, and the posterior auricular surface. Retroauricular incision was followed by extensive dissection of a cutaneous flap at the posterior surface of the ear reaching the perichondrium plan and dissection of the mastoid in the ear projection. Hemostasis was provided by direct cauterization of blood vessels.

The excess of the concha was treated by a partial conchal resection and the scaphoconchal angle was reduced using two conchomastoid nonabsorbable sutures. Restoration of the antihelical fold was obtained using three scaphoconchal nonabsorbable sutures. The lobule was repositioned using a dermoconchal suture, joining the lobule dermis to the lower portion of the concha. The retroauricular skin incision was closed with a continuous suture. After bandage was removed on the second day, the patient was asked to continuously use an elastic band during the first month and just during the night in the second month.

The same examiner tested the sensibility of ear preoperatively and 6 and 12 months after surgery using the PSSD. This unit consists of a transducer of force coupled to a computer and software capable of encoding an electrical signal into pressure, expressed in grams per squared millimeter (g/mm^2).

The examination with the PSSD consisted of the touch of one metal rod to the skin of ear (Fig. 56.2), anterior and posterior. The patient was in possession of a bell and was instructed to squeeze it when he/she felt the touch of the metal rod. Thus, the software recorded the perceived value of the pressure when the bell is activated (electrical signal). The test was repeated five times in each area and the average obtained corresponded to the cutaneous pressure threshold of that area (g/mm^2).

For the patient to understand the exam, a prior test was conducted on the dominant hand of the patient. During the test, the individuals remained comfortably in supine position on the examination table, in a quiet and isolated room. As a preliminary instruction, the patient was oriented to keep eyes closed to avoid confusion with visual sensation.

Each ear was tested in seven areas (Fig. 56.3), five on the anterior surface, root of the helix (area 1), medium helix (area 2), antihelix (area 3), concha (area 4), and lobule (area 5), and two on the posterior surface: retroauricular sulcus (area 6) and scaphoconchal sulcus (area 7). The distribution of sensory innervation over the ear was taken as a basis for choosing these areas, given by branches of the cervical plexus and the branches of V, VII, IX, and X cranial nerves.

On each area, the static one-point test was first performed, obtained by only one prong of the transducer, and then the dynamic one-point test, obtained by moving and pressing the transducer (one prong) on the ear skin. Statistical analysis of pressure measurements was performed by Wilcoxon signed-rank test.

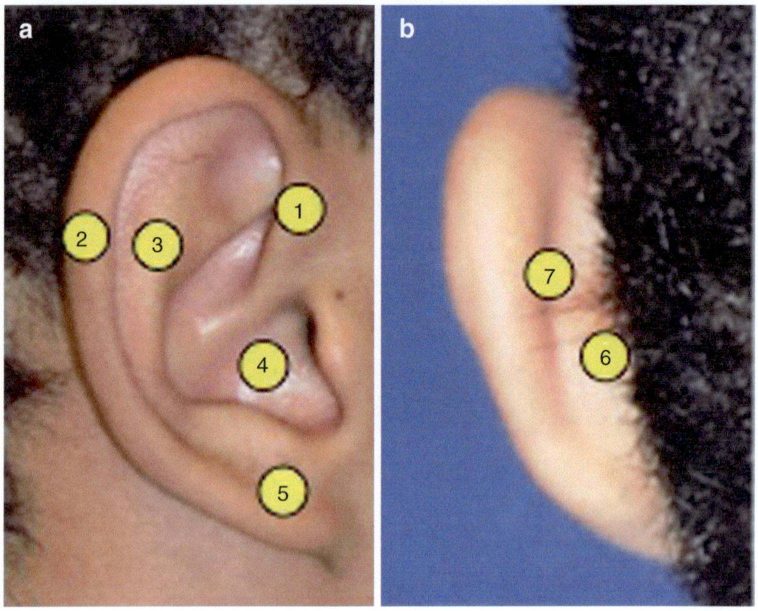

Fig. 56.3 Areas of the ear tested by PSSD. Anterior (**a**) *1* root of the helix, *2* medium helix, *3* anti-helix, *4* concha, *5* lobule. Posterior (**b**) *6* retro-auricular sulcus, *7* scaphoconchal sulcus

Tests of vibratory sensibility were made by a diapason of 128 Hz. Patients were tested with closed eyes and the vibrating diapason was touched on the same seven areas above for 5 s. Vibratory sensibility was considered preserved if patient felt the vibration in overtime. Study of hot/cold sensibility was performed by the contact of a test tube filled by hot water (40 °C) and another by cold water (5 °C). Hot/cold sensibility was considered preserved if patient felt the hot tube as a "hot sensation" and the cold tube as a "cold sensation."

The comparison and the evolution of the cutaneous pressure thresholds measurements on the preoperative and 6 and 12 months postoperative for the one point static and moving tests are represented in Figs. 56.4 and 56.5. The mean (M) of cutaneous pressure thresholds (g/mm^2) in the seven areas studied as well as the standard deviation (SD) and "*p* value" are described in Tables 56.1 and 56.2.

Vibratory and hot/cold sensibilities were considered preserved bilaterally in all 15 patients, without difference between preoperative and 6 or 12 months postoperative.

Tests to detect changes in sensibility of the skin were developed to assess and quantify sensory function in patients with neurological disease complaints or in potential risk to develop it [17–19]. They can be used to evaluate skin sensibility in many anatomical sites such as breast, abdomen, face, and members, including the hands and feet [11–15, 20, 21]. Such studies compare changes in skin sensibility before and after a medical or surgical intervention, and severity of some known diseases. For example, previous tests have evaluated the sensibility of the skin, breast, and nipple areola complex before and after mammaplasty and others studied the severity of neuropathy in the diabetic lower extremity [6, 11, 12].

Over time, there was a change in the instruments used to perform these sensitive tests [5]. In 1905, von Frey [22] developed an evaluation method through the use of horsehair attached to a stem, being very inaccurate and only with historical importance.

Semmes and Weinstein, in 1962 [23], created an indirect sensitive quantifying method for using nylon monofilaments with progressive diameters

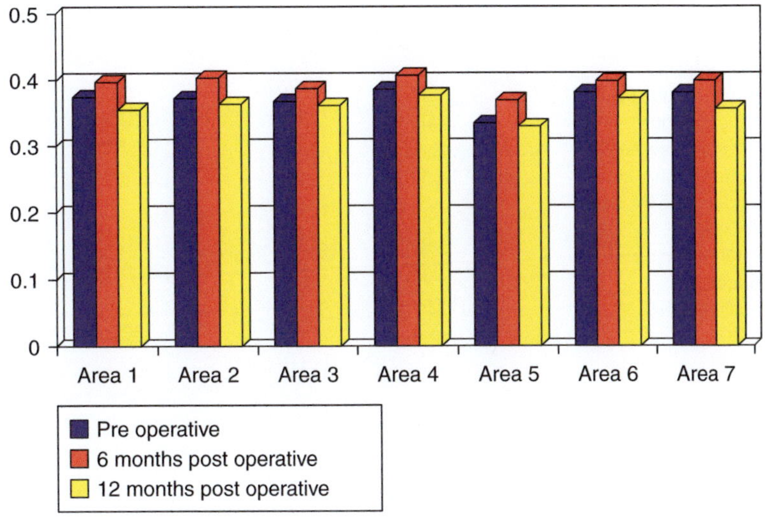

Fig. 56.4 Mean of the cutaneous pressure thresholds (g/mm^2) of the static one-point test (preoperative, 6 and 12 months postoperative)

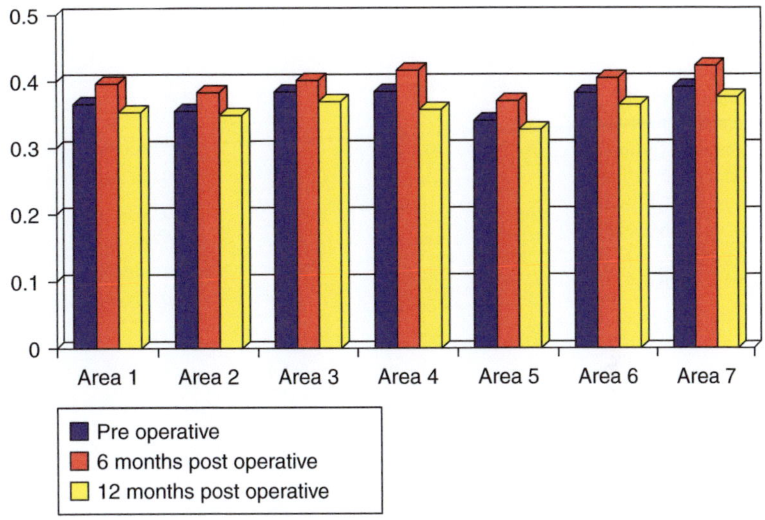

Fig. 56.5 Mean of the cutaneous pressure thresholds (g/mm^2) of the moving one-point test (preoperative, 6 and 12 months postoperative)

and attached to plastic rods, being widely disseminated for loss of sensibility assessment due to its simplicity, rapidity, and low cost. However, several criticisms have been made to the use of the Semmes-Weinstein monofilament. Since this is a discontinuous test, it provides only an estimate of the skin pressure thresholds, limiting the statistical analysis [5, 24, 25].

The objective tests to assess skin sensibility were used in plastic surgery by Dellon in 1983, by quantitative vibrometer, which also had some controversy [5, 26]. In 1989, Dellon et al. [9] developed a new method for skin sensibility quantification, the Pressure Specified Sensory Device™ (PSSD). The data obtained with the PSSD represent the true pressure threshold, provided directly in grams per millimeter squared (g/mm^2), which allows objective comparisons and statistical analysis tests. This method is more accurate than the Semmes-Weinstein monofilament because it is a continuous and direct measure and allows the study of slow and fast to adaptative fibers, being more complete for skin sensibility evaluation [5, 10].

Table 56.1 Static and moving one-point test – mean (M) of the cutaneous pressure thresholds (g/mm2), standard deviation (SD), and "*p*" value (preoperative and 6 months postoperative)

Area		Preoperative		6 months postoperative		
		M	SD	M	SD	*p*
Area 1	Static	0.3767	0.06244	0.3987	0.05958	0.043
	Moving	0.3653	0.05218	0.3947	0.056	0.0112
Area 2	Static	0.374	0.04854	0.4053	0.0545	0.0007
	Moving	0.3547	0.04091	0.3813	0.03989	0.0041
Area 3	Static	0.37	0.04955	0.3893	0.05051	0.0138
	Moving	0.382	0.0572	0.4007	0.04127	0.0402
Area 4	Static	0.388	0.05592	0.41	0.0393	0.0335
	Moving	0.3827	0.05317	0.414	0.05184	0.0002
Area 5	Static	0.3373	0.03542	0.372	0.03498	0.0002
	Moving	0.3393	0.04601	0.368	0.05102	0.0009
Area 6	Static	0.383	0.05676	0.40	0.04835	0.1
	Moving	0.38	0.06384	0.402	0.04715	0.0273
Area 7	Static	0.382	0.05524	0.4013	0.05722	0.0465
	Moving	0.3887	0.04637	0.4207	0.04193	0.0003

Table 56.2 Static and moving one-point test – mean (M) of the cutaneous pressure thresholds (g/mm2), standard deviation (SD), and "*p*" value (preoperative and 12 months postoperative)

Area		Preoperative		12 months postoperative		
		M	SD	M	SD	*p*
Area 1	Static	0.3767	0.06244	0.3567	0.04589	0.335
	Moving	0.3653	0.05218	0.3527	0.0469	0.1928
Area 2	Static	0.374	0.04854	0.3653	0.04569	0.114
	Moving	0.3547	0.04091	0.3473	0.03352	0.4561
Area 3	Static	0.37	0.04955	0.3635	0.04478	0.2359
	Moving	0.382	0.0572	0.3673	0.05324	0.0916
Area 4	Static	0.388	0.05592	0.378	0.04944	0.3271
	Moving	0.3827	0.05317	0.356	0.03114	0.0626
Area 5	Static	0.3373	0.03542	0.3313	0.01655	0.6456
	Moving	0.3393	0.04601	0.3253	0.01456	0.4718
Area 6	Static	0.383	0.05676	0.3747	0.04776	0.2353
	Moving	0.38	0.06384	0.362	0.05189	0.1967
Area 7	Static	0.382	0.05524	0.358	0.03263	0.1177
	Moving	0.3887	0.04637	0.3747	0.04257	0.1409

Evaluation of Cutaneous Sensibility of the Ear Before and After Otoplasty

During otoplasty, the dissection on the posterior ear skin and surroundings may cause many kinds of nerve injury. Injury to the sensory nerve fibers can lead to two patterns of chronic sequel: a decrease in sensibility or hypoesthesia (the patient feels less sensibility at the site) and increased sensibility or hyperesthesia (the perception is excessive or there is exaggerated sensibility in response to the stimuli).

Knowledge of normal sensibility is important for effective evaluation and treatment of sensitive disorders [7]. The objective registration of skin sensibility in various areas of the body – including breast, abdomen, face, hands, and feet – increases the scientific data and contributes to surgical techniques improvement, reducing nerve injuries to minimize nerve sensory loss. Many postoperative sensory deficits can be observed when strict analysis is made [11, 13, 14, 20].

Studies regarding ear sensibility are scarce in the medical literature. In 1990, Posnick et al. [27] assessed the skin sensibility in facial areas of healthy subjects innervated by supraorbital, infraorbital, mental, and greater auricular nerves, including the distal helix and ear lobule.

The cutaneous pressure thresholds in this study were measured using the Semmes-Weinstein monofilament, a nonquantitative method.

In 1994, Costas et al. [28] studied the sensibility on 13 regions of the face and neck of volunteers with no history of neuropathy, diabetes, trauma, or surgery on the face. The tested areas corresponded to the main sensory branches of the head and neck, including the greater auricular nerve (anterior and posterior branch), minor occipital nerve, and auriculotemporal nerve, but not directly evaluating the ear. Moreover, the cutaneous pressure thresholds measurements were also obtained with the Semmes-Weinstein monofilament. No study could be found assessing ear sensibility using a quantitative method like the PSSD or that compares objectively cutaneous pressure thresholds before and after otoplasty.

The authors' study compared preoperative and 6 months' postoperative sensibilities [16]. A higher cutaneous pressure thresholds (partial loss of sensation) related to slow adaptative fibers was observed (static one-point test), with statistically significant differences in six of seven areas tested, the exception being the static test on area 6 (posterior: retroauricular sulcus). Regarding to the dynamic point test (fast-adaptative fibers), the measurements demonstrated a higher thresholds, the difference being statistically significant on all areas tested. Therefore, there was reduction in ear tactile sensibility 6 months after otoplasty.

When comparing the preoperative and 12 months postoperative results, the cutaneous static pressure and the motion were similar. There were no statistically significant differences in all seven areas tested, for both tests. Thus, the sensory thresholds indicated that the ear tactile sensibility 12 months after otoplasty returned to levels similar to preoperative level, but not exactly identical.

Furthermore, vibratory and hot/cold sensibility was preserved bilaterally, without difference between preoperative level and at 6 or 12 months postoperative. Thus, the fibers responsible for conducting such sensibility were not affected by the otoplasty.

The best approach for assessment of cutaneous tactile sensibility should include the static pressure and motion sensation thresholds [7, 8] and this was observed in our study, reduction in ear tactile sensibility at 6 months after otoplasty, followed by return at 12 months after surgery [16].

These data can be used for the preparation of a more consistent informed consent term for otoplasty adding this information about change on postoperative level of ear sensibility, based on more scientific criteria. Also it is shown that the reduction in the ear sensibility after surgery is temporary and it is expected to return to similar levels to the preoperative, though not exactly identical ones.

Further studies are needed to assess techniques used for otoplasty, such as scraping the anterior cartilage and others with lesser extensive dissection of flaps, and see the impact on the pre- and postoperative sensation levels. It is possible to compare changes in ear sensibility among various otoplasty surgical techniques.

This study represented the first evaluation of ear tactile sensibility using a quantitative method that compared objectively cutaneous pressure thresholds before and after otoplasty. After otoplasty, there was initially a reduction on the ear tactile sensibility, followed by a return to similar levels to the preoperative. Documentation and assessment of auricular sensibility are important for clinical and surgical knowledge, and it helps accurate orientation to the patient on the postoperative follow-up.

References

1. Janis JE, Rohrich RJ, Gutowski KA. Otoplasty. Plast Reconstr Surg. 2005;115(4):60e–72e.
2. Hoehn JG, Ashruf S. Otoplasty: sequencing the operation for improved results. Plast Reconstr Surg. 2005; 115(1):5e–16e.
3. Kelley P, Hollier L, Stal S. Otoplasty: evaluation, technique, and review. J Craniofac Surg. 2003;14(5): 643–53.
4. Peker F, Celiköz B. Otoplasty: anterior scoring and posterior rolling technique in adults. Aesthetic Plast Surg. 2002;26(4):267–73.
5. Dellon AL. Invited discussion: sensibility of the breast following reduction mammaplasty. Ann Plast Surg. 2003;51(1):6–9.
6. Carvalho VF, Ferreira MC, Vieira SA, Ueda T. Cutaneous sensibility threshold in the feet of diabetic patients with pressure specified sensory device: an assessment of the neuropathy. Rev Assoc Med Bras. 2009;55(1):29–34.

7. Dellon AL. Evaluation of sensibility and re-education of sensation in the hand. Baltimore: Lippincott Williams & Wilkins; 2000.
8. Dellon AL. Somatosensory testing and rehabilitation. Baltimore: Lippincott Williams & Wilkins; 2000.
9. Dellon ES, Mourey MS, Dellon AL. Human pressure perception values of constant and moving one and two-point discrimination. Plast Reconstr Surg. 1992; 90(1):112–7.
10. Dellon ES, Crone S, Mourey R, Dellon AL. Comparison of the Semmes-Weinstein monofilaments with the pressure specified sensory device. Restor Neurol Neurosci. 1993;5(5):323–6.
11. Ferreira MC, Costa MP, Cunha MS, Sakae E, Fels KW. Sensibility of the breast after reduction mammaplasty. Ann Plast Surg. 2003;51(1):1–5.
12. Ferreira MC, Rodrigues L, Fels KW. New method for evaluation of cutaneous sensibility in diabetic feet: preliminary report. Rev Hosp Clin Fac Med Sao Paulo. 2004;59(5):286–90.
13. Fels KW, Cunha MS, Sturtz GP, Gemperli R, Ferreira MC. Evaluation of cutaneous abdominal wall sensibility after abdominoplasty. Aesthetic Plast Surg. 2005;29(2):78–82.
14. Fogaça WC, Ferreira MC, Dellon AL. Infraorbital nerve injury associated with zygoma fractures: documentation with neurosensory testing. Plast Reconstr Surg. 2004;113(3):834–8.
15. Fogaça WC, Sturtz GP, Surjan RC, Ferreira MC. Evaluation of cutaneous sensibility on infraorbital nerve area. J Craniofac Surg. 2005;16(6):953–6.
16. Coltro PS, Alves HR, Gallafrio ST, Busnardo FF, Ferreira MC. Sensibility of ear after otoplasty. Ann Plast Surg. 2011;68(2):120–4.
17. Yarnitsky D. Quantitative sensory testing. Muscle Nerve. 1997;20(2):198–204.
18. Dellon AL. From there to here: a personal viewpoint after three decades of neuropathy research. Clin Podiatr Med Surg. 2006;23(3):497–508.
19. Soomekh D. Quantitative sensory testing. Clin Podiatr Med Surg. 2006;23(3):545–57.
20. Mofid MM, Dellon AL, Elias JJ, Nahabedian MY. Quantitation of breast sensibility following reduction mammaplasty: a comparison of inferior and medial pedicle techniques. Plast Reconstr Surg. 2002;109(7): 2283–8.
21. Grime PD. A pilot study to determine the potential application of the pressure specified sensory device in the maxillofacial region. Br J Oral Maxillofac Surg. 1996;34(6):500–3.
22. Levin S, Pearsall G, Ruderman RJ. Von Frey's method of measuring pressure sensibility in the hand: an engineering analysis of the Weinstein-Semmes pressure aesthesiometer. J Hand Surg Am. 1978;3(3): 211–6.
23. Malgrange D, Richard JL, Leymarie F. Screening diabetic patients at risk for foot ulceration. A multi-centre hospital-based study in France. Diabetes Metab. 2003;29(3):261–8.
24. Dellon AL. Testing for facial sensibility. Plast Reconstr Surg. 1991;87(6):1140–1.
25. Posnick JC, Grossman JA. Facial sensibility testing: a clinical update. Plast Reconstr Surg. 2000;106(4): 892–4.
26. Dellon AL. The vibrometer. Plast Reconstr Surg. 1983;71(3):427–31.
27. Posnick JC, Zimbler AG, Grossman JA. Normal cutaneous sensibility of the face. Plast Reconstr Surg. 1990;86(3):429–33.
28. Costas PD, Heatley G, Seckel BR. Normal sensation of the human face and neck. Plast Reconstr Surg. 1994;93(6):1141–5.

Measurement of Postoperative Cephaloauricular Distance to Evaluate and Compare Results of Otoplasty

57

Stuart D. Richards

Introduction

Measurement of human proportions was most famously described by Leonardo da Vinci. His drawing of the Vitruvian man has been reproduced countless times. Vitruvian man was da Vinci's interpretation of the observations of Marcus Vitruvius Pollio (born c70–80 BC), a Roman writer and architect. He likened the symmetry of man to architecture in his book De architectura. Da Vinci further studied the human form, and in his drawing entitled "The facial proportions of a man in profile; study of soldiers and horses c1490-95 – 1503," Leonardo describes the relationship of the proportions of the ear. In his own words, "...The hollow of the cheek-bone occurs half-way between the tip of the nose and the top of the jaw-bone, which is the lower angle of the setting on of the ear...from the angle of the eye socket to the ear is as far as the length of the ear, or the third of the face."

The human ear grows throughout life. Eighty-five percent of growth takes place before the age of three with a further steady growth throughout life up to the seventh decade [1]. Adamson et al. measured the conchomastoid distance in 2,300 ears in children from birth to aged 16 and adults from 60 to 80. The conchomastoid distance increased up to an average of 2 cm at age ten, but changes little after this. Farkas [2] produced numerous papers on the anthropometry of the ear. Farkas found the average protrusion of the ear from the head if measured as an angle was around 20°.

Many authors have described measurement of the distance between the pinna and the cranium to measure postoperative outcome from otoplasty. Few authors have measured the projection of the ear as an angle, probably due to the ease of measuring distance versus angulation. The author would recommend measurement of the conchomastoid distance as the optimum method of defining outcome for the simple reason that it is the most commonly published method and therefore allows authors to compare their work.

The most widely quoted description of conchomastoid measurement was by McDowell in 1968 [3]. He measured the projection at three levels: the top of the helix, the Frankfort line, and the tail of the helix. Messner and Crysdale [4] added a fourth point, the superior line in 1996 (Fig. 57.1): The measurement of both ear projection and size requires the subject to be positioned in a standardized way. This is best done by ensuring the head is positioned so that the Frankfort horizontal is parallel to the floor. The Frankfort horizontal is a reference line that is primarily used for cephalometric analysis. It is drawn from the superior margin of the external auditory canal on lateral radiographs to the inferior border of the infraorbital rim and is familiar to medical photographers. They use this line to ensure correct orientation of the head before taking lateral views

S.D. Richards, M.D., FRCSEd (ORL-HNS)
Department of Otorhinolaryngology, ENT Department,
Rotherham NHS Foundation Trust,
Moorgate Road, Rotherham, S60 2UD, UK
e-mail: stuart.richards@rothgen.nhs.uk

M.A. Shiffman (ed.), *Advanced Cosmetic Otoplasty*,
DOI 10.1007/978-3-642-35431-1_57, © Springer-Verlag Berlin Heidelberg 2013

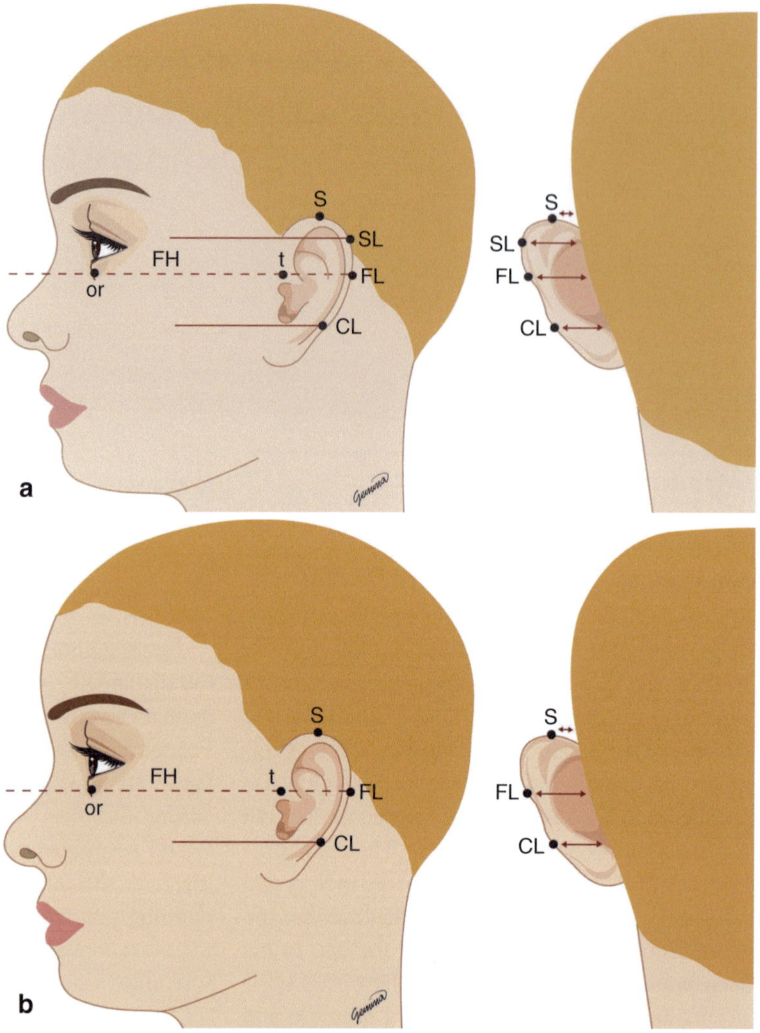

Fig. 57.1 Points for measurement of cephaloauricular distance. (**a**) Four-point measurement after Anna H. Messner: *S* superior point, *SL* superior line, *FL* Frankfort line, *CL* conchal line. (**b**) Three-point measurement after Allyn J. McDowell: top of the helix (*S*), Frankfort line (*FL*), tail of the helix (*CL*)

of the head [5]. Interestingly, Farkas [2] found that the Frankfort horizontal is not always at the same level on both sides; the left side is most commonly lower than the right by 4°.

Documentation through photography should be performed preoperatively for evaluation of postoperative results and for medicolegal reasons, with appropriate consent. Anterior-posterior and lateral views are recommended with care to ensure that the Frankfort horizontal is maintained in the horizontal plane.

McDowell proposed normal values for the three measurement points, which are consistent with the measurements taken by Adamson et al. (Table 57.1). Pilz et al. [6] and Messner and Crysdale [4] have both published data on postoperative outcome as measured by the conchomastoid distance.

Table 57.1 Normal measurements of cephaloauricular distances

Position on pinna	Measurement (mm)
Top of the helix	10–12
Frankfort line	16–18
Tail of the helix	20–22

Articles describing the objective assessment of postoperative results also compare the results by application of the McDowell and Wright criteria [3, 7–9]. These criteria are not truly objective, but do bear mention as they are so commonly quoted for comparing results. These criteria list six items

Table 57.2 Goals of otoplasty according to McDowell and Wright

1. All trace of protrusion in the upper one third of the ear must be corrected (Some remaining protrusion in the middle third or lower portions may be acceptable, provided the superior aspect is thoroughly corrected; however, the reverse does not hold true)
2. From the front view, the helix of both ears should be seen beyond the antihelix (at least down to the mid-ear and preferably all the way)
3. The helix should have a smooth and regular line throughout
4. The postauricular sulcus should not be markedly decreased or distorted
5. Protrusion should measure between 15 and 20 mm from the helix to the head
6. Position of the two ears (i.e., distance from the lateral border to the head) should be within 3 mm at any given point

against which the outcome can be measured. They consist of a mixture of subjective assessment and measurement of ear proportions (Table 57.2).

It is a fact that most articles on the postoperative results of otoplasty do not use consistent objective measurement. The author published a review of surgical outcomes in 2005 in which the use of the measurement of the cephaloauricular distance at the Frankfort horizontal [10] was advocated. The most scientifically useful method is to utilize the three-point measurement described by McDowell; however, to allow comparison to the available literature, measurement at the Frankfort horizontal is all that is required.

References

1. Adamson JE, Horton CE, Crawford HH. The growth pattern of the external ear. Plast Reconstr Surg. 1965;36(4):466–70.
2. Davis J. Aesthetic and reconstructive otoplasty. New York: Springer; 1987.
3. McDowell AJ. Goals in otoplasty for protruding ears. Plast Reconstr Surg. 1968;41(1):17–27.
4. Messner AH, Crysdale WS. Otoplasty. Clinical protocol and long-term results. Arch Otolaryngol Head Neck Surg. 1996;122(7):773–7.
5. Sorribes MM, Tos M. Nonsurgical treatment of prominent ears with the Auri method. Arch Otolaryngol Head Neck Surg. 2002;128(112):1369–76.
6. Pilz S, Hintringer T, Bauer M. Otoplasty using a spherical metal head dermabrader to form a retroauricular furrow: five-year results. Aesthetic Plast Surg. 1995;19(1):83–91.
7. Wright WK. Otoplasty goals and principles. Arch Otolaryngol. 1970;92(12):568–72.
8. Lee D, Bluestone CD. The Becker technique for otoplasty: modified and revisited with long-term outcomes. Laryngoscope. 2000;110(6):949–54.
9. Vital V, Printza A. Cartilage-sparing otoplasty: our experience. J Laryngol Otol. 2002;116(9):682–5.
10. Richards SD, Jebreel A, Capper R. Otoplasty: a review of the surgical techniques. Clin Otolaryngol. 2005;30(1):2–8.

Otoplasty: Focusing on Patient Benefit and Health-Related Quality of Life

58

Thomas Braun, Alexander Berghaus, and John Martin Hempel

The Subjective Point of View in Aesthetic Surgery

Unarguably, the main aim of every aesthetic surgery is to produce a subjective benefit for the patient. However, most publications about certain surgical procedures in aesthetic surgery focus on details of the operative technique from the surgeon's point of view and on the occurrence of complications, while the aesthetic outcome is usually graded by the surgeons themselves. From our own experience in surgery of the auricle, sometimes there is a huge discrepancy between the subjective perception of the surgical results by the patient and the evaluation by medical professionals. In a study performed in a large collective of patients having received auricular reconstruction [1], it was striking how patients with mediocre or even poor results from the surgeon's point of view were nonetheless absolutely satisfied, while on the other hand patients with excellent results did not experience a relevant subjective benefit from auricular reconstruction. A subgroup analysis revealed that patients with acquired auricular defects were twice more likely to be not satisfied with the results compared to patients with congenital deformities [1]. The authors have found it helpful to indicate this fact in preoperative counseling to prevent the development of false expectations in certain patients; this is an example how studies focusing on the patients' subjective point of view can have an impact on clinical practice.

However, it seems obvious that assessing satisfaction rates only is a too simple method. Recently, "health-related quality of life" (HRQOL) has established itself as a reasonable construct to measure subjective benefit from interventions in a standardized approach [2, 3]. Today, HRQOL is considered by many authors even to be the most important parameter in the evaluation of a therapy regime [3]. Measuring HRQOL is a valuable approach particularly in aesthetic surgery with its main aim being to produce a subjective benefit for the patient and with the difficulty to collect objective data that are often restricted to anthropometric variables. Although there is no gold standard for measuring HRQOL, it is generally agreed that HRQOL is a multidimensional item, which includes physical, psychological, and social aspects [3]. A still growing number of validated questionnaires have been developed to measure HRQOL. However, not all of them seem to be appropriate for the evaluation of aesthetic surgery, since they predominantly cover

T. Braun, M.D. (✉) • A. Berghaus, M.D.
J.M. Hempel, M.D.
Department of Otorhinolaryngology, Head and Neck Surgery, Ludwig Maximilian University, Munich, Germany

Klinik und Poliklinik für Hals-Nasen-Ohren-Heilkunde der Ludwig-Maximilians-Universität München, Marchioninistraße 15, Munich, D-81377, Germany
e-mail: thomas.braun@med.uni-muenchen.de; alexander.berghaus@med.uni-muenchen.de; john-martin.hempel@med.uni-muenchen.de

M.A. Shiffman (ed.), *Advanced Cosmetic Otoplasty*,
DOI 10.1007/978-3-642-35431-1_58, © Springer-Verlag Berlin Heidelberg 2013

too general aspects of an individual's health, like the ability to perform daily activities autonomously (e.g., The Short Form 36 Health Survey Questionnaire, SF-36 [4]). The authors have made good experiences with the Glasgow Benefit Inventory (GBI) developed by Stuart Gatehouse [5], a questionnaire which is well validated for otorhinolaryngological interventions and particularly for plastic surgery [6]. Another advantage is that also a validated version for children exists (Glasgow Children's Benefit Inventory, GCBI) [7]. Both questionnaires are sensitive tools for changes in health status following an intervention. The GBI consists of 18 questions covering different aspects of health-related quality of life. Answers are selected from a Likert scale ranging from 1 to 5. Raw data are processed into total GBI scores, which can range from −100 (maximal adverse effect of the operation) over 0 (no effect) to +100 (maximal positive effect). Additionally, subscores can be calculated: a general subscore, a social support score, and a physical health score [5, 6]. The GCBI is constructed as an analogue to the GBI but consists of 24 questions and is answered by the patient's parents; in addition to a total score (ranging from −100 to +100), the subscores emotion, physical health, learning, and vitality can be calculated [7].

Effects of Otoplasty on Patients' Health-Related Quality of Life

Prominent ears do not have any physiological disadvantages and are considered to be a minor auricular deformity. However, several studies show that the emotional stress caused by teasing due to an ear deformity leads to a decline in the patient's HRQOL, resulting in loss of self-confidence, social avoidance, and poor school or job performance [8–10]. Attractive individuals are judged to be socially more desirable and are expected to have better prospects for social and professional lives [11]. Accordingly, negative evaluation of personal attractiveness in children is associated with dysphoria [12]. Thus, since about 5 % of the population suffer from prominent ears, otoplasty is the most common aesthetic surgery in children and adolescents [13, 14].

Several studies using validated questionnaires show that otoplasty leads to improvements in self-esteem and behavior as well as reduced psychological anxiety or depression [15–18]. Bradbury et al. analyzed a collective of 30 children suffering from protruding ears (without using validated tools): 63 % reported an increase in happiness and confidence after otoplasty; 13 % reported improvement in social experience in terms of better integration with other children; 53 % reported teasing and bullying to have stopped postoperatively [19]. An analogous study by Cooper-Hobson and Jaffe yielded even more promising results: 97 % reported an increase in happiness and 92 % in self-confidence, 79 % noted improved social experience, and 100 % reported bullying reduced or stopped [20].

As pointed out above, HRQOL with its holistic approach is one of the most important parameters in the evaluation of a therapy regime. Remarkably, only few studies evaluating the effect of otoplasty on HRQOL using validated tools are available in the current medical literature.

Studies Using SF-36 to Measure HRQOL

The Short Form 36 Health Survey Questionnaire (SF-36) is a well-validated tool that measures eight aspects of health status: physical function, role limitations due to physical problems, role limitations due to emotional problems, social function, mental health, energy, pain, and health perception [4]. Klassen et al. [16] have been able to show that patients undergoing otoplasty ($n=41$) had reduced social functioning and mental health scores compared to normative data; after otoplasty, patients ($n=31$) reached values of the general population.

Studies Using GBI/GCBI to Measure HRQOL

Schwentner et al. conducted a study using the GBI in an adult population of five men and nine women having received otoplasty with modified techniques according to Stenström et al. [21]. A median GBI total score of 37.5 and a general

Table 58.1 GCI and GCBI total scores after otoplasty as published to the present date in comparison with selected data from other aesthetic operations in the head and neck area

Operation	Authors	Mean GBI/GCBI total score	Collective
Otoplasty	Schwentner et al. 2006 [21]	37.5 (median)	Adults
	Braun et al. 2010 [22]	30.6 (mean and median)	Adults
	Braun et al. 2010 [22]	24.1	Children
Auricular reconstruction	Braun et al. 2010 [1]	21.1	Adults
	Braun et al. 2010 [1]	27.7	Children
Cosmetic (septo)rhinoplasty	Robinson et al. 1996 [6]	24.0	Adults
	Draper et al. 2007 [23]	20.0	Adults
Cosmetic and functional (septo)rhinoplasty	McKiernan et al. 2001 [24]	58.3	Adults
	Chauhan et al. 2010 [25]	53.8	Adolescents

subscale score of 58.3 were found, while the medians of the social support and the physical health score were 0.0. No differences were found between male and female patients in total GBI scores or any subscores. Furthermore, no statistical differences were found between short (<3 years) and long (>3 years) follow-up periods. Schwentner et al. therefore conclude that otoplasty leads to a long-lasting improvement in patients' HRQOL.

Since analogous data in the main patient group, children and adolescents, were missing, we initiated a study to analyze the HRQOL after otoplasty in our own patients [22]. We almost invariably perform suture techniques for reasons stated later in this chapter. Sixty-two patients (27 men, 35 women) were assessed with the GBI. For the adults' cohort ($n=21$), the mean total GBI score was 30.6 and the mean general subscore 43.0, indicating a benefit from the operation. The social support and the physical health score were only marginally elevated (mean 7.9 and 9.5, respectively). The HRQOL was raised in 95.2 % of the adult patients (indicated by total GBI scores >0). Negative GBI scores or subscores were not found in a single case. As in the study by Schwentner et al. [21], statistical analysis showed no significant differences in the scores and subscores of male and female patients. 100.0 % of the adults were satisfied with the aesthetical result. 90.5 % would again decide in favor of the operation. For the children's cohort, the mean total GCBI score was 24.1. All GCBI subscores (emotion, physical health, learning, and vitality) were raised (mean 31.8, 16.5, 19.9, and 24.6, respectively). The HRQOL was raised in 95.1 % of the children (indicated by total GCBI scores >0). Same as in the adults' collective, no negative GCBI scores or subscores and no differences between male and female patients were found. 95.1 % of the parents and 95.1 % of the children were satisfied with the aesthetical result. 97.6 % of the parents and 92.7 % of the children would again decide in favor of the operation. GBI and GCBI scores of patients with short-term (<6 months) and long-term (>2 years) follow-up times did not show statistical differences. Therefore, the findings of Schwentner et al. were confirmed saying that subjective benefit from otoplasty seems to be stable over the time.

To put it in a nutshell, otoplasty can significantly increase the HRQOL of children and adults suffering from protruding ears, and it leads to a high rate of patient satisfaction. An advantage of standardized measurement of HRQOL after aesthetic surgery is that a comparison with other operative techniques or other fields of aesthetic surgery is possible. Table 58.1 shows that the extent of the effect of otoplasty on HRQOL is comparable to other purely aesthetic operations, like ear reconstruction or rhinoplasty, but lower than for operations with both a functional and aesthetic aim in the head and neck area.

When Should Otoplasty Be Performed?

Songu and Adibelli [26] conducted a survey in ten patients with a median age of 51.5 months and found that nine out of ten parents were "very" or "completely" satisfied with the result of otoplasty in their children; from their results, the authors recommend to perform otoplasty before the age of five, since they think that there may be significant benefit from an early intervention after the child has expressed some concern about the deformity.

From the authors' data, it can be concluded that children seem to take a larger benefit from otoplasty than adults: Whereas in the children's cohort all GCBI scores and subscores were significantly elevated, social support and physical health scores in the adults' cohort were affected insignificantly only [22]. It can be speculated that problems with participating in social life due to reduced self-confidence because of the protruding ears remain constant with increasing age and that physical health in adults is usually not affected by aesthetic operations. Also, with increasing age at the time of otoplasty, patients state that the timing of the operation was too late, most probably due to an increased period of time during which they are teased for the protruding ears. Patients who stated that the operation was performed too late had received surgery at the median age of 15.5, while the patients stating that the operation was performed at the right age had received surgery more than 5 years earlier.

Therefore, the recommendation can be given to operate before the beginning of puberty, if possible, and in cases of need as early as in the age around five.

Otoplasty: Patient Benefit Guaranteed?

The positive findings for the effect of otoplasty discussed above have to be attenuated for several reasons. Of course, neither subjective benefit from the operation nor satisfaction with the result can be guaranteed as for every aesthetic operation. Also, complications can occur to a considerable extent (e.g., [27, 28]). While minor complications like postoperative pain and hypersensitivity, relapse or asymmetry, thread granuloma, othematoma, or scar and small keloid formation, if handled adequately by the experienced surgeon, do not threaten the beneficial effect of otoplasty [22], auricular deformities after failed otoplasty often result in an appearance which is more annoying than the preoperative state of prominent ears.

The huge number of different techniques for correcting protruding ears can be grouped into three basic concepts: the cutting technique described by Converse [7], the scoring technique according to Stenström [29], and the pure suture techniques introduced by Mustardé [30]. Compared to all cutting or scoring techniques, the risk of undesired edges, defects, or deformities difficult to correct is lower with cartilage-sparing, suture techniques [14, 31, 32]. The authors therefore think otoplasty using suture technique is especially recommendable when focusing on patient benefit. In our own patients, we use to fold the antihelix with sutures according to Mustardé [30] and, if necessary, approximate the cavum conchae to the skull as described by Furnas [33] and Goldstein [34] and correct the earlobe position by a suspension suture following the recommendations of Crikelair, Siegert, and Weerda [35].

References

1. Braun T, Gratza S, Becker S, Schwentner I, Stelter K, Patscheider M, et al. Auricular reconstruction with porous polyethylene frameworks: outcome and patient benefit in 65 children and adults. Plast Reconstr Surg. 2010;126(4):1201–12.
2. Fischer D, Stewart AL, Bloch DA, Lorig K, Laurent D, Holman H. Capturing the patient's view of change as a clinical outcome measure. J Am Med Assoc. 1999;282(12):1157–62.
3. Guyatt GH, Feeny DH, Patrick DL. Measuring health-related quality of life. Ann Intern Med. 1993;118(8):622–9.
4. Jenkinson C, Coulter A, Wright L. Short form 36 (SF36) health survey questionnaire: normative data for adults of working age. BMJ. 1993;306(6890):1437–40.
5. Gatehouse S. The Glasgow health status questionnaires manual. Glasgow: MRC Institute of Hearing Research, Glasgow Royal Infirmary; 1998.
6. Robinson K, Gatehouse S, Browning GG. Measuring patient benefit from otorhinolaryngological surgery and therapy. Ann Otol Rhinol Laryngol. 1996;105(6):415–22.
7. Kubba H, Swan IR, Gatehouse S. The Glasgow Children's Benefit Inventory: a new instrument for assessing health-related benefit after an intervention. Ann Otol Rhinol Laryngol. 2004;113(12):980–6.

8. Horlock N, Vögelin E, Bradbury ET, Grobbelaar AO, Gault DT. Psychosocial outcome of patients after ear reconstruction: a retrospective study of 62 patients. Ann Plast Surg. 2005;54(5):517–24.
9. Kapp-Simon KA, Simon DJ, Kristovich S. Self-perception, social skills, adjustment, and inhibition in young adolescents with craniofacial anomalies. Cleft Palate Craniofac J. 1992;29(4):352–6.
10. Sheerin D, Macleod M, Kusumakar V. Psychosocial adjustment in children with port-wine stains and prominent ears. J Am Acad Child Adolesc Psychiatry. 1995;34(12):1637–47.
11. Dion K, Berscheid E, Walster E. What is beautiful is good. J Pers Soc Psychol. 1972;24(3):285–90.
12. McCabe M, Marwit SJ. Depressive symptomatology, perceptions of attractiveness, and body image in children. J Child Psychol Psychiatry. 1993;34(7):1117–24.
13. Adamson PA, Strecker HD. Otoplasty techniques. Facial Plast Surg. 1995;11(4):284–300.
14. Kelley P, Hollier L, Stal S. Otoplasty: evaluation, technique, and review. J Craniofac Surg. 2003;14(5): 643–53.
15. Gasques JA, Pereira De Godoy JM, Cruz EM. Psychosocial effects of otoplasty in children with prominent ears. Aesthetic Plast Surg. 2008;32(6): 910–4.
16. Klassen A, Jenkinson C, Fitzpatrick R, Goodacre T. Patients' health related quality of life before and after aesthetic surgery. Br J Plast Surg. 1996;49(7):433–8.
17. Sarwer DB, Pertschuk MJ, Wadden TA, Whitaker LA. Psychological investigations in cosmetic surgery: a look back and a look ahead. Plast Reconstr Surg. 1998;101(4):1136–42.
18. Sarwer DB, Wadden TA, Pertschuk MJ, Whitaker LA. The psychology of cosmetic surgery: a review and reconceptualization. Clin Psychol Rev. 1998;18(1):1–22.
19. Bradbury ET, Hewison J, Timmons MJ. Psychological and social outcome of prominent ear correction in children. Br J Plast Surg. 1992;45(2):97–100.
20. Cooper-Hobson G, Jaffe W. The benefits of otoplasty for children: further evidence to satisfy the modern NHS. J Plast Reconstr Aesthet Surg. 2009;62(2): 190–4.
21. Schwentner I, Schmutzhard J, Deibl M, Sprinzer GM. Health-related quality of life outcome of adult patients after otoplasty. J Craniofac Surg. 2006;17(4): 629–35.
22. Braun T, Hainzinger T, Stelter K, Krause E, Berghaus A, Hempel JM. Health-related quality of life, patient benefit, and clinical outcome after otoplasty using suture techniques in 62 children and adults. Plast Reconstr Surg. 2010;126(6):2115–24.
23. Draper B, Pfaff JJ, Pirkis J et al. Long-term effects of childhood abuse on the quality of life and health of older people: results from the Depression and Early Prevention of Suicide in General Practice Project. J Am Geriatr Soc. 2008;56:262–71.
24. McKiernan DC, Banfield G, Kumar R et al. Patient benefit from functional and cosmetic rhinoplasty. Clin Otolaryngol Allied Sci. 2001;26:50–2.
25. Chauhan N, Warner J, Adamson PA. Adolescent rhinoplasty: challenges and psychosocial and clinical outcomes. Aesthetic Plast Surg. 2010;34:510–16.
26. Songu M, Adibelli H. Otoplasty in children younger than 5 years of age. Int J Pediatr Otorhinolaryngol. 2010;74(3):292–6.
27. Limandjaja GC, Breugem CC, van der Mink Molen AB, Kon M. Complications of otoplasty: a literature review. J Plast Reconstr Aesthet Surg. 2009;62(1):19–27.
28. Olivier B, Mohammad H, Christian A, Akram R. Retrospective study of the long-term results of otoplasty using a modified Mustarde (cartilage-sparing) technique. J Otolaryngol Head Neck Surg. 2009; 38(3):340–7.
29. Stenström SJ. A "natural" technique for correction of congenitally prominent ears. Plast Reconstr Surg. 1963;32:509–18.
30. Mustardé JC. The correction of prominent ears using simple mattress sutures. Br J Plast Surg. 1963;16: 170–8.
31. Adamson PA, Mcgraw BL, Tropper GJ. Otoplasty: critical review of clinical results. Laryngoscope. 1991;101(8):883–8.
32. Mandal A, Bahia H, Ahmad T, Stewart KJ. Comparison of cartilage scoring and cartilage sparing otoplasty–A study of 203 cases. J Plast Reconstr Aesthet Surg. 2006;59(11):1170–6.
33. Furnas DW. Correction of prominent ears by conchamastoid sutures. Plast Reconstr Surg. 1968;42(3): 189–93.
34. Goldstein MA. The cosmetic and plastic surgery of the ear. Laryngoscope. 1908;18(10):826–51.
35. Weerda H. Surgery of the auricle. Stuttgart/New York: Thieme; 2007.

Psychosocial, Behavioral, and Emotional Effects Following Otoplasty

59

Raquel Aguilar Cuesta and Carmen Soto Beauregard

Introduction

Nowadays, physical appearances are of major importance because of the beauty ideal that constantly appears in the media and that has been increased by social networking in the Internet era. Better socioeconomic statuses allow the use of plastic surgery as an affordable method to improve physical appearances to achieve our society's ideal of beauty.

Surgical treatment of prominent ears is more than a simple cosmetic correction. On one hand, it is a plastic surgery, which implies that there should be a confidence-based physician-patient relationship. In this situation, the surgeon and the patient can reach an agreement about the preoperative expectations and the best postoperative results that can be achieved. This is important because in plastic surgery it is all about a "results contract." It is also very important to determine if there is a body dysmorphic disorder underlying patient's problem, because it is known that such patients will not feel better after the surgery even with the best technical results, so they may also need a psychiatric evaluation. But, on the other hand, in the case of protruding ears, as in other kinds of physical anomalies, there is an important psychosocial component that has to be considered.

It is difficult to establish a clear differentiation between the objective physical and subjective aspects, and although prominent ears are considered a minor defect with no physiological disadvantages, this defect is a frequent source of severe social and psychological problems. The aim of this chapter is to describe these factors and their relationships with otoplasty.

Otoplasty

Prominent Ears

Prominent ears are the most frequent congenital craniofacial malformation, with an incidence of near 5 % in the Caucasian population and both sexes affected equally [1, 2]. It is transmitted by an autosomal dominant pattern with variable penetrance. Eight percent of the patients [1] have familial antecedents. Environmental factors have also been implicated in its

R.A. Cuesta, M.D. (✉)
Department of Pediatrics and Pediatric Surgery,
Hospital Clínico Universitario de Valladolid,
C/Ramón y Cajal, 3, 47003 Valladolid, Spain
e-mail: raquelnita@gmail.com,

C.S. Beauregard, M.D., Ph.D.
Department of Pediatric Surgery,
Hospital Clínico San Carlos,
C/Prof. Martín Lagos s/n, 28040 Madrid, Spain
e-mail: cirped.hcsc@salud.madrid.org

M.A. Shiffman (ed.), *Advanced Cosmetic Otoplasty*,
DOI 10.1007/978-3-642-35431-1_59, © Springer-Verlag Berlin Heidelberg 2013

appearance, affecting the external auricular development which starts in the second trimester of gestation [2].

Prominent ears are defined as those more than 20 ± 4 mm from the skull or more than 21–30° from the temporomandibular plane.

The external ear is composed of five basic elements: the concha, helix, antihelix, tragus, and lobule. The alteration of one or, more frequently, a number of these components and the relationships between them produces the auricular anomalies. Thus, the most frequent causes of prominent ears are an insufficiently shaped or distinctive antihelix, hyperplasia of the cavum conchae, and lobular anomalies.

Also other factors contribute to accentuating the defect, such as a prominent mastoid apophysis or plagiocephaly. Identification of the type of protruding ears in each patient is the main step to obtaining satisfactory results. The next step is to choose the most appropriate timing for the correction. This should be based on a balance among the auricular development, the age at which the child could start to have psychosocial problems, and the age at which the child can carry out the postoperative care (bandaging, physical exercise restriction).

Based on these three factors, the majority of surgeons consider 7 years old to be the lower age limit [1]. At that age, the external auricular development is nearly completed, the child can be involved in the whole treatment process, and also is becoming conscious of the physical defects.

Surgical Technique

More than 200 surgical and nonsurgical techniques have been described for the treatment of this anomaly. Among the nonsurgical interventions, in 1990 Matsuo et al. [3] used malleable molds fixed with adhesive tape for the neonatal period, and in 2002 Sorribes and Tos [4] described a system based on the application of clips and adhesives that can be used from the neonatal period to the age of 5 with a success rate of 89 %.

The first otoplasty was performed by Ely in 1881 [5]. In 1903, Morestin [6] was the first surgeon to describe the concha-mastoid and Mustardé's sutures (used to conform the helical plicature), although they went unnoticed for many decades (Fig. 59.1). Stenstroem [7] described the technique of scraping and rasping cartilage to obtain and/or stabilize the helical plicature. Many variations of this technique have been described. Also, interventions with posterior auricular muscle repositioning have been carried out. Recently, Pereira-Filho et al. [8] have described prominent ear correction using a unique posterior auricular incision without skin resection that they call endoplasty, obtaining good results.

Whichever technique is chosen, the aims are the same: an adequate helical plication and a concha-mastoid distance within normal limits in order to obtain a natural and symmetrical aspect with as few signs of surgical intervention as possible.

Surgical Process

The patient is admitted to the hospital the day of surgery. The procedure is done under general anesthesia, and a combination of local anesthesia and sedation in adults can be used. When the surgical correction is concluded, an elastic bandage is set in place for a variable period of time depending on the surgeon's preference. The reason for this variation is that there have been a number of studies comparing different periods of time with no statistically significant differences [1]. Pediatric patients are discharged 1 day after the procedure in order to achieve better postoperative pain control and to avoid the occasional nausea and vomiting related to stimulation of the tympanic nerve cord, which is connected with the vomit center in the brainstem.

The nonabsorbable intradermal skin suture is removed at the external point 7–10 days postoperatively. The elastic bandage, diurnal and/or nocturnal, is left in place according to the surgeon's choice, ranging between 1 and 3 months in most cases.

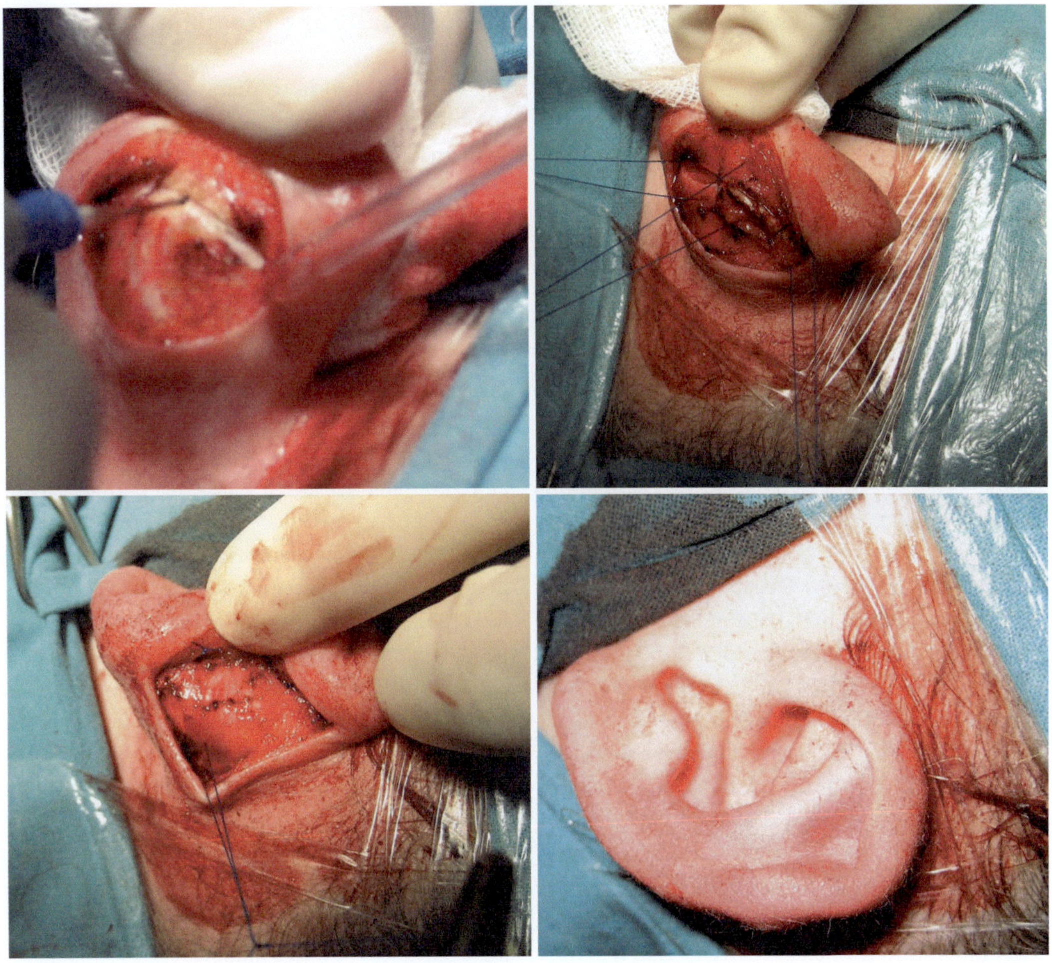

Fig. 59.1 Mustardé's otoplasty

Technical Results

The postoperative complications described for this surgical intervention are pain, bruises, surgical wound infection, suture-related complications such as extrusion of sutures or keloid formation, cartilage irregularities, and recurrence of the prominence. All of them are rare. Depending on the authors, the suture extrusion rate is 10 %, and the recurrence rate is between 5 and 10 % [1].

The surgical treatment of suture extrusion depends on the clinical course, but it is usually solved by removing the suture, without a higher rate of recurrence or need for redo-otoplasty.

Redo-otoplasty obtains successful results similar to the initial procedure.

Psychosocial, Behavioral, and Emotional Aspects

Social Cruelty

Pickhardt [9] defines social cruelty as "aggressively attacking another person with words or actions directed to injure the victim's well-being, to damage his standing, or simply to assert the aggressor's dominance." This occurs in the middle school years, in children around 9–13 years old, because of the destabilizing and challenging early adolescence period. Social cruelty is exhibited by teasing, excluding, bullying, rumoring, and ganging up. Aggressors are protected by the desire of adolescents to keep adults out, the "don't-tell-on-peers" code of secrecy and silence [9]. All of these forms of social cruelty play on an adolescent's deepest fears (the physical aspect in the case of the prominent ears).

Teasing is the act of making fun of a difference in others to criticize their traits, diminish their social standing, and set them apart socially. Humiliation is carried out with insults, making the victim feel inferior.

Exclusion is the refusal to let someone associate with others or join a group, playing with the fear of isolation.

Bullying is the act of verbally or physically intimidating, injuring, coercing, or dominating another person, acting thus in the fear of weakness.

Rumoring is to use gossip to spread lies or secrets about others that demean their social reputation and play with the fear of defamation.

Ganging up is to join and act against others to torment them, acting in fear of persecution.

Social cruelty produces anger, depression, feeling demeaned, fear, humiliation, isolation, hurt, and shame, and because it undermines the victim's social safety, it often reduces academic focus and school performance. So, of course, it can produce psychosocial and emotional problems in adult life. Social cruelty is also a symptom of an underlying emotional discomfort that largely originates in a common cause: the social dislocation and developmental insecurity of early adolescent change.

Early Adolescence

Early adolescence is a period of time that starts around the age of 9 and ends at around 13 years old. This is a very important period in which the child becomes an adult and involves many changes that makes the adolescent feels insecure. The early adolescent needs to find attachment and acceptance in an independent and unstable society of peers who are feeling insecure and vulnerable, too. It is this potent mix of insecurity, vulnerability, and need for social belonging in a more independent world of peers that is the cradle for social cruelty [9].

Social Cruelty and Prominent Ears

The most used form of social cruelty in the case of children with prominent ears is to tease them with insults and name calling. Its power arises from the adolescents' constant feelings of the danger of being publicly exposed because of some awkwardness or ineptitude. In fact, in this period, they have an enormous appearance anxiety, both boys and girls, because they are painfully self-conscious and self-critical about their physical appearance. They think that the others will detect and judge their defects harshly and turn against them. This makes them feel afraid and insecure. In some cases of children with prominent ears, we have also seen parents who have psychosocial disturbances because of their own experiences and come to consult us to prevent their child from suffering the same fate.

Teasing inflicts more damage when the victim believes that the degrading is true and then feels justly accused, so his or her self-esteem plummets. A specific characteristic of this form of social cruelty is that the motivation of the aggressor(s) can sometimes be hard to determine, because the teasers can say that they was just kidding, making the victim feel doubly teased, not only for taking the insult seriously, but also for overreacting and lacking a sufficient sense of humor.

The surgical correction of prominent ears should be carried out together with appropriate coaching strategies about handling teasing, which can reverse the victim's psychosocial and emotional disturbances. There are many strategies for fighting against teasing, basically based on not taking the teasing personally, for example, by pretending to misunderstand it, ignoring it, laughing at it, or agreeing with it.

However, for most cases of children with protruding ears, this is not enough, and they need surgical correction.

Psychosocial Results Following Otoplasty

There are many publications, papers, and studies of the benefits of otoplasty for prominent ears in terms of psychosocial repercussions, cosmetics results, and the degree of patient satisfaction . Most of them are based in comparing health-related quality of life scales before and after the surgical treatment, which show an important improvement in the quality of life for most patients [10, 11].

The authors published a "Satisfaction Survey of the Evolution of 238 Otoplasties" carried out at La Paz Hospital in Madrid in 2008 [1]. This study was made by sending a satisfaction questionnaire to 127 patients who underwent Mustardé's otoplasty for prominent ears during the years 2003–2006. The mean age was 8.15 ± 3.25 years (range, 1–15 years), with a follow-up period of 27.15 ± 13.62 months (range, 4–52 month). 38 % of the patients were old enough to want the surgery to correct a long-standing defect, having psychosocial disturbances, and in 32 % of them, there was also a reduction in school performance. All of them recovered their self-esteem after the procedure, even the patients who suffered total or partial recurrence (6.29 % of cases).

In the article published by Gasques et al. [5] on "Psychosocial Effects of Otoplasty in Children with Prominent Ears," it was noted that after surgical correction, the patients feel less anxiety and increased self-esteem, making important improvements and learning achievements in in-group and out-of-school activities.

Thus, the patients feel happier and report increased social integration probably related to the previously mentioned benefits of improved self-confidence, which makes them less vulnerable to social cruelty.

In a few cases, surgical correction does not have the benefits expected. Cooper-Hobson and Jaffe [10] reported in their study that this may be because of extremely high expectations, even with the best technical results. This can be avoided simply by having a good, trusting physician-patient relationship, because this allows the physician to understand the patient's expectations and to explain the results that can be achieved in each particular case.

Conclusions

Prominent ears, although considered a minor deformity causing no physiological problems, can be an important source of psychosocial, emotional, and behavioral problems. This situation is especially hurtful in the middle school years because of the extreme feelings of insecurity and vulnerability experienced in the early adolescent period, which can be prolonged into adulthood.

Surgical correction of prominent ears is an easy technique with a low risk of complications that has demonstrated improvement in the psychosocial, behavioral, and emotional problems related to these anomalies (Figs. 59.2 and 59.3).

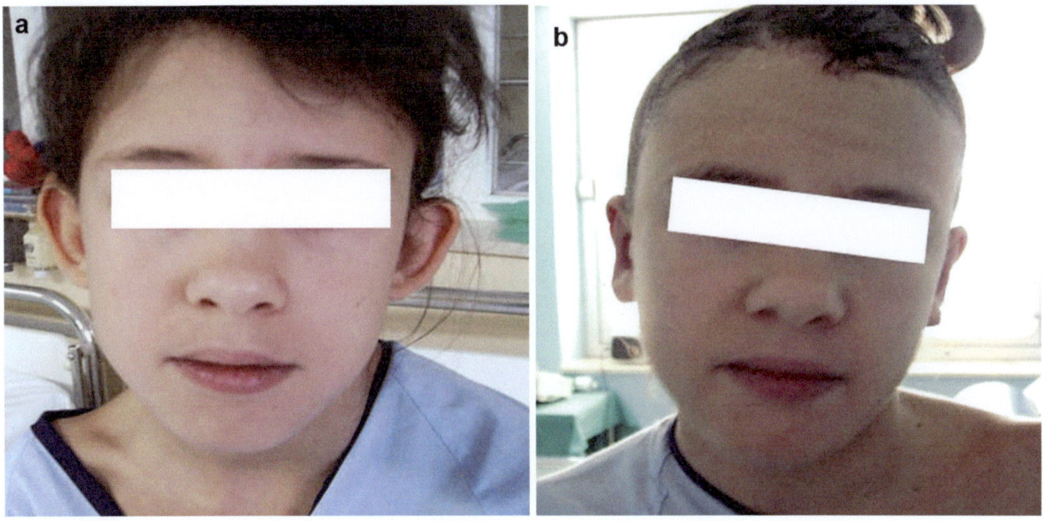

Fig. 59.2 (**a**) Preoperative. (**b**) Early postoperative results

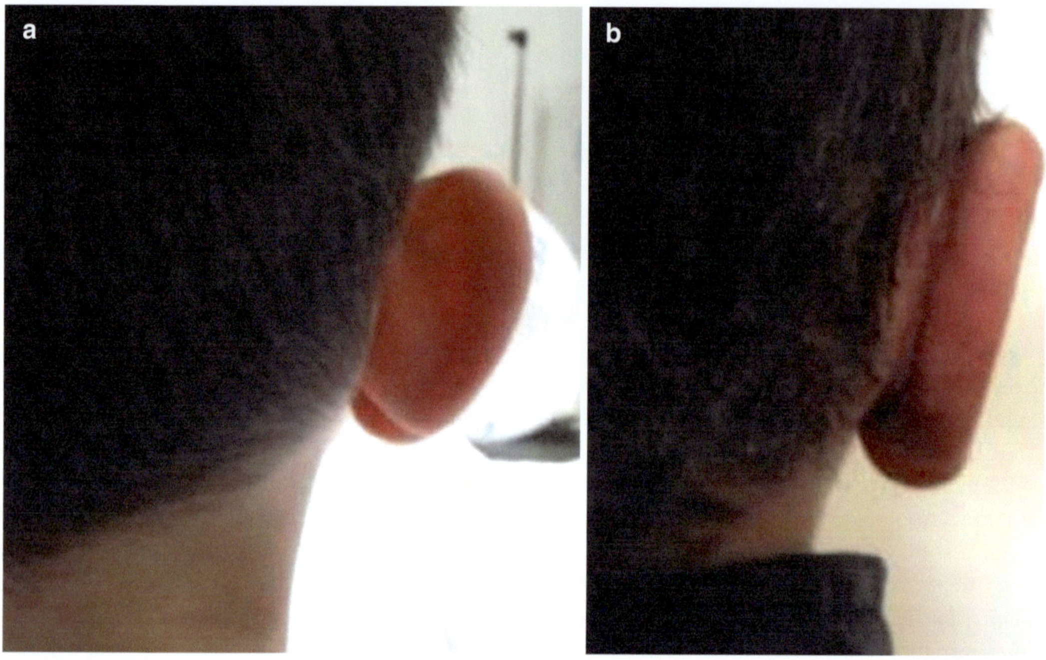

Fig. 59.3 (**a**) Before surgical correction. (**b**) 7 postoperative day

References

1. Aguilar R, Soto C, Barrena S, Díaz M, López JC, Ros Z, et al. Estudio de la evolución de 238 otoplastias mediante encuesta de satisfacción. Cir Pediatr. 2008; 21(2):104–6.
2. Braun T, Hainzinger T, Stelter K, Krause E, Berghaus A, Hempel JM. Health-related quality of life, patient benefit and clinical outcome after otoplasty using suture techniques in 62 children and adults. Plast Reconstr Surg. 2010;126(6):2115–24.
3. Matsuo K, Hayashi R, Kiyono M, Hirose T, Netsu Y. Nonsurgical correction of congenital auricular deformities. Clin Plast Surg. 1990;17(2):383–95.
4. Sorribes MM, Tos M. Nonsurgical treatment of prominent ears with the Auri method. Arch Otolaryngol Head Neck Surg. 2002;128(12):1369–76.
5. Ely ET. An operation for prominence of the auricles. Arch Otolaryngol. 1881;10:97.
6. Morestin H. De la reposition et du plissement cosmétiques du pavillon de l'oreille. Rev Orthop. 1903;4:394.
7. Stenstrom SJ. A "natural" technique for correction of congenitally prominent ears. Plast Reconstr Surg. 1969;42:189–201.
8. Pereira-Filho O, Eickhoff DR, Eickhoff DR, Bins-Ely J, Bins-Ely J, Granemann AS, et al. Novel approach to closed treatment of prominent ear without skin resection (endoplasty) of prominent ear without skin resection (endotoplasty). Plast Reconstr Surg. 2006;118(7 Suppl):55S.
9. Pickhardt C. Why good kids act cruel. The hidden truth about the pre-teen years. Naperville: Sourcebooks Inc; 2010.
10. Cooper-Hobson G, Jaffe WJ. The benefits of otoplasty for children: further evidence to satisfy the modern NHS. J Plast Reconstr Aesthet Surg. 2009;62(2):109–14.
11. Gasques JA, de Pereira Godoy JM, Cruz EM. Psychosocial effects of otoplasty in children with prominent ears. Aesthetic Plast Surg. 2008;32(6):910–4.

Part VII

Miscellaneous

Evolution of Consent and Alternatives to Traditional Consent Forms

60

Kayvan Shokrollahi and Adeyinka Molajo

Consent

Has my patient understood the procedure and agreed to treatment? If yes is the answer, then you have probably obtained legally valid consent from your patient. However, it is good practice – if not essential – to gain such consent in writing, and this is stipulated in hospital guidelines and protocols and sometimes the law. Consent forms provide a useful starting point for obtaining consent, but it plays mainly an evidentiary role and it has significant limitations:

> "I regard the consent form immediately before operation as pure window dressing….and designed to avoid the suggestion that a patient has not been told."
> Lord Popwell in Taylor v Shropshire HA 1998

Historical Perspective and the Importance of Consent

The first legal case pertaining to consent was settled way back in 1767 in the case of Slater v Baker and Stapleton, where surgery had been performed against the wishes of a patient, and has been evolving as a concept ever since.

Consent is said to be necessary to uphold patient autonomy as well as an ethical and professional duty, but importantly it will lead to improved clinical outcomes through better cooperation from patients. We should help patients to make decisions through good explanations and information resources.

Consenting patients in most hospitals revolves around the consent form, which is filled in by the surgeon outlining the relevant operation with stated risks and benefits. Patients express their consent by signing this document. Written consent is seen as the current gold standard, as other forms of consent that may be explicit (verbal) or implied are less robust and certainly unreliable if challenged.

Some difficulties with our current method of written consent include a "legalistic" approach, the timing is often immediately before or close to the operation, and the process tends to be negative by concentrating on risks and complications which can be significantly detrimental to patients' state of mind and anxiety in the run-up to surgery. It has been shown that patients take in very little of what they hear despite the best of explanations in this scenario. Furthermore, the consent form does not go very far in proving that patients actually understand or that they have capacity.

Many have attempted to improve consent within this framework by enhancing consent

K. Shokrollahi, BSc, MBChB, MSc, LLM, MRCS(Eng), FRCS(Plast) (✉)
Mersey Regional Burns and Plastic Surgery Unit, Ward 4d, Whiston Hospital, Warrington Rd, Liverpool L35 5DR, UK
e-mail: kshokrollahi@hotmail.com

A. Molajo, M.D., MRCS
Department of Plastic and Reconstructive Surgery, St Helens ad Knowsley NHS Trust, Whiston Hospital, Merseyside, UK
e-mail: adeyinka.molajo@gmail.com

M.A. Shiffman (ed.), *Advanced Cosmetic Otoplasty*,
DOI 10.1007/978-3-642-35431-1_60, © Springer-Verlag Berlin Heidelberg 2013

forms by making them procedure specific, providing improved patient information, and by obtaining consent in a clinic or office setting remote from the operating time. These may certainly improve aspects of the consent process, but to make a real difference, an entirely new and radical approach is required. Patients request treatment instead of consenting to treatment, and such a request-based method of consent has recently been published [1, 2]. The advantages are numerous and include a patient-centric and constructive approach, superior documentation of consent which for the first time demonstrates both capacity and informed consent in patients' own handwriting and vocabulary, speed (often completed prior to attendance for surgery), and flexibility (can be used selectively).

Request for Treatment (RFT)

Request for treatment, otherwise called patient-centered consent, is a type of written consent. As with traditional consent, it relies on a form, but this time it is a request form and it is completed by patients and finally signed by a surgeon accepting to undertake the procedure. It can be used in isolation as the method of consent or as dual consent (either permanently or as a transitional step to request-only consent). The forms used are very similar to traditional consent forms, but instead of "I consent to" the onus is "I request...." The name of the procedure as well as risks and complications are all written by patients in their own writing and vocabulary.

The RFT process puts some advantageous pressures on clinicians:

1. To provide excellent patient information resources
2. To communicate well and explain sufficiently such that patients are able to complete the request forms

However, these pressures lead to practice which is safe and patient-centric and leads to truly informed consent – the documentation of which should be beyond reproach.

A particular advantage to RFT is that it ensures that patient expectations are aligned with surgeon expectations. There is no doubt that the leading cause of complaints and litigation is a mismatch in this area. One learns a great deal at almost every consent episode of RFT – what patients expect to be the benefits of their surgery, for example, which is eye-opening at times. It is therefore an excellent early-warning system for unrealistic patients. If written consent is required as evidence in court, the RFT document written by the patient's own hand stating various risks is both a strong shield – in court – and indeed a psychological barrier to litigation and complaints in the first place.

There are many aspects of the author's practice for which RFT is routinely used, especially cosmetic practice. Routine and minor procedures will still benefit from its use, but surgeons will tailor its use to those areas where they perceive it to provide the greatest benefit. Example request forms can be found at www.rft.org.uk, and most surgeons will tailor these forms for their own requirements.

Consent for Otoplasty

The majority of patients undertaking otoplasty are children, and therefore parents will be consenting on behalf of their children rather than patients themselves. Prominent ears are viewed in different social and cultural lights in different ethnic and national groups, and this must be born in mind. The vast majority of patients with significant prominence are likely to experience negative psychological effects by about the age of six. I would recommend that the combination of "sensible" parents and children whom are either keen for surgery or indifferent about surgery are good candidates for surgery. Obviously a preference for intervention from the child is desirable, and surgery is scheduled for an appropriate time when the child is able to contribute to decision-making. A delay can also allow a less risky local anesthetic procedure at an older age. It is important to be cautious in children who demonstrate reluctance to surgery, and careful consideration is required before overriding the child's wishes in favor of parental wishes, although this is rare [3].

References

1. Shokrollahi K. Request for treatment: the evolution of consent. Review. Ann R Coll Surg Engl. 2010;92(2):93–100.
2. Request for treatment: Patient centred consent www.rft.org.uk. Accessed 5 Aug 2012
3. Shokrollahi K, Kaney S. Psychological considerations in patient selection for pinnaplasty. J Plast Reconstr Aesthet Surg. 2009;62(1):118.

Index

M.A. Shiffman (ed.), *Advanced Cosmetic Otoplasty*,
DOI 10.1007/978-3-642-35431-1, © Springer-Verlag Berlin Heidelberg 2013

D

T

U

V

W

Y

Z

MIX
Papier aus verantwortungsvollen Quellen
Paper from responsible sources
FSC® C105338

If you have any concerns about our products,
you can contact us on
ProductSafety@springernature.com

In case Publisher is established outside the EU,
the EU authorized representative is:
Springer Nature Customer Service Center GmbH
Europaplatz 3, 69115 Heidelberg, Germany

Printed by Libri Plureos GmbH
in Hamburg, Germany